AF746051

Practical Issues in Geriatrics

Series Editor
Stefania Maggi
Aging Branch
CNR-Neuroscience Institute
Padua
Italy

This practically oriented series presents state of the art knowledge on the principal diseases encountered in elderly patients and addresses all aspects of management, including current multidisciplinary diagnostic and therapeutic approaches. It is intended as an educational tool that will enhance the everyday clinical practice of both young geriatricians and residents and also assist other specialists who deal with aged patients. Each volume is designed to provide comprehensive information on the topic that it covers, and whenever appropriate the text is complemented by additional material of high educational and practical value, including informative video-clips, standardized diagnostic flow charts and descriptive clinical cases. Practical Issues in Geriatrics will be of value to the scientific and professional community worldwide, improving understanding of the many clinical and social issues in Geriatrics and assisting in the delivery of optimal clinical care.

More information about this series at http://www.springer.com/series/15090

Stefano Masiero • Ugo Carraro
Editors

Rehabilitation Medicine for Elderly Patients

Springer

Editors
Stefano Masiero
Department of Neuroscience
Physical Medicine and Rehabilitation Unit
University of Padua
Padua
Italy

Ugo Carraro
IRRCS, Fondazione Ospedale San Camillo
Venezia
Italy

ISSN 2509-6060 ISSN 2509-6079 (electronic)
Practical Issues in Geriatrics
ISBN 978-3-319-57405-9 ISBN 978-3-319-57406-6 (eBook)
DOI 10.1007/978-3-319-57406-6

Library of Congress Control Number: 2017952951

© Springer International Publishing AG 2018
This work is subject to copyright. All rights are reserved by the Publisher, whether the whole or part of the material is concerned, specifically the rights of translation, reprinting, reuse of illustrations, recitation, broadcasting, reproduction on microfilms or in any other physical way, and transmission or information storage and retrieval, electronic adaptation, computer software, or by similar or dissimilar methodology now known or hereafter developed.
The use of general descriptive names, registered names, trademarks, service marks, etc. in this publication does not imply, even in the absence of a specific statement, that such names are exempt from the relevant protective laws and regulations and therefore free for general use.
The publisher, the authors and the editors are safe to assume that the advice and information in this book are believed to be true and accurate at the date of publication. Neither the publisher nor the authors or the editors give a warranty, express or implied, with respect to the material contained herein or for any errors or omissions that may have been made. The publisher remains neutral with regard to jurisdictional claims in published maps and institutional affiliations.

Printed on acid-free paper

This Springer imprint is published by Springer Nature
The registered company is Springer International Publishing AG
The registered company address is: Gewerbestrasse 11, 6330 Cham, Switzerland

Foreword

In developed countries, people aged 65 years and over constitute 12–18% of the general population but account for around 30–40% of the consumption of healthcare services. The global increase in total numbers of older persons is astonishing; by the year 2025, there will be more than 800 million people aged 65 years and over in the world, two thirds of them in developing countries.

Physiological changes, multiple pathology, physical incapacity, concomitant mental disorders, and social disadvantage mean that special skills are required in the diagnosis and management of illness in old age. There is growing concern that our medical care system is not structured to effectively address complex chronic disease and multi-morbidity, which are both common in the geriatric population.

Since knowledge is power and today knowledge is essential, the more information we get, the better we will be able to work with older persons and their different conditions. *Healthy aging* remains a goal.

Rehabilitation Medicine for Elderly Patients is an excellent step in that direction. It provides a wide variety of in-depth knowledge about the disorders that affect older people, their prevention, and their treatment, because care of older persons is complex and involves the expertise of many different healthcare practitioners.

It has been written by a group of internationally well-known scientists, researchers, and highly skilled and informed practitioners and condenses the rapidly growing body of knowledge about aging, geriatric care, and rehabilitation, in 57 chapters, subdivided into three parts (Part I, aging; Part II, rehabilitation of the elderly; Part III, organization). It has been designed to inspire and inform the reader about the science and art of aged care.

The strengths of this generally excellent book, covering an important and sometimes neglected area of health in old age, lie in its thoughtful presentation of current approaches to clinical rehabilitation in older people. The goal is to assist all members of the healthcare team in better chronic care practice, by developing and enhancing interventions to prevent disease and postpone further disability.

Thus, it aims to be an innovative, comprehensive, and educational tool not only for international junior doctors but also for all healthcare providers, attracting them to think about the total patient; to consider the medical as well as the psychosocial, ethical, and complex interdisciplinary aspects of caring for elderly patients; and finally to enrich our knowledge, so as to be able to provide efficient and effective care to the rapidly growing population of older adults.

Putting together a book of this magnitude requires enormous effort by many people.

We wish to thank the internationally distinguished academics and recognized experts in their fields, who covered many different and sometimes innovative topics, brought their knowledge, research, experience and good judgment, thus ensuring the high scientific standard of the book. We have been particularly impressed by their excellent contributions!!

We have particularly appreciated the intensive and creative efforts and the contribution of the editors, Prof. S. Masiero and U. Carraro, whom we congratulate for bringing together the best minds and leaders in the field.

It is an honor and privilege for us to provide this foreword to the first edition of the book *Rehabilitation Medicine for Elderly Patients*, published by Springer in Practical Issues in Geriatrics, a series whose Editor in Chief is Prof. Stefania Maggi, current president of the European Union Geriatric Medicine Society (EUGMS).

Alain Delarque
European Society of Physical
and Rehabilitation Medicine (ESPRM)
Paiania, Greece

Xanthi Michail
ESPRM Special Interest Scientific
Paiania, Greece

PRM in Ageing Persons
Paiania, Greece

Preface

The world's older population is rapidly growing in number and proportion, and people over 60 years are expected to double in the next few decades (United Nations, Department of Economic and Social Affairs, Population Division (2015). *World Population Ageing, 2015*). The European continent is projected to remain for at least the next 50 years the world's area with the oldest population: by 2050 about 37% of Europeans is expected to be 60 or over (*Communication from the commission to the Council and the European parliament*, 2002).

Increased life expectancy which reflects, at least in part, the success of public health interventions has many implications: the growing number of older persons suffering of chronic diseases increases demands on the public healthcare system, costs for management, and social burden. Delirium, sarcopenia, frailty, balance disorders, falls, dizziness, and urinary incontinence are just some the most common medical conditions that occur among the elderly, diminish their quality of life (QOL), and contribute to their physical and cognitive decline, disability, and death. However, aging itself should not be considered negatively, and many interventions can be set up by the governments, communities, and families in order to promote health, participation, social inclusion, and security of older people and improve their QOL (*Policies and priority interventions for healthy ageing – WHO/Europe, 2012*). The elderly individuals, of whom 60–75% are healthy, 20–30% suffer from chronic diseases, and 2–10% are "frail," should benefit from health-related differentiated and targeted measures applied in the different contexts in which they live. It is in this regard that this book, *Rehabilitation Medicine for Elderly Patients*, offers insight into the complex world of older persons in their different conditions (healthy, frail, diseased, or dying) in the specialty of physical medicine and rehabilitation (PM&R), approaching matters from a variety of viewpoints. It represents the perspective of some international leaders in the field based on both updated literature review (including the chapters about biomedical and experimental approaches) and their practical clinical applications to ensure high-quality standards to the book contents.

Rehabilitation Medicine for Elderly Patients is organized into three parts: Part I is general and deals with many issues of elderly people such as sarcopenia, frailty, exercise, nutrition, new technologies, therapeutic modalities, etc.

Part II is on rehabilitation of the most commonly encountered diseases of seniors. Some innovative topics covered in this part are cognitive therapy, spinal lesions, sexual dysfunction rehabilitation, etc.

Part III is devoted to the description of different organizations of healthcare system for the elderly in European countries.

Rehabilitation Medicine for Elderly Patients is a comprehensive educational tool, simple, easy to read, clear, and written in a structured way. The idea of writing this book came primarily to help junior doctors who are about to embark on their studies and PM&R residents in learning the basic concepts of rehabilitation of older adults. However, it can also help physiatrists in reviewing the main topics in the field of rehabilitation, general practitioners, and physicians of other specialties in assisting patients with disabling conditions solve their health problems.

This is the first edition of *Rehabilitation Medicine for Elderly Patients*. We are aware that, like all first attempts, the book has limitations. Nonetheless, we hope it can be appreciated and will contribute an important resource for training and education in the field of PM&R of medical professionals and beyond.

Finally, we would like to thank all colleagues for their tireless efforts to complete on time their contributions to the book.

Padua, Italy — Stefano Masiero, MD
Venezia-Lido, Italy — Ugo Carraro, MD

Contents

Part I

Part II

Part III

Contributors

Pasquale Abete, MD, PhD Department of Translational Medical Sciences, University of Naples Federico II, Naples, Italy

Amedeo Amoresano M.D. Unità Operativa di Medicina Fisica e Riabilitazione Centro Protesi INAIL Vigorso di Budrio, Bologna, Italy

Gert Apich Physical Medicine and General Rehabilitation, KABEG LKH and Lymphklinik Wolfsberg, Wolfsberg, Austria

M. Ardia Dipartimento economia aziendale, sanità e sociale, Centro Competenze Anziani, Manno, Switzerland

Dipartimento economia aziendale, sanità e sociale, Scuola Universitaria Professionale della Svizzera Italiana (SUPSI), Manno, Switzerland

Iris D. Arnadottir Institute for Biomedical and Neural Engineering, Reykjavík University, School of Science and Engineering, Reykjavík, Iceland

C. Assenza Clinical Medicine and Translational Medicine Department, Tor Vergata University, Rome, Italy

A. Baba IRCCS Fondazione San Camillo Hospital, Venice, Italy

Alessio Baricich, MD Physical and Rehabilitative Medicine, Department of Health Sciences, University of Eastern Piedmont "A. Avogadro", Novara, Italy

Giulia Bellon Department of Neuroscience, Rehabilitation Unit, University of Padua, Padua, Italy

Laura Bernardi, MD Department of Neuroscience, Section of Rehabilitation, University of Padua, Padua, Italy

Y. Bertholom Il Paese di Oz – ANFFAS, Trento, Italy

Società Tecnico Scientifica Italiana di Terapia Occupazionale (SITO), Rome, Italy

Facoltà di Medicina & Chirugia, Università degli Studi di Modena & Reggio-Emilia, Modena, Italy

Paolo Boldrini, MD Department of Rehabilitation Medicine, ULSS9 Treviso – Ospedale Riabilitativo di Alta Specializzazione, Motta di Livenza, Italy

Simona Boncompagni CeSI – Center for Research on Aging & DNICS, Department of Neuroscience, Imaging and Clinical Sciences, University G. d'Annunzio, Chieti, Italy

Marko Bonjako Department of Physical Medicine and Rehabilitation, University of Padua, Padua, Italy

Francesca M. Bosco Department of Psychology, University of Turin, Turin, Italy

Isabelle Bourdel-Marchasson Department of Clinical Gerontology, CHU Bordeaux, Bordeaux, France

CNRS, RMSB, UMR 5536, Bordeaux, France

University Bordeaux, RMSB, UMR 5536, Bordeaux, France

Elisabeth Bourkel, PhD Centre for Memory and Mobility, Zitha, Luxembourg City, Luxembourg

Research & Development, ZithaSenior, Luxembourg City, Luxembourg

Roberto Bovo Neuroscience Department, Operative Unit of Otolaryngology, Padua University, Padua, Italy

Chiara Briani Department of Neuroscience, University of Padua, Padua, Italy

Stefano Brunelli Santa Lucia Hospital, Neurorehabilitation Unit, Rome, Italy

Antonella Brunello Department of Experimental and Clinical Oncology, Medical Oncology 1, Veneto Institute of Oncology – IRCCS, Padua, Italy

Francesco Cacciatore, MD, PhD Department of Translational Medical Sciences, University of Naples Federico II, Naples, Italy

Heart Transplant Unit, Azienda Ospedaliera Specialistica dei Colli, Naples, Italy

G. Caiata-Olgiati Dipartimento economia aziendale, sanità e sociale, Centro Competenze Anziani, Manno, Switzerland

Dipartimento economia aziendale, sanità e sociale, Scuola Universitaria Professionale della Svizzera Italiana (SUPSI), Manno, Switzerland

Caribù Center of Occupational Therapy, Biasca, Switzerland

Luca Calanca Division of Angiology, Heart and Vessel Department, University Hospital Lausanne, Lausanne, Switzerland

Ugo Carraro IRRCS, Fondazione Ospedale San Camillo, Venezia, Italy

Clara Casco Department of General Psychology, University of Padua, Padua, Italy

Leonora Castiglia, MD Department of Neuroscience, Section of Rehabilitation, University of Padua, Padua, Italy

Alessandro Castiglione Neuroscience Department, Operative Unit of Otolaryngology, Padua University, Padua, Italy

H.A. Cerrel Bazo Spinal Cord Injury and Severe Acquired Brain Injury Center, Rehabilitation Hospital at High Level of Specialization of Motta di Livenza, Treviso, Italy

Carlo Cisari, MD, PhD Physical and Rehabilitative Medicine, Department of Health Sciences, University of Eastern Piedmont "A. Avogadro", Novara, Italy

Enrica Convento, MSc Department of Ophthalmology, University of Padua, Padua, Italy

Valentina Copetti Department of Physical Medicine and Rehabilitation, University of Padua, Padua, Italy

Emanuela Covella Department of Medical and Surgical Specialties and Dentistry, University of Campania "Luigi Vanvitelli", Caserta, Italy

C. Crotti Center for Traditional & Complementary Medicine, Milan State University, Milan, Italy

A.G. Cutti Eng. Centro Protesi INAIL Vigorso di Budrio, Bologna, Italy

Elena Demertzis, MD Department of Neuroscience, Section of Rehabilitation, University of Padua, Padua, Italy

Erwan de Mones Otorhinolaryngology Department, CHU of Bordeaux, Bordeaux, France

Marina De Rui Department of Medicine, Geriatrics Division, University of Padua, Padua, Italy

Alessandra Del Felice, MD, PhD Department of Neuroscience, Section of Rehabilitation, University of Padua, Padua, Italy

Paolo Di Benedetto University Tor Vergata, Rome, Italy

Miriam Duso, MD University of Padua, Padua, Italy

Orthopedic Rehabilitation Unit, Neuroscience Department, Hospital of Padua, Padua, Italy

Kyle J. Edmunds Institute for Biomedical and Neural Engineering, Reykjavík University, School of Science and Engineering, Reykjavík, Iceland

Inge Ehlebracht-König Center of Rehabilitation Bad Eilsen, Bad Eilsen, Germany

Carine Federspiel, MD Centre for Memory and Mobility, Luxembourg City, Luxembourg

E. Ferlito Rehabilitation Unit, Department of Neurosciences, University of Padua, Padua, Italy

C. Foti Clinical Medicine and Translational Medicine Department, Tor Vergata University, Rome, Italy

Antonio Frizziero, MD, PhD Department of Physical Medicine and Rehabilitation, University of Padua, Padua, Italy

Walter R. Frontera, MD, PhD Departments of Physical Medicine, Rehabilitation and Sports Medicine and Physiology and Biophysics, University of Puerto Rico School of Medicine, San Juan, Puerto Rico

Andrea Furlan, MD, PhD Toronto Rehabilitation Institute – University Health Network, Toronto, ON, Canada

University of Toronto, Toronto, ON, Canada

Magnus K. Gíslason Institute for Biomedical and Neural Engineering, Reykjavík University, School of Science and Engineering, Reykjavík, Iceland

Paolo Gargiulo Institute for Biomedical and Neural Engineering, Reykjavík University, School of Science and Engineering, Reykjavík, Iceland

Landspítali, Reykjavík, Iceland

Giuseppe Gasparre Department of Physical Medicine and Rehabilitation, University of Padua, Padua, Italy

K. Gava Interdepartmental Research Center of Myology, University of Padua, Padua, Italy

Giovanni Gentile I.R.C.C.S. San Camillo Hospital, Venice, Italy

Francesca Gimigliano Department of Medical and Surgical Specialties and Dentistry, University of Campania "Luigi Vanvitelli", Caserta, Italy

Raffaele Gimigliano Department of Medical and Surgical Specialties and Dentistry, University of Campania "Luigi Vanvitelli", Caserta, Italy

C. Giordani Clinical Medicine and Translational Medicine Department, Tor Vergata University, Rome, Italy

L. Gobbo Neurorehabilitation Unit, Padua General Hospital, Padua, Italy

Emelyne Grech Speech Language Therapy Department, University of Bordeaux, Bordeaux, France

Guri Hagberg, MD Department of Research, Vestre Viken Hospital Trust, Bærum Hospital, Drammen, Norway

H.L. Hammond Società Tecnico Scientifica Italiana di Terapia Occupazionale (SITO), Rome, Italy

Facoltà di Medicina & Chirugia, Università degli Studi di Modena & Reggio-Emilia, Modena, Italy

Facoltà di Medicina & Chirugia, Claudiana Scuola Provinciale Superiore di Sanità, Bolzano, Italy

Centro di Terapia Occupazionale, Bologna, Italy

Christian Hofer Ludwig Boltzmann Institute of Electrical Stimulation and Physical Rehabilitation, Vienna, Austria

P. Ianes Presidio Ospedaliero "Villa Rosa" Pergine Valsugana (TN), Azienda Provinciale per i Servizi Sanitari Provincia Autonoma di Trento, Trento, Italy

Håkon Ihle-Hansen, MD Department of Research, Vestre Viken Hospital Trust, Bærum Hospital, Drammen, Norway

Hege Ihle-Hansen, MD, PhD Department of Research, Vestre Viken Hospital Trust, Bærum Hospital, Drammen, Norway

Domenico Intiso Unit of Physical Medicine and Rehabilitation, Unit of Neuro-rehabilitation, IRCCS "Casa Sollievo della Sofferenza", San Giovanni Rotondo, FG, Italy

Marco Invernizzi, MD, PhD Physical and Rehabilitative Medicine, Department of Health Sciences, University of Eastern Piedmont "A. Avogadro", Novara, Italy

Giovanni Iolascon Department of Medical and Surgical Specialties and Dentistry, University of Campania "Luigi Vanvitelli", Caserta, Italy

Silvia Iovino Division of Respiratory Pathophysiology, University-City Hospital of Padua, Padua, Italy

I. Johnson Occupational Therapy and Assistive Technology Service (DAT), S. M Nascente Rehabilitation Centre, Don Gnocchi Foundation, Milan, Italy

Helmut Kern Ludwig Boltzmann Institute of Electrical Stimulation and Physical Rehabilitation, Vienna, Austria

Juliane Lamprecht Institute of Rehabilitation Medicine, Martin Luther University Halle-Wittenberg, Halle (Saale), Germany

Stefano Lanzi Division of Angiology, Heart and Vessel Department, University Hospital Lausanne, Lausanne, Switzerland

V. Lazzari Rehabilitation Unit, Department of Neurosciences, University of Padua, Padua, Italy

E. Lena Clinical Medicine and Translational Medicine Department, Tor Vergata University, Rome, Italy

Stefan Loefler Ludwig Boltzmann Institute of Electrical Stimulation and Physical Rehabilitation, Vienna, Austria

Giuseppe Lombardi Department of Experimental and Clinical Oncology, Medical Oncology 1, Veneto Institute of Oncology – IRCCS, Padua, Italy

Enzo Manzato Department of Medicine, Geriatrics Division, University of Padua, Padua, Italy

Andrea Marcante I.R.C.C.S., Fondazione Ospedale San Camillo, Venezia-Lido, Italy

IRCCS Fondazione San Camillo Hospital, Venice, Italy

Andrea Marini University of Udine, Udine, Italy

Scientific Institute, IRCCS Eugenio Medea, Bosisio Parini, Italy

Alessandro Martini Neuroscience Department, Operative Unit of Otolaryngology, Padua University, Padua, Italy

Stefano Masiero Department of Neuroscience, Physical Medicine and Rehabilitation Unit, University of Padua, Padua, Italy

M. Mastrocostas Neurorehabilitation Unit, University of Padua, Padua, Italy

Kerstin Mattukat Institute of Rehabilitation Medicine, Martin Luther University Halle-Wittenberg, Halle (Saale), Germany

Winfried Mayr Center for Medical Physics and Biomedical Engineering, Medical University of Vienna, Vienna, Austria

Anna Mazzola Department of Medical and Surgical Specialties and Dentistry, Second University of Naples, Naples, Italy

Lucia Mazzolai Division of Angiology, Heart and Vessel Department, University Hospital Lausanne, Lausanne, Switzerland

Xanthi Michail, MD, PhD Emeritus Prof. of Rehabilitation Medicine, Faculty of Health & Caring Professions, Technological Educational Institute of Athens (TEI-A), Athens, Greece

Edoardo Midena, MD, PhD Department of Ophthalmology, University of Padua, Padua, Italy

Fondazione GB Bietti per l'Oftalmologia, IRCCS, Rome, Italy

Antimo Moretti Department of Medical and Surgical Specialties and Dentistry, University of Campania "Luigi Vanvitelli", Caserta, Italy

Giovanni Morone Santa Lucia Hospital, Neurorehabilitation Unit, Rome, Italy

Ragnhild Munthe-Kaas, MD Department of Research, Vestre Viken Hospital Trust, Bærum Hospital, Drammen, Norway

Antonio Musarò Institute Pasteur Cenci-Bolognetti; DAHFMO-Unit of Histology and Medical Embryology, IIM; Sapienza University of Rome, Rome, Italy

Center for Life Nano Science@Sapienza, Istituto Italiano di Tecnologia, Rome, Italy

A. Musumeci Department of Physical Medicine and Rehabilitation, University of Padua, Padua, Padua, Italy

Beatrice Nordio Division of Respiratory Pathophysiology, University-City Hospital of Padua, Padua, Italy

Luca Padua Department of Geriatrics, Neurosciences and Orthopaedics, Università Cattolica del Sacro Cuore, Rome, Italy

Don Carlo Gnocchi Onlus Foundation, Milan, Italy

Antonio Paoli, MD, PhD Nutrition and Exercise Physiology Laboratory, Department of Biomedical Sciences, University of Padua, Padua, Italy

Jannis V. Papathanasiou, MD, PhD Department of Kinesitherapy, Faculty of Public Health, Medical University of Sofia, Sofia, Bulgaria

Department of Medical Imaging, Allergology and Physiotherapy, Faculty of Dental Medicine, Medical University of Plovdiv, Plovdiv, Bulgaria

Alberto Parola Department of Psychology, University of Turin, Turin, Italy

Sophie Pautex Community and Geriatric and Palliative Care Unit, Primary Care Division, University Hospital Geneva, Geneva, Switzerland

Francesco Piccione I.R.C.C.S., Fondazione Ospedale San Camillo, Venezia-Lido, Italy

IRCCS Fondazione San Camillo Hospital, Venice, Italy

Andrea Pignataro Department of Physical Medicine and Rehabilitation, University of Padua, Padua, Italy

Rehabilitation Unit, Department of Neurosciences, University of Padua, Padua, Italy

Elisabetta Pilotto, MD Department of Ophthalmology, University of Padua, Padua, Italy

Marco Poletti Division of Respiratory Pathophysiology, University-City Hospital of Padua, Padua, Italy

Amber Pond Anatomy Department, Southern Illinois University, School of Medicine, Carbondale, IL, USA

C. Pozzi Department of Rehabilitation and Aged Care of the Ancelle Hospital, Cremona, Italy

Geriatric Research Group, Brescia, Italy

Facoltà di Medicina & Chirugia, Università Cattolica del Sacro Cuore, Rome, Italy

Feliciano Protasi CeSI – Center for Research on Aging & DNICS, Department of Neuroscience, Imaging and Clinical Sciences, University G. d'Annunzio, Chieti, Italy

Rosario Rizzuto Department of Biomedical Science, University of Padua, Padua, Italy

F. Romagnoli Centro Riabilitativo "Dalla Mano e Arto Superiore" Srl – CRIMAS, Parma, Italy

P. Ruggieri Department of Orthopedics and Orthopedic Oncology, University of Padua, Padua, Italy

P. Rumeau Telemedicine Activity, Pôle Gériatrie du CHU de Toulouse, Toulouse, France

Patrizio Sale, MD, PhD IRCCS Fondazione San Camillo, Venice, Italy

Department of Neuroscience, Rehabilitation Unit, University of Padua, Padua, Italia

Marco Sandri Department of Biomedical Science, University of Padua, Padua, Italy

F. Scarponi Neurorehabilitation Unit, USL Umbria 2, S. Giovanni Battista Hospital, Foligno, Perugia, Italy

Christoph Schäfer Clinic for Internal Medicine II, Department of Internal Medicine, Martin Luther University Halle-Wittenberg, Halle (Saale), Germany

Giuseppe Sergi Department of Medicine, Geriatrics Division, University of Padua, Padua, Italy

Cornel C. Sieber Direktor des Institut für Biomedizin des Alterns Friedrich-Alexander-Universität Erlangen-Nürnberg, Erlangen, Germany

U. Solimene World Health Organization (WHO) Coll. Center for Traditional & Complementary Medicine, Milan State University, Milan, Italy

Jean-Paul Steinmetz, PhD Centre for Memory and Mobility, Zitha, Luxembourg City, Luxembourg

Research & Development, ZithaSenior, Luxembourg City, Luxembourg

Luigi Tesio, MD Department of Biomedical Sciences for Health, Physical and Rehabilitation Medicine, Università degli Studi di Milano, Milan, Italy

Department of Neurorehabilitation Sciences, Istituto Auxologico Italiano, IRCCS, Milan, Italy

S. Tocco Centro Riabilitativo "Dalla Mano e Arto Superiore" Srl – CRIMAS, Parma, Italy

Marco Traballesi Santa Lucia Hospital, Neurorehabilitation Unit, Rome, Italy

C. Trevisan Department of Medicine, Geriatrics Division, University of Padua, Padua, Italy

G. Trovarelli Department of Orthopedics and Orthopedic Oncology, University of Padua, Padua, Italy

Marie Ursin, PhD Department of Research, Vestre Viken Hospital Trust, Bærum Hospital, Drammen, Norway

Marta Valente Department of Physical Medicine and Rehabilitation, University of Padua, Padua, Italy

Gennaro Verni Eng. Centro Protesi INAIL Vigorso di Budrio, Bologna, Italy

Nicola Veronese Department of Medicine, Geriatrics Division, University of Padua, Padua, Italy

Andrea Vianello Division of Respiratory Pathophysiology, University-City Hospital of Padua, Padua, Italy

Adriana Visonà Angiology Unit, San Giacomo Hospital, Castelfranco Veneto, TV, Italy

Italian Society for Angiology and Vascular Medicine (SIAPAV), Italy

European Society for Vascular Medicine (ESVM), Italy

Filippo Vittadini Department of Physical Medicine and Rehabilitation, University of Padua, Padua, Italy

Raphael Wittenberg Personal Social Services Research Unit, London School of Economics and Political Science, London, UK

Vittorina Zagonel Department of Experimental and Clinical Oncology, Medical Oncology 1, Veneto Institute of Oncology – IRCCS, Padua, Italy

Sandra Zampieri Ludwig Boltzmann Institute of Electrical Stimulation and Physical Rehabilitation, Vienna, Austria

Venetian Institute of Molecular Medicine, Padua, Italy

Department of Biomedical Science, University of Padua, Padua, Italy

M. Zampolini Neurorehabilitation Unit, USL Umbria 2, S. Giovanni Battista Hospital, Foligno, Perugia, Italy

Foligno Hospital, Via M. ArcamoneFoligno, Perugia, Italy

B.M. Zanforlini Department of Medicine, Geriatrics Division, University of Padua, Padua, Italy

H. Zatti Rehabilitation Unit, Department of Neurosciences, University of Padua, Padua, Italy

Part I

Physical Activity and Rehabilitation in Elderly

1

Walter R. Frontera

1.1 Aging Demographics

The World Health Organization has estimated that by the year 2050, the world's population over 60 years will double from about 11% in 2015 to 22% [1, 2]. This means that there will be approximately two billion people aged 60 or older living on the planet. Of these, approximately 20% or 400 million will be 80 years or older. In the year 2015, Japan was the only country in the world with 30% or more of the population in the 60 years or older group. The WHO is projecting that by the year 2050, more than 25 countries, including most countries in Europe, will have a population distribution very similar to that of Japan. For example, the percentage of Italians older than 60 years will increase from approximately 20% in 2010 to approximately 33% in the year 2050. This increase in the number of people in older age groups is associated with an increase in life expectancy. For example, in Japan, life expectancy at age 60 is 86 years and in at least 13 other countries life expectancy at age 60 is now 85 years (Table 1.1). Further, the number of centenarians is also increasing, and in several regions of the world, including Sardinia, Italy and Icaria, Greece, there are a disproportionately large number of people in this age group.

W.R. Frontera, MD, PhD
Departments of Physical Medicine, Rehabilitation and Sports Medicine and Physiology and Biophysics, University of Puerto Rico School of Medicine, San Juan, Puerto Rico
e-mail: walter.frontera@upr.edu

© Springer International Publishing AG 2018

S. Masiero, U. Carraro (eds.), *Rehabilitation Medicine for Elderly Patients*, Practical Issues in Geriatrics, DOI 10.1007/978-3-319-57406-6_1

Table 1.1 At 86 years, Japan's life expectancy is the longest in the world followed by the 13 countries listed in the table with a life expectancy of 85 years

Andorra
Australia
Canada
France
Israel
Italy
Luxembourg
Monaco
New Zealand
San Marino
Singapore
Spain
Switzerland

References [1] and [2]

The increase in the number of people in older age groups, per se, should not be considered a problem. However, aging is associated with an increased incidence of chronic health conditions and, perhaps more importantly, an increased prevalence of impairment and disability that may lead to a lower quality of life. Most of these impairments lead to a reduction in activity levels and restrict participation in personal, work-related, and social activities. One specific example is the age-associated loss of muscle mass and strength that is associated with a higher risk of falls and hospitalization. As a consequence, it has been estimated that the number of older people requiring rehabilitation and/or long-term care due to loss of functional independence will quadruple by 2050 [1]. The social, economic, and political implications of these demographic changes are enormous because, by 2050, 80% of older people will live in low- and middle-income countries. This is not a situation that governments should or could ignore and may require the reorganization of health care systems to accommodate the needs of this population. It is necessary to develop public and health policies that will address the needs of an aging society and for rehabilitation professionals to become an important part of the solution by generating new knowledge via research and educating others on the best strategy to address disability in society.

1.2 Functional Changes in Elderly

A decline in physical function and significant increases in the risk for disability and dependence are typical of advanced adult age [3]. In humans, a number of age-related changes in various biological systems contribute to this decline including, but not limited to, decreases in muscle and bone mass, increases in body fat, loss of brain volume and cognitive capacity, loss of cardiovascular and pulmonary reserves, impaired visual and hearing function, sleeping disorders, anxiety and depression, and changes in dietary habits leading to mal-/undernutrition. Some of these changes are directly associated with lower levels of habitual physical activity. Further, pain associated with musculoskeletal disorders is frequently reported by older men and women and is associated with a reduction in their habitual level of physical activity.

It is important to note that the prevalence of mobility limitations in elderly is high but it does not have to be considered a static condition. In other words, older people experience frequent changes in their level of independence transitioning between more functional to less functional states and vice versa. For example, several studies [4, 5] have shown that older men and women transition more frequently from intermittent to continuous mobility limitation than from no mobility limitation to intermittent mobility limitation. The dynamic nature of this condition is demonstrated by the fact that it is possible to recover mobility after being disabled for 3 months (40% recovery rate) or even for 6 months (30% recovery rate). These findings suggest that the road from impairment to activity limitation and restricted participation in elderly is a bidirectional process. This is precisely why rehabilitation, as a health and functionally oriented strategy, is so crucial to influence this process. Perhaps more importantly, the plastic nature of the process suggests specific opportunities to intervene, restore function, and recover independence [4–6]. The habitual level of physical activity, an increase in various types of physical activity including work-related and leisure activity, and more structured exercise training programs have been shown to be modifiers of this process.

A very important determinant of functionality and independence is skeletal muscle function. Muscle strength is a strong predictor of severe mobility limitation, slow gait speed, increased fall risk, risk of hospitalization, and high mortality rate. For example, older adults with low muscle strength have a 2.6 fold greater risk of severe mobility limitation, 4.3 fold greater risk for slow gait speed, and a 2.1 fold greater risk of mortality compared to older adults with high muscle strength [7]. The loss of muscle strength in elderly cannot be explained only by the characteristic presence of skeletal muscle wasting or atrophy. During the last two decades, several studies have shown that other factors such as changes in central nervous system drive and activation, peripheral nerve dysfunction, alterations in the structure and function of the neuromuscular junction, fat infiltration of muscle, and a number of complex cellular and molecular changes at the level of single muscle fibers and individual myofilaments such as myosin impair muscle force generation, velocity of movement, and power production [8]. It is interesting to note that the well-described loss of muscle strength in older men and women appears to be less in those that have maintained a higher level of physical activity throughout their lives [9, 10]. This is true even in the presence of obesity and highlights the importance of habitual physical activity in this process. Thus, it is reasonable to suggest that different levels of reduced activity including a sedentary lifestyle, inactivity, and/or immobilization contribute to age-related changes and that these changes do not have to be considered inevitable consequences of the biological process of aging. It is interesting to note that sedentary behaviors such as driving a car and watching television are being considered independent risk factors equivalent to the more traditional ones such as cigarette smoking. Finally, scientific evidence suggests that interventions such as those including physical activity and appropriate nutritional support are safe and beneficial and can enhance the functional capacity of even very old frail people. (Sarcopenia will be discussed in another chapter of this book.)

1.3 Physical Activity vs. Exercise

It should not come as a surprise that part of the solution to the functional decline and muscular dysfunction associated with advanced adult age is an increase in physical activity and/or exercise training. Many rehabilitation interventions are characterized by increases in one or the other and sometimes both. However, it is important to make a distinction between these two related but different concepts. For the purpose of this chapter, physical activity will be defined as any bodily movement produced by skeletal muscles that result in energy expenditure [11]. Furthermore, physical activity can be subdivided depending on associated characteristics, for example, into household (e.g., gardening), leisure-time or recreational (e.g., walking), occupational (e.g., climbing stairs on the job), or sports-related activity (a game of soccer with friends on a Saturday afternoon). In many research studies however, all types of physical activity are combined into a single estimate of daily energy expenditure making the interpretation of the results more difficult. Exercise, on the other hand, will be considered as subset of physical activity that is planned, structured, and repetitive and has as an objective, the improvement or maintenance of physical fitness. This is the subtype of physical activity used in many rehabilitation programs and clinical intervention studies. Finally, fitness is a set of attributes that are health related (e.g., muscle strength, cardiorespiratory endurance, body composition, flexibility) or skill related (agility, balance, coordination) and can be measured with specific tests. One example of a health-related fitness test is the duration of exercise on a treadmill test. Physical fitness is an attribute influenced, but not entirely determined, by behaviors such as the level of physical activity and exercise training. The distinction between physical activity, exercise, and fitness, although not always clear and/or possible, is of practical value when evaluating the scientific literature on this topic. This brief review is more focused on physical activity while other chapters in this volume discuss exercise in more detail.

1.4 Measuring Physical Activity

Some brief comments about assessing physical activity are needed here. The measurement of the level of physical activity in humans requires valid and reliable instruments that are simple enough to be used in epidemiological studies and at the same time flexible enough to be adjusted to the challenges of impaired mobility that is prevalent in older adults. One of the more traditional methods is the questionnaire. Many studies have used a set of standard questions that examine the type, frequency, intensity, and duration of physical activity in a certain period of time. The results can be used to estimate average daily energy expenditure. These self-report instruments, although easy to administer and appropriate when a large number of individuals are included in a study, depend on the memory of the participant and can be subject to bias and influenced by the participant's psychological status and the training of the interviewer (see reference [12] for review).

More objective measures of physical activity include double-labeled water (considered by many as the gold standard to measure energy expenditure over time), metabolic chambers (expensive facilities that are available only in very few specialized research centers), and accelerometers (devices that measure acceleration and estimate total amount of activity). The latter have received significant attention because they are wearable (usually at the level of the waist), easy to use, and relatively inexpensive, capture real-time data, can be used over multiple days (usually 7 days), and have been validated in several research studies and in various populations including older adults [13]. Because of recent advances in this technology, it is likely that this measurement instrument will continue to be used in research, in the clinic, and by those individuals who monitor their daily activity.

1.5 The Importance of Physical Activity in the Prevention of Chronic Disease

During the last 60 years, a large number of scientific studies have evaluated the association between the level of physical activity (leisure time, occupational, total) and the incidence and prevalence of several chronic diseases. These studies are of particular relevance for the aging population because the incidence of these chronic noncommunicable diseases is high in older men and women and increases with age. Some of these diseases are associated with a high mortality rate particularly in older people. Furthermore, the level of leisure-time aerobic physical activity among individuals with chronic disease has been shown to be very low [14]. This is particularly true in patients with comorbidities or more than one chronic illness. Taken together, the main conclusion supported by these studies is that a high level of habitual physical activity significantly reduces the risk and incidence of many chronic noncommunicable diseases.

The hypothesis that a higher level of daily physical activity of work is inversely related to coronary heart disease was tested for the first time by investigators in London, England [15]. Since that classical study by Morris and collaborators, hundreds of other studies have confirmed that same hypothesis in various age groups and in several countries. Furthermore, the same hypothesis has been tested with similar results in various studies looking at other chronic conditions. Many studies, although not all, have included both, men and women, and people older than 60 years of age. A higher level of physical activity has been shown to be associated with a reduction in the risk of developing heart disease, hypertension, obesity, type 2 diabetes, osteoporosis, several forms of cancer (including colon, breast, lung, esophageal adenocarcinoma, liver, gastric cardia, head and neck, and other types of cancer) [16], sarcopenia, and sarcopenic obesity. It is important to note that these studies have controlled for the potential confounding influence of other risk factors such as body mass index, smoking status, alcohol intake, education, race, and sex.

Further, it is interesting to note that associations similar to the above have been reported between the incidence of some of these conditions and the level of physical fitness. Specific tests are used for each fitness attribute mentioned above (see page 7). In most of the studies on the prevention of chronic illness, fitness has been defined as the duration of exercise in a treadmill test or metabolic equivalent (MET level). In other words, a higher level of cardiorespiratory fitness is associated with a lower incidence of several chronic illnesses. Although the level of physical activity impacts cardiorespiratory fitness, other factors such as the genotype of the individual are considered independent determinants of fitness. Finally, some studies have shown a reduction in mortality associated with both lung and digestive cancers among individuals with high levels of cardiorespiratory fitness. In most cases, the biological mechanism underlying these relationships is not understood, but it is important to know that activity and/or fitness can influence not only the incidence of a chronic condition but also its clinical outcome or mortality (Fig. 1.1).

One of the most devastating conditions associated with age is an increased incidence of mental health problems such as depression and anxiety as well as a decline in cognitive function. It is fair to say that the consensus based on scientific research is that a high level of physical activity is positively associated with human well-being and good mental health. Epidemiological studies have shown that people that have a high level of habitual physical activity have lower levels of mild to moderate depression and anxiety. On the other hand, the prevalence of cognitive impairment in the general population increases with age. Again, high levels of habitual physical activity are associated with a reduced risk of cognitive decline, dementia, and Alzheimer's disease in later life [17]. The strength of this association between physical activity and cognitive function is supported by both cross-sectional and longitudinal studies. It appears that the underlying mechanism explaining this protective effect is vascular in nature and includes an increase in brain perfusion as well as the ability of cerebral blood vessels to respond to demand.

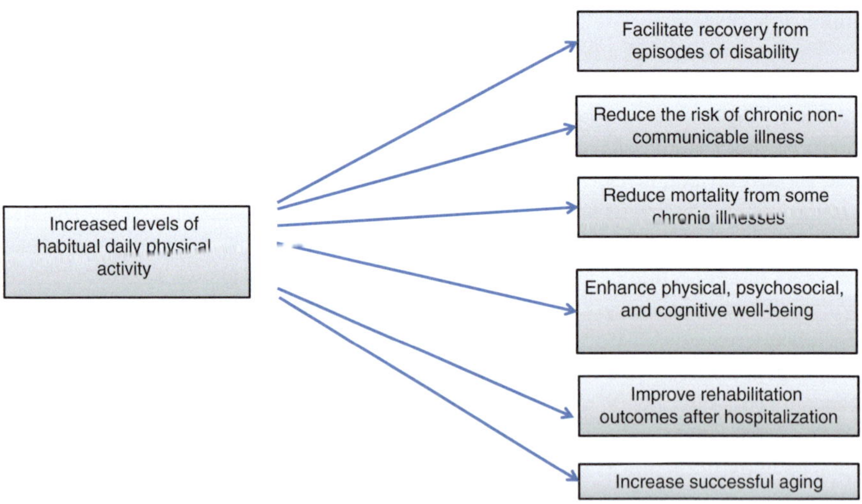

Fig. 1.1 Increased levels of habitual physical activity is associated with positive health-related and functional outcomes

1.6 Level of Regular Physical Activity in Older Men and Women

Notwithstanding the abundant evidence demonstrating that appropriate levels of physical activity contribute to the prevention of many disabling chronic illnesses in older people, most members of this age group in our society do not reach the levels of physical activity needed to obtain the health-related benefits associated with physical activity. For example, in the United States, the percent of adults engaging in leisure-time physical activity decreases with age in both men and women [18]. In fact, only 20–30% of men and 11–20% of women performed 30 min of light to moderate physical activity 5 times per week or 20 min of vigorous activity 3 times per week. As mentioned above, the presence of one or more chronic illness (such as arthritis, hypertension, diabetes, obesity, stroke, and others) is associated with low levels of leisure-time physical activity [14]. The participation in any leisure-time strengthening activity is even lower in older people ranging from 6 to 14% depending on the sex. It seems that those who need physical activity the most are less likely to engage in it. This situation is not limited to the United States as reports from the WHO show a high level of sedentary lifestyle in many countries. These and other observations suggest that we need to better understand those factors that motivate people to be physically active and design ways to change human behavior by enhancing adherence to a lifestyle that includes appropriate levels of physical activity (Fig. 1.2).

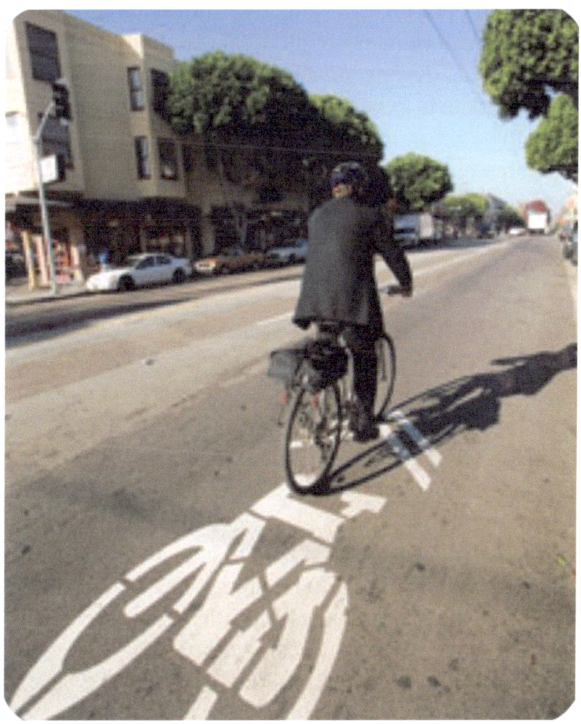

Fig. 1.2 Physical activity incorporated into our daily routine and encouraged by the presence of a bicycle lane (From: Centers for Disease Control and Prevention. *Strategies to Prevent Obesity and Other Chronic Diseases: The CDC Guide to Strategies to Increase Physical Activity in the Community.* Atlanta: US Department of Health and Human Services, 2011)

1.7 Determinants of Levels of Physical Activity

The interest and ability of a person to engage in physical activity is determined by many factors. For example, the presence of medical conditions (controlled and uncontrolled) that limit mobility and endurance, symptoms such as musculoskeletal pain and general fatigue, the use of medications that may cause side effects such as dizziness or muscle dysfunction, and the presence of a permanent physical impairment like the loss of a limb can limit a person's capacity to perform physical activity and his/her motivation to be physically active. This is particularly true if the activity must be performed outdoors where the presence of uneven terrain, weather conditions, and the fear of falling act as deterrents. Rehabilitation interventions must be designed with the goal of limiting the impact of these factors allowing a higher level of physical activity. Medical interventions as well as environmental modifications may be necessary. These can contribute to the maintenance of a higher functional capacity as these two factors, physical activity and function, relate to each other.

Other nonmedical factors that may enhance an individual's level of physical activity include a high level of support and encouragement provided by family members, the presence of friends and neighbors during the activity with whom they can interact socially, the absence of crime in the neighborhood, and the presence of a racially diverse population. In addition, environmental factors such as walkability of streets, access to parks and similar facilities, physical barriers such as inappropriate sidewalks and absence of bridges or elevated pathways, heavy traffic, and aesthetics such as the presence of attractive surroundings and nature have been shown to be important determinants of physical activity [19]. Finally, the use of assistive devices and products may significantly enhance an individual's mobility (see the list of the top 50 products to be included in WHO's Priority Assistive Products List in: http://www.who.int/phi/implementation/assistive_technology/global_survey-apl/en/). More research is needed to understand how the use of these devices contributes to the type of energy expenditure and physical activity associated with desirable health outcomes.

1.8 Benefits of Increasing Physical Activity During Rehabilitation

Scientific research shows that older men are more susceptible to the negative effects of inactivity and deconditioning associated with bed rest than younger men [20]. For the purpose of this chapter, deconditioning is defined as the process by which inactivity or a sedentary lifestyle results in a reduction in physiological and functional capacity or fitness. Older men and women lose more muscle mass and function after bed rest but also maintain their capacity to respond well to rehabilitation. In most, if not all, circumstances, the process of rehabilitation includes an increase in the daily level of physical activity. This process should begin very early after injury or the onset of an illness, a principle that applies to all ages but may be particularly important in elderly. The increase in physical activity is needed even during a stay in a hospital-based intensive care unit because it contributes to increasing early mobility, preventing complications, and enhancing functional outcomes. Indeed, the degree of mobility or walking as determined using accelerometry during hospitalization can be a good predictor of rehabilitation outcomes [21].

An increase in physical activity may also be recommended in persons living in institutions for long-term care who are not independent enough to function in a community setting. To minimize risks such as falls, this increase in daily physical activity must be supervised. Finally, many people living independently in their communities may benefit from an increase in daily physical activity. Although these recommendations may include an exercise (see above definition of physical activity vs. exercise) training program, this is not a requirement. Encouraging persons to become engaged in more activities at home and in the community is a way to accomplish this goal. In general, all persons should accumulate a total of 150 min of moderate physical activity per week. Simple changes in their lifestyle such as participating in a gardening activity, climbing stairs more frequently, performing household duties, or walking to the grocery store instead of driving may be enough to achieve this goal.

A consistent observation across epidemiological studies is that the level of daily physical activity in the community is an independent factor that contributes to successful aging [22]. This appears to be particularly true when high levels of physical activity are combined with a high quality diet like the Mediterranean diet. The geography of a country may contribute to this because the level of daily physical activity is spontaneously higher in islanders compared to those who live in continental areas. It would be interesting to know if increasing the level of physical activity in an environment that encourages or facilitates physical activity can be a means of enhancing functional capacity.

1.9 Concluding Remarks

Physical activity, defined as any bodily movement resulting in energy expenditure, is an important determinant of functional capacity and health. This is particularly true in a growing segment of the population across the world, older men and women. The benefits of a high level of habitual and daily physical activity (generally defined as 150 min of moderate intensity activity per week) include the prevention of many noncommunicable diseases and the reduction in mortality associated with several chronic illnesses. Furthermore, an increase in physical activity is an important component of most rehabilitation interventions. Rehabilitation professionals must work to remove barriers to physical activity and motivate individuals in any clinical service setting and in the community to change their behavior by increasing their level of physical activity. The benefits of such a change far outweigh the risks and will help us overcome the deleterious effects of a sedentary lifestyle, at any age!

Key Points
- An increase in human life expectancy has characterized the last century.
- Aging is associated with reductions in physiological and functional capacities and quality of life.
- An increase in level of physical activity has been shown to increase functional capacity, prevent many chronic noncommunicable diseases, and contribute to the rehabilitation of older persons after injury or illness.
- Behavioral and environmental strategies are needed to encourage the general population to accumulate 150 min of moderate intensity physical activity every week.

References

1. www.who.org. Accessed 13 May 2016
2. World Health Organization (2015) World report on ageing and health
3. Brady AO, Straight CR, Evans EM (2014) Body composition, muscle capacity, and physical function in older adults: an integrated conceptual model. J Aging Phys Act 22:441–452
4. Gill TM, Allore HG, Hardy SE, Guo Z (2006) The dynamic nature of mobility disability in older persons. J Am Geriatr Soc 54:248–254
5. Hardy SE, Dubin JA, Holford TR, Gill TM (2005) Transitions between states of disability and independence among older persons. Am J Epidemiol 161:575–584
6. Hardy SE, Gill TM (2004) Recovery from disability among community-dwelling older persons. JAMA 291:1596–1602
7. Manini TM (2011) Development of physical disability in older adults. Curr Aging Sci 4:184–191
8. Frontera WR, Rodriguez Zayas A, Rodríguez N (2012) Human aging muscle: understanding sarcopenia at the single muscle fiber level. PM&R Clin NA 23:201–207
9. Ryu M, Jo J, Lee Y, Chung Y-S, Kim K-M, Baek W-C (2013) Association of physical activity with sarcopenia and sarcopenic obesity in community-dwelling older adults: the Fourth Korea National Health and Nutrition Examination Survey. Age Ageing 42:734–740
10. Mijnarends DM, Koster A, Schols JMGA, Meijers JMM, Halfens RJG, Gudnason V, Eiriksdottir G, Siggeirsdottir K, Sigurdsson S, Jónsson PV, Meirelles O, Haris T (2016) Physical activity and incidence of sarcopenia: the population-based AGES-Reykjavik Study. Age Ageing. doi:10.1093/ageing/afw090
11. Caspersen CJ, Powell KE, Christenson GM (1985) Physical activity, exercise, and physical fitness: definitions and distinctions for health-related research. Public Health Rep 100:126–131
12. Loyen A, Van Hecke L, Verloigne M, Hendriksen I, Lakerveld J, Steene-Johannessen J, Vuillemin A, Koster A, Donnelly A, Ekelund U, Deforche B, De Bourdeaudhuij I, Brug J, van der Ploeg HP, DEDIPAC consortium (2016) Variation in population levels of physical activity in European adults according to cross-European studies: a systematic literature review within DEDIPAC. Int J Behav Nutr Phys Act 13:72
13. Strath SJ, Pfeiffer KA, Whitt-Glover MC (2012) Accelerometer use with children, older adults, and adults with functional limitations. Med Sci Sports Exerc 44(1 Suppl 1):S77–S85
14. Brawner CA, Churilla JR, Keteyian SJ (2016) Prevalence of physical activity is lower among individuals with chronic disease. Med Sci Sports Exerc 48:1062–1067
15. Morris JN, Heady JA, Raffle PAB, Roberts CG, Parks JW (1953) Coronary heart-disease and physical activity of work. Lancet 262:1053–1057
16. Moore SC, Lee IM, Weiderpass E, Campbell PT, Sampson JN, Kitahara CM et al (2016) Association of leisure-time physical activity with risk of 26 types of cancer in 1.44 million adults of physical disability in older adults. JAMA Int Med (online May 16, 2016)

17. Davenport MH, Hogan DB, Eskes GA, Longman RS, Poulin MJ (2012) Cerebrovascular reserve; the link between fitness and cognitive function? Exerc Sports Sci Rev 40:153–158
18. Bassuk SS, Manson JE (2003) Physical activity and cardiovascular disease prevention in women: how much is good enough? Exerc Sports Sci Rev 31:176–181
19. Van Holle V, Van Cauwenberg J, Gheysen F, Van Dyck D, Deforce B, Van de Weghe N, De Bourdeaudhuij I (2016) The association between Belgian older adults' physical functioning and physical activity: what is the moderating role of the physical environment? PLoS One 11(2):e0148398
20. Pišot R, Marusic U, Biolo G, Mazzucco S, Lazzer S, Grassi B, Regianni C, Toniolo L, di Prampero PE, Passaro A, Narici M, Mohammed S, Rittweger J, Gasparini M, Blenkuš MG, Šimunič B (2016) Greater loss in muscle mass and function but smaller metabolic alterations in older compared with younger men following 2 wk of bed rest and recovery. J Appl Physiol 120:922–929
21. Fisher SR, Graham JE, Ottenbacher KJ, Deer R, Ostir GV (2016) Inpatient walking activity to predict readmission in older adults. Arch Phys Med Rehabil. doi:10.1016/j.apmr.2015.09.029
22. Mariolis A, Foscolou A, Tyrovolas S, Piscopo S, Valacchi G, Tsakountakis N, Zeimbekis A, Bountziouka V, Gotsis E, Metallinos G, Tyrovola D, Tur J-A, Matalas A-L, Lionis C, Polychronopoulos E, Panagiotakos D, for the MEDIS study group (2016) Successful aging among elders living in the Mani continental region vs. insular areas of the Mediterranean: the MEDIS study. Aging Dis 7:285–294

Aging Brain and Neurological Changes

2

Håkon Ihle-Hansen and Hege Ihle-Hansen

Aging is inevitable, but aging well is not. Keeping the brain robust is an essential part of health.

2.1 Introduction

The aging process involves all the body's cells and tissues but does not happen with equal speed in all tissues. Normal brain aging is characterized by a reduction in cognitive abilities, particularly in the domains of executive function, processing speed, and episodic memory. Both structural and functional changes in the central nerve system are linked to the decline, but it is still uncertain whether and how the cognitive decline is caused by the brain changes.

2.2 The Aging Brain: Structural Changes in Normal Aging

2.2.1 Basic Anatomy

To understand and predict the age-specific changes in an aging brain, it is important to know the principle and structure of the brain. The central nerve system (CNS), the spinal cord and the brain, are divided into gray and white matter. In the gray matter, we mostly find the cell bodies of the neurons, while the white matter consists of long myelinated axons.

The CNS's main task is to convey signals. The neurons build large complex circuits with each other. Neurons are contacted and communicate with each other

H. Ihle-Hansen, MD (✉) • H. Ihle-Hansen, MD, PhD
Department of Research, Vestre Viken Hospital Trust, Bærum Hospital,
3004 Drammen, Norway
e-mail: haaihl@vestreviken.no; hege.ihle-hansen@vestreviken.no

© Springer International Publishing AG 2018

S. Masiero, U. Carraro (eds.), *Rehabilitation Medicine for Elderly Patients*,
Practical Issues in Geriatrics, DOI 10.1007/978-3-319-57406-6_2

Anatomic part	Function
Soma	Cell body of a neuron
Neurite	Any process extending from the body of a neuron
Axon	A neurite, that often project to another region. Specialized to conduct axons potential. A neuron has in general one axon, which again can have a lot of branches
Dendrite	A local neurite. The number of dendrite correlates with the input. Primary function receiving axonal input.

Fig. 2.1 Anatomic parts of the neuron and their function

through synapses, a chemical transmission, in which a signal is transferred to the next cell in the signal path. It is believed that our intelligence, memory, emotions, and behavior are stored and regulated through activity and interplay in these complex circuits. A modern conception views the function of the nervous system partly in terms of stimulus-response chains and partly in terms of intrinsically generated activity patterns, meaning spontaneous cell-generated activity.

The neurons are electrically excitable cells consisting of soma and neurites (one axon and dendrites). Neuron geometry is associated with functions: number of synapse, signal patterns, location remove and pattern of connection (Fig. 2.1).

Most neurons send signals via their axons, although some of them are capable of dendrite-to-dendrite communication.

2.2.2 Basic Physiology

The cell communicates through the action potential (AP). Prerequisite to develop an action potential are ion channels, a lipid bilayer and a potential across the membrane. Action potentials are generated by voltage-gated ion channels embedded in the membrane. These channels are shut when the membrane potential is near the membrane potential of the cell, but they rapidly begin to open if the membrane potential increases to a precisely defined threshold value. The shift in membrane polarity leads aging to inactivity in the ion channels. This is the start of the repolarization phase, ending with the cell again assuming its steady-state condition. The AP propagates along the neuron's axon toward its ends and thereby connects with other neuronal synapses, motor cells or glands.

As the AP reached the axonal end, the electrical potential is transformed into chemical signals. This happens in the synapse. The AP leads to release of neurotransmitters, which are stored in presynaptic vesicles, into the synaptic cleft. Then the neurotransmitters diffuse to the postsynaptic membrane (on the dendrite), bind to a receptor, and induce a signal that can be excited or inhibited. In other words, synaptic inputs to a neuron cause the membrane to depolarize or hyperpolarize.

A chemical synaptic transmission provides flexibility and provides the opportunity to a wide range of chemical transmitters and receptors in a single synapse.

Formation of the synapses and the plasticity of the synapses changes over time and during the normal aging. Biochemical changes seem to play an important role in the aging brain. Alteration in syntheses and turnover of neurotransmitters has been observed. The reduction of dopamine synthesis and dopamine receptors has been linked to motility disturbance and change in cognitive flexibility. Alterations in calcium regulation, glutamate, and serotonin are also described. Calcium plays an important role in neuronal firing and propagation of AP. Glutamate is an excitatory neurotransmitter, and it is a documented age-related decrease, especially in the parietal gray matter and basal ganglia. Interconnections of neuronal network are involved in human cognition and mental life and are thought to represent a cognitive reserve. The neuronal degeneration is part of the normal aging process.

2.2.3 Synaptic Plasticity

Through learning we can build, strengthen, or remodel the circuits. This leads to structural and biochemical changes, as a response to increase or decrease in their activity, with the development of new synapses and up- and downregulations of neurotransmitters, receptors, and ion channels.

Synapses are capable of forming memory traces by means of long-lasting increase in signal transmission between two neurons—a change in synaptic strength. One of the most interesting and studied forms of neural memory is the long-term potentiation, which was first described back in 1973, but is still not fully understood. The phenomenon is characterized by the fact that the neurotransmitter glutamate acts on a special type of receptor known as the NMDA receptor. The NMDA receptor has an "associative" property: if the two cells involved in the synapse are both activated at approximately the same time, a channel opens that permits calcium to flow into the target cell. A second messenger induces a cascade that ultimately leads to an increase in the number of glutamate receptors on the target cell, thereby increasing the effective strength of the synapse. This change in strength can last for weeks.

2.2.4 Structural Changes

The reason why the brain atrophies or shrinks in size with age is not completely understood.

It is assumed that normal healthy aging is associated with numerous structural, chemical, gene expression and functional changes. Downregulation and genetic and environmental factors are central concepts, and there is a thin line between normal aging and pathology. Over the past decade, the introduction of new radiological modalities has made it possible to measure brain volume and in some part brain activity in healthy aging individuals. Gray matter as well as white matter volume decreases with age. Some regions are especially vulnerable to gray matter loss, such as insula and superior parietal gyri. On the other hand, some regions are spared to this decrease in gray matter, such as the occipital cortex surrounding the calcarine sulcus and the cingulate gyrus. The decrease in volume is assumed not to be driven by loss of neurons or cell death, but through a decrease in spine density and synaptic alterations.

Age-related cognitive decline varies among older persons. Factors involved in this variability include genetics, education, occupational engagement, comorbidities and co-medications. In addition, lifestyle factors like nutrition, smoking, alcohol use, and physical activity and vascular risk factor have an impact on this decline.

Amyloid plaques, which are linked to Alzheimer's disease (AD), are supposed not to be found in a healthy brain. On the contrary, neurofibrillary tangles may be present in some regions and part of a normal aging process. The number of tangles in a cell is relatively low in a healthy brain and only located in amygdala, entorhinal cortex, the olfactory nucleus and parahippocampal gyrus. Findings of tangles in other specific locations may however indicate pathology.

DNA damage accumulates with age, leading to reduced expression of genes that are involved in learning, memory, and behavioral pattern. DNA damage is partly induced by oxidative stress, also linked to mitochondrial dysfunction. Environmental and lifestyle factors lead to vascular changes with potential disturbance in the cerebral blood flood and blood-brain barrier.

2.2.5 Neuroplasticity

The brain is a dynamic organ that has a natural ability to adapt and change with time, called brain plasticity or neuroplasticity. Even after a CNS injury, the brain changes by setting up new connections and paths between neurons, building new and strengthening existing circuits. We now know that the brain can create new neurons in some parts of the brain, although the extent and purpose of this is still uncertain.

Plasticity of the brain occurs at every stage of development throughout the life cycle. Plasticity is more likely to occur when there is stimulation of the neural system, meaning that the brain must be active to adapt. Development of new neuronal network through exposure to a stimulating environment leads to structural changes and improved skills. These changes do not occur quickly; the recovery goes on for months and sometimes years.

Education, occupation and cognitive activity have been found to be associated with higher cognitive performance and delay of cognitive impairments. A lifetime intellectual enrichment is thought to represent a preventive intervention for cognitive decline and dementia. By keeping the cognitive activity constant throughout the lifespan, we may protect the brain and delay the onset of cognitive impairments for 5 years! Specific training is linked to both faster response and general cognitive improvement.

There is a growing body of evidence regarding the benefit of exercise in terms of neuroplasticity and the ability of the brain to self-repair. In particular, goal-based exercises and aerobic exercises increase synaptic strength (increasing neurotransmission, receptor density, and dendritic spine formation) and improve brain health by increasing trophic factors, blood flow, immune system, neurogenesis, and metabolism. Therefore, the strengthening of the circuitry of basal ganglia, cortex, thalamus, cerebellum and brainstem results in improved motor and cognitive behavior, mood and motivation.

2.3 The Aging Brain: Functional Changes

2.3.1 Cognitive Decline

The decline in cognitive function is thought to begin around the age of 50. Age-related reductions in brain volume are approximately 0.5% every year and may start even earlier. Temporal and frontal lobes seem to be more vulnerable and have some higher degree of changes, but the clinical impact of these changes is not known. In addition, it seems like the rate of atrophy may increase in older age.

Aerobic exercise may promote neuroplasticity and slow the progression of age-related neural changes. Structured exercise has been shown to improve attention, executive function, psychomotor speed and episodic memory. Sleep is of benefit for the brain, where it seems like a good night's sleep helps to clear the brain.

2.3.2 Dementia Is Not Part of the Normal Aging

Alzheimer's disease (AD) is considered to be a disease and not part of the normal aging. Dementia due to AD is expected to become much more prevalent in the years to come. AD is characterized by an accumulation of protein waste products including amyloid that triggers inflammation that over several years leads to a loss of brain cells. A number of cascade interactions are thought to cause neuron loss where mitochondrial dysfunction or altered energy supply contribute to the neurodegeneration.

There is no cure for AD today, so we have to focus on early detection and prevention. Cardiovascular disease is known to be a risk factor for dementia and cognitive decline, and targeting vascular risk factors may preserve brain health. Especially midlife elevations in blood pressure have been shown to predict dementia later in the life span. Hypertension is associated with both cognitive decline and structural brain changes like atrophy and degraded white matter connectivity. Carriers of APOEε4 allele with additional cardiovascular disease seem to have higher risk for cognitive decline than those without.

2.4 Conclusions

2.4.1 Preserve Brain Health!

The process of aging is inevitable, but with a healthy way of life, it may be possible to delay the process. Evidence points out education, intellectually activity, cardiovascular risk control, physical activity, healthy environment, and social activity as key elements to preserve brain health.

Key Points

- Through normal aging there is a reduction in cognitive abilities, particularly in the domains of executive function, processing speed, and episodic memory.
- The brain is adaptive and impressionable throughout life.
- Intellectual enrichment prevents cognitive decline.
- Physical exercise and a healthy way of life may promote neuroplasticity.

3 Age-Related Changes in Body Composition and Energy Metabolism

G. Sergi, C. Trevisan, B.M. Zanforlini, N. Veronese, and E. Manzato

3.1 Introduction

In the geriatric population, rehabilitation care is important in preventing or limiting mobility impairment and loss of self-sufficiency, which raise the risk of comorbidities, frailty, and mortality [1]. The exercise workload to adopt in rehabilitation programs needs to be adapted to each patient's characteristics and to the physiological, age-related changes in their body composition and energy metabolism, as illustrated in Fig. 3.1. The musculoskeletal changes generally seen in old age concern fat-free mass, fat mass, and bone mass, with a gradual loss of muscle bulk and strength, a gain and redistribution of adipose tissue, and the onset of joint stiffness and declining bone mineral density [2]. Among the multiple factors influencing these changes, endocrine, immunological, and inflammatory mediators have a fundamental role: together with the age-related decline in cardiovascular and pulmonary performance, they give rise to significant changes in energy metabolism and particularly in resting metabolic rate and maximal aerobic capacity. This chapter briefly describes the main physiological age-related changes in body composition and energy metabolism to consider when dealing with elderly people, with a view to providing physicians with the information needed to adapt the load of any rehabilitation programs to the real functional capacity of geriatric patients.

G. Sergi (✉) • C. Trevisan • B.M. Zanforlini • N. Veronese • E. Manzato
Department of Medicine, Geriatrics Division, University of Padua, Padua, Italy
e-mail: giuseppe.sergi@unipd.it

© Springer International Publishing AG 2018

S. Masiero, U. Carraro (eds.), *Rehabilitation Medicine for Elderly Patients*, Practical Issues in Geriatrics, DOI 10.1007/978-3-319-57406-6_3

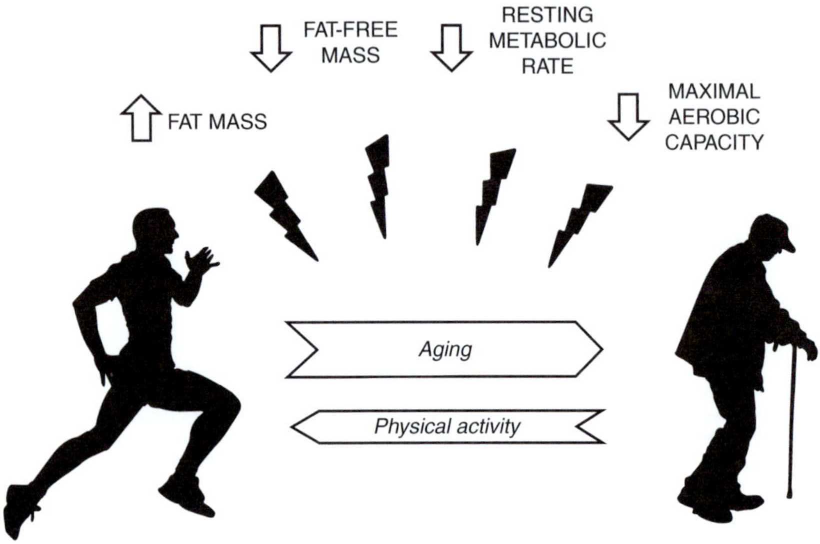

Fig. 3.1 Age-related changes in body composition and energy metabolism

3.2 Body Composition and Aging

Physiological changes in body composition may influence physical performance in older age. Lean mass, and appendicular muscle mass in particular, undergoes quantitative and qualitative changes with aging. The reduction in skeletal muscle mass has been estimated at 8% every 10 years between 40 and 70 years of age, after which this phenomenon seems to speed up, with a loss of 15% or more per decade [2, 3]. This ultimately gives rise to a roughly 40% difference in muscle volume between individuals 20 and 60 years of age [4]. Some of the factors that may influence these changes include an inadequate dietary protein intake, oxidative stress, vitamin D deficiency, hormonal dysregulation (with low levels of GH, IGF-1, and androgens), and inflammatory states [5, 6]. The loss of muscle mass particularly concerns the fast-twitch glycolytic muscle fibers (type IIb), which may be lost or partially replaced by slow-twitch muscle fibers (type I). This conversion affects the muscle's energy metabolism and physical performance because type II fibers are involved in short exercises demanding power and speed, not in long-endurance activities [7]. To describe the age-related reduction in muscle mass and the associated decline in muscle function, Rosenberg coined the term "sarcopenia," a condition characterized by a progressive mobility impairment and loss of physical performance [8]. Like lean mass, fat also undergoes peculiar physiological changes with aging. The proportion of adipose tissue tends to increase in older people, who reported 10% more body fat than younger people [9]. Older people's fat mass tends to deposit mainly in the visceral compartment, generating hormonal and inflammatory pathways associated with negative metabolic and cardiovascular outcomes, and thus limiting their endurance and physical performance [10]. In older age, adipose tissue also tends to infiltrate the muscle fibers, thereby accelerating muscle loss through encumbrance and lipotoxicity mechanisms [11]. Estimating changes in fat and lean mass with such noninvasive methods such as dual X-ray absorptiometry and bioelectrical impedance analysis [12, 13] thus represents the first step when planning tailored rehabilitation programs.

3.3 Changes in Resting Energy Rate

The resting metabolic rate (RMR) represents the energy needed to maintain basic body functions in a state of rest. Using a calorimetric method, it has been estimated at around 50–65% of the total daily energy expenditure. The RMR gradually decreases with aging, due mainly to changes in body composition (and especially the reduction in fat-free mass) but also to changes in tissue energy metabolism [14]. Skeletal muscle metabolism, in particular, has been recognized as one of the most relevant factors influencing the RMR [15]. However, regardless of the impact of body composition on the RMR decline over time, the effect of aging per se as a factor capable of influencing the RMR has been confirmed by several studies [14, 16], which identified a 4.6% lower RMR in the middle-aged than in younger adults, irrespective of body size, body composition, and physical activity [16]. Moreover, other factors can contribute to influencing resting energy expenditure in older people, as well as age and the proportion of lean mass. Patients undergoing rehabilitation, in fact, often suffer from various comorbidities and have a history of neurohormonal dysregulation, fasting, mobility problems and body temperature alterations—all variables that may affect their RMR. These factors therefore need to be considered before initiating any rehabilitation programs. The potential effect of physical exercise in increasing an individual's RMR and daily energy requirement must be considered too, in order to ensure an adequate energy intake for patients under rehabilitation.

3.4 Maximal Aerobic Capacity and Metabolic Equivalent in Aging

The maximal aerobic capacity (VO_2max) is the highest rate of oxygen uptake and distribution to the peripheral tissue that a cardiorespiratory system can cope with during exercise, beyond which there is no increase even if more effort is made. Like the RMR, VO_2max values may be influenced by numerous factors, including age, gender, body composition, and training. Aging has a strong impact on VO_2max, which can decline by 10% per decade beyond the age of 50 years [17], depending on cardiopulmonary fitness and exercising behavior but also due to age-related changes in skeletal muscle mass, with the related loss of muscle fibers and decline in oxidative function [18]. A more standardized index of cardiopulmonary performance has been introduced to express individual tolerance of physical activity for clinical purposes, namely, metabolic equivalents (METs), defined as the ratio between the work metabolic rate and the RMR. Under maximal workload, this measure expresses how many times an individual's energy metabolism could be increased to cover the body's needs in maximal effort. While younger adults achieve METs of around 11, elderly people generally reach values of 6–8 METs, compatible with a moderate physical activity level [19]. The decrease in METs in maximal effort begins from the age of 40 years and is accelerated by certain subclinical conditions or a sedentary lifestyle [20]. Although measuring METs in older people fails to take age-related changes in body composition and energy metabolism into account [19], their use can facilitate the estimation of an individual's tolerance of exercise and cardiorespiratory reserves. A low capacity for exercise, judging from a low METs count in maximal oxygen uptake, is a significant predictor of cardiovascular disease and mortality, with each increase of 1 METs corresponding to a 10% lower mortality risk [21]. Aerobic capacity is therefore another factor to consider when planning safe rehabilitation programs for older people.

3.5 Approaches to Rehabilitation for Elderly Patients

Age-related changes in body composition and energy metabolism need to be taken into account when planning rehabilitation programs for older people. Patients needing rehabilitation have often suffered from medical conditions that may have exacerbated the age-related reduction in their metabolic performance and accelerated the functional decline of skeletal muscle mass. Such physiological and pathological changes mainly affect the individual's maximal aerobic capacity, giving rise to a lower exercise tolerance. This decline can be countered, however, by rehabilitation aiming to improve older patient's physical performance, which often leads to an increase in their energy needs. Estimating body composition and maximal aerobic capacity could therefore represent fundamental steps in the design of rehabilitation programs tailored to each patient's characteristics.

Key Points

- Rehabilitation programs in advanced age have to consider the physiological modifications in body composition and energy metabolism.
- Older people tend to present reduced skeletal muscle mass and increased adipose tissue.
- Resting metabolic rate and maximal aerobic capacity gradually decrease with aging.

References

1. Metter EJ, Talbot LA, Schrager M, Conwit R (2002) Skeletal muscle strength as a predictor of all-cause mortality in healthy men. J Gerontol A Biol Sci Med Sci 57:B359–B365
2. Goodpaster BH, Park SW, Harris TB, Kritchevsky SB, Nevitt M, Schwartz AV et al (2006) The loss of skeletal muscle strength, mass, and quality in older adults: the health, aging and body composition study. J Gerontol A Biol Sci Med Sci 61:1059–1064
3. Grimby G, Saltin B (1983) The ageing muscle. Clin Physiol 3:209–218
4. Porter MM, Vandervoort AA, Lexell J (1995) Aging of human muscle: structure, function and adaptability. Scand J Med Sci Sports 5:129–142
5. Morley JE (2012) Sarcopenia in the elderly. Fam Pract 29(Suppl 1):i44–i48. doi:10.1093/fampra/cmr063
6. Brüünsgaard H, Pedersen BK (2003) Age-related inflammatory cytokines and disease. Immunol Allergy Clin N Am 23:15–39
7. Toji H, Kaneko M (2007) Effects of aging on force, velocity, and power in the elbow flexors of males. J Physiol Anthropol 26:587–592
8. Rosenberg IH, Roubenoff R (1995) Stalking sarcopenia. Ann Intern Med 123:727–728
9. Coin A, Sergi G, Minicuci N, Giannini S, Barbiero E, Manzato E et al (2008) Fat-free mass and fat mass reference values by dual-energy X-ray absorptiometry (DEXA) in a 20–80 year-old Italian population. Clin Nutr 27:87–94. doi:10.1016/j.clnu.2007.10.008
10. Riechman SE, Schoen RE, Weissfeld JL, Thaete FL, Kriska AM (2002) Association of physical activity and visceral adipose tissue in older women and men. Obes Res 10:1065–1073. doi:10.1038/oby.2002.144
11. Goodpaster BH, Carlson CL, Visser M, Kelley DE, Scherzinger A, Harris TB et al (2001) Attenuation of skeletal muscle and strength in the elderly: the Health ABC Study. J Appl Physiol 90:2157–2165
12. Saragat B, Buffa R, Mereu E, De Rui M, Coin A, Sergi G et al (2014) Specific bioelectrical impedance vector reference values for assessing body composition in the Italian elderly. Exp Gerontol 50:52–56. doi:10.1016/j.exger.2013.11.016
13. Haarbo J, Gotfredsen A, Hassager C, Christiansen C (1991) Validation of body composition by dual energy X-ray absorptiometry (DEXA). Clin Physiol 11:331–341
14. Fukagawa NK, Bandini LG, Young JB (1990) Effect of age on body composition and resting metabolic rate. Am J Phys 259:E233–E238
15. Zurlo F, Larson K, Bogardus C, Ravussin E (1990) Skeletal muscle metabolism is a major determinant of resting energy expenditure. J Clin Invest 86:1423–1427. doi:10.1172/JCI114857
16. Klausen B, Toubro S, Astrup A (1997) Age and sex effects on energy expenditure. Am J Clin Nutr 65:895–907
17. Pimentel AE, Gentile CL, Tanaka H, Seals DR, Gates PE (2003) Greater rate of decline in maximal aerobic capacity with age in endurance-trained than in sedentary men. J Appl Physiol 94:2406–2413. doi:10.1152/japplphysiol.00774.2002
18. Jackson AS, Beard EF, Wier LT, Ross RM, Stuteville JE, Blair SN (1995) Changes in aerobic power of men, ages 25–70 yr. Med Sci Sports Exerc 27:113–120
19. Sergi G, Coin A, Sarti S, Perissinotto E, Peloso M, Mulone S et al (2010) Resting VO2, maximal VO2 and metabolic equivalents in free-living healthy elderly women. Clin Nutr 29:84–88. doi:10.1016/j.clnu.2009.07.010
20. Morris CK, Myers J, Froelicher VF, Kawaguchi T, Ueshima K, Hideg A (1993) Nomogram based on metabolic equivalents and age for assessing aerobic exercise capacity in men. J Am Coll Cardiol 22:175–182
21. McAuley P, Myers J, Abella J, Froelicher V (2006) Evaluation of a specific activity questionnaire to predict mortality in men referred for exercise testing. Am Heart J 151:890.e1–890.e7. doi:10.1016/j.ahj.2005.09.017

Sarcopenia and Aging

4

Marco Invernizzi, Alessio Baricich, and Carlo Cisari

4.1 Aging

Aging is a physiological time-dependent process, resulting in a decline in organ function that can in the last lead to death. Changes in environment, nutrition, and medical care have extended the expected survival age for humans; thus, it has become crucial to understand the mechanisms and consequences of age. Research has recently gained crucial insight into the processes and underlying molecular mechanisms of aging. Lastly, a strong correlation between aging and common chronic diseases like cardiovascular disorders, cancer, diabetes, and neurodegenerative pathologies has been clearly demonstrated.

Several mechanisms have been proposed to explain the complexity of the aging process. Recently they have been grouped in seven pillars of age-related research and nine hallmarks of aging, mostly connected between each other. They resume the most important pathophysiological mechanisms underlying this complex condition [1].

These nine hallmarks of aging are the following: genomic instability, telomere attrition, epigenetic alterations, loss of proteostasis, deregulated nutrient sensing, mitochondrial dysfunction, cellular senescence, stem cell exhaustion, and altered intercellular communication. Notably, they can be grouped into three main categories: the primary hallmarks that cause damage to cellular functions, antagonistic hallmarks in the response to such damage, and, finally, integrative hallmarks that are the result of clinical phenotype, which ultimately contribute to the clinical effects of aging as seen in physiological loss of reserve, organ decline, and reduced function [1].

M. Invernizzi, MD, PhD • A. Baricich, MD • C. Cisari, MD, PhD (✉)
Physical and Rehabilitative Medicine, Department of Health Sciences, University of Eastern Piedmont "A. Avogadro", Novara, Italy
e-mail: marco.invernizzi@med.uniupo.it; cisari50@gmail.com

© Springer International Publishing AG 2018

S. Masiero, U. Carraro (eds.), *Rehabilitation Medicine for Elderly Patients*,
Practical Issues in Geriatrics, DOI 10.1007/978-3-319-57406-6_4

4.2 Sarcopenia: Definition, Etiology, and Staging

In the last 20 years, there has been a growing clinical and scientific interest in the role of disability related to the loss of muscle mass and strength in the elderly. In 1989, Irwin Rosenberg proposed the term "sarcopenia" (Greek "sarx" or flesh + "penia" or loss) to describe this age-related decrease in muscle mass [1, 2]. Sarcopenia has since been defined as the loss of skeletal muscle mass and strength that occurs with advancing age [3]. However, a widely accepted definition of sarcopenia suitable for use in research and clinical practice is still lacking, and only recently a consensus paper of the European Working Group on Sarcopenia in Older People defined Sarcopenia as "a decrease in muscle mass and function (strength and mobility)" [4]. This syndrome is characterized by a progressive and generalized loss of skeletal muscle mass and strength with a risk of adverse outcomes such as physical disability, poor quality of life, and death [5, 6]. Mentioning only muscle mass is not sufficient and may limit the real clinical value of this definition. Thus, both low muscle mass and function are fundamental criteria for sarcopenia diagnosis mainly because of the nonlinear relationship between muscle mass and strength [6].

Because of the different etiologies and due to the fact that in some individuals a clear and single cause cannot be identified, it has been proposed to divide sarcopenia in primary (or age related), when no other cause is evident but ageing itself, and secondary when one or more other causes are evident. A similar approach has been used to define the stages of sarcopenia, reflecting its severity, so as to provide a better clinical management of this condition. Several classes of sarcopenia have been proposed, ranging from pre-sarcopenia, characterized by low muscle mass without impact on muscle strength or physical performance, to sarcopenia, characterized by low muscle mass, in addition to low muscle strength or low physical performance, up to severe sarcopenia (low muscle mass, low muscle strength, and low physical performance). Staging is a helpful tool not only to define better treatment strategies and outcomes but also in research study design [4, 7].

In Table 4.1, the main sarcopenia definitions and diagnostic criteria are resumed.

4.3 The Pathophysiology of Sarcopenia

The skeletal and the muscular systems are tightly intertwined, and bone fragility is known to depend on several pathogenetic mechanisms leading to bone mass loss and reduction of bone strength, a condition widely known as osteoporosis. Interestingly, the degenerative processes leading to osteoporosis and sarcopenia show many common pathogenic pathways. Aging skeletal muscle tissue undergoes some important structural and functional modifications regarding mass, viscoelastic properties, fiber-type expression, and innervation. All these modifications lead to the pathogenesis of the sarcopenic state, which is complex and multifactorial. Alongside with external factors such as nutritional status and lower mobility, there are internal factors such as endocrine function, variation in the rate of apoptosis, micro-injuries, variability in recovery, and mitochondrial dysfunction sustaining the development of sarcopenia [2, 3].

Table 4.1 Summary of sarcopenia definitions and diagnostic criteria

Organization	Definition	Diagnostic criteria to identify muscle mass loss	Diagnostic criteria to characterize functional status
Sarcopenia Working Group of the European Union Geriatric Medicine Society	"Sarcopenia is a syndrome characterized by progressive and generalized loss of skeletal muscle mass and strength with a risk of adverse outcomes such as physical disability poor quality of life and death"	MM measured by CT, MRI, DXA, BIA, or total body potassium counting using appropriate cut points [4]	Poor hand grip strength, knee flection/extension, or peak expiratory flow Low physical performance identified by the impaired short physical performance battery or gait speed or TUG or stair climb power test
European Society of Parenteral and Enteral Nutrition Clinician Nutrition and Metabolism Special Interest Group	"Sarcopenia is a condition characterized by loss of muscle mass and muscle strength"	% of MM measured via BIA, at least 2 SDs below mean for sex- and race-matched adults aged 18–39 years	Low physical performance defined as gait speed <0.8 m/s during a 4-min walking test
International Working Group on Sarcopenia	"Sarcopenia is the age-associated loss of skeletal muscle mass and function"	Low appendicular MM corrected for height defined as ≤ 7.23 kg/m^2 in men and ≤ 5.67 kg/m^2 in women, measured via DXA	Low physical performance defined as gait speed <1 m/s during a 4-m walking test
Society of Sarcopenia Cachexia and Wasting Disorders	"Sarcopenia with limited mobility"	Low appendicular MM corrected for height defined as at least 2 SDs below mean for sex- and race-matched adults aged 20–30 years	Low physical performance defined as gait speed <1 m/s or walking distance <400 m during a 6-min walk

Adapted from Peterson et al. [7]

CT computed tomography, *MRI* magnetic resonance imaging, *MM* muscle mass, *DXA* dual energy X-ray absorptiometry, *BIA* bioelectrical impedance analysis, *TUG* timed get-up-and-go test, *SD* standard deviation

The main mechanisms underlying sarcopenia are resumed as follows:

- *Muscle cross sectional area (CSA) reduction:* loss of both slow and fast motor units, with an accelerated loss of fast motor units.
- *Myosteatosis*
- *Muscle denervation* due to age-related neurodegenerative processes, in particular reduction of spinal alpha motor neurons, peripheral nerve fibers and alterations of their myelin sheaths, neuromuscular junctions, and synaptic vesicles.

- *Increased protein degradation/decreased protein synthesis.* Inflammatory cytokines (IL-6 and TNF-alpha) and endocrine factors (GH and IGF-I) are strictly involved in this process.
- *Increased oxidative damage* altering and damaging cell components, particularly mitochondria and DNA sequences.
- *Reduced tissue regeneration* due to myogenic regulatory factors (MRF) negatively influencing satellite cells activity [3].

4.4 Sarcopenia Assessment

In order to evaluate and define sarcopenia, skeletal muscle mass and its function should be objectively quantified. The two measurable variables are skeletal muscle mass and strength; however the challenge is to determine how best to measure them in an accurate and consistent way. Below, the main techniques to assess muscle mass and strength will be briefly described. Cost, availability, and ease of use can determine whether the techniques are better suited to clinical practice or for research purposes [4].

4.4.1 Muscle Mass

- *Computed tomography (CT) and magnetic resonance imaging (MRI).* They are considered the gold standards for estimating muscle mass in research because of their precision in discriminating fat and other soft tissues. However, because of the high cost and limited access, their use is highly limited in routine clinical practice.
- *Dual energy X-ray absorptiometry (DXA).* DXA is a whole-body scan, mainly used for bone mineral density evaluation but able to assess also lean muscle mass. DXA exposes the patient to minimal radiation and is the preferred alternative method to CT and MRI for research and clinical use.
- *Bioimpedance analysis (BIA).* BIA estimates the volume of fat and lean body mass. BIA is inexpensive, easy to use, readily reproducible, and appropriate for both ambulatory and bedridden patients. Moreover BIA results have a good correlation with MRI; thus, BIA might be a good portable alternative to DXA and CT and MRI.
- *Anthropometric measures.* They are used mainly in ambulatory setting, calculating mid-upper arm circumference and skinfold thickness, to assess muscle mass. However they are not recommended for sarcopenia diagnosis because of their low reproducibility [4].

4.4.2 Muscle Strength

- *Handgrip strength.* It has a stronger predictive power on outcomes, disability, and ADL than muscle mass evaluation, being strongly related to lower limb muscle power and calf CSA. Thus, it is a good simple measure of muscle strength being recommended for both research and clinical purposes.

- *Knee flexion/extension.* Knee flexion techniques are suitable for research purposes; however their use in clinical practice is limited by the need for special equipment.
- *Peak expiratory flow (PEF).* It measures the strength of respiratory muscles. Although it is a cheap, simple, and widely accessible technique, it cannot be recommended as an isolated measure to determine sarcopenia [4].

4.5 Sarcopenia: Epidemiology and Outcomes

The prevalence of sarcopenia is reported as 5–13% in the population aged 60–70, reaching 11–50% in people aged more than 80. Considering the rise in the number of people worldwide aged more than 60 (up to 2 billion in 2050), even with a conservative estimate of prevalence, sarcopenia will affect more than 200 million in the next 40 years [4]. As previously described, sarcopenia determines functional and phenotypic modifications resulting in loss of muscle mass and strength. The increased risks of mobility loss and injury resulting from loss of muscle mass and strength are part of a vicious cycle which is amplified with age, leading to reduced autonomy, falls, fractures, and consequent disability [4, 7]. In 2000, US healthcare costs directly attributed to sarcopenia were estimated $18.5 billion, mainly related to decreased functional status, autonomy [8], falls increase [5], disability [9], and mortality [7, 10]. Moreover, in the clinical setting, sarcopenic patients suffer from greater infectious complications, prolonged duration of mechanical ventilation, longer hospitalization, increased readmission to the hospital, greater need for rehabilitation care after hospital discharge, and higher mortality compared to age-matched non-sarcopenic patients [7, 11, 12]. Thus, the loss of muscle mass and strength has a devastating impact on the overall health of a subject, being a major risk factor for disability, morbidity, and mortality. In addition to reductions in performance, the intermediate consequences of muscle loss include reductions in metabolic rate and aerobic capacity. The loss of power and endurance increases the difficulties associated with procuring adequate nutrition and increases the effort required to undertake exercise. The combination of nutritional loss and reduced physical activity levels results in further loss of muscle mass and power, exacerbating the process of sarcopenia. The resulting decrements in power, endurance, and physical performance, if unchecked, subsequently lead to a loss of independence which may or may not be preceded by injury or illness, for example, a fall and/or fracture [4, 7].

4.6 Sarcopenia and Frailty

Potential definitions of frailty abound, being often synonymous with disability, comorbidity, or advanced old age. However the "risk concept" distinguishes frailty from disability. Thus, frailty is defined as "a geriatric syndrome resulting from age-related cumulative declines across multiple physiologic systems, with impaired homeostatic reserve and a reduced capacity of the organism to withstand stress, thus increasing vulnerability to adverse health outcomes including falls, hospitalization, institutionalization and mortality" [3, 4, 13, 14]. Moreover frailty is a progressive process with a latent phase. The progression in the frailty ladder reflects decline in homeostasis mechanisms which results in constant loss of performance leading to a cascade of dysregulation in multiple systems. The "frailty cycle" may be triggered by separate or joint effects like lack of physical exercise, inadequate nutrition, unhealthy environment, injuries, disease, age- and/or obesity-related hormonal alterations, inflammation, and polypharmacy [3].

Interestingly, frailty and sarcopenia overlap; most frail elderly people are sarcopenic, and some older people with sarcopenia are also frail. Moreover, as previously stated, skeletal and muscular systems are tightly intertwined, and the degenerative processes leading to osteoporosis and sarcopenia show many common pathogenic pathways. However, the general concept of frailty goes beyond physical factors to encompass psychological and social dimensions as well, including cognitive status, social support, and other environmental factors [13–15].

Key Points

- **Aging** is a physiological time-dependent process, resulting in a decline in organ functions that can in the last lead to death. The main pathophysiological mechanisms have been recently grouped in seven pillars of age-related research and nine hallmarks of aging, mostly connected with each other.
- **Sarcopenia** can be defined as "a decrease in muscle mass and function (strength and mobility)." It can be divided in primary (or age related) and secondary sarcopenia and staged in pre-sarcopenia, sarcopenia, and severe sarcopenia.
- **Mechanism underlying sarcopenia** are CSA reduction, myosteatosis, age-related muscle denervation, increased protein degradation/decreased protein synthesis, increased inflammatory cytokine expression (IL-6 and TNF-alpha), decreased GH and IGF-I production, increased oxidative damage, and reduced tissue regeneration.
- **Sarcopenia** has a negative impact on functional status, autonomy, falls, disability, and mortality. In the clinical setting, sarcopenic patients suffer from greater infectious complications, prolonged duration of mechanical ventilation, longer hospitalization, increased readmission to the hospital, greater need for rehabilitation care after hospital discharge, and higher mortality.
- **Frailty** is defined as "a geriatric syndrome resulting from age-related cumulative declines across multiple physiologic systems, with impaired homeostatic reserve and a reduced capacity of the organism to withstand stress, thus increasing vulnerability to adverse health outcomes including falls, hospitalization, institutionalization, and mortality."

References

1. Aunan JR, Watson MM, Hagland HR et al (2016) Molecular and biologicalhallmarks of ageing. Br J Surg 103:e29–e46
2. Lang T, Streeper T, Cawthon P et al (2009) Sarcopenia: etiology, clinicalconsequences, intervention, and assessment. Osteoporos Int 21(4):543–559
3. Buch A, Carmeli E, Boker LK et al (2016) Muscle function and fat content in relation to sarcopenia, obesity and frailty of old age – an overview. Exp Gerontol 76:25–32
4. Cruz-Jentoft AJ, Baeyens JP, Bauer JM et al (2010) Sarcopenia: European consensus on definition and diagnosis: Report of the European Working Group on sarcopenia in older people. Age Ageing 39(4):412–423
5. Delmonico MJ, Harris TB, Lee JS et al (2007) Alternative definitions of sarcopenia, lower extremity performance, and functional impairment with aging in older men and women. J Am Geriatr Soc 55:769–774
6. Goodpaster BH, Park SW, Harris TB et al (2006) The loss of skeletal muscle strength, mass, and quality in older adults: the health, aging and body composition study. J Gerontol A Biol Sci Med Sci 61:1059–1064
7. Peterson SJ, Braunschweig CA (2016) Prevalence of sarcopenia and associated outcomes in the clinical setting. Nutr Clin Pract 31(1):40–48
8. Newman AB, Kupelian V, Visser M et al (2003) Sarcopenia: alternative definitions and associations with lower extremity function. J Am Geriatr Soc 51(11):1602–1609
9. Janssen I, Heymsfield SB, Ross R (2002) Low relative skeletal muscle mass (sarcopenia) in older persons is associated with functional impairment and physical disability. J Am Geriatr Soc 50(5):889–896
10. Bigaard J, Frederiksen K, Tjønneland A et al (2004) Body fat and fat-free mass and all-cause mortality. Obes Res 12(7):1042–1049
11. Gariballa S, Alessa A (2013) Sarcopenia: prevalence and prognostic significance in hospitalized patients. Clin Nutr 32(5):772–776
12. Moisey LL, Mourtzakis M, Cotton BA (2013) Skeletal muscle predicts ventilator-free days, ICU-free days, and mortality in elderly ICU patients. Crit Care 17(5):R206
13. Bauer JM, Sieber CC (2008) Sarcopenia and frailty: a clinician's controversial point of view. Exp Gerontol 43:674–678
14. Fried LP, Tangen CM, Walston J (2001) Frailty in older adults: evidence for a phenotype. J Gerontol A Biol Sci Med Sci 56:M146–M156
15. Rizzoli R, Reginster JY, Arnal JF et al (2013) Quality of life in sarcopenia and frailty. Calcif Tissue Int 93(2):101–120

Physical Exercise and Aging

5

Antonio Paoli

5.1 Introduction

Independence and improvement of quality of life in elderly people are needed in an increasing aging society. The population of the developed countries is aging quickly, and, especially during the past century, life expectancy rapidly increased due to many factors, including decrease in infant mortality, rising living standards, improved lifestyles, better education, and mainly advances in health care. Several studies showed the positive effects of physical exercise (PE) on physical and mental health during the lifetime [1]. An active lifestyle, including a regular physical activity during the aging process, is, therefore, a major challenge for public and health care systems to maintain a good health and physical fitness in the aging population [2].

Physical exercise is therefore a key factor for a healthy aging process. But, aside the general consideration about the healthy effects of PE [2], it is important to specify which kind of PE should be prescribed and with which effects.

5.2 Physical Exercise Is Multifaceted

PE is classically divided in endurance training (ET) (low load-high repetitive stimulus) and strength training (ST) (high load-low repetitive). These two training modalities represent, as a matter of fact, the extremes of a continuum options with many variables that affecting load, duration, frequency, rest, and mode of contraction. Moreover ET and RT could be mixed in very different ways [3, 4]. Understanding the metabolic and molecular pathway involved in the human body response to PE is

A. Paoli, MD, PhD
Nutrition and Exercise Physiology Laboratory, Department of Biomedical Sciences, University of Padua, Padua, Italy
e-mail: antonio.paoli@unipd.it

© Springer International Publishing AG 2018

S. Masiero, U. Carraro (eds.), *Rehabilitation Medicine for Elderly Patients*, Practical Issues in Geriatrics, DOI 10.1007/978-3-319-57406-6_5

Table 5.1 Effects of aerobic and resistance exercise on different variables

	Aerobic/ endurance	Resistance/ strength
Skeletal muscle morphological and physiological adaptations		
Muscle hypertrophy	≅	↑↑↑
Muscle CSA	≅↑	↑↑↑
Myofibrillar protein synthesis	≅↑	↑↑↑
Mitochondrial protein synthesis	↑↑	↑
Capillarization	↑↑	↑
Mitochondrial number, size, and function	↑↑↑	≅↑
Exercise performance		
Muscle strength (power)	≅	↑
Lactate buffer capacity	↑↑	↑↑
VO_2max	↑↑↑	≅↑
Neural adaptation	↑	↑↑↑
Endurance capacity	↑↑↑	≅
Anaerobic capacity	↑	↑↑

mandatory to create tailored programs for healthy and unhealthy subjects and especially for elderly.

Classical endurance training protocols usually induce an increase in VO_2max (maximal oxygen consumption) that is related to a complex cascade of effects that results in modifications in both cardiovascular system and trained skeletal muscles. In skeletal muscle, ET stimulates a shift from IIX heavy chain myosin phenotype to IIa and I types. Compared to IIx-type fibers, I-type fiber showed an increase of oxidative characteristics, such as muscle capillarity, muscle mitochondrial volume, and mitochondrial density, and oxidative enzymes: enzymes of the Krebs cycle and oxidative phosphorylation such as SDH (succinate dehydrogenase), CS (citrate synthase), and Cytox (cytochrome *c* oxidase) (see Table 5.1).

Regarding morphological changes muscle fiber cross-sectional area is generally poor or not affected by endurance-type exercise except when exercised muscles were immobilized. Endurance training also leads to a shift in metabolism stimulating to a higher lipid utilization as fuel and to an increase in IMCL (intramyocellular lipid) and glycogen stores.

Instead classic strength training protocols influence mainly muscle and muscle fiber cross-sectional area. It is important to underline that the earliest adaptation during a ST protocol belongs to a modification of neuromuscular function [5]; this mechanism allows strength increase with little or null structural adjustments, thus a more economical adaptation. After few weeks ST stimulates the increase of muscle cross-sectional area due mainly to an increase in the number of myofibrils, notably of the fast fiber types (type IIA and type IIX) [6]. Training affects also the shifts from one type of myosin heavy chain (MHC) to another; these changes are related to the characteristics of training [6–8]. Even though mitochondria and capillaries are little affected by ST and mitochondrial volumes and capillary densities are low in strength-trained athletes, the role of mitochondria in muscle mass maintaining has been recently highlighted [9].

With the onset of the sixth decade in life, there is a gradual increases of many degenerative processes (described elsewhere in this book); these processes cause a decrease of muscle power (dynapenia) [10] and muscle mass (sarcopenia) [11, 12]. These modifications are related both to neural (e.g., loss of alpha motoneurons) and morphological changes (e.g., reduced number and size of muscle fibers) [10].

General muscular weakness is highly associated with impaired mobility and an increased risk for falls in the elderly; for this reason RT is a key point for improving elderly's quality of life [13]. As a matter of fact, lower limb muscle weakness was identified as the main intrinsic fall-risk factor in the elderly [14]. It is interesting to observe that although the age-related decline in muscle strength is associated with skeletal muscle mass loss, other studies reported a greater decline in muscle strength compared to muscle size [15].

Even though exercise cannot completely prevent aging-related loss of strength, due mainly to the modification of the neuromuscular system, RT showed great age-related changes. Many studies in the last years, starting from the seminal paper of Frontera et al. [16], showed the importance of RT on muscle mass maintenance over years. While the calculated loss of strength is 1.3% by year after 52 years of age [17], other researches showed that from 60 years old to 72 years old, there is a decline of isokinetic knee extensor torque of −24% and in quadriceps cross-sectional area (CSA) of −16%. On the contrary only 12 weeks of high intensity RT (80% of 1 RM) leads to a 16% increase in isokinetic torque and 11% in knee extensor CSA [18].

Unfortunately PE is often prescribed by physicians in a very "low-intensity," "low-volume" manner [10]. It is of paramount importance when developing RT programs, considering all the various training variables such as frequency, duration, exercises, sets, recovery, intensity, repetitions, and type of contractions (see Table 5.2). Adverse events in healthy elderly are very rare. Most adverse events are usually related to musculoskeletal problems, but serious adverse events were very rare and appear not to be directly related to the exercise program. Anyway subjects

Table 5.2 Different training variables in endurance exercise and resistance training

Endurance training		Resistance training	
Variable	Examples	Variable	Examples
Duration (total duration of training)	Minutes, hours	Muscle contraction type	Eccentric, concentric, isometric
Intensity (relative effort)	% Maximal heart rate (HR_{max}) % Heart rate reserve (HR_{res}) % Maximal oxygen consumption (VO_2max)	Type of load	Barbell, dumbbell, elastics, calisthenics, weight machines
Type of exercise (exercise modalities)	Running, cycling, rowing	Volume	Sets × repetitions
		Training structure	Total body, split routine, numbers of muscle area
		Rest between sets	Seconds, minutes
		Speed of movement	Slow, explosive
		Training frequency (amount of times per week)	

at risk of RT's induced adverse events should undergo to a complete specialized health screening. These subjects are those with high-grade hypertension, diabetic neuropathy, and/or retinopathy, with ischemic and cerebrovascular heart diseases and heart failure.

5.3 PE Frequency

At least 2 (from 2 to 4) days per week were recommended. Two/three times of endurance training and two sessions of RT. The most common approach is 2 times a week of ET and 1–2 times a week of RT; in our opinion 2 times a week for ET and 2 times for RT should be an adequate frequency. Another solution could be 3 times a week on alternating days (e.g., Monday, Wednesday, and Friday) of RT + ET, the so-called circuit training [3, 4, 19, 20]; all the above methodologies are performed as a "total body" routine. An alternative approach exercise session with the "total body" is the so-called "split routine" where routine is performed 2–3 times per week. In this methodology subjects are exercising selected muscle groups on 1 or 2 days per week, while the remaining are exercised on a separate 1 or 2 days per week (e.g., chest, arms, and limbs on Monday; back, shoulder, and hamstring on Wednesday; ET on Tuesday and Thursday). When performing only RT, the typically split routine could be A, B, and C, where A is training the chest and biceps, B the lower limbs and shoulder, C the back and triceps.

5.4 PE Duration

Generally speaking the duration of a single training session should not exceed the 60' [21] with interset rest range from 1 to 2.5/3 min depending on the load used, the number of reps, the muscle area involved, and the speed of movement.

5.5 PE Exercises

Resistance exercises can be classified, according to the number of joints involved, as multi-joint (MJ) or single-joint (SJ) exercises. MJ exercises are those in which more than one joint is involved during the exercise (e.g., chest press and leg press). SJ exercises are those where only one joint is involved (e.g., bicep curls and leg extensions). Although MJ and SJ have many differences, there is no precise guideline indicating which one is more suitable for different outcomes. We demonstrated that MJ exercises are able to increase the resting energy expenditure compared to an equal load SJ exercise [20].

Older adults should be encouraged to perform, where possible, MJ (MJ are more "functional" compared to SJ) although SJ exercises could be also performed. Also resistance exercise machines (e.g., leg press machines) could be recommended for the beginner instead of free weights (barbells and dumbbells) if the ratio between instructors and trainees is <1.

5.6 Number of Repetitions and Sets and Derived Variables

The number of repetition is linked mainly to the load and the aim of exercise. Higher loads lifted mean lower reps performed. Clearly, in accordance with the Hill law, higher loads constrain a slower movement [22, 23]. It is well known that the number of repetitions increases as training intensity decreases; the effects of the different loads on muscle architecture are outside the limits of this chapter, but, in general, the more efficient reps range for muscle hypertrophy was defined between 6 and 10 reps, with a median of 8, even though recent findings challenged this old knowledge [24, 25]. Also, different speeds influence load effects on muscle [26]; a voluntary slow movement with higher loads affects different molecular pathway linked to muscle hypertrophy [27].

5.7 Intensity

While in ET intensity is simply well defined by the percentage of VO_2max or percentage of HR, for RT the *scenario* is more complex: in RT loads, speed and rest periods define the intensity; thus in RT this is a parameter more complex to calculate and still under discussion [28] (Table 5.3).

Table 5.3 Different activities and variables for PE in elderly

Parameter	Endurance training	Resistance training	Balance training	Flexibility training
Mode	Movement that does not impose excessive joint stress: walking, water-based exercise, and stationary-cycle exercise for those with joint problems	Dynamic strength training using the major muscle groups. Free weights, machine, elastic resistance bends, and calisthenics exercises	Neuromuscular training combining balance, agility, and proprioceptive exercises. Exercises with perturbations of center of gravity	Exercises that maintain or increase flexibility; static stretching for major muscle groups
Intensity	Using the Borg RPE (0–10) scale: from 5 to 8 (from moderate to vigorous)	Using the Borg RPE (0–10) scale: from 5 to 8 (from moderate to vigorous)	No indications	Using the Borg RPE (0–10) scale: from 5 to 6 (moderate)
Duration	For moderate intensity at least 30 min per day; for vigorous at least 20 min per day	At least 1 set for each exercise (is preferable 2 or 3 sets) for 10–15 repetitions per exercise	No indications	One set for each exercise; 15–30 s each bout of stretch
Frequency	Moderate intensity: 5 days per week; vigorous intensity: 3 days per week	Minimum 2 days per week	Minimum 2 days per week	Minimum 2 days per week

Adapted from American College of Sports Medicine position stand. Exercise and physical activity for older adults. Med Sci Sports Exerc. (2009) [29]

Conclusions

Physical activity is a key factor for a healthy aging. It is of paramount importance for the physician to understand the different mechanisms underlying the positive effects of PE on the different health-related outcomes. At the same time, it is fundamental for health professionals to know how different types of exercises differently affect different metabolic and physiological outcomes in the elderly to use exercise as a poly-pill.

Key Points

- PE is a key factor for a healthy aging.
- Both endurance training and resistance training are fundamental to maintain and enhance elderly's quality of life.
- PE could reduce the relative risk for disability and noncommunicable diseases.
- PE should be prescribed with the correct dose (intensity and volume) to achieve better results.

References

1. Witard OC, McGlory C, Hamilton DL, Phillips SM (2016) Growing older with health and vitality: a nexus of physical activity, exercise and nutrition. Biogerontology 17(3):529–546
2. Evans WJ (1999) Exercise training guidelines for the elderly. Med Sci Sports Exerc 31(1):12–17
3. Paoli A, Pacelli F, Bargossi AM, Marcolin G, Guzzinati S, Neri M et al (2010) Effects of three distinct protocols of fitness training on body composition, strength and blood lactate. J Sports Med Phys Fitness 50(1):43–51
4. Paoli A, Pacelli QF, Moro T, Marcolin G, Neri M, Battaglia G et al (2013) Effects of high-intensity circuit training, low-intensity circuit training and endurance training on blood pressure and lipoproteins in middle-aged overweight men. Lipids Health Dis 12(1):131
5. Sale DG (1988) Neural adaptation to resistance training. Med Sci Sports Exerc 20(5 Suppl):S135–S145
6. Schiaffino S, Reggiani C (2011) Fiber types in mammalian skeletal muscles. Physiol Rev 91(4):1447–1531
7. Paoli A, Pacelli QF, Cancellara P, Toniolo L, Moro T, Canato M et al (2016) Protein supplementation does not further increase latissimus dorsi muscle fiber hypertrophy after eight weeks of resistance training in novice subjects, but partially counteracts the fast-to-slow muscle fiber transition. Forum Nutr 8(6). pii: E331 (not Forum Nutr)
8. Reggiani C (2015) Not all disuse protocols are equal: new insight into the signalling pathways to muscle atrophy. J Physiol 593(24):5227–5228
9. Reggiani C (2015) Regulation of muscle mass: a new role for mitochondria? J Physiol 593(8):1761–1762
10. Law TD, Clark LA, Clark BC (2016) Resistance exercise to prevent and manage sarcopenia and dynapenia. Annu Rev Gerontol Geriatr 36(1):205–228
11. Wang C, Bai L (2012) Sarcopenia in the elderly: basic and clinical issues. Geriatr Gerontol Int 12(3):388–396
12. Walston JD (2012) Sarcopenia in older adults. Curr Opin Rheumatol 24(6):623–627

13. Aagaard P, Suetta C, Caserotti P, Magnusson SP, Kjaer M (2010) Role of the nervous system in sarcopenia and muscle atrophy with aging: strength training as a countermeasure. Scand J Med Sci Sports 20(1):49–64
14. Hurley BF, Roth SM (2000) Strength training in the elderly: effects on risk factors for age-related diseases. Sports Med (Auckland, NZ) 30(4):249–268
15. Frontera WR, Hughes VA, Fielding RA et al (2000) Aging of skeletal muscle: a 12-yr longitudinal study. J Appl Physiol (1985) 88(4):1321–1326
16. Frontera WR, Meredith CN, O'Reilly KP et al (1988) Strength conditioning in older men: skeletal muscle hypertrophy and improved function. J Appl Physiol (1985) 64(3):1038–1044
17. Vandervoort AA, McComas AJ (1986) Contractile changes in opposing muscles of the human ankle joint with aging. J Appl Physiol (1985) 61(1):361–367
18. Borde R, Hortobagyi T, Granacher U (2015) Dose-response relationships of resistance training in healthy old adults: a systematic review and meta-analysis. Sports Med 45(12):1693–1720
19. Paoli A, Moro T, Bianco A (2014) Lift weights to fight overweight. Clin Physiol Funct Imaging 35(1):1–6
20. Paoli A (2011) Different metabolic response to single-joint or multiple-joint resistance training of similar total volume. Acta Physiol 203(688):243
21. Paoli A, Neri M, Bianco A (2013) Principi di Metodologia del Fitness. Elika, Ed., Cesena
22. Hill AV (1949) The heat of activation and the heat of shortening in a muscle twitch. Proc R Soc Lond B Biol Sci 136(883):195–211
23. Hill AV (1913) The heat-production in prolonged contractions of an isolated frog's muscle. J Physiol 47(4-5):305–324
24. Morton RW, Oikawa SY, Wavell CG et al (2016) Neither load nor systemic hormones determine resistance training-mediated hypertrophy or strength gains in resistance-trained young men. J Appl Physiol (1985) 121(1):129–138
25. Burd NA, Mitchell CJ, Churchward-Venne TA, Phillips SM (2012) Bigger weights may not beget bigger muscles: evidence from acute muscle protein synthetic responses after resistance exercise. Appl Physiol Nutr Metab 37(3):551–554
26. Sakuma K, Yamaguchi A (2010) Molecular mechanisms in aging and current strategies to counteract sarcopenia. Curr Aging Sci 3(2):90–101
27. Tran QT, Docherty D, Behm D (2006) The effects of varying time under tension and volume load on acute neuromuscular responses. Eur J Appl Physiol 98(4):402–410
28. Fisher J, Steele J, Smith D (2016) High-and low-load resistance training: interpretation and practical application of current research findings. Sports Med 47(3):393–400
29. American College of Sports Medicine, Chodzko-Zajko WJ, Proctor DN, Fiatarone Singh MA et al (2009) American College of Sports Medicine position stand. Exercise and physical activity for older adults. Med Sci Sports Exerc 41(7):1510–1530

Safe Antiaging Full-Body In-Bed Gym and FES for Lazy Persons: Home In-Bed Exercises for Fighting Muscle Weakness in Advanced Age

6

U. Carraro, K. Gava, A. Musumeci, A. Baba, F. Piccione, and A. Marcante

6.1 Introduction

Elderly persons, due to advanced age or associated diseases, spend only a small amount of time for daily physical activity, contributing to limit their independence up to force them to bed and to hospitalization for long periods. Immobility is associated with neuromuscular weakness, functional limitations, thromboembolism, and high costs [1–3]. All progressive muscle contractile impairments (including advanced age-related muscle power decline) need permanent management. Besides eventual pharmacological treatment, a home-based physical exercise approach is helpful. Awaiting the development of implantable devices for muscle stimulation, as effective as pacemakers for cardiac arrhythmias or cochlear implants for hearing loss, education of lazy patients to home physical exercises during and after hospitalization could be an effective, low-cost alternative.

Inspired by the proven capability to recover skeletal muscle contractility and strength by home-based functional electrical stimulation (h-bFES) even in the worse cases of neuromuscular traumatic injuries, [4–8] and guided by common sense, we suggest for sedentary persons a short (15–20 min) daily sequence of 12 easy-to-perform physical exercises that may be performed in bed (full-body in-bed gym). Full-body in-bed gym is an extension to all body muscles of the well-established in-bed cardio-circulation-ventilation physiotherapy approaches.

U. Carraro (✉) • A. Baba • F. Piccione • A. Marcante
IRCCS Fondazione San Camillo Hospital, Venice, Italy
e-mail: ugo.carraro@ospedalesancamillo.net; ugo.carraro@unipd.it

K. Gava
Interdepartmental Research Center of Myology, University of Padua, Padua, Italy

A. Musumeci
Rehabilitation Unit, Department of Neuroscience, University – General Hospital of Padua, Padua, Italy
e-mail: alfredomusumeci@yahoo.com

© Springer International Publishing AG 2018

S. Masiero, U. Carraro (eds.), *Rehabilitation Medicine for Elderly Patients*, Practical Issues in Geriatrics, DOI 10.1007/978-3-319-57406-6_6

6.2 Suggested Exercises

Active persons, able to make 25 consecutive push-ups in 3 min, do not need the following exercises, but sedentary people may gradually start, after asking their family physician's advice, with five repetitions of each suggested exercise. The next week they may add groups of five additional repetitions up to 30. Exercises are showed and fully detailed in the legend of Figs. 6.1, 6.2, 6.3, 6.4, 6.5, 6.6, 6.7, 6.8, 6.9, 6.10, 6.11, and 6.12. The daily routine exercises may last from 10 (in the beginning) to 30 min (for complete session in accustomed persons).

6.3 Conclusions

If sedentary persons, without major comorbidities but with rest-related muscle weakness, challenge themselves, avoiding stress, in a few days of full-body in-bed gym, they may increase their muscle strength, fatigue resistance, and independence in daily life activities. Cautious in-bed gym may help patient's recovery after the acute phase of hospitalization, prevent the risk of thromboembolism after surgical interventions, and concur to reduce arterial hypertension [9]. Full-body in-bed gym could mitigate the bad mood that is usually associated to mobility limitations, strengthening patients' confidence in recovering partial or total independence, thus reducing the risk of accidental falls [10]. However, if elderly persons cannot, or are reluctant to, perform physical exercises, functional electrical stimulation (FES) may mimic them and be almost equally useful [2–6]. In conclusion, it is never too early and it is never too late to increase daily levels of volitional or FES-induced muscle contractions!

6.4 Antiaging Total-Body In-Bed Gym

Figures 6.1, 6.2, 6.3, 6.4, 6.5, 6.6, 6.7, 6.8, 6.9, 6.10, 6.11, and 6.12 show the series of safe and easy exercises that elderly persons could perform staying next to bed. Figure 6.1a, b suggests to start every morning the total-body in-bed routine with flexions and extensions of the ankles; Fig. 6.2a, b demonstrates that leg and abdomen muscle could be activated by cycling movements; Fig. 6.3a, b shows arm up and arm down exercise. Notice, please, that hand muscles are also activated; Fig. 6.4 shows how deep breathing could be performed; Fig. 6.5a, b show forward bending exercise; Fig. 6.6 suggests how to raise your pelvis to activate back muscles, glutei, and posterior leg muscles; Fig. 6.7a–d demonstrates neck torsions; Fig. 6.8 suggests to lift the upper part of the body in sitting position to exercise arm muscles; Fig. 6.9a, b, demonstrates how to lift the legs in sitting position to strength quadriceps muscles; Figs. 6.10 and 6.11 show how to stand up and get up on the toes, respectively. Figure 6.12 shows push-up (for active persons). A video may be downloaded from the link: http://www.bio.unipd.it/bam/video/InterviewCarraro-tutorial.mp4

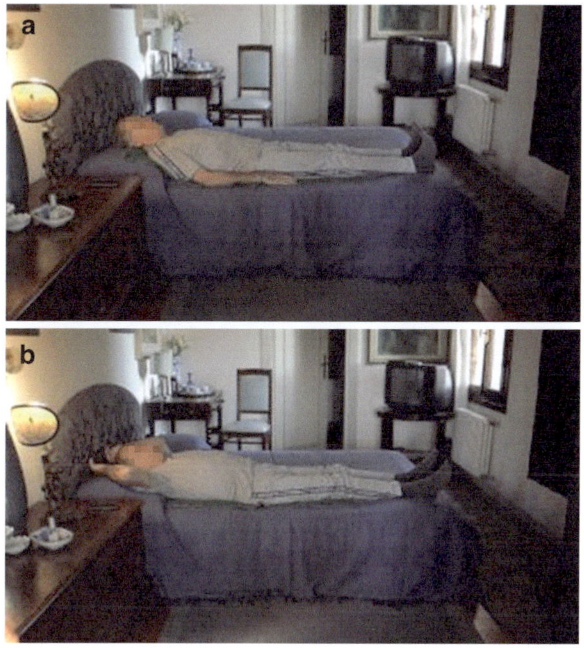

Fig. 6.1 (**a**, **b**) Flexion and extension of the ankles

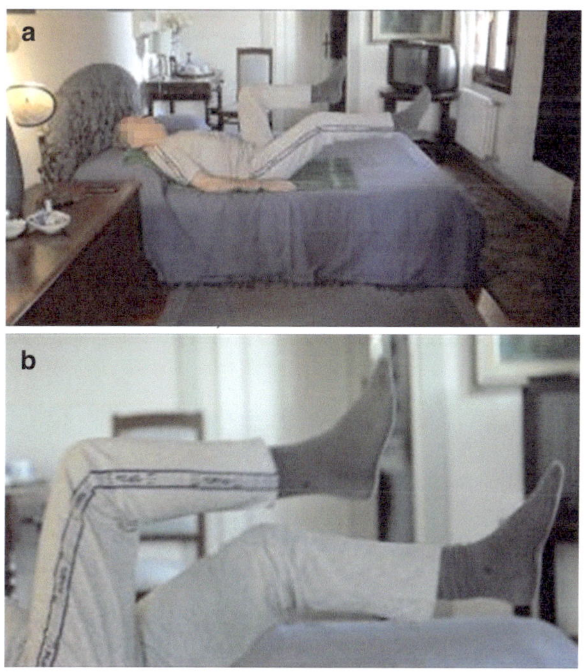

Fig. 6.2 (**a**, **b**) Cycling movements

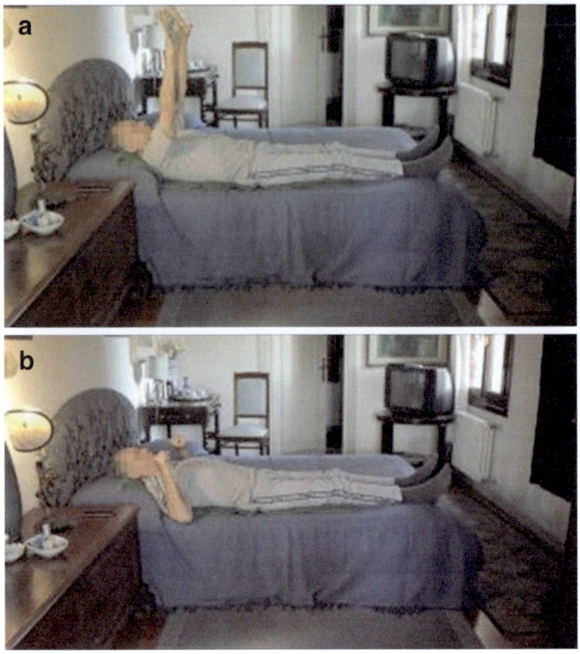

Fig. 6.3 (**a**, **b**) Arms up and arms down

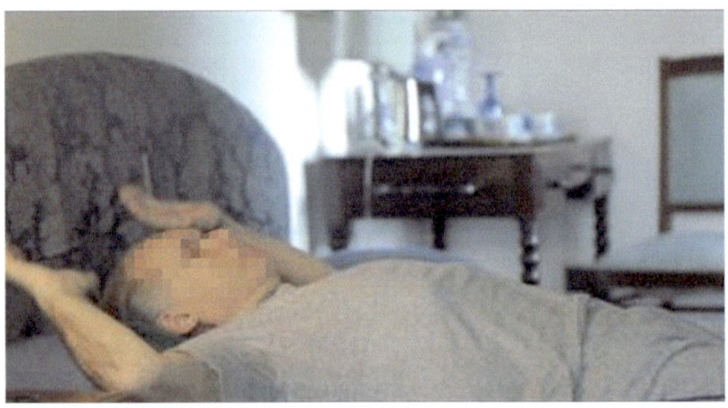

Fig. 6.4 Deep breathing

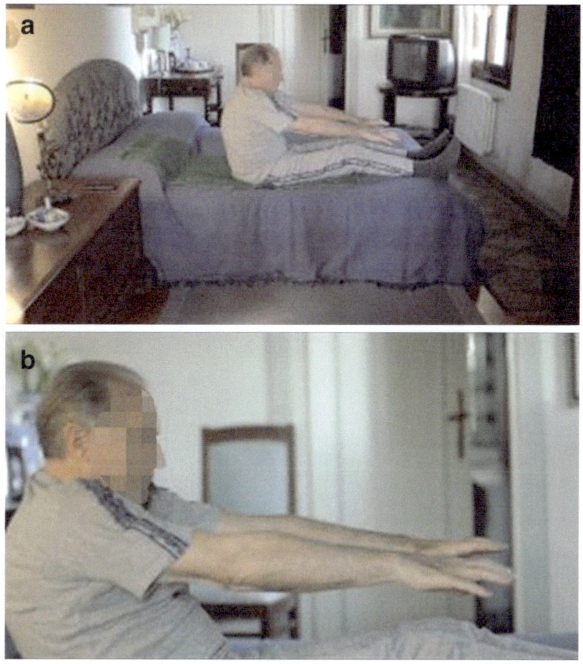

Fig. 6.5 (**a**, **b**) Forward bending

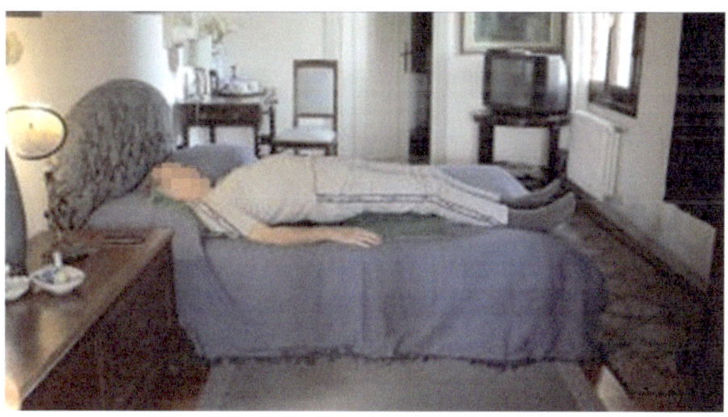

Fig. 6.6 To raise the pelvis

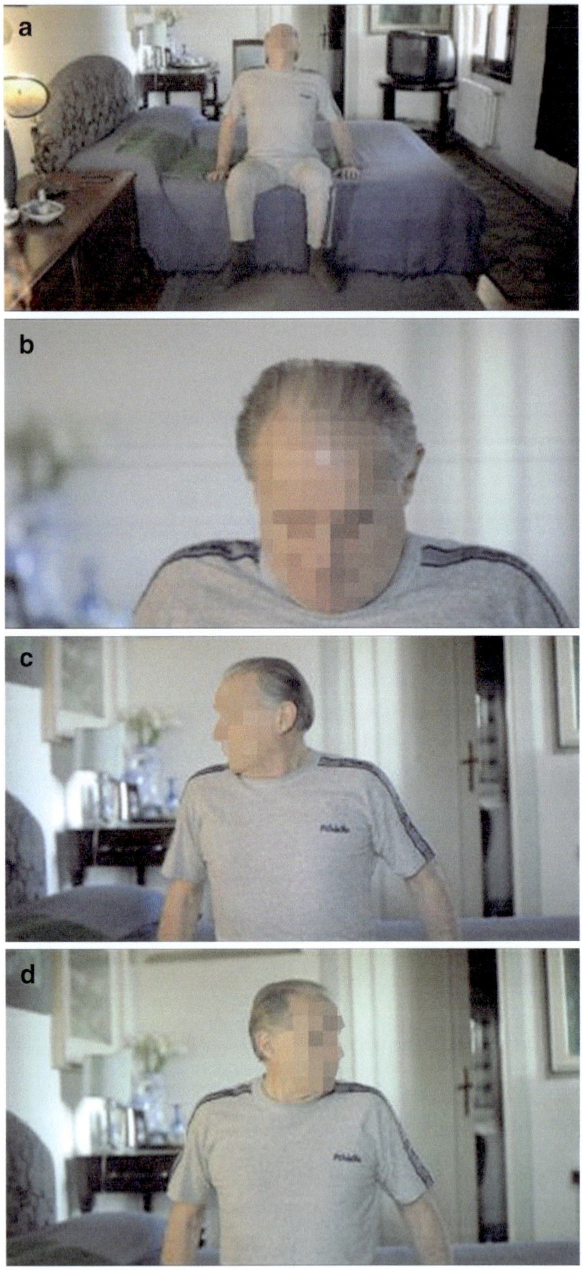

Fig. 6.7 (**a**–**d**) Neck torsions

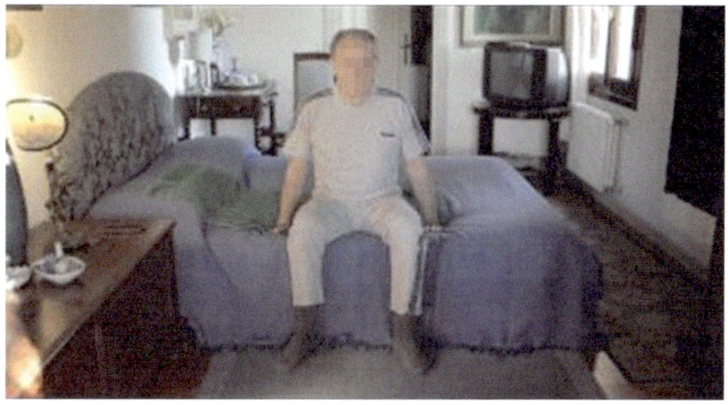

Fig. 6.8 Sit up

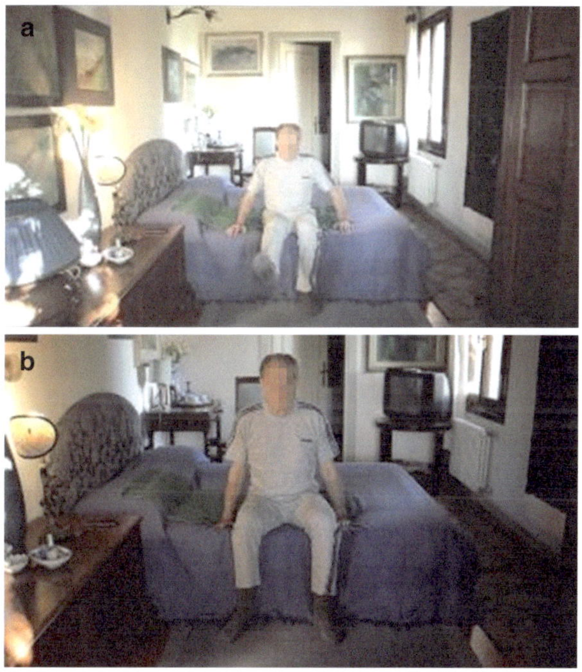

Fig. 6.9 (**a**, **b**) Lift the legs when in sitting position

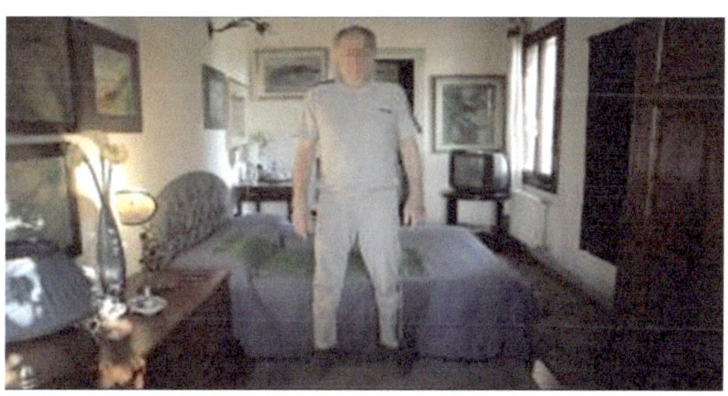

Fig. 6.10 Stand up

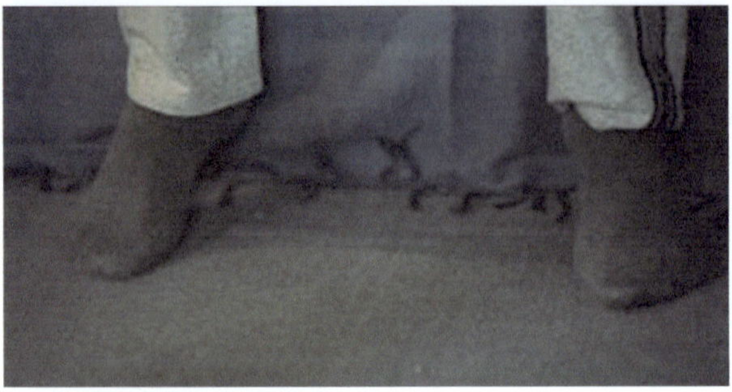

Fig. 6.11 Get up on toes

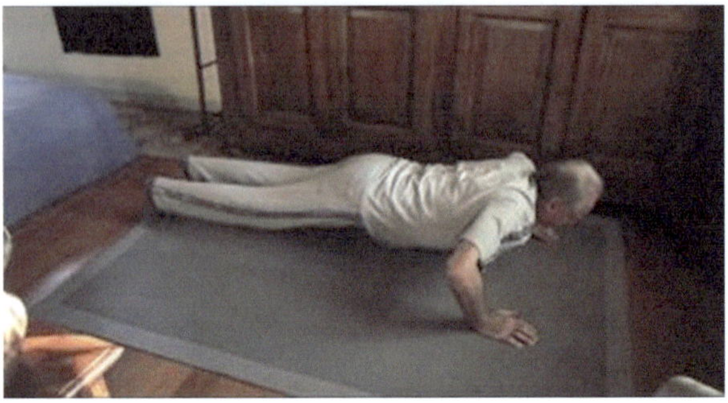

Fig. 6.12 Push-up (for the active person)

If elderly persons cannot, or are reluctant to, perform physical exercises, functional electrical stimulation may mimic them and be almost equally useful (see Chap. 8, Section C in this book, and Refs. [3–8]).

Key Points

- Full-body in-bed gym is an extension to all body muscles of the well-established cardio-circulatory-ventilation in-bed management.
- Elderly patients may develop severe limitations to their independence after immobilization or bed-ridding.
- Instructing and supporting patients to perform daily in-bed exercises are an effective and low-cost measure to limit disability and improve physical and mental being of older patients.
- When full-body in-bed gym is not indicated or persons are reluctant to do it, functional electrical stimulation can be an alternative.

References

1. Hopkins RO, Mitchell L, Thomsen GE, Schafer M, Link M, Brown SM (2016) Implementing a mobility program to minimize post-intensive care syndrome. AACN Adv Crit Care 27:187–203
2. Camillo CA, Osadnik CR, van Remoortel H, Burtin C, Janssens W, Troosters T (2016) Effect of "add-on" interventions on exercise training in individuals with COPD: a systematic review. ERJ Open Res 2
3. Czyrny JJ, Kaplan RE, Wilding GE, Purdy CH, Hirsh J (2016) Electrical foot stimulation: a potential new method of deep venous thrombosis prophylaxis. ERJ Open Res 2(1). pii: 00078-2015. Review. Erratum in Vascular. 2010 Mar–Apr;18(2):121
4. Kern H, Carraro U, Adami N, Biral D, Hofer C, Forstner C, Mödlin M, Vogelauer M, Pond A, Boncompagni S, Paolini C, Mayr W, Protasi F, Zampieri S (2010) Home-based functional electrical stimulation rescues permanently denervated muscles in paraplegic patients with complete lower motor neuron lesion. Neurorehabil Neural Repair 24:709–721. doi:10.1177/1545968310366129. Epub 2010 May 11
5. Carraro U, Kern H, Gava P, Hofer C, Loefler S, Gargiulo P, Mosole S, Zampieri S, Gobbo RB, Piccione P, Marcante A, Baba A, Schils S, Pond A, Gava F (2015) Biology of muscle atrophy and of its recovery by FES in aging and mobility impairments: roots and by-products. Eur J Transl Myol 25:211–230
6. Kern H, Barberi L, Löfler S, Sbardella S, Burggraf S, Fruhmann H, Carraro U, Mosole S, Sarabon N, Vogelauer M, Mayr W, Krenn M, Cvecka J, Romanello V, Pietrangelo L, Protasi F, Sandri M, Zampieri S, Musaro A (2014) Electrical stimulation counteracts muscle decline in seniors. Front Aging Neurosci 6:189. doi:10.3389/fnagi.2014.00189. eCollection 2014
7. Carraro U, Kern H, Gava P et al (2016) Recovery from muscle weakness by exercise and FES: lessons from Masters, active or sedentary seniors and SCI patients. Aging Clin Exp Res Sep 3. [Epub ahead of print] Review
8. Zampieri S, Mosole S, Löfler S et al (2015) Physical exercise in aging: nine weeks of leg press or electrical stimulation training in 70 years old sedentary elderly people. Eur J Transl Myol 25:237–242. doi:10.4081/ejtm.2015.5374
9. Börjesson M, Onerup A, Lundqvist S, Dahlöf B (2016) Physical activity and exercise lower blood pressure in individuals with hypertension: narrative review of 27 RCTs. Br J Sports Med Jan 19. pii: bjsports-2015-095786. doi:10.1136/bjsports-2015-095786
10. Carneiro LS, Fonseca AM, Serrão P, Mota MP, Vasconcelos-Raposo J, Vieira-Coelho MA (2016) Impact of physical exercise on catechol-O-methyltransferase activity in depressive patients: a preliminary communication. J Affect Disord 193:117–122. doi:10.1016/j.jad.2015.12.035. [Epub ahead of print]

Motivation and Rehabilitation in Older Patients

7

Carine Federspiel and Jean-Paul Steinmetz

Physical and rehabilitation medicine (PRM) aims restoring functional ability and quality of life of patients suffering from physical, cognitive, and/or psychological impairments. A disabling condition with no known cure chronically limits the patient in his functions and may disable the patient from completing most basic activities of daily living. In general, the patient's goal is to be pain-free and to attain a previous level of independence, thus to leave the rehabilitation institution as soon as possible [1]. Generally, patients are characterized by multiple morbidities and thus may be deficient in cognition, nutrition, muscle strength, and affectivity or have an unfavorable social living situation. In the geriatric context, the emphasis of PRM is not primarily put on the full restoration of all of these functions to a previous (premorbid) level but rather on reestablishing in the patient an appropriate level of quality of life. Thus and in our understanding, PRM should focus on providing the necessary support to the patient to maximize functionality (in the widest sense) within the limitations placed upon him by the disabling condition. Consequently, restoring a level of independence in the patient's activities of daily living allowing him to experience adequate levels of quality of life is crucial.

To achieve this goal, patient involvement is the prerequisite. It is generally accepted that compliance to rehabilitation has a positive influence on rehabilitation outcomes [2] with factors compromising motivation (e.g., cognitive or mood disorders) increasing the length of the rehabilitation [1, 3, 4]. Motivation is a complex construct and depends on many factors. Intrinsic factors such as self-efficacy beliefs, personal needs and preferences, pain, affectivity (dysthymia/depression), fear, weakness, and cognitive deficits or extrinsic factors such as unfamiliar surroundings, contextual support, and incentives given by the therapists or the family influence motivation directly or indirectly [5]. Self-efficacy, initially defined by Bandura

C. Federspiel, MD • J.-P. Steinmetz, PhD (✉)
Centre for Memory and Mobility - ZithaSenior, Luxembourg City, Luxembourg
e-mail: carine.federspiel@zitha.lu; jean-paul.steinmetz@zitha.lu

© Springer International Publishing AG 2018

S. Masiero, U. Carraro (eds.), *Rehabilitation Medicine for Elderly Patients*, Practical Issues in Geriatrics, DOI 10.1007/978-3-319-57406-6_7

[6], is a person's belief in his or her capabilities to have control over or to influence a (personal) situation or an event. Previous research found that sense of control in people and their age is negatively related, with older persons experiencing generally less control [7, 8]. Beliefs in one's own capabilities (i.e., self-efficacy) are thought to govern cognition, emotions, and behavior and are crucial to determine to what extent a patient feels motivated. In PRM it is thus important to identify potential sources of self-efficacy enhancing information to help strengthen those beliefs [9]. To enhance motivation and corresponding behaviors (i.e., participation in rehabilitation activities), several factors are relevant: the patient's personality, patient's active participation in the development of the interdisciplinary rehabilitation program, definition of relevant goals to be achieved during rehabilitation, encouragement and support from the therapists, empowerment of the patient, and the rehabilitation environment in general [1, 10, 11]. Moreover, providing information about the necessity of certain exercises or therapies (i.e., patient education) may furthermore be beneficial in generating patient motivation to engage in rehabilitation [11]. Detrimental effects of lack of motivation have been discussed in the literature. Findings suggest that if patients are perceived as unmotivated by the therapist, the clinician is less likely to support and encourage him/her. Thus, motivated patients are differently treated than unmotivated ones, especially if the unmotivated patient is old [11]. Therapists play a vital role in positively influencing their patients to actively participate in therapy. An interpersonal relationship characterized by respect and trust may easily be established between the therapist and the motivated patient but takes time and effort to be established with patients lacking motivation. That is, therapists must develop an important amount of sensitivity toward their patients enabling the therapist to recognize cognitive and mood disorders threatening positive rehabilitation outcomes in their patient [4]. As a positive consequence, rehabilitation interventions can promptly be adapted according to the mental and physical state of the patient.

After more than a decade of clinical practice in geriatric rehabilitation, our general experience is that the acquisition of knowledge of the patient's preferences prior the critical health event and the patient's personality (e.g., through contacts with the family) is beneficial in determining a tailored intervention program. Tailored intervention programs are ideally developed by an interdisciplinary team composed of various healthcare professionals. A multidisciplinary team can be composed of a geriatrician and/or a specialist in rehabilitation medicine, an occupational therapist, a physiotherapist, a psychologist, a speech therapist, a social worker, and a nursing staff. This interdisciplinary composition is an important key toward a better understanding, evaluation, adaptation, and scheduling of individualized rehabilitation interventions. Monitoring physical and mental capacities and the social condition of the old patients helps us in approaching the very personal interests of each patient on different levels. Thus and, for example, assessing (e.g., through semi-structured interviews) and integrating systematically individual biographic elements in the development of tailored interventions is useful in enhancing compliance among patients as interventions may be better focused and adapted to the individual patient. Furthermore, spending time with the patient and trying to build up an empathetic relationship to make the patient feel comfortable and welcome may furthermore positively affect compliance and consequently, rehabilitation outcomes [12]. We conclude that exploring the construct of motivation is fundamental in the work with older adults and should hence be systematically considered in geriatric rehabilitation units as it figures as a key mediator of the success or the failure of a rehabilitation program.

References

1. Resnick B (2002) Geriatric rehabilitation: the influence of efficacy beliefs and motivation. Rehabil Nurs 27:152–159
2. Duncan PW, Horner RD, Reker DM, Samsa GP, Hoenig H, Hamilton B, LaClair BJ, Dudley TK (2002) Adherence to postacute rehabilitation guidelines is associated with functional recovery in stroke. Stroke 33:167–178. doi:10.1161/hs0102.101014
3. Kerr T (2000) Depression in the elderly. Adv Phys Ther Phys Ther Assist 11:38–39
4. Givens JL, Sanft TB, Marcantonio ER (2008) Functional recovery after hip fracture: the combined effects of depressive symptoms, cognitive impairment, and delirium. J Am Geriatr Soc 56:1075–1079. doi:10.1111/j.1532-5415.2008.01711.x
5. So C, Pierluissi E (2012) Attitudes and expectations regarding exercise in the hospital of hospitalized older adults: a qualitative study. J Am Geriatr Soc 60:713–718. doi:10.1111/j.1532-5415.2012.03900.x
6. Bandura A (1977) Self-efficacy: toward a unifying theory of behavioral change. Psychol Rev 84:191–215
7. Wolinsky FD, Wyrwich KW, Babu AN, Kroenke K, Tierney WM (2003) Age, aging, and the sense of control among older adults: a longitudinal reconsideration. J Gerontol B Psychol Sci Soc Sci 58:S212–S220. doi:10.1093/geronb/58.4.S212
8. Wolinsky FD, Stump TE (1996) Age and the sense of control among older adults. J Gerontol B Psychol Sci Soc Sci 51:S217–S220
9. Buckman M (2016) A systemic literature review exploring the effects of occupational therapy rehabilitation and motivation on geriatric patients. Honors Major Theses Pap. 7
10. Resnick B (1996) Motivation in geriatric rehabilitation. ResearchGate 28:41–45
11. Maclean N, Pound P, Wolfe C, Rudd A (2002) The concept of patient motivation a qualitative analysis of stroke professionals' attitudes. Stroke 33:444–448. doi:10.1161/hs0202.102367
12. Maclean N, Pound P (2000) A critical review of the concept of patient motivation in the literature on physical rehabilitation. Soc Sci Med 50:495–506. doi:10.1016/S0277-9536(99)00334-2

Bed Rest Syndrome

8

F. Scarponi and M. Zampolini

8.1 Introduction

Since Hippocrates' time, traditional medicine has intended bed rest as: "In every movement of the body, whenever one begins to endure pain, it will be relieved by rest" [1]. The harmful effects of prolonged bed rest only started to be studied in the late twentieth century [2, 3].

Bed rest does not have specific positive effects yet causes numerous physiologic adaptations in all organ systems, often with negative consequences [3]. However, there are no studies that clearly show the benefit of avoiding bed rest, and in a recent meta-analysis the conclusion of the authors is: "*There are no RCTs or controlled trials that provide evidence for, or against, staying in bed for at least four weeks after symptom onset in patients with aneurysmal SAH*" [4]. Furthermore, neither does lateral positioning lead to a clear benefit in critically ill patients [5].

Although being bedridden might be an inevitable situation in some clinical conditions, in aging patients due to frailty and muscle loss, too much bed rest could worsen the effects, due to increased protein degradation (cachexia), decreased rate of muscle protein synthesis (inactivity), or an alteration in both (sarcopenia) [6]. Recently, a review has shown that the aetiology of these conditions is not completely understood but involves some common processes, such as the dysregulation of inflammatory pathways, which seems to be important, and several biomarkers and combinations of biomarkers have been suggested as measures of frailty [7].

F. Scarponi
Neurorehabilitation Unit, USL Umbria 2, Foligno Hospital,
Via. M. Arcamone, Foligno, Perugia 06034, Italy

M. Zampolini (✉)
Department of Rehabilitation, USL UMBRIA 2, Foligno Hospital, Via M. Arcamone,
Foligno, Perugia 006034, Italy
e-mail: mzampolini@gmail.com; mauro.zampolini@uslumbria2.it

© Springer International Publishing AG 2018

S. Masiero, U. Carraro (eds.), *Rehabilitation Medicine for Elderly Patients*,
Practical Issues in Geriatrics, DOI 10.1007/978-3-319-57406-6_8

In older people frailty is a syndrome of lower strength, endurance, and physiological functions that increase an individual's vulnerability and risk of mortality. Due to frailty, people can lose their independence leading to the condition of being bedridden with assistance required even for "minor" acute events and consequent increased risk of sarcopenia, cachexia, and atrophy. This overlap of geriatric syndromes may be relevant in the development of damage caused by being in a bedridden condition. In fact, frailty sarcopenia and cachexia can combine to form a vicious circle: strength, endurance, and physical activity are lower, the total energy expenditure diminished, with a subsequent chronic undernutrition that maintains sarcopenia [8].

8.1.1 Effects of Bed Rest

Prolonged bedrest is associated with several time-dependent effects. The effects of being bedridden have an impact on the whole organism, and a good knowledge of every physiological mechanism involved is recommended for the physician. Table 8.1 summarizes the fundamental aspects for the principal body systems.

Table 8.1 Effects of prolonged bed rest

Cardiovascular system	Increased resting heart rate
	Venous thrombosis
	Early increased cardiac stroke
Respiratory system	Reduced tidal volume
	Potential permanent restrictive pulmonary disease due to fixed contractures of the costovertebral joints
	Reduced FVC and FEV1
	Loss of elastic recoil as a result of structural changes within the lungs
	Tendency for mucus to pool in the lower part of the airway
	Collapse of airways and small areas of lung tissue (atelectasis), which reduces the area available for gaseous exchange
Musculoskeletal system	Atrophy of postural muscles, leading to an increased risk of falls and disability [15]
	Reduction of bone mass in the spine and lower limbs
Gastrointestinal system	Decreased gastric bicarbonate secretion and increased acidity within the stomach
	Symptoms associated with gastroesophageal reflux disease (GERD)
	Increased transit time and constipation
Urinary system	Release of ANP and increased diuresis
	Transient increase in plasma and urinary urea, a decrease in plasma creatinine, and no change in urinary creatinine
	Rise of urinary calcium excretion
	Incomplete emptying and urinary stasis, due to weakened abdominal and pelvic floor musculature
	Renal and bladder stones and infections
Skin	Higher risk of pressure sores

Table 8.1 (continued)

Endocrine system	Depressed levels of aldosterone and antidiuretic hormone
	Sodium loss during diuresis and hyponatremia with subsequent increased plasma renin activity and increased plasma aldosterone levels
	Progressive loss of potassium in the urine due to aldosterone secretion
	Increased cortisol secretion, onset of insulin resistance, impaired glucose tolerance, and the subsequent development of type 2 diabetes
Central and peripheral nervous system	Dysfunctions in mental status (confusion, sleep disorders, drowsiness)
	Difficulties in posture and balance in sitting and standing position
	Development of polyneuropathies

8.2 Prevention of Bed Rest Syndrome

Patients in the intensive care unit (ICU) could be the paradigm of the management of bed rest via mobilization. They are often sedated, critical/frail patients, with obvious difficulty in changing position, sitting or walking. Immobilization in complex patients in the ICU, together with systemic inflammation, is a strong independent risk factor for the development of intensive care unit-acquired weakness (ICUAW) [9].

Evidence indicates that functionally significant joint limitations are shown by more than a third of patients admitted to ICU for over 2 weeks.

It is noteworthy that enough damage to create the basis for a decubitus ulcer is done after as little as 2 h of immobility. Susceptibility to pressure ulcers comes from a combination of external factors (pressure, friction, shear force, and moisture) and internal factors (e.g., fever, malnutrition, anemia, and endothelial dysfunction).

Although a few years ago, early physical rehabilitation of critically ill patients was considered unsafe, in the last decade growing literature has shown the safety and feasibility of mobilizing ICU patients to prevent impairments, adverse events, in-hospital infections, and functional limitations [10].

In order to address these aspects, components of the ABCDE bundle include: Awaken from sedation, Breathe independently without a ventilator, Choice of sedation, Delirium management, and Early mobilization [11].

While preliminary data regarding early mobilization of ICU patients has been shown to be safe, feasible, and beneficial, in one multicenter, observational Italian study, postural changes and early mobilization were prescribed in about two thirds of the cases, suggesting that these treatments are not yet widely practiced [12].

In this study, despite mobilization being included within the nurses' activities in some cases, in almost all cases the physiotherapist was indicated for an average of 38 min/day.

Since mobilization is not always possible, another tool to prevent bed rest syndrome is limiting development of sarcopenia by implementing nutrition with essential amino acids (EAA). The benefit of EAA in these conditions is not completely understood but could stimulate anabolic processes in skeletal muscles, thus helping to preserve them. In some papers, EAA supplementation leads to stimulation of the production of lean body mass in older women and is associated in maintaining strength of plantar flexion and going upstairs, muscle mass, and motor coordination [8].

Probably, the most effective strategy to mitigate the impact of bed rest on the development of sarcopenia is adequate nutrition and/or the utilization of resistance exercise [13].

Another strategy is the utilization of "low magnitude mechanical signals (LMMS)" that seem to improve the strength and endurance of hip and knee muscles [8]. Furthermore, in experimental studies LMMS are anabolic to bone if applied at a high frequency (15–90 Hz) and could be useful in preventing osteoporosis caused by bed rest [14]. Further future studies are clearly necessary to understand the efficacy of these strategies in preventing the consequences of bed rest syndrome.

Conclusions

Evidence indicates that physiopathological mechanisms of bedridden conditions start very early after immobilization and can lead to prolonged and severe consequences that are often difficult to heal, painful, and impact negatively on the individual's quality of life. Preventing such damage must be considered part of clinical routine. Care should be provided by a multiprofessional team with skills and expertise in medicine, nursing, and physiotherapy.

As specifically recommended also in the acute phase of very critical patients, the minimum provision of interventions is repeated postural changes during the day (every 2–3 h) as well as joint mobilization.

Key Points

- Physiopathological mechanisms of bed rest syndrome are time dependent; few hours of immobilization are enough to begin a cascade of modifications that can lead to impairments for several weeks or months.
- Immobilization could overlap with geriatric syndromes, with heavier impact on functional recovery.
- Bed rest syndrome involves various physiological systems.
- Bedridden condition should be discouraged when there're no rational motivations to reduce mobility of patients, even in critical conditions.
- Care must be provided by a multiprofessional team with skills in medicine, nursing, and physiotherapy.
- Essential interventions are early mobilization, change positioning every 2–3 h, facilitating awakeness, and promote weaning from mechanical ventilation.
- If mobilization isn't possible, a dietary intake of EAA or other solutions could be considerate.

References

1. Hippocrates (1849) The genuine works of Hippocrates. The Sydenham Society, London
2. Convertino VA (1997) Cardiovascular consequences of bed rest: effect on maximal oxygen uptake. Med Sci Sports Exerc 29(2):191–196
3. Allen C, Glasziou P, Del Mar C (1999) Bed rest: a potentially harmful treatment needing more careful evaluation. Lancet 354(9186):1229–1233
4. Ma Z, Wang Q, Liu M (2013) Early versus delayed mobilisation for aneurysmal subarachnoid haemorrhage. Cochrane Database Syst Rev 5:CD008346. doi:10.1002/14651858.CD008346.pub2
5. Hewitt N, Bucknall T, Faraone NM (2016) Lateral positioning for critically ill adult patients. Cochrane Database Syst Rev 5:CD007205
6. Evans WJ (2010) Skeletal muscle loss: cachexia, sarcopenia, and inactivity. Am J Clin Nutr 91(4):1123S–1127S
7. Partridge JS, Harari D, Dhesi JK (2012) Frailty in the older surgical patient: a review. Age Ageing 41(2):142–147
8. Coker RH, Wolfe RR (2012) Bedrest and sarcopenia. Curr Opin Clin Nutr Metab Care 15(1):7–11
9. Meduri GU, Schwingshackl A, Hermans G (2016) Prolonged glucocorticoid treatment in ARDS: impact on intensive care unit-acquired weakness. Front Pediatr 4:69
10. Needham DM (2008) Mobilizing patients in the intensive care unit: improving neuromuscular weakness and physical function. JAMA 300(14):1685–1690
11. Dang SL (2013) ABCDEs of ICU: early mobility. Crit Care Nurs Q 36(2):163–168
12. Bartolo M et al (2016) Early rehabilitation for severe acquired brain injury in intensive care unit: multicenter observational study. Eur J Phys Rehabil Med 52(1):90–100
13. Glover EI, Phillips SM (2010) Resistance exercise and appropriate nutrition to counteract muscle wasting and promote muscle hypertrophy. Curr Opin Clin Nutr Metab Care 13(6):630–634. doi:10.1097/MCO.0b013e32833f1ae5
14. Rubin C, Judex S, Qin YX (2006) Low-level mechanical signals and their potential as a non-pharmacological intervention for osteoporosis. Age Ageing 35(Suppl 2):ii32–ii36
15. Ikezoe T et al (2012) Effects of age and inactivity due to prolonged bed rest on atrophy of trunk muscles. Eur J Appl Physiol 112(1):43–48. Epub 2011 Apr 7

Exercise for Frail Older Adults

9

A. Musumeci, A. Pignataro, E. Ferlito, V. Lazzari, H. Zatti, and S. Masiero

9.1 Introduction

Frailty is a geriatric syndrome characterized by an increased vulnerability of older persons to the external stressors and decreased ability to regain physiological functions after a destabilizing event [1–3]. It is highly prevalent in people older than 65 years (7–16.3%) and can increase up to 25% in people over 85 years [4–6]. Data about frailty are variable from country to country, and no clear differences have been demonstrated between both sexes [7]. Frailty is one of the most important causes of adverse outcomes and premature mortality of older patient [1]. Frail adults have reduced strength and endurance; they are more dependent, prone to falls, and susceptible to be admitted to nursing home residencies.

Pre-frailty is a silent precursor of frailty, in which the presence of psychological stressors, acute diseases, or traumatic injuries predisposes to the development of frailty.

Pathogenesis of frailty is still unclear and different hypotheses have been proposed. Fried speculated that fragility could be the consequence of malnutrition and sarcopenia [8, 9]. According to Rockwood, instead, frailty is the result of the accumulation of many non-related deficits (e.g., gait difficulties, cognitive and sphincteric disorders, etc.) [10]. Some authors have also hypothesized that inflammation may determine muscle deterioration and consequent frailty [3, 11]. Sociodemographic (e.g., poverty or living alone) and psychological factors (e.g., depression), the polypharmacy, and several other clinical conditions (e.g., insulin resistance and diabetes) have also been implicated as determinants of the frailty status [12].

A. Musumeci (✉) • A. Pignataro • E. Ferlito • V. Lazzari • H. Zatti • S. Masiero
Rehabilitation Unit, Department of Neurosciences, University of Padua, Padua, Italy
e-mail: alfredomusumeci@yahoo.com; andreapignataro88@gmail.com;
erika.ferlito@sanita.padova.it; valentina.lazzari@sanita.padova.it; hilariz@hotmail.it;
stef.masiero@unipd.it

© Springer International Publishing AG 2018

S. Masiero, U. Carraro (eds.), *Rehabilitation Medicine for Elderly Patients*,
Practical Issues in Geriatrics, DOI 10.1007/978-3-319-57406-6_9

9.2 Balance and Gait in Frail Older People

Aging process may cause several modifications in muscle strength, postural control, balance, and gait, which are considered the main components of frailty.

Human stability is the intrinsic capacity to maintain, reach, or regain a state of balance. Balance control involves many systems and requires an optimal integration of external information that pass through the sense organs. A balance decline, due to somatosensory system progressive impairment, occurs as early as 40 years of age, and older people do not easily adapt to perturbations [13, 14]. An increase of dorsal kyphosis is common in elderly and may result in further imbalance between the gravity center and the supporting base, increasing the risk of falls (Fig. 9.1).

Moreover, flexed posture determines an overload to the lower limbs and to the spine.

Gait also changes during aging, as a consequence of a reduction in muscular capacity, sensory function, and neural processing [13]. Muscle weakness of hip

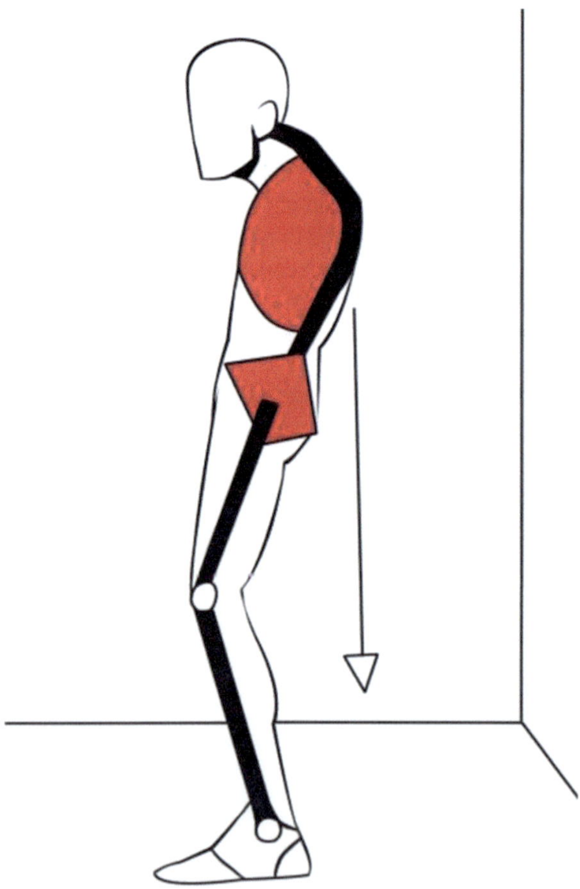

Fig. 9.1 This figure shows the imbalance between the gravity center and the supporting base in older adults

abductors and adductors has been reported, and a greater instability of elderly people when initiating stepping has been reported in elderly people [15]. Older adults tend to slow their walking speed and to show a slower reaction to external stimuli [15–21]. The loss of plantar cutaneous sensation is another important factor leading to impairment of motor control [21].

9.3 Frailty Measurement

Identifying frail older people is the first and essential step in rehabilitation. Multiple scales have been developed, but the most common are the Fried frailty phenotype assessment and the frailty index of accumulative deficits (FI-CD) index. According to Fried's criteria, frailty is defined by the presence of three or more criteria and pre-frail state by the presence of one or two of the following: shrinking (unintentional weight loss of 4.5 kg or more in the last year), weakness (low grip strength), exhaustion, slowness (slow walking speed), and low physical activity. Fried's criteria are also predictive of adverse clinical outcomes, including mortality. They are, however, not commonly used for routine assessment and cannot be routinely applied in acutely ill or severely disabled patients; moreover, they do not include the psychosocial components [3].

FI-CD requires the aggregation of 30 or more symptoms, co-morbidities, diseases and disabilities, or any health deficiency: a greater number of deficits mean higher frailty and risk of adverse events in both hospital and community settings [10, 13].

9.4 Physiotherapy in Frail Older Adult

Frailty is a modifiable dynamic process that can be prevented and even reversed by early identification and treatment of pre-frail older adults. Specific strategies could be therefore be used in order to attain this goal, and the best results seem to be obtained by combining exercise and nutritional supplementation [22].

Scientific literature showed that regular physical activity reduces the risk of developing cardiovascular and metabolic diseases, obesity, cognitive decay, osteoporosis, and muscular atrophy as well as the risk of falls in both healthy and frail elderly people [23]. There is, however, a great variety among the studies concerning the number of patients enrolled, degree of frailty, training programs, and assessments.

Generally, the more a person is physically active, the better will be its physical performances. This is due mainly to a better adjustment in the hemodynamic (a more efficient distribution of oxygen and nutrients to the tissues) and in the motor coordination in response to environmental changes [23–26].

International guidelines highlighted the importance of multimodal interventions that combine strength activities, cardio conditioning workout, and balance and functional exercises. Nevertheless—although the scientific community unanimously promotes regular physical activity of elderly people—participation to exercise programs progressively decreases during aging and, concomitantly, the desire to participate. This is the reason why it is important to define a personalized exercise program, responding to subject's own features and expectations (taking into account the level of previous physical activity), its social engagement, and the support of caregivers.

Various exercise modalities have been proven to be effective in older patients, but the combination of strength, resistance, power, coordination, proprioception, and balance and aerobic training is the most beneficial.

The effect of exercise on falls was studied in terms of incidence, and risk of falls and fear of falling were studied, but results were controversial.

The exercise has a positive influence on body and muscle composition, is beneficial for mobility, and improves older patients' functional abilities [27]. Therefore, it is always important, when starting a training program, to find the appropriate level of dosage, intensity, frequency of an exercise, as well as the correct level of progression; physical exercise should always be administered and scheduled according to the goals and the physical fitness of the subject.

9.5 Strength Training and Aerobic Exercise

An exercise program should last 3–4 months in average, with a maximum frequency of 3 sessions/week of at least 45 min each. Every session must include a phase within the aerobic threshold, related to daily life activities, such as walking, cycling, climbing stairs, or recreational activities (exercises with a ball) and a part dedicated to the muscular strengthening, using free weights, elastic resistance, etc.

The exercise intensity is variable, according to the exercise experience and physical fitness of each subject.

Repetition maximum (1RM) is the maximum force that can be developed in one maximal contraction. 1RM test is generally employed to measure the intensity of an exercise. There is not a common agreement in the literature, on the amount of intensity to be adopted during an exercise; however, the majority of authors suggest that the intensity should be light or moderate (20–30% 1RM) and slowly increased progressively (i.e., it can be obtained by increasing the percentage of 1RM up to a maximum of 80% 1RM or the number of repetitions from 8 to 15 repetitions for one series). An increase in exercise intensity is allowed no more than once every 4 weeks, or when the series is perceived as easy to perform. Currently, there is no evidence on the muscular groups to train; several recent studies focused their attention on the plantar flexors, since a loss of strength in this group is associated with a reduction of walking speed while an increase to an improvement in balance. No risk in executing muscular strength training has been shown; however, some minor musculoskeletal symptoms have been reported (e.g., diffuse arthralgia, joint and muscle swelling, fatigue, or even muscular sprain, especially in those subjects who started from very debilitated or sedentary conditions) (Figs. 9.2 and 9.3).

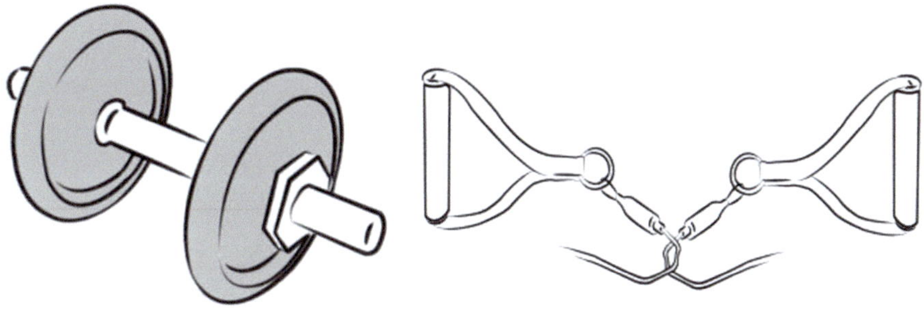

Fig. 9.2 This figure shows some tools that are commonly used for strength and power training. Dumbbells, a type of free weight, can be used for reinforcement of the upper limbs. Elastic bands and elastic tubes can be used for strength training of both upper and lower limbs

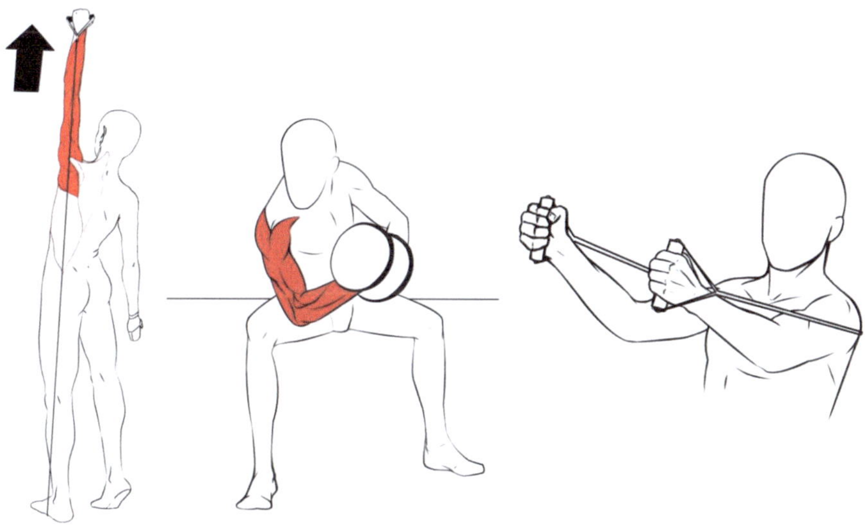

Fig. 9.3 Examples of exercises using dumbbells and elastic bands

The risk of serious adverse events after cardiopulmonary training is low for both moderate and elevated efforts, and it is higher during the first weeks of training. This training determines central and peripheral circulatory adjustments and aims to increase the musculoskeletal system's ability to produce energy through the oxidative pathways. The first week cardiopulmonary training should start from 5 to 10 min of activity per session and then progressively increase up to 15–30 min.

The methods for controlling training intensity are different. The most frequently employed are the heart rate, which should be kept between 70% and 80% of the maximum heart rate (HRmax) in order to maintain oxidative metabolism, or self-monitoring scales, which evaluate the perceived fatigue, in which the intensity should be between moderate and well tolerated (12–14 on the 20 point Borg scale) (Figs. 9.4, 9.5, and 9.6).

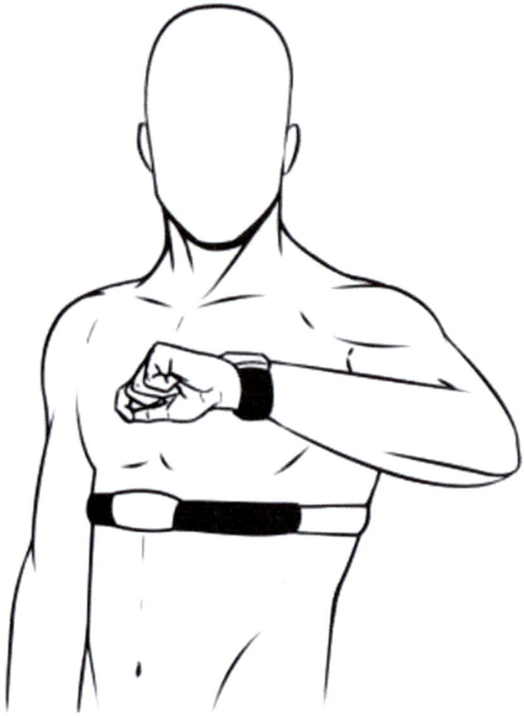

Fig. 9.4 Cardiopulmonary training. Watch or chest strap are simple, wearable tools used to monitor heart rate and the intensity during exercises

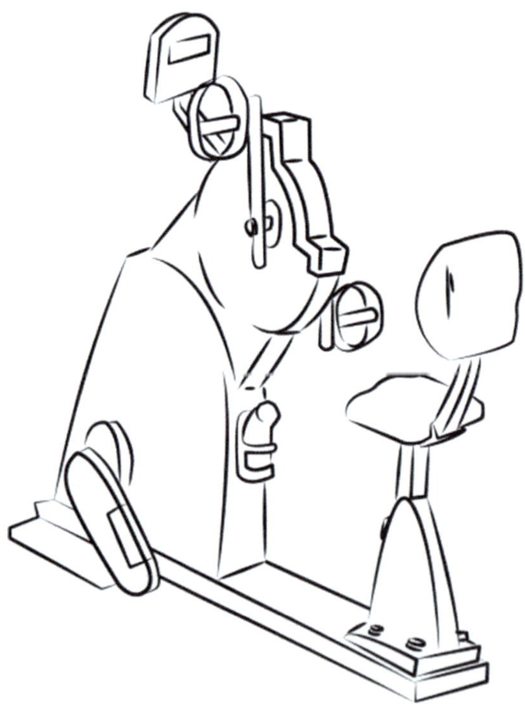

Fig. 9.5 The ergometer is a machine used for cardiopulmonary training that allows measuring the work performed by exercising

9.6 Balance

Balance exercises are mainly functional and progressively difficult, allowing the body to develop anticipatory abilities, in relation to different tasks or environmental situations.

In order to improve their balance, subjects must exercise themselves against an external force consequent to their movements or applied from outside.

Examples of exercise interventions are walking and tandem walking, cycling, proprioceptive static and dynamic exercises (e.g., using balance balls), strength exercises, and computerized balance training with visual feedback, coordination exercises, dance, tai chi, and yoga. Exercises can be proposed either singularly or combined. Different tools are used to improve balance and postural control such as proprioceptive or unstable surfaces and systems using computerized visual or acoustic feedback (Fig. 9.6).

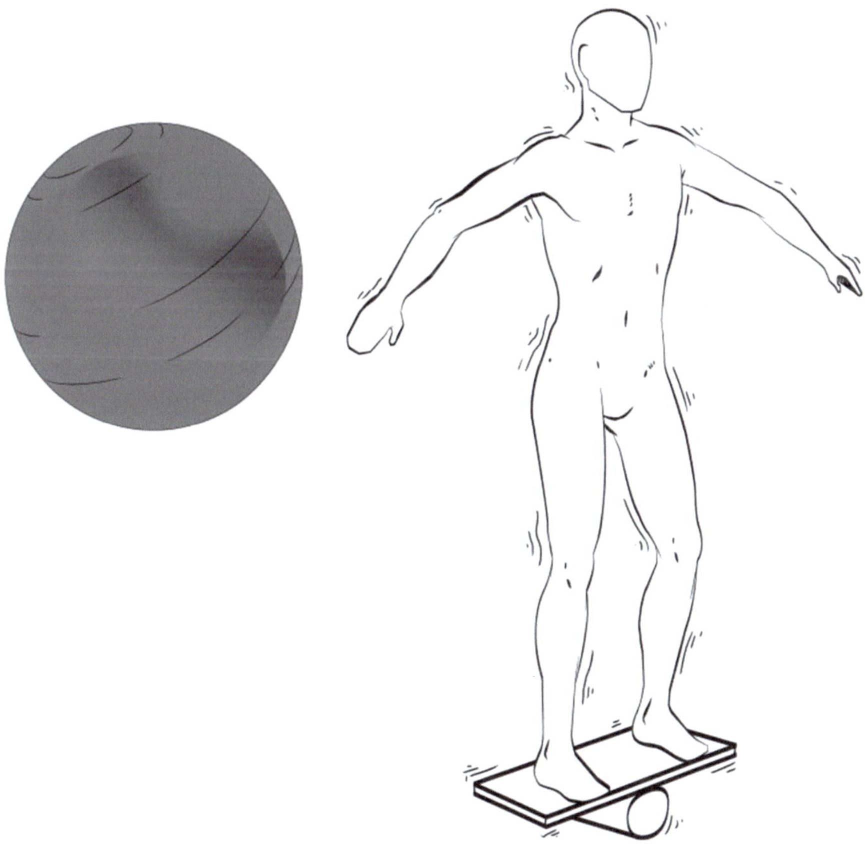

Fig. 9.6 Unstable surfaces (balance pillows, boards, or balls) are commonly used to improve balance and postural control

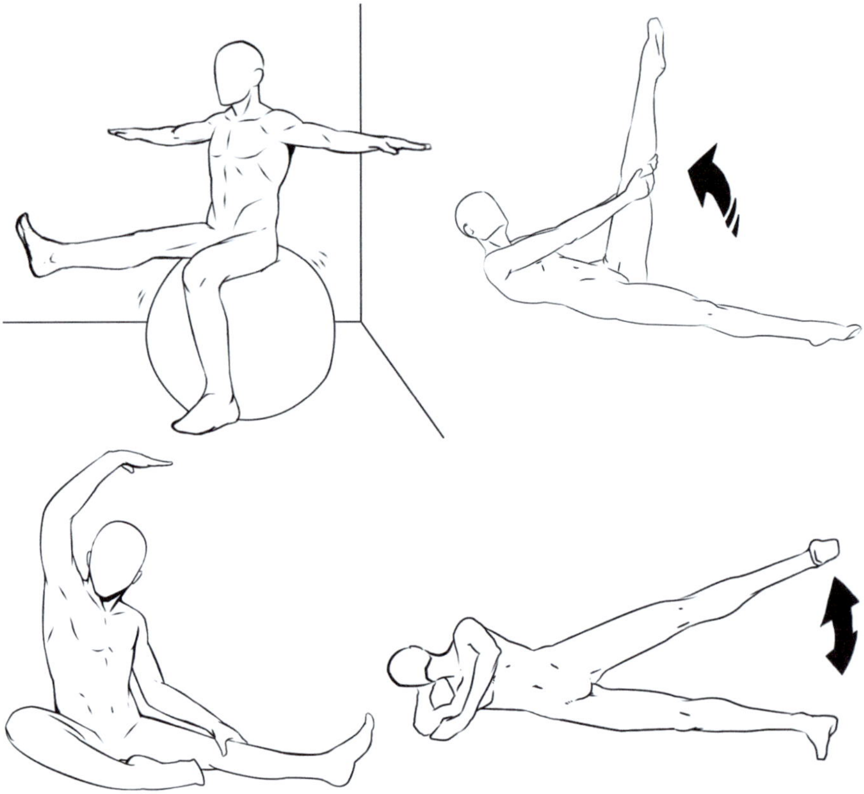

Fig. 9.7 These figures show some examples of useful exercises for postural control

Duration of the exercises ranges from a minimum of 4 weeks to a maximum of 12 months, with sessions taking place from twice a week up to once a day. The most common frequency is three times a week. Duration of the single session varies from 3 to 90 min, with a major frequency of 60 min.

Stretching and coordination exercises can also be useful in older patients. Coordination exercises aim to prepare older patients in managing external disturbing forces and allow a better control of the center of gravity during walking, thus reducing the risk of falls (Figs. 9.7 and 9.8) [28].

Both the aforementioned training typologies should be performed during the training session, and the exercise proposal should be functional to daily life activities as much as possible [27–31].

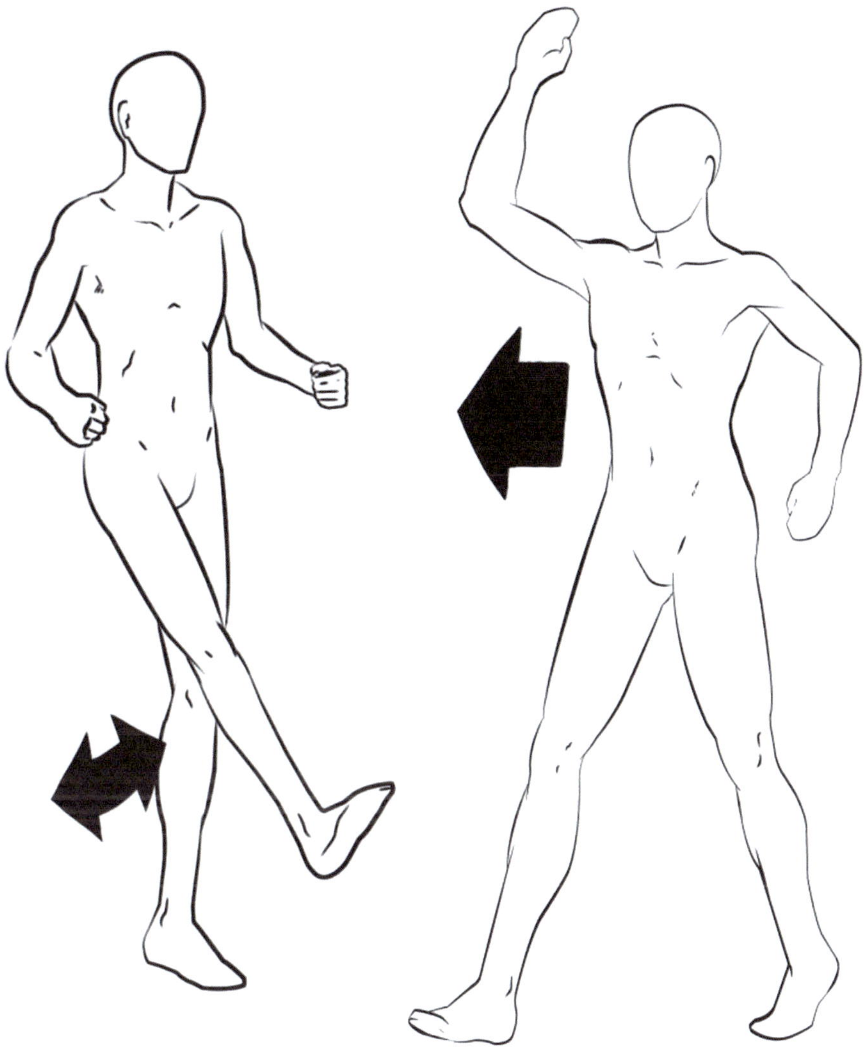

Fig. 9.8 Examples of coordination exercises: moving upper and lower limbs at the same time while walking

9.7 Promotion to Participation

Senior patient tends to become sedentary with age, as well as to progressively lose the will to perform physical exercise. Older people are frequently less motivated to improve their physical conditions and more interested in maintaining the residual abilities they possess. Therefore, they need to be encouraged by social workers, healthcare professionals, families, and friends. The most common barriers to participation to physical activities are the economic cost, lack of time, physical limitations, and the frequent need to ask third parties for assistance to perform the exercises or to reach the gym. Social or communicative factors may also limit participation (e.g., the necessity to dress in a particular way or difficulties in verbal expression).

In order to encourage patient's involvement, the exercise proposition should consist of low-cost activities, the training session should prove to be pleasant and funny, and the trainee should be often reassured of the safety and the harmlessness of the activity he is performing. Moreover, it would be better if the activity could become a moment of social sharing.

A significant factor related to the adhesion to an exercise program and its maintenance in the long term is the increase of independence (self-efficacy). Self-efficacy is one's belief he can succeed in doing specific tasks. It is therefore important for the trainee to perceive his improvement in performing exercises into a safe context and to be confirmed by the operator.

Another factor that favors the participation is witnessing how the activity is bringing positive results in relation to the predetermined goals: for example, on a functional level in the everyday activity, both in terms of quantity (being able to walk for longer) and in terms of quality (less fatigue in climbing the stairs), or even at a social level (new relationships created in the group activity).

When managing elderly patients, it is therefore essential to consider the pivotal role of the caregiver. He has a significant role in motivating older patients to continue physical activities. He plays a very important role in patient's health, functionality, well-being, and quality of life. He also represents the crucial partner for seniors' care, especially if frail, and in management of his life both inside and outside home. According to the World Health Organization, the cooperation between the professionals and the caregivers should be the base of the assistance to the elderly person. In particular, many are so far the studies on the economic, social, and personal burden the caregiver and patient's family have to bear for patient's management. The main characteristics of the patient perceived as highly affecting the caregiver's life are the risk of falls, depressive symptoms, and behavioral problems. It needs to be highlighted that the bigger the responsibility load (e.g., cohabitation, patient's disability, the presence of only one caregiver, etc.) for the caregiver, the higher the probabilities of patient's frequent hospitalization or institutionalization are.

Assessing patient and level of autonomy is therefore not sufficient, as we have to consider the context where he lives, his personal characteristics, and if the persons who look after him are eager to collaborate. Helping the caregiver to understand the benefits of an exercise program for the patient, also in terms of reduction of the risk of falls and increase or support of his residual abilities, could prove a successful strategy [32].

Conclusions

Frailty is a very complex and impactful condition for an older adult. Early identification of frailty conditions and pre-frail status is important to reduce adverse outcomes and premature mortality of older patient.

Although the best training program still remains unclear, international guidelines highlighted the importance of reversing pre-frail and frail status, using a multimodal exercise approach, possibly in a fun and pleasant contest. Exercise interventions have many advantages: they can improve frail adult's quality of life, balance, and mobility reduce the risk of institutionalization and hospitalization.

The caregiver is a very important figure in frail adult's life and should be involved in the intervention, in order to facilitate patient's participation and to reduce his own burden in caring the patient.

Acknowledgments Figures courtesy of Monteverde Filippo and Sette Beatrice, Liceo Artistico Selvatico, Padua, Italy.

Key Points

- Frailty and pre-frailty rehabilitation can be reversed by multimodal exercises.
- An adequate evaluation and, subsequently, a targeted exercise program are very important to attain goals.
- Exercise proposal focuses on functional, strength, aerobic, balance, and proprioceptive exercises.
- The role of the caregiver is very important in promoting and maintaining a physical active style of life of older adults.

References

1. Vaupel JW (2010) Biodemography of human ageing. Nature 464(7288):536–542
2. Kuzuya M (2012) Process of physical disability among older adults—contribution of frailty in the super-aged society. Nagoya J Med Sci 74(1–2):31–37
3. Chen X, Mao G, Leng SX (2014) Frailty syndrome: an overview. Clin Interv Aging 9:433–441
4. Lang PO, Michel JP, Zekry D (2009) Frailty syndrome: a transitional state in a dynamic process. Gerontology 55(5):539–549
5. Garcia-Garcia FJ, Gutierrez Avila G, Alfaro-Acha A et al (2011) The prevalence of frailty syndrome in an older population from Spain. The Toledo Study for Healthy Aging. J Nutr Health Aging 15:852–865
6. Sanchez-Garcia S, Sanchez-Arenas R, Garcia-Pena C et al (2014) Frailty among community-dwelling elderly Mexican people: prevalence and association with sociodemographic characteristics, health state and the use of health services. Geriatr Gerontol Int 14(2):395–402
7. Romero-Ortuno R, Fouwheather T, Jagger C (2014) Cross-national disparities in sex differences in life expectancy and without frailty. Age Aging 43:222–228
8. Clegg A, Young J, Iliffe S et al (2013) Frailty in elderly people. Lancet 381(9868):752–762
9. Fried LP, Tangen CM, Walston J et al (2001) Frailty in older adults: evidence for a phenotype. J Gerontol A Biol Sci Med Sci 56(3):M146–M156
10. Mitnitski AB, Mogilner AJ, Rockwood K (2001) Accumulation of deficits as a proxy measure of aging. Sci World J 1:323–336
11. Gielen E, Verschueren S, O'Neill TW et al (2012) Musculoskeletal frailty: a geriatric syndrome at the core of fracture occurrence in older age. Calcif Tissue Int 91(3):161–177
12. Heuberger RA (2011) The frailty syndrome: a comprehensive review. J Nutr Gerontol Geriatr 30(4):315–368

13. Nitz JC, Low Choy NL (2008) Falling is not just for older women: support for pre-emptive prevention intervention before 60. Climacteric 11:461–466
14. Huxham F, Goldie P, Patela A (2001) Theoretical considerations in balance assessment. Aust J Physiother 47:89–100
15. Tinetti ME, Williams CS (1988) The effect of falls and fall injuries on functioning in community-dwelling older persons. J Gerontol A Biol Sci Med Sci 53:M112–M119
16. Rogers MW, Mille ML (2003) Lateral stability and falls in older people. Exerc Sport Sci Rev 31:182–187
17. Maki BE, Edmondstone MA, McIlroy WE (2000) Age-related differences in laterally directed compensatory stepping behavior. J Gerontol A Biol Sci Med Sci 55(5):M270–M277
18. Lazaro M, Gonzalez A, Latorre G et al (2011) Postural stability in the elderly: fallers versus non fallers. Eur Geriatr Med 2:1–5
19. Maki BE, Mcilroy WE (2006) Control of rapid limb movements for balance recovery: age-related changes and implications for fall prevention. Age Ageing 35(S2):ii12–ii18
20. Maki BE, Zecevic A, Bateni H et al (2001) Cognitive demands of executing rapid postural reactions: does aging impede attentional switching? NeuroReport 12:3583–3587
21. Do MC, Bussel B, Breniere Y (1990) Influence of plantar cutaneous afferents on early compensatory reactions to forward fall. Exp Brain Res 79:319–324
22. Kim H, Suzuki T, Kim M et al (2015) Effects of exercise and milk fat globule membrane (MFGM) supplementation on body composition, physical function, and hematological parameters in community-dwelling frail Japanese women: a randomized double blind, placebo-controlled, follow-up trial. PLoS One 10(2):e0116256
23. McPhee JS, French DP, Jackson D et al (2016) Physical activity in older age: perspectives for healthy ageing and frailty. Biogerontology 17(3):567–580
24. Department of Health UK (2011) Start active, stay active: UK physical activity guidelines. Department of Health, London, UK. http://www.dh.gov.uk/health/category/publications/
25. Health USDo (2009) Physical activity guidelines advisory committee report, 2008. To the secretary of health and human services part A: executive summary. Nutr Rev 67:114–120
26. Tak E, Kuiper R, Chorus A, Hopman-Rock M (2013) Prevention of onset and progression of basic ADL disability by physical activity in community dwelling older adults: a meta-analysis. Ageing Res Rev 12:329–338
27. Beijersbergen CM, Granacher U, Vandervoort AA et al (2013) The biomechanical mechanism of how strength and power training improves walking speed in old adults remains unknown. Ageing Res Rev 12:618–627
28. Stenroth L, Sillanpaa E, McPhee JS et al (2015) Plantarflexor muscle-tendon properties are associated with mobility in healthy older adults. J Gerontol A Biol Sci Med Sci 70(8):996–1002
29. Pereira A, Izquierdo M, Silva AJ et al (2012) Effects of high-speed power training on functional capacity and muscle performance in older women. Exp Gerontol 47:250–255
30. Cadore EL, Rodriguez Manas L, Sinclair A, Izquierdo M (2013) Effects of different exercise interventions on risk of falls, gait ability, and balance in physically frail older adults: a systematic review. Rejuvenation Res 16(2):105–114
31. De Labra C, Guimaraes-Pinheiro C, Maseda A et al (2015) Effects of physical exercise interventions in frail older adults: a systematic review of randomized controlled trials. BMC Geriatr 15:154
32. De Almeida Mello J, Macq J, Van Durme T et al (2016) The determinants of informal caregiver's burden in the care of frail older persons: a dynamic and role-related perspective. Aging Ment Health 1–6

Physical Therapy Modalities for Older Persons

10

A. Musumeci, J.V. Papathanasiou, E. Lena, C. Assenza, C. Giordani, C. Foti, L. Gobbo, and S. Masiero

10.1 Introduction

This chapter aims to introduce the reader to the knowledge of physical therapy modalities (PM) commonly employed by healthcare professionals for the treatment of elderly diseases. PM use physical agents to unleash a chain reaction of biological modifications in body tissues that produce specific therapeutic effects. The most important physical agents used in PM are thermal, mechanic, electric, and electromagnetic. Their efficacy is based on the knowledge of their mechanisms of action, dosages and modalities of administration, and their proper use. Common indications for PM are musculoskeletal pain treatment, reduction of muscle contractures, spasms, inflammation and edema, facilitate wound healing, etc. In the geriatric population, PM are often used in conjunction with other manual therapies and prescribed in cycles with a variable number of sessions within a rehabilitation program [1, 2].

A. Musumeci (✉) • L. Gobbo • S. Masiero
Neurorehabilitation Unit, Padua General Hospital, Padua, Italy
e-mail: alfredomusumeci@yahoo.com; luca.gobbo@sanita.padova.it; stef.masiero@unipd.it

J.V. Papathanasiou
Department of Kinesitherapy, Faculty of Public Health, Medical University of Sofia, Sofia, Bulgaria

Department of Medical Imaging, Allergology and Physiotherapy, Faculty of Dental Medicine, Medical University of Plovdiv, Plovdiv, Bulgaria

E. Lena • C. Assenza • C. Giordani • C. Foti
Clinical Medicine and Translational Medicine Department, Tor Vergata University, Rome, Italy

© Springer International Publishing AG 2018

S. Masiero, U. Carraro (eds.), *Rehabilitation Medicine for Elderly Patients*, Practical Issues in Geriatrics, DOI 10.1007/978-3-319-57406-6_10

10.2 Thermotherapy

Thermotherapy is the application of heating (heat therapy) and cooling agents (cryotherapy) for muscle, joint, and soft tissue disorders. The goal of thermotherapy is to increase tissue temperature in a targeted region in order to induce the desired biological response in a specific tissue. Thermotherapy has many effects: it enhances tissue metabolism, modifies cell permeability, increases collagen tissue distensibility, and has hemodynamic effects. Moreover, it can alter nerve fibers' excitability, thus reducing pain sensation and muscle spasms.

Heat therapy conveys thermal energy to the body through conduction, convection, and radiation. Heat is typically applied by placing a warming device on the relevant part or the entire human body.

Superficial tissues are heated using many different tools, such as mud packs, hot packs, heat wraps, wax baths, hot water, saunas, and steam baths.

Cryotherapy is often used to reduce the metabolic demand, edema, inflammation, and bleeding after muscle and soft tissue injuries. It is commonly applied through ice packs, towels, massage, gel packs, etc.

Both heat and cold therapies can be used in the inpatient and outpatient setting and at home [3].

10.2.1 Heat

10.2.1.1 Paraffin Bath

Liquid paraffin, also known as *paraffinum liquidum*, transfers thermal energy through conduction but, as soon as it solidifies, also determines a mechanical compression on the part.

The paraffin bath is a mixture of paraffin and mineral oil that is kept and heated to a temperature of 50–55 °C. The patient dips into paraffin the injured extremity for a couple of seconds then remove it, thus allowing paraffin to harden; this action is repeated daily from six to twelve times. The next step is to put the heated part into a plastic bag and wrap it with several towels for 20–30 min. The procedure ends by removing the hardened wax [4].

The topical action of the paraffin relieves pain symptoms and reduces edema, muscle spasms, and contractures of the hand and foot joints, mainly in osteoarthritis. Contraindications to its usage are pulmonary or cardiac failure, intolerance to paraffin, open wounds, or skin infections.

10.2.1.2 Infrared Radiations

The infrared are electromagnetic radiations (wavelength from 760 nm to 1 mm) produced by natural (e.g., sun) or artificial (luminous or nonluminous) sources. Luminous sources (wavelength from 760 to 1400 nm) emit near infrared (NIR), visible light, and UVA. The higher is the temperature of the source, the higher the frequency, and the shorter the wavelength.

Most home devices, commonly used in PM, emit NIR radiations. NIR deliver energy to the cells causing vasodilatation, an increment in blood flow of the skin and local warming. The infrared have a maximum depth of penetration of 1 cm.

Infrared lamps have biostimulating and healing effects and are used for relieving muscle and joint's pain; treatment usually lasts from 10 to 30 min. Indications for use of NIR are pain treatment in osteoarthritis, muscle spasms, and contractions, as a means to warm the muscle prior to physical exercises, massage, or manual therapy, or for ulcer treatment (associated with UVA).

Contraindications are fever and cardiac diseases [5].

10.2.1.3 Shortwave Diathermy

Shortwave diathermy (*dia* = through, *thermy* = heat) uses high-frequency electromagnetic energy generated by a condenser (capacitive field) or by coils (induction field), to produce molecular vibration and to heat the part to be treated. Shortwave diathermy produces a radiofrequency at 27.12 MHz and can be applied in a continuous (CSWD) or a pulsed (PSWT) mode; it can penetrate about 3 cm deep. CSWD uses thermal effect in muscles and superficial joints; in PSWT nonthermal effects are predominant.

Shortwave diathermy main effects are the increase in cell membrane permeability, the improvement of mitochondrial function, the modulation of enzymatic activity, the increase in tissue distensibility, etc.

Indications for CSWD treatment are degenerative rheumatic diseases, low back pain (subacute or chronic), musculoskeletal injuries (strains, tendinopathies, tenosynovitis, bursitis, sprains), and muscle contractures.

CSWD is contraindicated in people using pacemakers, audio or metal prostheses, pregnant women, people with active bleeding, osteoporosis and neoplasms. Moreover, it should be cautiously used in patients with altered thermal and pain sensibility [6]. Duration of treatment is 20–30 min and can be repeated for 2 weeks.

In PSWT the mean power delivered to the tissue is relatively low, and the peak power is commonly 150–200 W. PSWT may be effective in restoring the cell membrane potential and ionic transport of musculoskeletal and soft tissues during the inflammatory and repair phases. In fact, its primary target seems to be the cell membrane and the ion transport across it. Treatment should not last more than 20 min.

PSWT is indicated in the presence of edema or hematoma; it enhances tissue healing and osteogenesis.

Contraindications are acute vascular (arterial or venous) diseases, pacemaker, pregnancy, recent hemorrhage, malignancy, active tuberculosis, and recent radiation therapy in the region to be treated (≤6 months) (Table 10.1).

Table 10.1 Tissue absorption according to different PM treatment (Adapted from www.electrotherapy.org/modality/ultrasound-therapy)

Physical modality	Tissue absorption	Action
Infrared radiations	Superficial	Muscle, joint, ulcer
Continuous shortwave	Deep	Muscle, joint
Pulsed shortwave	Wet, ionic	Muscle, nerve, edema, hematoma
Laser	Superficial vascular	Muscle, nerve, tendon, joint, open wounds
Ultrasound	Dense collagen, deep	Ligament, tendon, fascia, joint capsule, fibrotic muscle

10.2.2 Cold

Local application of cold (cryotherapy) decreases blood flow by activating a vasoconstrictive reflex and reduces inflammation and the metabolic request of hypoxic tissues. Moreover, it has a topical anesthetic effect by reducing the activation threshold of tissue nociceptors, the conduction velocity of nerves, and muscle spindle fiber activity.

Cold therapy improves pain symptoms and reduces local edema and inflammation; it is also effective in reducing muscle spasms and contractures and in the treatment of sprains, strains, contusions, tendonitis, etc. For all these reasons, cryotherapy is commonly used after acute injuries and articular diseases.

10.3 Laser Therapy

"Laser" is the acronym for "light amplification by stimulated emission of radiation." Laser therapy transfers energy within the tissues, thus modulating the biological processes (photobiomodulation) according to "the Arndt-Schultz law": low dosage photonic energy stimulates the biological processes (photobiostimulative effect), whereas, on the contrary, high dosage energy has an inhibitory effect (photobioinhibitive effect).

Lasers can be classified, according to the wavelength/max output power and the ability to damage exposed persons, into four classes of risk: from the lowest (class I: no hazard) to the highest (class IV: severe risk for the eyes and skin). Most therapeutic lasers are class III (low-level, cold, or low-power lasers) and deliver limited amount of energy and power (≤500 mW). However, they are not as effective as high power lasers (class IV therapeutic lasers).

The laser therapy effects are analgesic, anti-inflammatory (it stimulates the release of beta-endorphins), and reparative (regenerative action on deep structures by inducing the protein synthesis and increasing blood flow). The physiological effects are:

- biostimulation (increase of cell metabolism)
- blood circulation improvement and vasodilatation
- increased ATP production
- wound healing stimulation
- increased collagen production
- enhanced macrophage activity
- modification of nerve conduction (velocity)

Lasers are commonly applied through a connector maniple, if small areas are to be treated (Fig. 10.1), or through scanning technique, when dealing with wider areas (Fig. 10.2).

Common indications of laser therapy are musculoskeletal pain symptoms, inflammatory diseases of tendons and soft tissue, enthesopathies, edema, and pressure sores (Table 10.1).

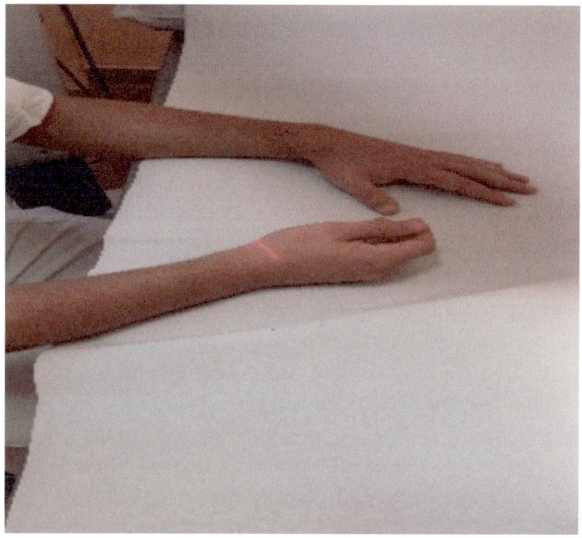

Fig. 10.1 Laser application using scanning technique

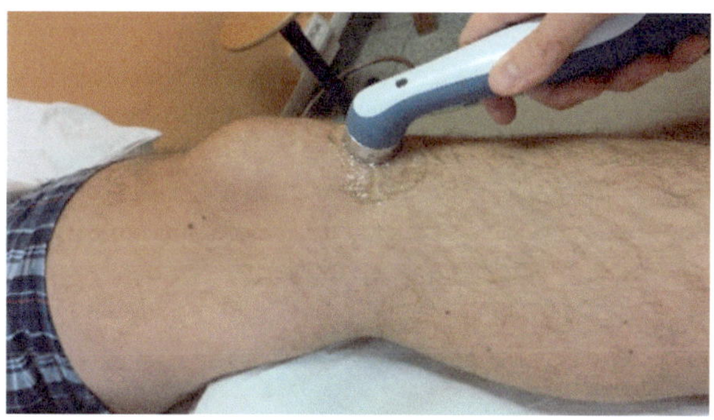

Fig. 10.2 US therapy applied directly on the knee

10.3.1 Low-Level Laser Therapy (LLLT)

LLLT (wavelength from 600 to 1000 nm) uses red beam or NIR lasers. It consists of different procedures and is performed by different methods.

It is useful in relieving pain of rheumatic diseases, osteoarthritis, neck or nonspecific chronic low back pain, tendinopathies, and joint disorders. Usual treatment lasts from 5 to 10 min [7–12].

10.3.2 High Dose: High Power Laser Therapy

High power lasers are used to stimulate tissue healing, but they can also improve pain from osteoarthritis, carpal tunnel syndrome, epicondylitis, sprains or strains, and muscle disorders.

10.4 Therapeutic Ultrasound

Ultrasound (US) is a mechanical wave that, passing through the body, transfers its energy to the tissues, causing molecular vibration. US determines thermal and nonthermal effects; nonthermal effects are attributed to a combination of cavitation and shear stress (see also the paragraph on Thermotherapy). Cavitation leads to the formation of reactive oxygen species and stimulates cell repair during the inflammatory phase. Shear stress include the radiation pressure, radiation force, and acoustic streaming; the latter phenomenon changes cell diffusion rate, permeability, and membrane potentials. Thermal effects improve nerve transmission speed, increase blood flow rate, and reduce edema. From all the above, it is clear that therapeutic US is mainly used to promote tissue healing and improve the quality of tissue repair.

The frequencies used in US therapy are typically between 1.0 and 3.0 MHz. Depth of penetration is dependent on the frequency of the US machine. Therapeutic US can be applied as pulsed or continuous therapy, either directly, using a transducer and a conductive gel (Fig. 10.2), or indirectly transferred, through immersion of the transducer in water (Fig. 10.3). The penetration of US is better in tissues rich in collagen content (i.e., ligaments, tendons, fascias, joints, and fibrotic muscles) (Table 10.1) [13–16].

US treatment lasts approximately from 5 to 15 min and is repeated from one to three times a week; patient should never feel pain during therapy. Many clinicians use of pulsed US to treat, once or even twice daily, acute conditions. In this case, therapy lasts from 6 to 8 days until symptoms subside. In subacute or chronic conditions, patients can be treated every other day.

Indications for therapeutic US are osteoarthritis, rheumatic diseases, joint or tendon inflammation, soft tissue injuries, sprains or strains, myositis ossificans, nerve entrapments (brachialgia, sciatalgia), and muscle spasms.

Contraindications for US treatment are cardiac diseases, deep vein thrombosis, pregnancy, malignancy, and metal implants [17].

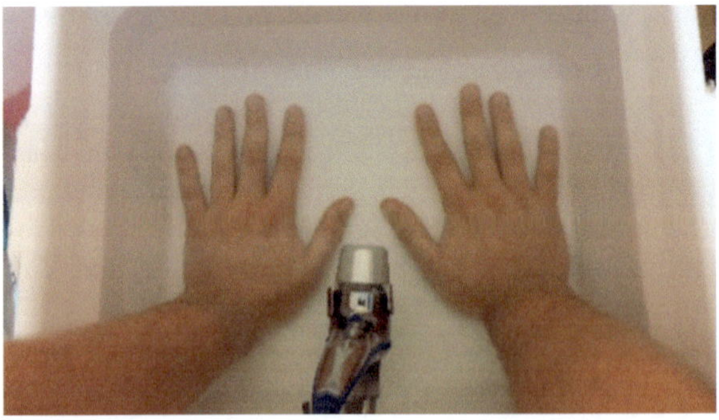

Fig. 10.3 US therapy through immersion technique is used for irregular surfaces

Table 10.2 Physical characteristics of ESWT

ESWT type	Pressure (bar)	Pulse duration	Pressure field	Penetration depth
Radial	1–10	0.2–0.5 ms	Radial, divergent	Small, superficial
Focused	100–1000	0.2 μs	Focused	Large

10.5 Extracorporeal Shockwave Therapy (ESWT)

Shockwaves are high-energy acoustic waves that travel faster than conventional sound wave. The more energy is applied, the more the shockwave will penetrate the tissue, determining a rapid expansion of the gases solved in blood and lymphatic fluids. Expanding gas molecules causes an increased pressure on the dysfunctional tissues, determining a phenomenon called "cavitation" in which voids quickly collapse on themselves generating an implosion (shockwave) in the tissue. Healthy tissues are not affected by the shockwaves because they can easily absorb their energy.

Shockwaves action on musculoskeletal system can determine:

- Cell permeability modifications
- Osteoblasts stimulation
- Osteogenic action
- Growth factors production
- Increase in type I and III collagen synthesis
- Vasoactive effects

Shockwaves can be focused or radial; they have different physical characteristic, are generated with different techniques (radial shockwaves are produced by a pneumatic system; focused shockwaves can be produced by electrohydraulic, electromagnetic, and piezoelectric shockwave generators), and use different parameters used for therapeutic penetration in the tissues (Table 10.2).

ESWT has been proven as effective and safe for treatment of musculoskeletal diseases [18, 19]. Radial shockwaves can be used in case of myofascial pain syndromes or spasticity.

Focused shockwaves seem to have a more favorable outcome in relieving deep pain or chronic tendinitis [20, 21]; they can also be used in the occurrence of:

- Tendinopathies (plantar fasciitis, ulnar and radial epicondylopathy, rotator cuff tendinitis with or without calcifications, adductor syndrome, etc.)
- Impaired bone healing function (delayed healing, stress fractures, early stage of avascular bone necrosis, etc.)
- Muscular pathologies (myofascial syndrome, excluded fibromyalgia excluded)
- Impaired wound healing
- Spasticity

10.6 Whole Body Vibration (WBV)

WBV has gained popularity in geriatric rehabilitation in the past decade. It is considered a passive exercise modality in which patients lay, sit, or stand on a platform that delivers vibration stimuli to the rest of the body. The vibration signals activate the sensory receptors by changing the length of the muscle-tendon complex and causing reflexive activation of motor units. However, the biological and mechanical effects of WBV are not completely understood.

WBV may induce positive effects on leg muscle strength, improving postural control and functional mobility among elderly adults, particularly frailer ones. Vibration therapy can also be used in multiple sclerosis, neuropathies, osteoporosis, and in case of pain (e.g., in women with fibromyalgia syndrome). WBV has also shown some positive effects on gait and balance in Parkinson disease [22–24].

Contraindications of WBV therapy are acute inflammations, infections, acute arthritis, severe cardiovascular diseases, heart failure, pacemaker, deep vein thrombosis, leg ulcers, pregnancy, spasticity, vertigo, severe headache, acute tendonitis, acute back pain, gliding spondylolisthesis, fractures, metal implants, severe osteoporosis, musculoskeletal metastatic tumors, serious ocular diseases, and fresh wounds.

10.7 Magnetotherapy

Magnetotherapy consists in applying artificial magnetic fields that are generated by electrical currents to the human body. Artificial magnetic fields used in PM have similar intensity to the earth's, but with higher frequencies and longer time of application.

Magnetotherapy acts on cell membranes by the modification of cell permeability and the increase of intracellular metabolic exchanges; it has a biostimulating effect (increasing nucleic acid synthesis, cell metabolism, and the oxygen consumption) and an analgesic effect (suppressing the peripheral nociceptive stimuli, enhancing the production and the release of pain-inhibiting substances, and increasing peripheral blood circulation). Magnetotherapy also acts on autonomic system increasing the catecholamine or acetylcholine level and promotes bone trophysm by stimulating the bony callous formation. Therefore, the effects of magnetotherapy can be analgesic, anti-inflammatory, anti-edematous, and reparative.

Artificial magnets can be electromagnets that work when connected to electricity, pulsed electromagnets generated by a brief pulse of electric current and connected to a coil (Fig. 10.4), or permanent magnets. Magnetic fields are used with low or high intensity, in the ambulatory care or home setting for several hours per

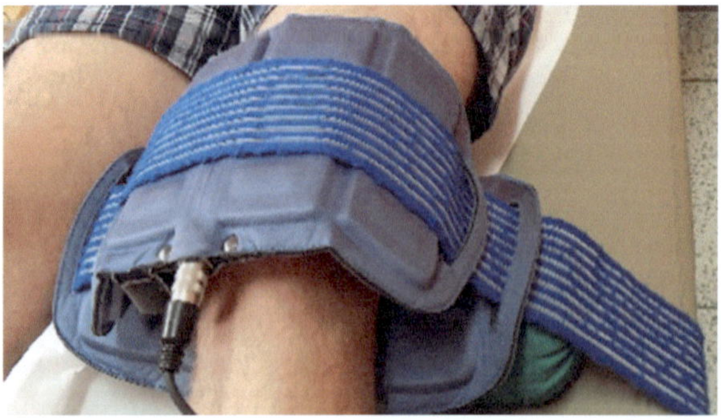

Fig. 10.4 Portable magnetotherapy with pulsed magnetic fields

day. Instrument settings should be adjusted according to patient's reactions; however, an increase in pain symptoms could signify a positive response to treatment.

Common indications for magnetotherapy are osteopenia, delayed fracture healing, posttraumatic algodystrophy, inflammatory or degenerative arthropathy, trophic ulcers, etc.

Contraindications are pacemaker, hemorrhage, pregnancy, acute infection, and malignancy.

10.8 Electrotherapy

All electrical modalities used in Physical and Rehabilitation Medicine (PRM) take the electrical current flowing from a wall outlet and modify that current to produce a specific, desired physiologic effect in human biologic tissue [25]. Electrotherapeutic devices regardless of whether they deliver alternating (AC), direct (DC), or pulsatile (PC) through electrodes attached to the skin are transcutaneous electrical stimulators. When they introduced into biologic tissue, they are capable of producing specific physiologic changes [26]. The term waveform indicates a graphic representation of the shape, direction, amplitude, duration, and pulse frequency of the electrical current being produced by the electrotherapeutic device, as displayed by an oscilloscope [27].

Waveform shapes (Fig. 10.5) can be:

- Rectangular
- Square
- Spike
- Sinusoidal (sine)

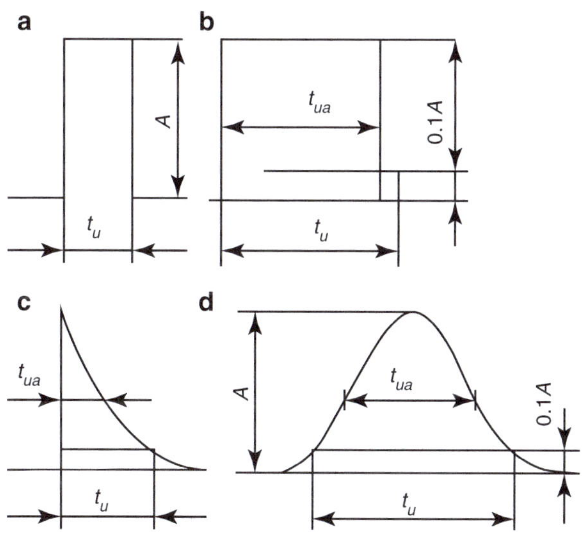

Fig. 10.5 Waveform shapes of pulsatile currents

Knowledge of the electric properties of cells, intercellular and intracellular communication, bioelectric potentials, tissue currents, strain-generated electric potentials, and biologic effects of other nonionizing energy will be essential for the PRM specialists in order to use present and future electrical modalities for maximum clinical benefit [26].

Today PRM specialists are using electrical currents in an effort to provide a quick and effective pain management, tissue healing, and neuromuscular stimulation. The treatment protocol must be tailored toward influencing the problems identified in the evaluation. Although electrotherapeutical procedures can provide dramatic results at times, this is the exception rather than the rule. Electrotherapy should not be used in a "shotgun" approach if we are to maximize the effectiveness of this modality. Usual electrotherapy treatment lasts 30 min for each session; it can be repeated two or three times a week for a total of 10/12 sessions [28–30].

10.8.1 Iontophoresis

Iontophoresis is a therapeutic procedure that involves the introduction of various ionized drugs into the skin by means of a direct electrical current for the purpose of transporting chemicals across the membrane [31]. Iontophoresis has several advantages is a painless, sterile, and noninvasive procedure that provides a high degree of compliance, acceptability, and has a positive effect on the healing process. *On the same time, it provides a high degree of patient compliance and acceptability, and it has been demonstrated to have a positive effect on the healing process.* A primary advantage of iontophoresis is the ability to provide both a spiked and sustained release of a drug, thus reducing the possibility of developing a tolerance to the drug [32]. Transdermal iontophoresis delivers medication at a constant rate so that the effective plasma concentration remains within a therapeutic window for an extended period of time. Clinically, iontophoresis is used in the treatment of inflammatory musculoskeletal conditions, for analgesic effects, scar modification, wound healing and in treating edema, calcium deposits, and hyperhidrosis. The effectiveness of iontophoresis is directly related to the medication administered or the solution used for ion transfer. Each medication has its own effect, regardless of the method of application [33].

Contraindications of iontophoresis are pacemakers, epilepsy, malignancy, metal implants, gastritis or active stomach ulcer (hydrocortisone), skin sensitivity reactions, skin wounds, asthma (mecholyl), and sensitivity to metals (zinc, copper, magnesium) and seafood (iodine). The most common complication associated with iontophoresis is a chemical burn, which usually occurs as a result of the direct current itself and not as a result of the ion being used in treatment. Heat burns may occur as a result of high resistance to current flow created by poor contact of the electrodes with the skin. During the treatment, the PRM specialist should closely supervise the patient, looking for either abnormal localized reactions of the skin or systemic reactions [34].

10.8.2 Neuromuscular Electrostimulation (NMES)

NMES also known as electrical muscle stimulation (EMS), or electromyostimulation, is a noninvasive method that, using the excitability of muscle cells, allows to induce muscle contraction by an electric current; this method can be applied either to a normally innervated muscle or to a denervated muscle [35].

The NMES is able to determine an increase in muscle strength. There are, however, uncertainties about the mechanisms, which are the basis of the changes that this kind of stimulation is able to determine [36]. Although NMES represents an artificial means of muscle activation that goes beyond the processes associated with the will, there is evidence showing how it can induce neuronal adaptations related to the force. And in fact it can be highlighted that there are improvements in strength that precede in time, the changes of the muscle size; a lower training intensity required, compared with that necessary for a voluntary training; and an increase in strength of the contralateral untrained limb accompanying the increase in strength of the limb treated with NMES (phenomenon of cross education) [37, 38]. The therapeutic use of NMES is also important to limit the feelings of discomfort that may affect patient compliance to therapy. The problem linked to the tolerability of the treatment for the patient was object of many studies: the results showed large variability of response in order to the different types of current; therefore, the choice of the type of current must be determined case by case in order to obtain the maximum validity of the contraction with minimal discomfort [28, 39]. In addition, to get the maximum benefits from the NMES, the intensity of current used must be enough to evoke relatively intense contractions. However, the minimum dosages of the currents, which determine the appropriate contraction forces for an effective muscle training, have yet to be determined.

In older adults the NMES can be integrated in rehabilitation programs of various conditions: atrophy ex non-usu, increase and maintenance range of motion, reduction of edema, muscle spasm or spasticity, increase muscle mass in sports and rehabilitation of the pelvic floor, muscle weakness in chronic progressive diseases or as a lower limbs strength training tool within rehabilitation programs in patients who are totally or partially immobilized, and prevention of venous thrombosis.

The main contraindications to the use of NMES are pacemaker, pregnancy, phlebitis, myositis, myasthenia, muscular dystrophy, and skin wounds [40]. Today many people confuse transcutaneous electrical nerve stimulation (TENS) with NEMS. NEMS and TENS devices look similar, with both using long electric lead wires and electrodes. TENS is for blocking pain, where NEMS is for stimulating muscles.

10.8.3 Transcutaneous Electrical Nerve Stimulation (TENS)

TENS is a non-pharmacological method, which is widely used for the management of acute and chronic pain in a variety of conditions. TENS is a noninvasive, inexpensive, and safe intervention, defined by the American PRM Association as the application of an electrical stimulation to the skin for pain management. The Food and Drug Administration (FDA) has approved TENS as a method of pain alleviation and classified it as class II device in 1972 [41]. The most popular theory to explain the mechanism of action of TENS is "gate control theory" of pain proposed by Melzack and Wall in 1965. They suggested that TENS stimulates large-diameter A-β fibers inducing an inhibition of substantia gelatinosa interneurons, localized in the spinal cord. The result is a repression of smaller A-δ and C pain fibers, with consequent presynaptic inhibition of the T-cells, closing of the "gate," and control of pain perception [42]. In 1977, Mayer et al. investigated the "opioid theory" as a second explanation for the mechanism of action of TENS. They hypothesized that naloxone, an opioid receptor antagonist, blocks the analgesia produced by low-frequency electroacupuncture (<10 Hz), suggesting that it works through the release of endorphins [43].

TENS devices are small portable contraptions powered by rechargeable or replaceable batteries, based on a one- or two-channel mode (Fig. 10.6). The unit is usually connected to the skin using two or more electrodes. A typical battery-operated TENS unit is able to modulate pulse width, frequency, and intensity. Generally TENS is applied at high frequency (>50 Hz) with an intensity below motor contraction (sensory intensity) or low frequency (<10 Hz) with an intensity that produces motor contraction.

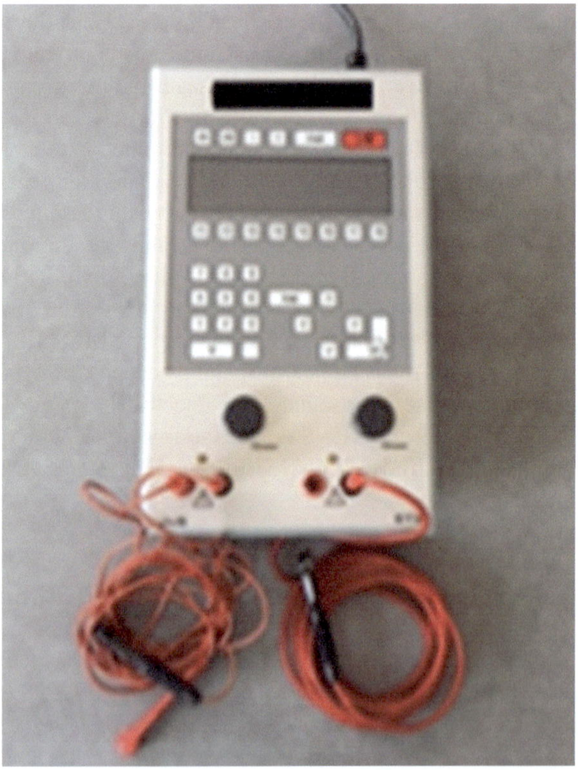

Fig. 10.6 TENS device

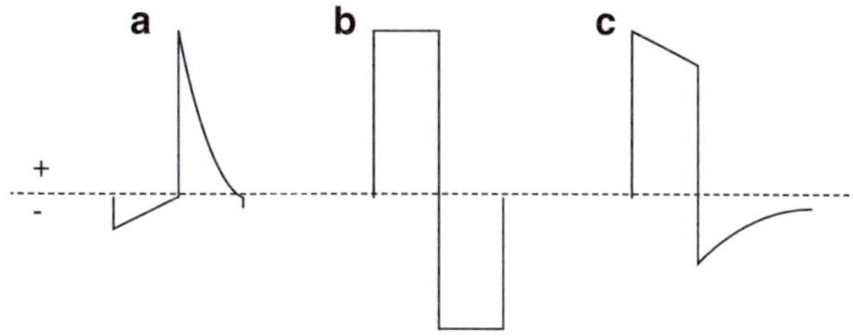

Fig. 10.7 (**a**) Spike wave, (**b**) symmetric rectangular wave, (**c**) asymmetric rectangular wave

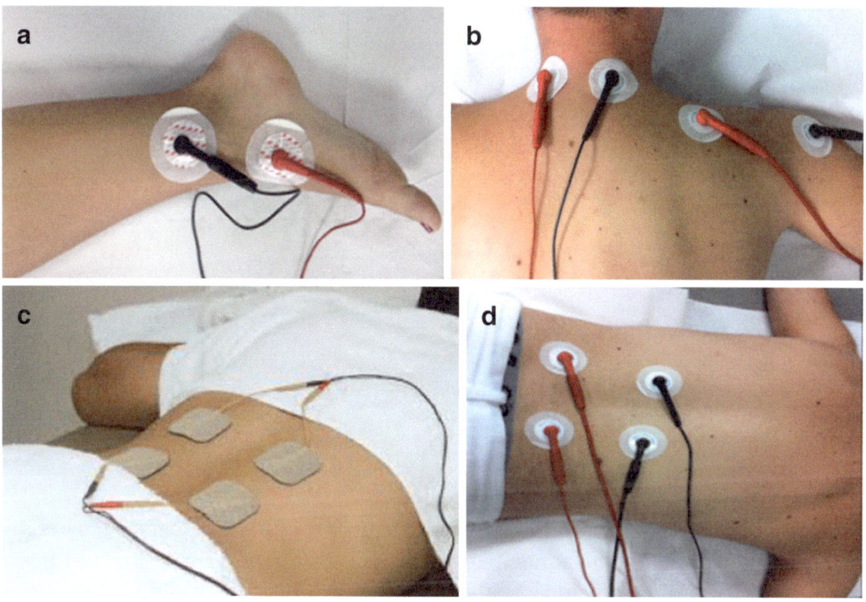

Fig. 10.8 (**a**) Trigger points for ankle pain, (**b**) trigger points for cervico-brachial pain syndrome, (**c**) longitudinal disposition, (**d**) crossed disposition

Electrodes of 4–30 cm^2 size can deliver current as biphasic, spike (Fig. 10.7a) or rectangular, symmetric (Fig. 10.7b), or asymmetric (Fig. 10.7c) waveform. The presence of the negative wave prevents accommodation of nervous fibers so that current cannot induce membrane damages.

The correct placement of the electrodes represents one of the reasons of the successful treatment. The correct sites of application depend on the variety of clinical and individual conditions. The electrodes can be positioned on trigger points (Fig. 10.8a, b), tender points, peripheral nerve, dermatomes, spinal nerve roots, motor points, and acupuncture points. Depending on the location of the painful area, the electrodes can be placed transversely, longitudinally (Fig. 10.8c), in a crossed manner (Fig. 10.8d), contralaterally, in a transarticular, or in a "Y" piggyback position [44, 45].

Table 10.3 Common treatment modes of TENS for pain relief

Mode	TENS characteristics	Advantages	Disadvantages	Duration of treatment
Conventional	Frequency: 10–100 Hz Intensity: low to medium	Comfortable Fast action (10–15 min) Acute or chronic pain	Accommodation	30 min to hours
Strong low rate or acupuncture like	Frequency: 10 Hz Intensity: high	Medium lasting pain relief	Muscle spasms Fatigue	30–60 min
Brief intense	Frequency: 60–150 Hz Intensity: high	Fast action Long lasting (6 h) Accommodation: rare	May not be effective for chronic pain Muscle spasms	15–30 min
Burst	Frequency: 60–100 Hz Intensity: low to high	Long lasting analgesia More comfortable than low-frequency TENS Small adaptation	Pain Fatigue	30–60 min
Modulated	Frequency: Pulse duration and amplitude are modulated Intensity: low to high	Comfortable Fast action Small adaptation Acute or chronic pain	May have shorter lasting effects May be uncomfortable	20–40 min
Hyperstimulation	Frequency: 1–100 Hz Intensity: high	Comfortable Accommodation: rare	Slow acting	20–60 min

TENS can be effective in management of acute post-operative pain. Many high-quality studies have demonstrated the analgesic effect of TENS in acute post-operative pain and the advantage of simple positioning of the electrodes sidelong the surgical wound. The reported placebo effect of TENS is between 20% and 40% and the analgesic effect between 70% and 85%.

Nowadays, the main indications of TENS include: sports injuries, acute neck pain, low back pain, dysmenorrhea, etc. In adulthood, TENS is used in pain related to TMJ disorders and during the dental treatment of root canal and dental extraction. Several studies evaluated the role of TENS in the treatment of chronic pain, in particular in rheumatoid arthritis, myofascial pain, neuropathic pain, and low back pain [46–48]. TENS can also improve obstetric, oncologic, and cardiac pain. Treatment modes of TENS for pain relief are resumed in Table 10.3 (Fig. 10.9).

TENS is contraindicated in patients with cardiovascular problems (cardiac pacemaker), venous or arterial thrombosis, cancer, various dermatological conditions, bleeding disorders and in pregnant women. In patients with epilepsy, TENS should be used carefully; the electrodes should not be positioned over the neck or head [49]. Recently, a new type of transcutaneous electrical stimulator has gained popularity that uses current intensities too small to excite peripheral nerves. The most common term used to describe these generators is microcurrent electrical nerve

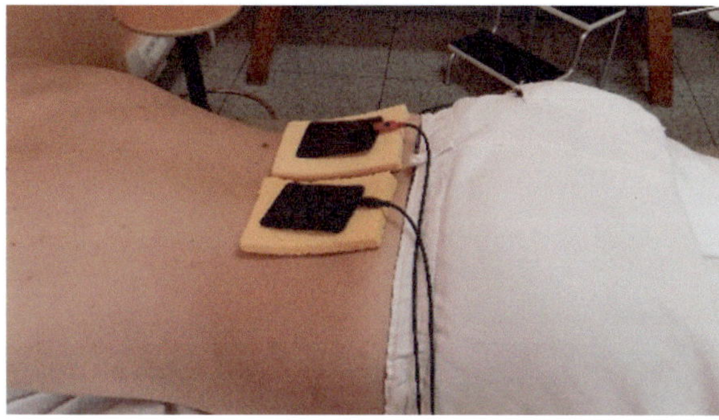

Fig. 10.9 TENS treatment for lumbar pain

stimulators (MENS). Most recently the term MENS has been replaced by the new term low-intensity stimulation (LIS) [50].

Electroacupuncture uses low-frequency, high intensity electrical stimulation, applied on the traditional acupuncture points, to determine muscle contraction and pain relief. This technique is commonly used for acute musculoskeletal disorders [51].

10.8.4 Interferential Current (IC)

The use of IFC has been introduced by an Austrian scientist, Ho Nemec, who suggested the concept and its therapeutic use.

To produce IFC two generators are used. One generator has a slightly slower or faster frequency than the other one, and they simultaneously begin producing current. Initially, the electric waves will be constructively summated; however, because the frequencies of the two waves differ, they gradually will get out of phase and become destructively summated. When any waveforms are out of phase but are combined in the same location, the waves will cause a beat effect. The blending of the waves is caused by the constructive and destructive interference patterns of the waves and is called heterodyne.

The biological effects of IFC are mediated by endorphins, enkephalins, and pain gate mechanisms [52, 53]. When applying IFC, the PRM specialist should select the frequencies to create a beat frequency corresponding to his or her choices of frequency when using other stimulators. Frequencies of 0–10 pulses per second (pps) can be used to produce small pulsating contractions of innervated muscle. Frequencies of 20–50 pps should be high enough to produce tetanic contractions of innervated muscle, 50–120 pps for pain management, and 1 pps for pain relief. Despite the deeper penetration, higher pulse rates, and greater intensities of IFC, it is proven that compared with other forms of electrical stimulation with different waveforms, it is less effective.

The main indications of IFC are in muscle spasms, in nonunion fractures, in reducing of spasticity, in edema, and in wound healing. The effectiveness of IFC in management of acute and chronic pain is explained with activation of the

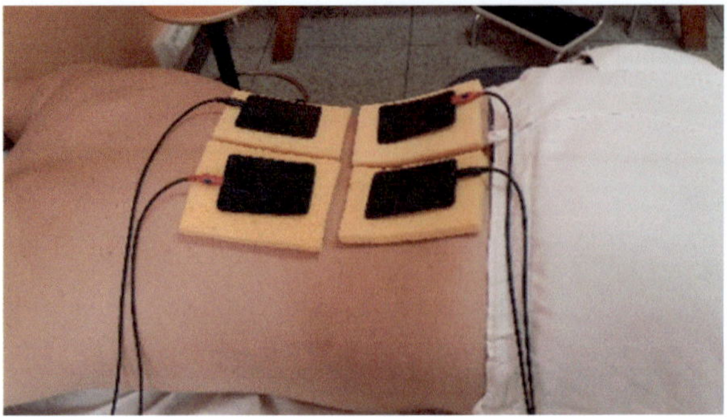

Fig. 10.10 Interferential current treatment for lumbar pain

larger-diameter peripheral nerve fibers to subsequently neuromodulate pain through a spinal gating mechanism.

Contraindications of IFC are the same as TENS (Fig. 10.10) [54].

Key Points

- Physical modalities use physical agents to produce biological modifications in body tissues and elderly patients' mobility, function, and quality of life.
- Most physical modalities are used to relieve pain in musculoskeletal diseases or to stimulate tissue healing.
- Common contraindications of physical modalities are cardiac diseases, acute arterial or venous diseases, pregnancy, fever, infections, and malignancy.

References

1. Perret D, Rim J, Adrian C (2006) A Geriatrician's guide to the use of the physical modalities in the treatment of pain and dysfunction. Clin Geriatr Med 22:331–354
2. Rakel B, Barr JO (2003) Physical modalities in chronic pain management. Nurs Clin North Am 38(3):477–494
3. Malanga GA, Yan N, Stark J (2015) Mechanisms and efficacy of heat and cold therapies for musculoskeletal injury. Postgrad Med 127(1):57–65
4. Dilek B, Gözüm M, Şahin E et al (2013) Efficacy of paraffin bath therapy in hand osteoarthritis: a single-blinded randomized controlled trial. Arch Phys Med Rehabil 94(4):642–649
5. Gale GD, Rothbart PJ, Li Y (2006) Infrared therapy for chronic low back pain: a randomized, controlled trial. Pain Res Manag 11(3):193–196
6. Draper D, Knight KL (2008) Therapeutic modalities: the art and science. Lippincott Williams & Wilkins, Philadelphia
7. Hegedus B, Viharos L, Gervain M, Galfi M (2009) The effect of low-level laser in knee osteoarthritis: a double blind, randomized, placebo-controlled trial. Photomed Laser Surg 27(4):577–584
8. Ozdemir F, Birtane M, Kokino S (2001) The clinical efficacy of low power laser therapy on pain and function in cervical osteoarthritis. Clin Rheumatol 20:181–184

9. Simunovic Z, Trobonjaca T, Trobonjaca Z (1998) Treatment of medial and lateral epicondylitis—tennis and golfer's elbow—with low laser therapy: a multicenter double-blind, placebo-controlled study on 324 patients. J Clin Laser Med Surg 16:145–151
10. World Association of Laser Therapy (2016) Recommended treatment doses for low level laser therapy. http://waltza.co.za/wpcontent/uploads/2012/08Dose_table_904nm_for_Low_Level_Laser_Therapy_WALT-2010.pdf. Accessed 9 Aug 2016
11. Haslerud S, Magnussen LH, Joensen J et al (2014) The efficacy of low-level laser therapy for shoulder tendinopathy: a systematic review and meta-analysis of randomized controlled trials. Physiother Res Int 20(2):108–125
12. Huang Z, Ma J, Chen J et al (2015) The effectiveness of low-level laser therapy for nonspecific chronic low back pain: a systematic review and meta-analysis. Arthritis Res Ther 17:360
13. Watson T (2008) Ultrasound in contemporary physiotherapy practice. Ultrasonics 48(4):321–329
14. http://www.nycc.edu/webdocs/ic/IQA/IQAFiles/Protocols/Chapter4/TherapeuticUltrasound4_3.pdf
15. Armagan O, Bakilan F, Ozgen M et al (2014) Effects of placebo-controlled continuous and pulsed ultrasound treatments on carpal tunnel syndrome: a randomized trial. Clinics (Sao Paulo) 69(8):524–528
16. Falconer J, Hayes KW, Chang RW (1990) Therapeutic ultrasound in the treatment of musculoskeletal conditions. Arthritis Care Res 3:85–91
17. Miller DL, Smith NB, Bailey MR et al (2012) Overview of therapeutic ultrasound applications and safety considerations. J Ultrasound Med 31(4):623–634
18. Lee JY, Kim SN, Lee IS et al (2014) Effects of extracorporeal shock wave therapy on spasticity in patients after brain injury: a meta-analysis. J Phys Ther Sci 26(10):1641–1647
19. Schmitz C, Császár NB, Milz S et al (2015) Efficacy and safety of extracorporeal shock wave therapy for orthopedic conditions: a systematic review on studies listed in the PEDro database. Br Med Bull 116:115–138
20. Van der Worp H, van den Akker-Scheek I, van Schie H, Zwerver J (2013) ESWT for tendinopathy: technology and clinical implications. Knee Surg Sports Traumatol Arthrosc 21(6):1451–1458
21. https://www.shockwavetherapy.org/fileadmin/user_upload/dokumente/PDFs/Formulare/ismst-consensus-statement-indications-2015.pdf
22. Sitjà-Rabert M, Martínez-Zapata MJ, Fort-Vanmeerhaeghe A et al (2011) Whole body vibration for older persons: an open randomized, multicentre, parallel, clinical trial. BMC Geriatr 11:89
23. Sitjà Rabert M, Rigau Comas D, Fort Vanmeerhaeghe A (2012) Whole-body vibration training for patients with neurodegenerative disease. Cochrane Database Syst Rev (2):CD009097
24. Lau RW, Liao LR, Yu F et al (2011) The effects of whole body vibration therapy on bone mineral density and leg muscle strength in older adults: a systematic review and meta-analysis. Clin Rehabil 25(11):975–988
25. Sadil V, Sadil S (1994) Electrotherapy. Wien Med Wochenschr 144:509–520
26. Robinson KR (1985) The responses of cells to electrical fields: a review. J Cell Biol 101:2023–2027
27. Knight KL, Draper DO (2012) Therapeutic modalities: the art and science, 2nd edn. Lippincott Williams & Wilkins, Baltimore
28. Maffiuletti NA, Minetto MA, Farina D, Bottinelli R (2011) Electrical stimulation for neuromuscular testing and training: state-of-the art and unresolved issues. Eur J Appl Physiol 111(10):2391–2397
29. Watson T (2000) The role of electrotherapy in contemporary physiotherapy practice. Man Ther 5:132–141
30. Troev T, Papathanasiou J (2016) Essentials of physical and rehabilitation medicine for undergraduate medical students, 1st edn. Lax Book
31. LeDuc S (1903) Electric ions and their use in medicine. Rebman, Liverpool

32. YN K, Naik A, Garrison J, Guy RH (2004) Iontophoretic drug delivery. Adv Drug Deliv Rev 56:619–658
33. Costello CT, Jeske AH (1995) Iontophoresis: applications in transdermal medication delivery. Phys Ther 75(6):554–563
34. Sieg A, Wascotte V (2009) Diagnostic and therapeutic applications of iontophoresis. J Drug Target 17:690–700
35. Albensi C, Scarpini C, Foti C (2016) Electrical muscle stimulation. In: Troev T, Papathanasiou J (eds) Essentials of physical and rehabilitation medicine for undergraduate medical students. Plovdiv, pp 63–73
36. Enoka RM (1988) Muscle strength and its development. New perspectives. Sports Med 6(3):146–168
37. Enoka R (2002) Neuromechanics of kinesiology. Human Kinetics Publisher, Champaign, IL
38. McMiken DF, Todd-Smith M, Thompson C (1983) Strengthening of human quadriceps muscles by cutaneous electrical stimulation. Scand J Rehabil Med 15(1):25–28
39. Delitto A, Rose SJ (1986) Comparative comfort of three waveforms used in electrically eliciting quadriceps femoris muscle contractions. Phys Ther 66(11):1704–1707
40. Jones S, Man WD, Gao W et al (2016) Neuromuscular electrical stimulation for muscle weakness in adults with advanced disease. Cochrane Database Syst Rev 10:CD009419
41. Sluka KA, Walsh D (2003) Transcutaneous electrical nerve stimulation: basic science mechanisms and clinical effectiveness. J Pain 4(3):109–121
42. Melzack R, Wall PD (1965) Pain mechanisms: a new theory. Science 150(3699):971–979
43. Mayer D, Price D, Rafii A (1977) Antagonism of acupuncture analgesia in man by the narcotic antagonist naloxone. Brain Res 121(2):368–372
44. Lena E, Assenza C, Giordani L, Foti C (2016) Transcutaneous Electrical Nerve Stimulation (TENS). In: Troev T, Papathanasiou J (eds) Essentials of physical and rehabilitation medicine for undergraduate medical students. Plovdiv, pp 57–63
45. Caruso I, Foti C (2005) TENS Mezzi fisici up to date, pp 158–168
46. Johnson MI, Paley CA, Howe TE, Sluka KA (2015) Transcutaneous electrical nerve stimulation for acute pain. Cochrane Database Syst Rev 6:CD006142
47. Carroll D, Moore RA, McQuay HJ, Fairman F, Tramèr M, Leijon G (2001) Transcutaneous electrical nerve stimulation (TENS) for chronic pain. Cochrane Database Syst Rev 3:CD003222
48. Deyo RA, Walsh NE, Martin DC, Schoenfeld LS, Ramamurthy S (1990) A controlled trial of TENS and exercise for chronic low back pain. N Engl J Med 322:1627–1634
49. Mannheimer C, Emanuelsson H, Waagstein F (1990) The effect of transcutaneous electrical nerve stimulation (TENS) on catecholamine metabolism during pacing-induced angina pectoris and the influence of naloxone. Pain 41:27–34
50. Zuim PR, Garcia AR, Turcio KH, Hamata MM (2006) Evaluation of microcurrent electrical nerve stimulation (MENS) effectiveness on muscle pain in temporomandibular disorders patients. J Appl Oral Sci 14(1):61–66
51. Zhang R, Lao L, Ren K, Berman BM (2014) Mechanisms of acupuncture-electroacupuncture on persistent pain. Anesthesiology 120(2):482–503
52. Gundog M, Atamaz F, Kanyilmaz S et al (2012) Interferential current therapy in patients with knee osteoarthritis: comparison of the effectiveness of different amplitude-modulated frequencies. Am J Phys Med Rehabil 91(2):107–113
53. Rocha CS, Lanferdini FJ, Kolberg C et al (2012) Interferential therapy effect on mechanical pain threshold and isometric torque after delayed onset muscle soreness induction in human hamstrings. J Sports Sci 30(8):733–742
54. Atamaz FC, Durmaz B, Baydar M et al (2012) Comparison of the efficacy of transcutaneous electrical nerve stimulation, interferential currents, and shortwave diathermy in knee osteoarthritis: a double-blind, randomized, controlled, multicenter study. Arch Phys Med Rehabil 93(5):748–756

Functional Electrical Stimulation of Skeletal Muscles in Aging and Premature Aging

11

Helmut Kern, Ugo Carraro, Stefan Loefler, Christian Hofer, Sandra Zampieri, Winfried Mayr, Simona Boncompagni, Feliciano Protasi, Rosario Rizzuto, Marco Sandri, Antonio Musarò, Stefano Masiero, Amber Pond, Francesco Piccione, and Andrea Marcante

H. Kern • S. Loefler • C. Hofer
Ludwig Boltzmann Institute of Electrical Stimulation and Physical Rehabilitation, Vienna, Austria
e-mail: helmut@kern-reha.at; wil.pys.kern-forschung@wienkav.at

U. Carraro (✉) • F. Piccione • A. Marcante
I.R.C.C.S., Fondazione Ospedale San Camillo, Via Alberoni 70, 30126 Venezia-Lido, Italy
e-mail: ugo.carraro@ospedalesancamillo.net; ugo.carraro@unipd.it

S. Zampieri
Ludwig Boltzmann Institute of Electrical Stimulation and Physical Rehabilitation, Vienna, Austria

Venetian Institute of Molecular Medicine, Padua, Italy

Department of Biomedical Science, University of Padua, Padua, Italy

W. Mayr
Center for Medical Physics and Biomedical Engineering, Medical University of Vienna, Vienna, Austria

S. Boncompagni • F. Protasi
CeSI – Center for Research on Aging and DNICS, Department of Neuroscience, Imaging and Clinical Sciences, University G. d'Annunzio, Chieti, Italy

R. Rizzuto • M. Sandri
Department of Biomedical Science, University of Padua, Padua, Italy

© Springer International Publishing AG 2018

S. Masiero, U. Carraro (eds.), *Rehabilitation Medicine for Elderly Patients*, Practical Issues in Geriatrics, DOI 10.1007/978-3-319-57406-6_11

A. Musarò
Institute Pasteur Cenci-Bolognetti; DAHFMO-Unit of Histology and Medical Embryology, IIM; Sapienza University of Rome, Rome, Italy

Center for Life Nano Science@Sapienza, Istituto Italiano di Tecnologia, Rome, Italy

S. Masiero
Rehabilitation Unit, Department of Neuroscience, University – General Hospital of Padua, Padua, Italy
e-mail: stef.masiero@unipd.it

A. Pond
Anatomy Department, Southern Illinois University, School of Medicine, Carbondale, IL, USA

11.1 Structural and Molecular Markers of Muscle Weakness and of Recovery Induced by h-b FES

Helmut Kern, Stefan Loefler, Christian Hofer, Sandra Zampieri, Winfried Mayr, Simona Boncompagni, Feliciano Protasi, Rosario Rizzuto, Marco Sandri, Antonio Musarò, Stefano Masiero, Amber Pond, Francesco Piccione, Andrea Marcante, Ugo Carraro

Aging is an unavoidable process, if lethal diseases do not prematurely end survival. A final evidence of this obvious concept has been recently provided by Gava et al. [1], describing the power decay of the series of world records obtained by master athletes (from 30 to 100 years). Skeletal muscle power begins to decline at the age of 30 years and continues, almost linearly, to zero at the age of 110 years. During aging, many factors contribute to the decline of the skeletal muscle, including subclinical and reversible muscle denervation/reinnervation [2]. Recently, we added evidence that denervation contributes to atrophy and slowness of aged muscles by comparing muscles of lifelong active seniors to those of sedentary elderly people. We found that the sportsmen have more muscle mass and slow fiber groupings, providing in this way evidence that physical activity maintains slow motoneurons, which reinnervate muscle fibers [3–5]. A premature muscle atrophy/degeneration occurs in irreversible and complete *conus* and *cauda equina* syndrome consequent to a lumbar/sacral spinal cord injury, determining a complete loss of muscle fibers within 5–8 years [6–8].

The impact of muscle denervation on aging skeletal muscle fibers is a relatively orphan topic [9, 10]. This is related in part to the difficulties in determining by molecular approaches whether motoneurons release chemical neurotrophic agents to the muscle fibers of the motor units. It is well known that such mechanism contributes to neuromuscular junction development and maintenance. However, if and which chemical trophic factors influence the synchronized expression of the hundreds of nuclei belonging to a single muscle fiber remains a subject of hypotheses. The synchronized spread of muscle action potential seems to be, on the contrary, a more rational mechanism [11]. On the other hands, the conclusions of recent reviews

[8, 9, 12] are that FES is poorly used in rehabilitation of elderly patients. Aging skeletal muscle presents both a loss of muscle mass and a conspicuous reduction in myofiber plasticity [9, 12–14] and alterations in muscle-specific transcriptional mechanisms. During the aging process, protein synthetic rates decrease, and an increase in protein degradation follows [15, 16], affecting muscle fibers [17]. It is generally recognized that an ineffective damage repair is a contributory cause of functional impairment during aging [18–20] and promotes the detrimental replacement of functional contractile muscle with fibrous tissue [17]. Volitional physical exercise can reverse these damaging processes. Interestingly, it has been shown that both acute and prolonged resistance exercises stimulate the proliferation of satellite cells in healthy sedentary elderly subjects [21]. This fact may be explained by the increased levels of myostatin, a negative regulator of muscle mass. An increase in autophagy in the muscle of athletic people has been reported, suggesting that exercise may activate an important system that detoxifies muscle cells [22]. Another important factor that is associated with physical exercise is insulin-like growth factor 1 (IGF-1) [23]. The evidence suggests that training and regular exercise can increase muscle strength and attenuate sarcopenia by modulating expression of autophagy, myokines (IL-6), and IGF-1 [24].

Unfortunately, elderly people may be unable or reluctant to adequately participate in physical exercise. We therefore suggested that FES could be an alternative approach. A stimulator for neuromuscular electrical stimulation (ES), which especially suits elderly people requirements, was designed. As detailed in Kern et al. [15], older persons were exposed to regular neuromuscular ES training for a period of 9 weeks, starting two times a week for the first 3 weeks and then switching to three times a week for the next 6 weeks, for a total amount of 24 training sessions (3 × 10 min for each session). After detailed instructions, ES training was performed by the subjects themselves at home, using a two-channel custom-built battery-powered stimulator [25]. The subjects applied two conductive rubber electrodes (9 × 14 cm, 126 cm^2) which were attached to the skin by wet sponge on the anterior thigh on both sides (left/right). The electrode pairs for the left and right thigh were connected to the two channels of the stimulator. This allowed independent activation of the left and right thigh muscles, which were alternatively stimulated. Each repetition (muscle contraction) was evoked by a 3.5 s train (60 Hz) of electrical pulses (rectangular, biphasic, width 0.6 ms). Consecutive contractions of the same thigh were separated by 4.5 s off intervals. In this study, constant voltage stimulation devices were applied. The subjects were also instructed to increase the stimulation intensity until their maximal tolerance was reached. Using this intensity, a full knee extension was achieved in all subjects. Nevertheless, the applied current and voltage were recorded by the stimulation device for each training session (the mean stimulation current was 128 ± 16 mA and voltage of 39 ± 14 V). The outcome was an increase in muscle strength, associated with an increase of fast fibers, which are the first to respond to ES and are related to the power of the skeletal muscle [14, 15]. We found that ES increases expression of IGF-1, the markers of satellite cell proliferation and extracellular matrix remodeling, downregulating the expression of proteases [14, 58]. There is also a collagen remodeling during both volitional physical exercise and ES. Three different forms of collagen are upregulated in electrically stimulated muscle [14, 15], but the increase in collagen does not likely stimulate fibrosis, as is shown by both morphological evidence and the increase in expression of miR29 [26]. The INTERREG IVa project recruited sedentary seniors with a normal lifestyle who were trained for 9 weeks with ES. Functional tests of trained subjects showed that ES induced improvements of leg muscle strength and mobility [27, 28]. ES significantly increased the size of fast-type muscle fibers and the number of Pax7- and NCAM-positive satellite cells. Moreover, no signs of muscle damage and/or inflammation were observed in muscle biopsies [14, 15]. Altogether, the results here summarized demonstrate that physical exercise, either voluntary or induced by ES, improves the functional performance of aging muscles. Of course, physical training can't stop the aging process, but ES is a safe home-based method that is able to counteract atrophy of fast-type muscle fibers.

Age-related muscle power decline is partially attributable to a loss of innervation, and it can be delayed by a lifelong high-level activity [3–5]. Diseases involving permanent denervation show a similar, but premature, aging process and a much more severe muscle deterioration. Despite doubts and criticisms of related literature [29, 30], we have shown that, with appropriate protocols, h-b FES can even inhibit degeneration of denervated muscle and even reverse it [31–33]. Therefore, the use of h-b FES should be extended in critical care units, rehabilitation centers, and nursing facilities and at home of elderly persons in presence of peripheral nerve lesions to improve hopefully muscle reinnervation [34–37].

11.2 FES for Partially Denervated Muscle and FES Protocols for Training of Denervated–Degenerated Skeletal Muscle

Helmut Kern, Christian Hofer, Stefan Loefler, Sandra Zampieri, Winfried Mayr, Simona Boncompagni, Feliciano Protasi, Amber Pond, Francesco Piccione, Andrea Marcante, Ugo Carraro

Functional electrical stimulation (FES) was introduced more than 50 years ago to identify those applications of electrical currents to organs and tissues of humans and other large mammals to obtain responses mimicking and/or restoring lost functions [38]. Spinal cord injury causes loss of functions and muscle wasting, which are especially severe after lower motor neuron (LMN) lesions. During the last decades, a great attention has been paid to denervated muscles, numerous studies focusing on the changes in gross anatomy, mechanical properties, and potential for reinnervation of skeletal muscle when the lesions involve the LMN. Results in literature are at best contradictory, and claims suggest that electrical stimulation of partially denervated muscles may even interfere with nerve regeneration [7]. During the last decade, we studied the effects of physical exercise induced by FES in spinal cord injury (SCI) with complete *conus* and *cauda equina* syndrome, in which denervated leg muscles are permanently and completely disconnected from the nervous system.

Denervated human muscles become refractory to the electrical stimulation developed by the common electrical devices and undergo ultrastructural disorganization within few months, while severe atrophy with nuclear clumping and fibro-fatty degeneration appears within 3 and 6 years [8, 9]. To counteract these progressive changes, a novel therapy concept for paraplegic patients with complete LMN denervation was developed in Vienna: the home-based FES (h-b FES) for denervated–degenerated muscles. New electrodes and a safe stimulator have been designed to reverse severe atrophy by delivering high-intensity (up to 2.4 J) and long-duration impulses (up to 150 ms) to stimulate contractions in long-term denervated skeletal muscle fibers. A specific clinical assessment and training, based on sound evidence from animal experiments, was developed at the Wilhelminenspital in Vienna, Austria. After 2-year training using h-b FES, the patient showed (1) significant increase of muscle mass and myofiber size with striking improvements of the muscle ultrastructural organization; (2) recovery of tetanic contractility with significant increase in muscle force output, during electrical stimulation; and (3) capacity to perform FES-assisted stand-up and stepping-in-place exercise. In conclusion h-b FES of permanent denervated muscle is an effective home therapy that results in rescue of muscle perfusion, mass, and function. Additional benefits are reduced leg edema, prophylaxis of thromboembolism, and enhanced cushioning effect for seating [32]. In our clinical experiences, nerve regrowth is not inhibited by FES of partially denervated muscles. On the contrary, we observed sensory or motor reinnervation (or both) during the application of high intensive stimulation training even 2–5 years after injury [39]. The complex response of muscle tissue to denervation is one of the most studied processes in muscle physiology and pathology. One of the important conclusions of pioneering studies is that, after a certain period of time (6 months in the rodents), denervated muscle undergoes some irreversible changes that inhibit its full restoration even after reinnervation. Findings from different experimental models, including free autotransplant, led to the same conclusion: after 2–7 months of denervation the restorative capacity of the muscle declines progressively in rat [40]. These observations were translated to the macroscopic behavior of the denervated human muscle and its potential for reinnervation, establishing a dogma that continues to negatively influence clinical management of denervated muscle. Despite countless published results [41], our recent studies in animal models and humans are enlightening several unrecognized characteristics and behaviors of the complex processes that occur during permanent LMN denervation of the human muscle tissue. These results are strengthening the rational basis of FES to maintain/recover permanently LMN denervated muscles. Some of the effects of long-lasting (in terms of years) LMN denervation of the human muscle we recently described were unexpected. In contrast to the well-known rodent model, the LMN denervated human muscle presents simple atrophy up to 1 year after SCI [7]. On the other hand, the characteristic denervation-induced muscle fiber disorganization in the atrophying muscle, documented by electron microscopy, occurs much earlier [7]. The ultrastructural disorganization of the muscle fibers that appears much earlier than severe atrophy in both animal models [42, 43] and humans [6, 7, 32, 44] explains the early functional impairments of the LMN denervated muscle. Until today, muscles of the extremities in *conus* and *cauda equina* syndrome were commonly not treated with FES, because it was widely recognized that long-term and completely denervated muscles cannot be effectively stimulated. On the other hand, our studies in animal models and humans indicate that (1) severe atrophy does not occur in rats for at least 3–4 months [40, 41]; (2) in rabbit, the degeneration of muscle tissue does not appear in the first year after denervation [43]; and (3) muscle tissue degeneration starts from the third year onward, in humans [32, 33, 42, 44]. Our findings that the long-term denervated rat muscle maintains L-type Ca2+ current and gene expression of the related proteins longer than functional contractile machineries [45] provide the molecular, structural, and functional rationale of a rehabilitation training for human permanently denervated muscles, which was developed as a result of empirical clinical observations [32]. The FES device stimulates muscle fibers in the absence of nerve endings and after prolonged denervation, determining (1) restoration of muscle fiber ultrastructure, (2) recovery of conduction velocity of the excitation–contraction apparatus up to a level that allows tetanic contraction, and (3) the maintenance/recovery of muscle mass and fiber size. Before this, electrical stimulation was believed to be effective only when started very early after LMN lesion, and FES was used only to delay muscle atrophy, since long-term denervated muscles (6 months onward) do not respond, when stimulated by surface electrodes and standard commercial electrical stimulators developed for innervated muscles. The results of the EU RISE Project [32, 33, 42, 44], and of the related animal research [43, 45], provide different perspectives.

11.2.1 Stimulation Devices and Electrodes

During the last 20 years, clinicians and engineers developed in Vienna novel rehabilitation concepts for paraplegic patients with complete LMN denervation of the lower extremity due to complete lesion of the *conus* and *cauda equina*. To counteract the progressive changes that transform muscle into an unexcitable tissue, these new rehabilitation managements became possible due to the development and optimization of new stimulation devices for h-b FES. They have been specifically designed to reverse longstanding and severe atrophy of LMN denervated muscles by delivering high-intensity and long-duration impulses that can directly elicit contraction of denervated skeletal muscle fibers in absence of functional neuromuscular endplates. These new stimulators and the large surface electrodes needed to cover large denervated muscles were developed by the Center of Medical Physics and Biomedical Engineering at the Medical University of Vienna, Austria [46–48]. Based on these prototypes, an electrical stimulator for denervated muscle is now commercially available, the "Stimulette den2x" of the Schuhfried Medizintechnik GmbH, Vienna, Austria [49]. Patients were provided with stimulators and electrodes in order to perform stimulation at home for 5 days per week. Large (180 cm^2) electrodes (Schuhfried Medizintechnik GmbH, Mödling, Austria) made of conductive polyurethane were placed on the skin surface using a wet sponge cloth (early training) and fixed via elastic textile cuffs. As soon as the skin was accustomed to the necessary high current density, gel was used under the polyurethane electrodes to achieve minimal transition impedance. The electrodes were flexible enough to maintain evenly distributed pressure to the uneven and moving skin, thus providing homogeneous current distribution throughout the entire contact area. In parallel, specific clinical assessments and training settings were developed at the Wilhelminenspital Wien, Austria [50–54].

11.2.2 Training Protocol

Details of the four phases of this rehabilitation strategy are summarized in Table 11.1 and Fig. 11.1. The rehabilitation training for complete denervated muscles was validated by the clinical outcome, strongly supported by the results obtained from light and electron microscopy muscle biopsies' analyses performed in Padua and Chieti Universities (Italy), respectively, and described by Kern et al.

Table 11.1 FES training of relatively short-term denervated (1–2 years) human muscles (Adapted from Kern et al. Neurorehabil Neural Repair. (2010); 24:709–21)

Training time (months)	Functional class	Stimulation parameters	Training parameters
3–4	I or II	120 ms **ID**/500 ms **IP**; 5 s **SD**/2 s **SP** 40 ms **ID**/10 ms **IP**; 3 s **SD**/3 s **SP**	5 × 3 min 5 d/week 3 × 3 min 5 d/week
5–6	II or III	120 ms **ID**/400–500 ms **IP**; 5 s **SD**/1 s **SP** 40 ms **ID**/10 ms **IP**; 3 s **SD**/3 s **SP**	5 × 4 min 5 d/week 3 × 3 min 5 d/week
6–8	III	120 ms **ID**/400 ms **IP**; 5 s **SD**/1 s **SP** 40 ms **ID**/10 ms **IP**; 3 s **SD**/3 s **SP**	5 × 4 min 5 d/week 3–4 × 3 min 5 d/week + ankle weight 2×/week
8	III or IV	120 ms **ID**/400 ms **IP**; 5 s **SD**/1 s **SP** 40 ms **ID**/10 ms **IP**; continues + switch	5 × 4 min 5 d/week Stand-up–sit-down exercise Stand-up–stepping–sit-down exercise
16	V	120 ms **ID**/400 ms **IP**; 5 s **SD**/1 s **SP** 40 ms **ID**/10 ms **IP**; continues + switch	5 × 4 min 5 d/week Walking exercise

Functional Classes
0 No torque measureable, no contraction/twitch visible
I No torque measureable, but contraction/twitch visible
II Torque measured between 0.1 and 2.9 Nm
III Torque measured more than 3.0 Nm, but not able to stand
IV Able to stand in parallel bars/standing frame
V Able to walk with an aid
ID impulse duration, *IP* impulse pause, *SD* stimulation duration, *SP* stimulation pause, *d* days, *rep* repetition in one set of stimulation

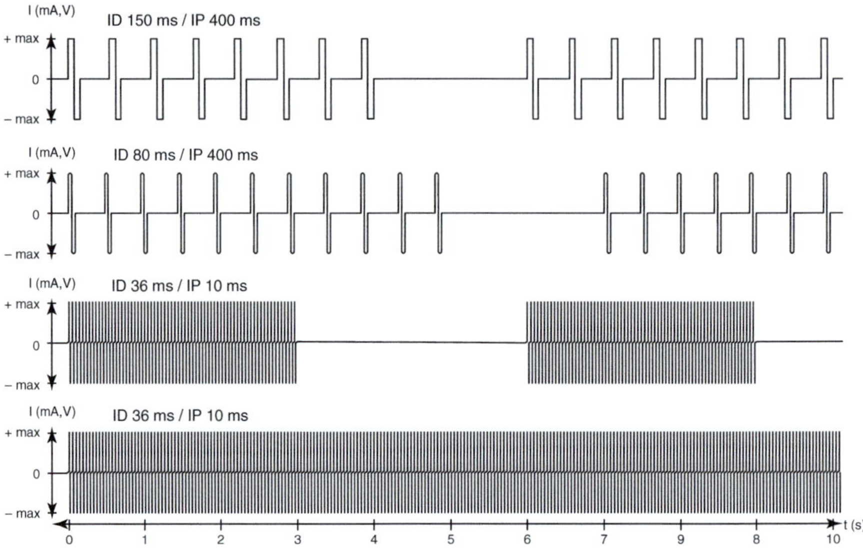

Fig. 11.1 Parameters for progressive home-based functional electrical stimulation (h-b FES) training of long-term fully denervated human muscles. Figure shows a sample of a progressive FES training according to the described training in Table 11.1. It starts with bursts of a stimulation duration (SD) of 4 s and a stimulation pause (SP) of 2 s containing impulses with an impulse duration (ID) of 150 ms and an impulse pause (IP) of 400 ms for 4 months (it can be reduced if the time of denervation is under 6 months) to activate poor denervated muscle fibers. According to the enhanced activation, the ID can be reduced to 80 ms and SD increased to 5 s for another 4 months approximately. The next training phase implements tetanic bursts of 3 s SD and 3 s SP with impulses of 36 ms ID and 10 ms IP to increase muscle fiber diameter, muscle mass, density, and force, with leg extensions with and without additional weights on the ankles of the patients. If a good condition is achieved, depending not only to the training but also to the time span of denervation, standing, stepping-in-place, and walking exercises can be performed with continuous stimulation (controlled by an external switch) with 36 ms ID and 10 ms IP

in his longitudinal prospective study [32]. The training strategy consisted of two progressive stimulation programs (Fig. 11.1), and positive changes and effects of FES on structural, functional, histological, and ultrastructural parameters were described in detail by Kern et al. in 2010 [32]. FES treatment can be integrated into daily life of patients without too much interference on their daily activities. The reduction of leg edema [55], the improved cosmetic appearance of lower extremities, the enhanced cushioning effect for seating, and the ability to perform home exercises are additional effects of FES. We are thus confident that it will be possible to translate into a wider population of diseased subjects and to aged people the knowledge of our interdisciplinary group of European scientists and clinicians. In fact, current studies suggest that electrical stimulation of the LMN denervated muscles could be extended to patients with incomplete lesions or elderly persons and could reduce secondary complications related to disuse and impaired blood perfusion (reduction in bone density, risk of bone fracture, decubitus ulcers, and thromboembolism) [55–57].

Key Points

- Elderly and mobility-impaired patients may develop severe limitations to their independence after arm and leg immobilization or being bedridden.
- Education and support of patients to perform daily exercises in the hospital and then at home is an effective and low-cost measure to limit disability and improve physical and mental being of older patients, but when persons are reluctant or hampered to perform volitional exercise, functional electrical stimulation in the hospital and then at home is an alternative worth to be tested in many patients.
- Section 11.1 discusses structural and molecular markers of muscle weakness and protocols of FES-induced recovery in aging and neuromuscular impairments.
- Section 11.2 presents detailed protocols of h-b FES for denervated–degenerated muscles.

References

1. Gava P, Kern H, Carraro U (2015) Age-associated power decline from running, jumping, and throwing male masters world records. Exp Aging Res 41:115–135
2. McKinnon NB, Connelly DM, Rice CL et al (2016) Neuromuscular contributions to the age-related reduction in muscle power: mechanisms and potential role of high velocity power training. Ageing Res Rev 35:147–154
3. Mosole S, Rossini K, Kern H et al (2013) Significant increase of vastus lateralis reinnervation in 70-year sportsmen with a lifelong history of high-level exercise. Eur J Transl Myol Basic Appl Myol 23:117–122
4. Mosole S, Carraro U, Kern H et al (2014) Long-term high-level exercise promotes muscle reinnervation with age. J Neuropathol Exp Neurol 73:284–294
5. Mosole S, Carraro U, Kern H et al (2016) Use it or lose it: tonic activity of slow motoneurons promotes their survival and preferentially increases slow fiber-type groupings in muscles of old lifelong recreational sportsmen. Eur J Transl Myol Basic Appl Myol 26:339–346
6. Kern H, Carraro U, Adami N, Hofer C, Loefler S, Vogelauer M, Mayr W, Rupp R, Zampieri S (2010) One year of home-based Functional Electrical Stimulation (FES) in complete lower motor neuron paraplegia: recovery of tetanic contractility drives the structural improvements of denervated muscle. Neurol Res 32:5–12
7. Kern H, Boncompagni S, Rossini K, Mayr W et al (2004) Long-term denervation in humans causes degeneration of both contractile and excitation-contraction coupling apparatus that can be reversed by functional electrical stimulation (FES). A role for myofiber regeneration? J Neuropathol Exp Neurol 63:919–931
8. Hepple RT, Rice CL (2015) Innervation and neuromuscular control in ageing skeletal muscle. J Physiol 594(8):1965–1978
9. Carraro U, Kern H, Gava P et al (2016) Recovery from muscle weakness by exercise and FES: lessons from masters, active or sedentary seniors and SCI patients. Aging Clin Exp Res:1–12
10. Carraro U, Kern H (2016) Severely atrophic human muscle fibers with nuclear misplacement survive many years of permanent denervation. Eur J Transl Myol 26(2):5894
11. Lømo T (2014) The response of denervated muscle to long-term stimulation (1985, revisited here in 2014). Eur J Transl Myol Basic Appl Myol 24:13–19
12. Mitchell WK, Williams J, Atherton P et al (2012) Sarcopenia, dynapenia, and the impact of advancing age on human skeletal muscle size and strength; a quantitative review. Front Physiol 3:260

13. Zampieri S, Mosole S, Löfler S et al (2015) Physical exercise in aging: nine weeks of leg press or electrical stimulation training in 70 years old sedentary elderly people. Eur J Transl Myol Basic Appl Myol 25:237–242
14. Zampieri S, Pietrangelo L, Loefler S et al (2015) Lifelong physical exercise delays age-associated skeletal muscle decline. J Gerontol A Biol Sci Med Sci 70:163–173
15. Kern H, Barberi L, Löfler S et al (2014) Electrical stimulation counteracts muscle decline in seniors. Front Aging Neurosci 6:189
16. Carnio S, LoVerso F, Baraibar MA et al (2014) Autophagy impairment in muscle induces neuromuscular junction degeneration and precocious aging. Cell Rep 8:1509–1521
17. Barberi L, Scicchitano BM, Musarò A (2015) Molecular and cellular mechanisms of muscle aging and sarcopenia and effects of electrical stimulation in seniors. Eur J Transl Myol Basic Appl Myol 25:231–236
18. Scicchitano BM, Rizzuto E, Musarò A (2009) Counteracting muscle wasting in aging and neuromuscular diseases: the critical role of IGF-1. Aging 1(5):451–457
19. Vinciguerra M, Musaro A, Rosenthal N (2010) Regulation of muscle atrophy in aging and disease. Adv Exp Med Biol 694:211–233
20. Carosio S, Berardinelli MG, Aucello M, Musarò A (2011) Impact of ageing on muscle cell regeneration. Ageing Res Rev 10:35–42
21. Musarò A (2014) The basis of muscle regeneration. Adv Biol 2014:1–16
22. Sandri M, Barberi L, Bijlsma AY et al (2013) Signalling pathways regulating muscle mass in ageing skeletal muscle: the role of the IGF1-Akt-mTOR-FoxO pathway. Biogerontology 14:303–323
23. Adamo ML, Farrar RP (2006) Resistance training, and IGF involvement in the maintenance of muscle mass during the aging process. Ageing Res Rev 5:310–331
24. Pelosi L, Berardinelli MG, De Pasquale L (2015) Functional and morphological improvement of dystrophic muscle by Interleukin 6 receptor blockade. EBioMedicine 2:274–275
25. Krenn M, Haller M, Bijak M et al (2011) Safe neuromuscular electrical stimulator designed for the elderly. Artif Organs 35:253–256
26. He Y, Huang C, Lin X, Li J (2013) MicroRNA-29 family, a crucial therapeutic target for fibrosis diseases. Biochimie 95:1355–1359
27. Cvecka J, Tirpakova V, Sedliak M et al (2015) Physical activity in elderly. Eur J Transl Myol Basic Appl Myol 25:249–252
28. Sarabon N, Löfler S, Hosszu G, Hofer C (2015) Mobility test protocols for the elderly: a methodological note. Eur J Transl Myol Basic Appl Myol 25:253–256
29. Hughes AM, Burridge JH, Demain SH et al (2014) Translation of evidence-based assistive technologies into stroke rehabilitation: users' perceptions of the barriers and opportunities. BMC Health Serv Res 14:124
30. Bersch I, Tesini S, Bersch U, Frotzler A (2015) Functional electrical stimulation in spinal cord injury: clinical evidence versus daily practice. Artif Organs 39:849–854
31. Kern H, Hofer C, Moedlin M et al (2002) Denervated muscle in humans: limitations and problems of currently used functional electrical stimulation training protocols. Artif Organs 26:216–218
32. Kern H, Carraro U, Adami N, Biral D, Hofer C, Forstner C, Mödlin M, Vogelauer M, Pond A, Boncompagni S, Paolini C, Mayr W, Protasi F, Zampieri S (2010) Home-based functional electrical stimulation rescues permanently denervated muscles in paraplegic patients with complete lower motor neuron lesion. Neurorehabil Neural Repair 24:709–721. doi:10.1177/1545968310366129
33. Kern H, Carraro U (2014) Home-based Functional Electrical Stimulation (h-b FES) for long-term denervated human muscle: history, basics, results and perspectives of the Vienna Rehabilitation Strategy. Eur J Transl Myol Basic Appl Myol 24:27–40
34. Willand MP (2015) Electrical stimulation enhances reinnervation after nerve injury. Eur J Transl Myol 25(4):243–248. doi:10.4081/ejtm.2015.5243. Review
35. Catapano J, Willand MP, Zhang JJ et al (2016) Retrograde labeling of regenerating motor and sensory neurons using silicone caps. J Neurosci Methods 259:122–128. doi:10.1016/j.jneumeth.2015.11.020.

36. Willand MP, Nguyen MA, Borschel GH, Gordon T (2016) Electrical stimulation to promote peripheral nerve regeneration. Neurorehabil Neural Repair 30(5):490–496
37. Willand MP, Rosa E, Michalski B et al (2016) Electrical muscle stimulation elevates intramuscular BDNF and GDNF mRNA following peripheral nerve injury and repair in rats. Neuroscience 334:93–104
38. Coste CA, Mayr W, Bijak M, Musarò A, Carraro U (2016) FES in Europe and beyond: current translational research. Eur J Transl Myol Basic Appl Myol 26(4):6369. http://www.pagepress-journals.org/index.php/bam/article/view/6369/6187
39. Rossato E, Marziali A, Carraro U et al (2009) Rise2-Italy Project: muscle FES after peripheral nerve lesions. Basic Appl Myol 19:169–172
40. Carlson BM (2014) The biology of long-term denervated skeletal muscle. Eur J Transl Myol 24:3293
41. Midrio M (2006) The denervated muscle: facts and hypotheses. A historical review. Eur J Appl Physiol 98:1–21
42. Boncompagni S, Kern H, Rossini K et al (2007) Structural differentiation of skeletal muscle fibers in the absence of innervation in humans. Proc Natl Acad Sci U S A 104:19339–19344
43. Ashley Z, Sutherland H, Lanmüller H et al (2007) Atrophy, but not necrosis, in rabbit skeletal muscle denervated for periods up to one year. Am J Physiol Cell Physiol 292:440–451
44. Rossini K, Zanin ME, Carraro U (2002) To stage and quantify regenerative myogenesis in human long-term permanent denervated muscle. Basic Appl Myol 12:277–286
45. Squecco R, Carraro U, Kern H et al (2009) Despite lost contractility, a sub-population of rat muscle fibers maintains an assessable excitation-contraction coupling mechanism after long-standing denervation. J Neuropathol Exp Neurol 68:1256–1268
46. Kern H, Hofer C, Mayr W, Carraro U (2009) European Project RISE: partners, protocols, demography. Basic Appl Myol/Eur J Transl Myol 19:211–216
47. Hofer C, Forstener C, Moedlin M et al (2005) In vivo assessment of conduction velocity and refractory period of denervatd muscle fibers. Artif Organs 29:436–439
48. Hofer C, Mayr W, Stöhr H et al (2002) A stimulator for functional activation of denervated muscles. Artif Organs 26:276–279
49. Dr. Schuhfried Medizintechnik GMBH (2012) The "stimulette den2x" is a compact, high performance two-channel electrotherapy device that was developed to be used exclusively for stimulating denervated muscles. http://www.schuhfriedmed.at/en/stimulette-en/stimulette-den2x-2/
50. Lehmkühl LD, Dimitrijevic MR, Zidar J (1988) Lumbosacral evoked potential (LSEPs) and cortical somatosensory evoked potentials (SEPs) in patients with lesions of the conus medullaris and cauda equina. Electroencephalogr Clin Neurophysiol 71:161–169
51. Gutrecht JA (1994) Sympathetic skin response. J Clin Neurophysiol 11:519–524
52. Kern H, Ch H, Mayr W et al (2012) Elektrostimulation komplett denervierter Muskulatur. In: Fialka-Moser V (ed) Kompendium der Physikalischen Medizin und Rehabilitation. Springer, Vienna, pp 445–456
53. Kern H, Hofer C, Mayr W (2008) Protocols for clinical work package of the European Project RISE. Basic Appl Myol 18:39–44
54. Pieber K, Herceg M, Paternostro-Sluga T, Schuhfried O (2015) Optimizing stimulation parameters in functional electrical stimulation of denervated muscles: a cross-sectional study. J Neuroeng Rehabil 12:51. doi:10.1186/s12984-015-0046-0
55. Bizzarini E, Zampa A, Malisan C et al (2009) Epidemiology and FES of Conus-Cauda Syndrome in Friuli Venezia Giulia: data of the spinal unit of udine and report of a difficult-to-stimulate case. Basic Appl Myol 19:163–168
56. Czyrny JJ, Kaplan RE, Wilding GE et al (2016) Electrical foot stimulation: a potential new method of deep venous thrombosis prophylaxis. ERJ Open Res 2(1):20–27
57. Carraro U, Sandri M, Zampieri S (2015) Patologia Generale del Tessuto Muscolare Scheletrico. In: Pontieri GM, Russo MA, Frati L (eds) Patologia Generale. Piccin Nuova Libraria spa, Padova, pp 1523–42. ISBN 978-88-299-2036-5
58. Barberi L, Scicchitano BM, De Rossi M et al (2013) Age-dependent alteration in muscle regeneration: the critical role of tissue niche. Biogerontology 14:273–292

12 The Contribution of Occupational Therapy: A Profession in Support of the Elderly

Mary Ardia, Yann Bertholom, Giovanna Caiata-Olgiati, Christian Pozzi, and Heather L. Hammond

M. Ardia
Dipartimento economia aziendale, sanità e sociale, Centro Competenze Anziani, Manno, Switzerland

Dipartimento economia aziendale, sanità e sociale, Scuola Universitaria Professionale della Svizzera Italiana (SUPSI), Manno, Switzerland
e-mail: mary.ardia@bluewin.ch

Y. Bertholom (✉)
Il Paese di Oz - ANFFAS, Trento, Italy

Società Tecnico Scientifica Italiana di Terapia Occupazionale (SITO), Rome, Italy

Facoltà di Medicina & Chirugia, Università degli Studi di Modena & Reggio-Emilia, Modena, Italy
e-mail: presidente.sito@terapiaoccupazionale.it

G. Caiata-Olgiati
Dipartimento economia aziendale, sanità e sociale, Centro Competenze Anziani, Manno, Switzerland

Dipartimento economia aziendale, sanità e sociale, Scuola Universitaria Professionale della Svizzera Italiana (SUPSI), Manno, Switzerland

Caribù Center of Occupational Therapy, Biasca, Switzerland
e-mail: giovanna.caiata@gmail.com

C. Pozzi
Department of Rehabilitation and Aged Care of the Ancelle Hospital, Cremona, Italy

Geriatric Research Group, Brescia, Italy

Facoltà di Medicina & Chirugia, Università Cattolica del Sacro Cuore, Rome, Italy
e-mail: christianpozzi81@libero.it

© Springer International Publishing AG 2018

S. Masiero, U. Carraro (eds.), *Rehabilitation Medicine for Elderly Patients*, Practical Issues in Geriatrics, DOI 10.1007/978-3-319-57406-6_12

H.L. Hammond
Società Tecnico Scientifica Italiana di Terapia Occupazionale (SITO), Rome, Italy

Facoltà di Medicina and Chirugia, Università degli Studi di Modena and Reggio-Emilia, Modena, Italy

Facoltà di Medicina and Chirugia, Claudiana Scuola Provinciale Superiore di Sanità, Bolzano, Italy

Centro di Terapia Occupazionale, Bologna, Italy
e-mail: h_hammond@Hotmail.com

12.1 Background

Occupational therapists, by virtue of their name (at least in English) and their history, have always been concerned with occupation, also called "meaningful activity." This concern has taken two forms: occupation as means and occupation as goal. The former, often captured under the rubric "therapeutic use of activity," has been a focus of occupational therapy[1] (OT) for most, if not all, of its history.

The latter, however, captured under the rubric "occupation-based practice," only became a major focus of practice at the end of the twentieth century. For much of its history, OT's use of occupation, or meaningful activity, was from within a medical paradigm, with the aim to improve outcomes for individuals suffering from diseases or disorders through the therapeutic use of activity [1].

12.2 Introduction

An elderly person carries with them their sense of being and doing, even with the risk of unexpected fragility [2] that comes with aging, and the limitations associated with it. Every elderly person has their own personal life course that has contributed to their current situation by the very nature of their past decisions. For example, as we see in the ecological model [3], the way in which each person experiences aging changes according to differences found in everyday situations, social and economical status, gender, and type of housing. The positive and negative events that shape the normal trajectory of life is modeled by the cultural environment, composed of socioeconomic conditions, career choices, health status, family relationships, and friendships.

Becoming aware early of this—that these factors need to be faced in life—creates an opportunity for an ongoing preparedness through a process of experiential engagement.

[1] "Occupational Therapy" is the term used in Italy and in Anglo-Saxon countries. *Ergoterapia/Ergothérapie* is the term used in Switzerland and in various other countries. The two terms, however, refer to the same health-care profession. It is derived from the Greek term *ergein* (do, work, act). In textbooks both terminologies can be found.

12.3 The Salutogenic Model and Occupational Therapy

Modifying one's lifestyle in the salutogenic [4] perspective enhances one's own sense of self, finding the resources and the capacity for a productive transformation, fruitful even in old age.

One can easily understand that the value of looking ahead, to both see yourself and what is beyond, is an internal, personal development that involves receptive listening. According to the salutogenesis theory, everyone has some creativity and ability to grow, even when faced with social isolation, or being under-stimulated, which may take away their desire to continue engaging in life. This valuable ability to self-reflect helps people to successfully understand others and be understood themselves. This personal ideal is a motivator to help actualize and contribute to their quality of life and their overall well-being. This transforms and shapes the meaningfulness of activities that the elderly person needs or wants to do, not only in the present time but also for the future.

So the salutogenic approach can be a theoretical basis for health promotion in the "health-ease versus disease" continuum to ensure that the person will become evermore the protagonist of their personal health project.

This perspective is at the heart of occupational therapy (OT).

The philosophy of modern geriatrics teaches that the care plan of the elderly person should include a careful, multidimensional analysis that covers both the biomedical and the psychological, cognitive, functional, social, personal [5], and spiritual aspects. It is crucial for health-care professionals to have a holistic view of the complexities [6] of the person in a therapeutic relationship built on direct contact and trust.

Consequently, each rehabilitative, preventative, informative, and salutogenic approach of OT fits well with palliative care too, in effectively supporting the aging process. The concept of "healing" is similar in that it involves a process of adaptation, a coming to terms with and accepting of things and events as they are, and not being in another state of mind, but instead discovering the breadth of personal resources that one has at their disposal. This mindfulness transforms the situation into a process of self-awareness that has direct and immediate effects on health and well-being [7].

By spending a few words on palliative care, it is useful to reiterate that the emphasis changes from "cure" to "care." This sensitive and welcoming approach changes, therefore, the care plan to include empathy and trust and collaboration with the elderly person and their family.

12.4 The Role of Occupational Therapy in Elderly Care

Occupational therapists take into account this fragility and solitude of the elderly, who find themselves at the crossroad between their past life and the onset of disease. Occupational therapists emphasize the expectations on the part of the family, society, and the elderly person themselves, as to what is their reality in aging. This enables the elderly to appreciate the things that give them enjoyment and are meaningful to them, despite their disability.

OT has always known this fact in dealing with people and their everyday problems, strengthening their autonomy and will to live. OT supports the elderly in their needs and desires, by helping them maintain their roles in society and therefore their place in life. OT restores identity and makes elderly clients feel that they are first seen as a person by health-care practitioners, so that they are still viewed as someone who participates, who takes decisions, and who lives moments to the fullest, authentically, even in the brevity of life (when symptoms prevent them from completing complex tasks due to a lack of energy or because the activity could aggravate their already precarious health even further) [8]. The elderly person is set at the center of their therapeutic process so that the likelihood that their personal goals are achieved increases. For OT, this relationship is essential, which brings meaning and planning to tasks, anticipates potential complications, maintains motivation, helps preserve important relationships, promotes compensatory and rehabilitative strategies, and fosters the right environment. This way the elderly client is able to engage in and maintain their roles and responsibilities, denoted in OT as their "occupational performance." The professional skills of OT also include the ability to measure results in terms of satisfaction in their participation.

Naturally, we cannot just dwell on the person with their needs and desires, maintaining and/or regaining their independence, since each person is placed in a physical and social context of limited resources. The occupational therapist must collaborate in an interprofessional and consultative process [9]. As described in the code of ethics of the World Federation of Occupational Therapists, there is a recognized need for interdisciplinary collaboration that respects the specific contributions of other professional groups [10]. A consultative process means that there is interprofessional, simultaneous, collaborative agreement [11] between the programming of daily and weekly activities of the client and their family to ensure a healthy work/rest balance and a conservation of energy.

12.5 The Scope of Occupational Therapy Assessment and Intervention

The elderly client learns strategies and techniques to lighten the load of occupations (meaningful activities) during the day and is taught ergonomics applicable to them to avoid pain and overload and to prevent falls. They are also taught (or re-taught) how to complete everyday tasks that they need and want to do, as well as being taught how to promote and/or maintain cognitive functions (memory, attention, concentration, problem-solving, etc.). The resumption of leisure activities is encouraged, such as participating in hobbies and physical activities that were once of interest to the elderly client, as well as generating new interests that better suit their current realties. Expressive, creative activities may be suggested as well with the goal of finding and communicating a personal sense of being, so that confidence and self-esteem may grow [9].

As can be seen, finding the right balance between the person, their environment and occupations are essential to promote the well-being of elderly clients during typical, everyday situations. This is true across all care settings, from acute care to being discharged home or to a long-term care facility. In summary, the Person-Environment-Occupation (PEO) theoretical model by Dr. Mary Law [12] and colleagues follows the holistic view of helping the client, along with their family and friends, to engage in an active therapeutic process.

The occupational therapist demonstrates clinical reasoning by taking into account the scientific literature in the geriatric field. The knowledge translation (KT) of scientific information is a multistage process that includes the collection, evaluation, summary, and sharing of scientific knowledge on a specific topic to the end user. Best practice is sought to inspire the professional practice to provide material to be discussed with the person and to determine together the application of the best practice techniques that are presented in the literature. In fact, the Canadian Institutes of Health Research defines knowledge translation as a dynamic and iterative process to include "… the exchange, synthesis and ethically-sound application of knowledge - within a complex system of interactions among researchers and users - to accelerate the capture of the benefits of research … through improved health, more effective services and products, and a strengthened health-care system" [9].

KT has always been a principle that is naturally integrated into the objectives of OT clinical practice via the consistent interaction with their clients and families [13].

According to the broad and solid scientific basis, the importance of having an occupational therapist within each rehabilitation team is clearly evidenced. Their specific knowledge can contribute and enrich the team by implementing the human aspect and interdisciplinary nature of the care plan. By including OT in the therapeutic and diagnostic treatment plan, their specific professional competences will favor the continuity of care throughout the network of services, supporting the elderly and their family during strenuous periods of adaptations and changes in routines that are necessary due to a disease or illness.

For these reasons, OT will provide a sound assessment practice, with the aim of identifying a truly individualized therapeutic project adapted to every level of difficulty of each client.

Conclusion

OT, therefore, is a powerful therapeutic discipline: preventing occupational deprivation (complete loss of participating in activity, with a gradual and inexorable social isolation) and the subsequent sensory deprivation. The profession seeks to avoid/reduce the client's dependency on social assistance and therefore the economic costs associated with it.

OT uses rigorous conceptual models from the scientific point of view, but with flexibility from the practical point of view. The therapeutic process begins with a discussion centered on the narrative of the client's own personal and occupational history, and then, through clinical reasoning, it will proceed to the core of OT:

going from assessment to occupational rehabilitation. This is explicit in the recovery and reinforcement of "a group of activities that have a personal meaning, that are culturally important and support the person to participate in a given social context" [14]. "Occupation is always evaluated and interpreted within a given context" [14]. This statement leads us to emphasize, in conclusion, one of the themes that is the cornerstone of OT: occupation does not have meaning when it is placed out of context, in an artificial or contrived way, but must always be incorporated simultaneously into various types of environments [14].

OT will not only become an explorer of the person's abilities but will support, to the fullest potential, the personal search inside each client for their own personal resources and capabilities to reinvent themselves. This allows the elderly person to find and/or recover the needed energy for the resolution of problems related to their occupations.

References

1. Polatajko H (2015) Occupation-based practice, client centered practice: an occupational therapy imperative. Giornale Italiano di Terapia Occupazionale 15:8
2. Regione Toscana (2013) La fragilità nell'anziano: Linea Guida. Accessed online on 21/06/2016 from: http://www.snlg-iss.it/cms/files/LG_Fragilita_anziano_2013.pdf
3. Richard L, Barthélémy L, Tremblay MC, Pin S, Gauvin L (2013) Interventions de prévention et promotion de la santé pour les aînés: modèle écologique. Guide d'aide à l'action franco-québécois. Inpes, coll. Santé en action, Saint-Denis, France, p 112
4. Simonelli I, Simonelli F (2010) Atlante concettuale della salutogenesi (modelli e teorie di riferimento per generare salute). Franco Angeli, Milan, Italy
5. Pozzi C, Bertholom Y (2015) Migliorare la pratica. Giornale Italiano di Terapia Occupazionale, n° 13
6. Benkirane R (2002) La teoria della complessità. Bollati Boringhieri, Torino, Italy
7. Boyce B (2011) The healing power of mindfulness. Accessed online 21/06/2016 from: http://www.mindful.org/the-healing-power-of-mindfulness/
8. Latini CM (2015) II bisogno occupazionale nel fine della vita. Quando un terapista occupazionale diventa palliativista. Giornale Italiano di Terapia Occupazionale, n° 15
9. Ardia M, Boffelli L, Caiata-Olgiati G, Capra B, Di Serio C, Ferrari F, Kunz O, Stock-Bernasconi K, Vukic T, Wangler K (2016) Ergoterapia e oncologia/oncoreha Dal to cure al to care: Affrontare i problemi quotidiani, accrescere l'autonomia e la voglia di vivere, accompagnare nei bisogni, desideri, mantenere i ruoli, adattare il luogo di vita. Poster presented at the "Lega Contro il Cancro" Event, Ticino, Switzerland
10. World Federation of Occupational Therapists (WFOT) (2004) Code of ethics. Accessed online on 22/06/2016 from: http://www.wfot.org/ResourceCentre.aspx
11. Interprofessional Education Collaborative Expert Panel (2011) Core competencies for interprofessional collaborative practice: report of an expert panel. Interprofessional Education Collaborative, Washington, DC
12. Law M, Cooper B, Strong SS, Rigby P, Letts L (1996) The person-environment-occupation model: a Transactive approach to occupational performance. Can J Occup Ther 63(1):9–23
13. Cramm H, White C (2011) KT and OT: a context for knowledge translation for occupational therapy. OT Now 13(6):24–26
14. Whiteford GE (2010) Occupation in context. In: Turner A et al (eds) Occupational therapy and physical dysfunction- enabling occupation. Churchill Livingstone – Elsevier, Stratford, United Kingdom, pp 135–147

Sitography

Associazione Italiana dei Terapisti Occupazionali (AITO): www.aito.it
Società Tecnico/Scientifica Italiana di Terapia Occupazionale (SITO): www.aito.it/sito
World Federation of Occupational Therapists (WFOT): www.wfot.org
Council of Occupational Therapists for the European Countries (COTEC): www.cotec-europe.org
European Network of Occupational Therapy in Higher Education (ENOTHE): www.enothe.hva.nl

Mary Ardia is an OT at the "Centro Competenze Anziani" in Manno, Switzerland, and is a lecturer for the Department of Business Economics, Health, and Social Care at the "Scuola Universitaria Professionale della Svizzera Italiana" (SUSPI). She specializes in palliative care and also works in private practice.

Yann Bertholom is an OT at the rehabilitation center of "Il Paese di Oz - ANFFAS" in Trento, Italy, and is the president of the Italian Scientific Society of Occupational Therapy (SITO). He is a lecturer for the Undergraduate Occupational Therapy program at the "University of Modena and Reggio Emilia" (UNIMORE).

Giovanna Caiata-Olgiati is an OT at the "Centro Competenze Anziani" in Manno, Switzerland, and is a lecturer for the Department of Business Economics, Health, and Social Care at the "Scuola Universitaria Professionale della Svizzera Italiana" (SUSPI). She also works at the "Caribù Center" of Occupational Therapy in Biasca, Switzerland.

Christian Pozzi is an OT at the "Ancelle" Rehabilitation Hospital in Cremona, Italy, and works with the Geriatric Research Group in Brescia, Italy. He teaches at the "Sacro Cuore" Catholic University in Rome, Italy.

Heather L. Hammond is an OT at the "Centro di Terapia Occupazionale" in Bologna, Italy. She is a lecturer for the Undergraduate Occupational Therapy programs at the "University of Modena and Reggio Emilia" (UNIMORE) and at the "Claudiana Scuola Provinciale Superiore di Sanità" in Bolzano, Italy. She is also a board member of the Italian Scientific Society of Occupational Therapy (SITO).

The Hand and the Occupational Therapy 13

F. Romagnoli and S. Tocco

The hand is the primary tool with which the human being relates with its environment and other living beings. Some see the hand as an extension of the brain, as both evolved into highly specialized organs throughout the ages. The insurgence of pathologies or trauma sustained to the distal aspect of the upper quadrant can have extremely negative repercussions on a person's life.

The hand, seen as the ultimate extension of the upper extremity, is in fact anatomically and functionally connected to everyday gestures. For this reason, specialized therapy of the hand was developed since the 1970s in the USA by a group of therapists which later formed the American Society of Hand Therapists (ASHT).

Muenzen and colleagues coined the official definition of hand therapy in 2002: "It is the **art** and **science** of rehabilitation of the upper quadrant of the human body. Hand therapy is a **merging of OCCUPATIONAL THERAPY and PHYSICAL THERAPY** theory and practice that combines comprehensive knowledge of the upper quarter, body function, and activity. Using specialized skills in assessment and treatment, hand therapists promote the goals of prevention of dysfunction, restoration of function and/or reversal of progression of pathology in order to enhance life participation in life situations for individuals with upper quarter disease or injury" [1].

Occupational therapists (OTs) represent 70% of all hand therapists worldwide [2]. Among other professional competencies and skills, OTs are able to analyze activities, gestures, and performances of daily living. They also enable participation by modifying a person's environment or adapting objects of daily living. This ability in OTs is essential to adequately administer personalized hand and upper extremity treatment according to the patient's specific needs.

Pathologies seen by occupational therapists working in hand rehabilitation are orthopedic, neurological, and rheumatoid based, and they are treated using an evidence-based medicine approach.

F. Romagnoli (✉) • S. Tocco
Centro Riabilitativo "Dalla Mano e Arto Superiore" Srl - CRIMAS, Parma, Italy
e-mail: fretheelf@gmail.com; silvio.tocco@libero.it

© Springer International Publishing AG 2018

S. Masiero, U. Carraro (eds.), *Rehabilitation Medicine for Elderly Patients*,
Practical Issues in Geriatrics, DOI 10.1007/978-3-319-57406-6_13

For orthopedic patients, OTs collaborate with hand surgeons during the immediate postoperative phase for wound care, edema control, and custom-made positioning orthoses, all of which have the goal of preventing unwanted joint stiffness or other complications.

For neurological disorders, OTs fabricate custom-made static orthoses that aim to prevent soft tissue contractures or dynamic models to compensate for muscle weakness of temporary paralysis. Recently, hand therapists alike have introduced sensory and motor re-learning techniques to rehabilitate the somatosensory cortex in central and peripheral nervous pathologies.

Finally, for the rheumatoid population, the OT is professionally equipped to slow down degeneration of joints and other soft tissues. Preventatively, OTs fabricate orthotic devices that rest inflamed joints or sustain weak joints. They also address joint protection techniques and energy conservation strategies with rheumatoid patients. If deformities have developed in hands or other parts of the body, orthotic intervention is also employed. During rehabilitation, exercises are performed to maintain proper fine and gross motor gestures following surgical procedures or even during conservative treatment. Activities of daily living (ADLs) are also assessed, and compensatory strategies are selected with the patient, as a client-centered approach is mandatory in this population since more than just hands are at stake with rheumatoid disease.

Overall treatment is based on published protocols, but an accurate functional evaluation is done using objective and subjective outcome measures such as goniometry, dynamometry, manual testing, sensory evaluation, functional assessment batteries, and self-administered validated questionnaires.

To conclude, these are some of the techniques used by OTs in hand rehabilitation:

- Static and mobilization orthotic fabrication using low-temperature thermoplastics (LLTP), neoprene, and synthetic casting materials.
- Bottom-up and top-down activities selected with the patient to initially improve active and passive range of motion and muscle strength, to later address coordination, proprioception, and sensory problems.
- Some therapeutic modalities are also employed by OTs working in hand rehabilitation such as thermal and cryotherapy, respectively, to prepare tissues for activities and ultimately cooling them once therapy sessions are ended; joint mobilization, neurogliding, and scar massage are necessary in some occasions along with functional or kinesio taping.

13.1 Hand Therapy

Hand therapy, which presents many facets, is provided by either physical or occupational therapists. These latter professionals will use a rehabilitation program based on activity analysis. This client-centered approach is based on graded meaningful activity that will address functional problems of the upper limb, whether it be joint motion limitation (Fig. 13.1a, b); decreased strength (Fig. 13.2); incoordination

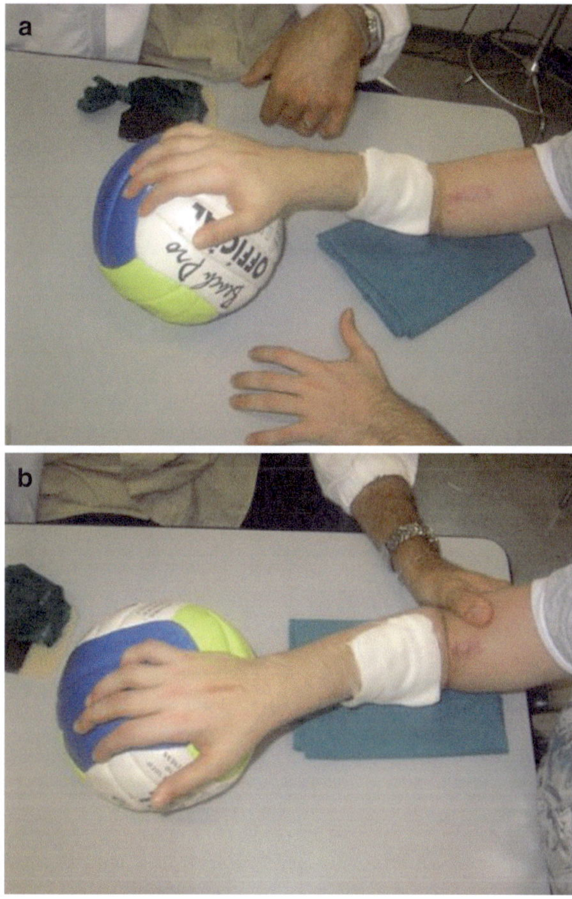

Fig. 13.1 Wrist exercises for flexion-extension (**a**) and prono-supination (**b**) with a ball

(Fig. 13.3); reduced or hypersensitivity of a finger, limb, or even a scar; or any other pathology or trauma-related problem.

Any chosen activity is graded according to the patient's function and improvement. Activity usually begins with simple exercises such as grasping objects of different sizes or shapes in the case of joint motion limitation (Fig. 13.4) or gripping handles of various resistances (Fig. 13.5) and grasping techniques. The patient later moves toward more complex activities such as assembling a simple furniture item (Fig. 13.3) to baking a cake to finally simulate real work or leisure activities, which are meaningful to the patient.

Ultimately, occupational therapy in the field of hand therapy aims at enabling patients through active or assisted exercises or activity which is meaningful to the patients and will allow them to minimize or eliminate impairment. In some cases where there is temporary (i.e., sport injury) (Fig. 13.6a, b) or permanent impairment, such as in degenerative diseases or amputees, the occupational therapist can also opt for an adaptive solution.

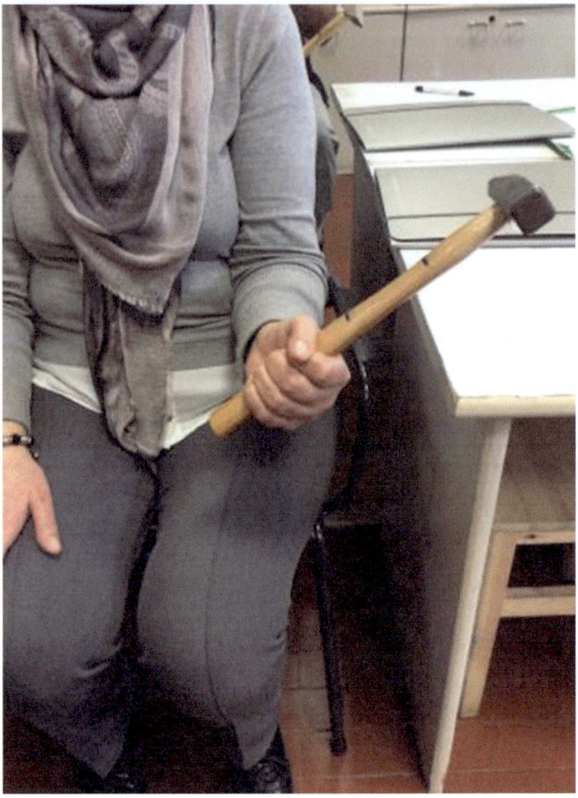

Fig. 13.2 Forearm rotation reinforcement with hammer

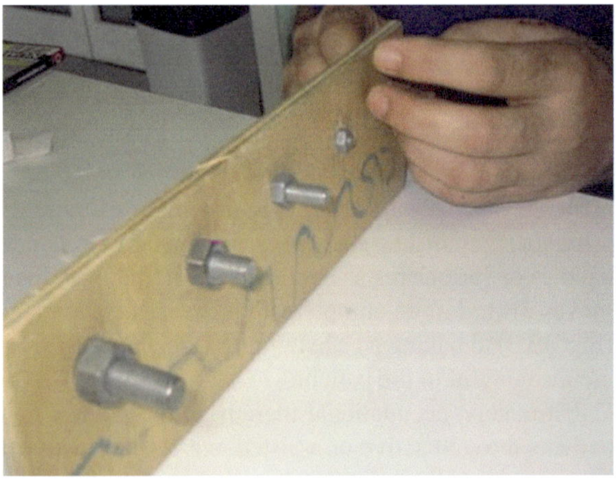

Fig. 13.3 Bolt screwing

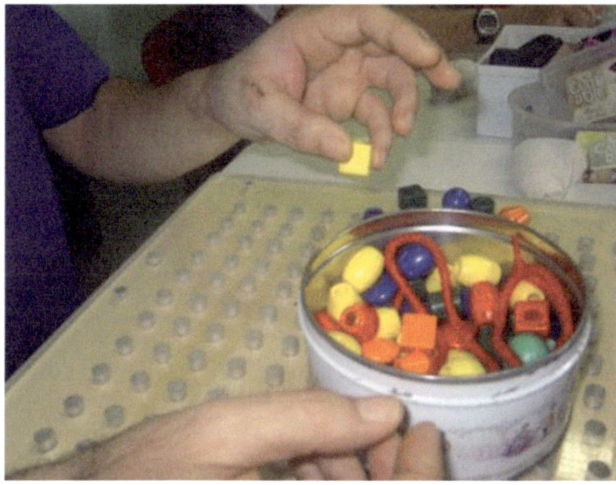

Fig. 13.4 Tip-to-tip grasp with beads

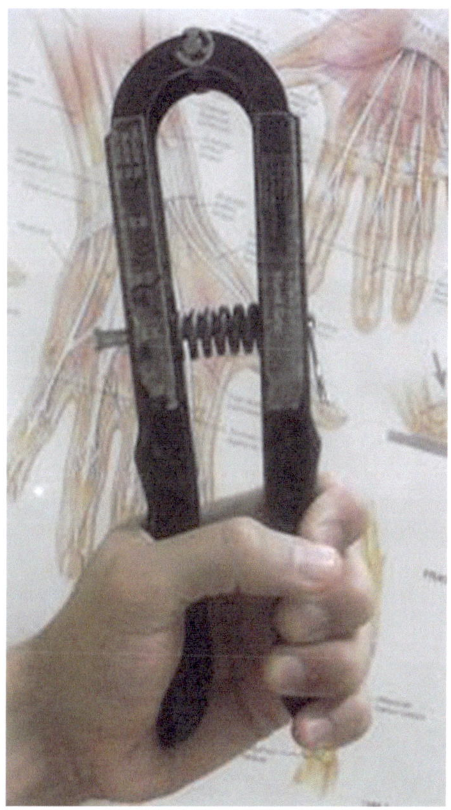

Fig. 13.5 Graded griping exercises

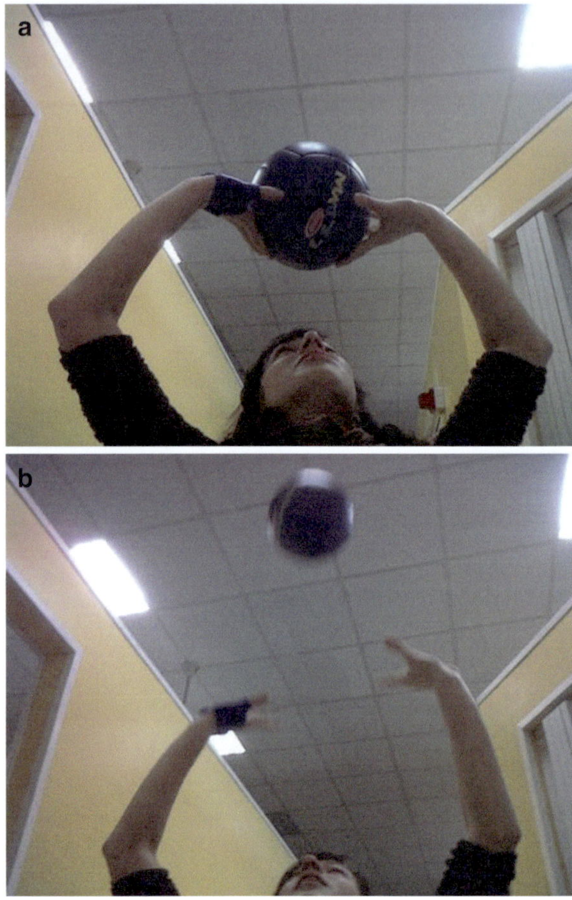

Fig. 13.6 (**a**, **b**) Thumb orthosis assisting volleyball player, avoiding pain and other thumb injuries

References

1. Muenzen PM et al (2002) A new practice analysis of hand therapy. JHT 3:215–225
2. IFSH2014 membership survey report

Frail Elderly Persons and Smart Home Technologies

14

I. Johnson and P. Ianes

14.1 Introduction

During earlier days, when different generations lived together, it was easier to take care of each other in situations of need. Grandparents used to take care of their grandchildren when parents were absent, and if a grandparent needed assistance with daily activities, there was always somebody there to help him/her. Today, the family structure has completely changed. Families are split apart, sometimes in the same city, sometimes in the same nation, but more often than before in different nations due to recent globalization. More people live alone or in small family structures which is a challenge for the social network. In addition, people live a longer life, part of it with possible disabilities [1, 2]. Specific Assistive Technology Information centers could be an answer to the needs of frail elderly persons living alone in their homes, but it is only part of the equation: technology works out well if it is combined with an individuals' strong motivation to use it, and of course, individuals must be able to afford it [3] (Fig. 14.1).

The home environment is a place where people ought to feel comfortable, a place which should be organized according to their lifestyle preferences, and a place where they should feel protected and safe. Unfortunately this is not always the case. We know, for example, that the home environment is a high-risk place for falls, especially among the elderly population with diminished performance in cognition, balance, and sensory-motor capacity [4–6]. The use of smart home technology could be an alternative to reduce the loss of everyday function resulting from aging or disabilities [7, 8] (Fig. 14.2).

I. Johnson (✉)
Occupational Therapy and Assistive Technology Service (DAT), S. M Nascente Rehabilitation Centre, Don Gnocchi Foundation, Milan, Italy
e-mail: ingela.johnson@siva.it

P. Ianes
Presidio Ospedaliero "Villa Rosa" Pergine Valsugana (TN), Azienda Provinciale per i Servizi Sanitari Provincia Autonoma di Trento, Trento, Italy
e-mail: patriziaianes@yahoo.ca

© Springer International Publishing AG 2018

S. Masiero, U. Carraro (eds.), *Rehabilitation Medicine for Elderly Patients*, Practical Issues in Geriatrics, DOI 10.1007/978-3-319-57406-6_14

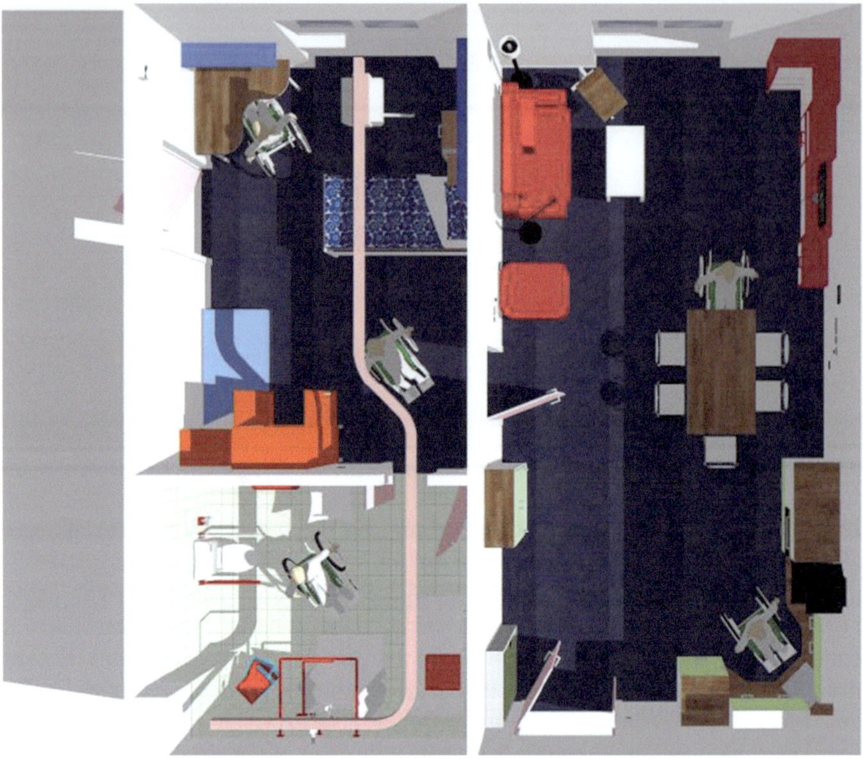

Fig. 14.1 AUSILIA: Assisted unit for simulating independent living activities, collaboration between the University of Trento and Azienda Provinciale per i Servizi Sanitari Provincia Autonoma di Trento, Italy, www.ausilia.tn.it

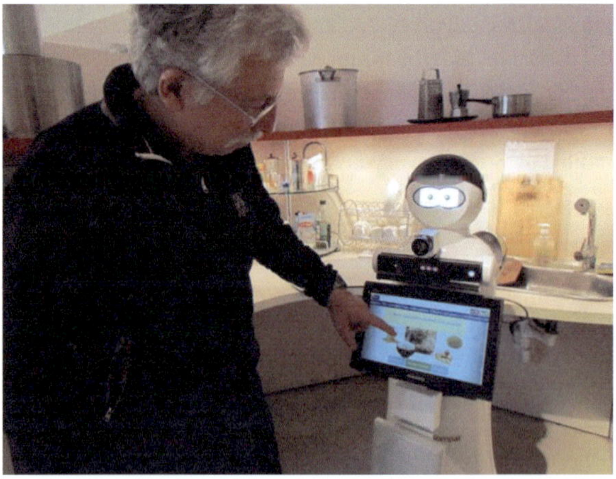

Fig. 14.2 User interacting with a robot in the smart home at the DAT center

14.2 Clinical Cases

Sue is a 78-year-old woman living alone since her husband died some years ago. Her two adult daughters are living in the same city not far away from her. Two years ago Sue was diagnosed with Alzheimer's disease. Since then she spends most days in the nearby day center where she can participate in social activities and eat cooked meals. At home she often wakes up in the middle of the night to go to the bathroom. Her daughters decided that it would be convenient to install some security measures in order to reduce the risk of falling. So when Sue gets up from her bed, the light automatically turns on providing a pathway to the bathroom. This way she will be able to reach the bathroom safely, where the water turns on/off automatically, as does the toilet flush. The lights then automatically provide a pathway back to bed.

Anne is a 68-year-old woman, divorced 10 years ago. She is living with her daughter and her 6-year-old grandson. Her daughter works during the day and her grandson goes to school. Anne has arthritis and spends most of the day alone. In the morning she needs a lot of time to get up since her joints are stiff and aching. To facilitate her independence, she has a remote control to turn on the light, open the curtains and windows, and change the bed position. The remote control also acts as a hands-free phone, allowing her to call her sister before getting out of bed.

Martin is a 72-year-old single man who recently had an accident while going by bicycle to the local post office. A car cut him off and Martin fell on the ground, resulting in a mild traumatic brain injury. He was brought to hospital and had a period of rehabilitation, but at discharge still had potential for further recovery. Martin lives far away from the rehabilitation center and was unable to organize transportation for outpatient services. He was offered a home training program from the rehabilitation center. Each morning he connects online for a 45-min rehabilitation training session with the occupational therapist at the center who uses strategy training to assist him to overcome the problems he encounters when performing daily activities.

In the above aforementioned situations, the occupational therapist helps the person prioritize everyday activities that need to be carried out in the home environment, but that the person is unable to perform, performs with difficulty, or is not satisfied with the way it is performed [9]. When the person does not have the capacity to adapt himself to the environment, the environment must be adapted to his/her personal needs. Thus environmental adaptations and technological solutions are an important part of the rehabilitation process, and occupational therapy interventions play a crucial role in working with the individuals to identify the most appropriate technology for them, promoting independent living in the proper home. Determining the best match between the person's needs and technology is essential so that the person feels comfortable with the solution and the risk of abandonment of technology is diminished. Since advanced technology is a result of the effort of different professionals, it is necessary to work in an interdisciplinary team to find the best technical and functional solution. Researchers and inventors must work alongside occupational therapists, rehabilitation clinicians, counselors, sociologists, and architects, to develop

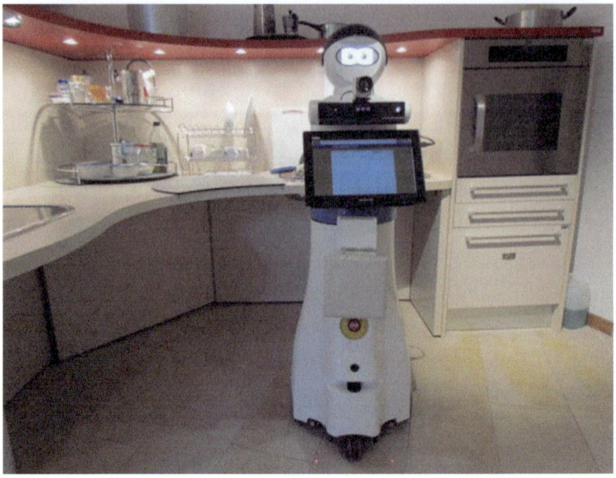

Fig. 14.3 Robot of the ENRICHME project in the kitchen at the DAT center

solutions that respect the unique sovereignty of the home environment and to ensure connections to an accessible community, where electronic wayfinders and wearable task management systems may facilitate outdoor activities [7, 8].

Conclusions

Advanced technology in the homes or smart home applications are surely of interest to minimize risks in activities, to perform everyday tasks in an easier way, or to pursue health-related tasks (telemedicine) [7, 8]. A new field which is still at research level is the use of robots or humanoids in the home environments as assistants in activities of everyday living [10, 11] (Fig. 14.3).

References

1. Center for policy on ageing (CPA), Changing family structures and their impact on the care of older people [WWW document]. URL http://www.cpa.org.uk/information/reviews/CPA-Rapid-Review-Changing-family-structures.pdf
2. Weicht B (2013) The making of the elderly constructing the subject of care. J Aging Stud 27(2):188–197
3. Scherer MJ, Sax C, Vanbeirvliet A, Cushman LA, Scherer JV (2005) Predictors of assistive technology use: the importance of personal and psychosocial factors. Disabil Rehabil 27(21):1321–1331
4. Lord SR, Menz HB, Sherrington C (2006) Home environment risk factors for falls in older people and the efficacy of home modifications. Age Ageing 35(Suppl 2):ii55–ii59
5. Soriano TA, DeCherrie LV, Thomas DC (2007) Falls in the community-dwelling older adult: a review for primary-care providers. Clin Interv Aging 2(4):545–554
6. Tinetti ME, Speechley M, Ginter SF (1988) Risk factors for falls among elderly persons living in the community. N Engl J Med 319(26):1701–1707
7. Dewsbury G, Linskell J (2011) Smart home technology for safety and functional independence: the UK experience. NeuroRehabilitation 28(3):249–260

8. Gentry T (2009) Smart homes for people with neurological disability: state of the art. NeuroRehabilitation 25(3):209–217
9. Townsend EA, Polatajko HJ (2007) Enabling occupation II: advancing an occupational therapy vision for health, well-being & justice through occupation. CAOT – ACE, Ottawa
10. Thrun S (2004) Toward a framework for human-robot interaction. Hum Comput Interact 19(1):9–24
11. European Commission. Horizon 2020 – PHC19. ENRICHME project [WWW document]. URL http://www.enrichme.eu

Thermal Rehabilitation of Geriatric Patients

15

C. Crotti and U. Solimene

15.1 Introduction

While being one of the oldest known treatment methods, thermal rehabilitation medicine has not been acknowledged as much as it deserves by the scientific community. Thermal healthcare includes three steps: prevention, care, and rehabilitation. These steps are integrated with a new focus on health and well-being. Following this approach, we expect that hundreds of thousands of people will recognize stays at thermal facilities as an option to protect their physical integrity and achieve a well-being status.

Hydrotherapy is the use of water in various physical conditions and with different chemical compositions through the implementation of a variety of methods, aimed at treating and preventing health problems, as well as at preserving good health.

Hydrotherapy should be divided into two parts in consideration of its development as a whole: one of these—called, more appropriately, crenotherapy (from the Greek *krene*, which means "source")—uses the specific chemical properties of so-called mineral waters, while the other basically leverages on the physical properties of water.

C. Crotti
Center for Traditional & Complementary Medicine, Milan State University, Milan, Italy
e-mail: crcrott@tin.it

U. Solimene (✉)
World Health Organization (WHO) Coll. Center for Traditional & Complementary Medicine, Milan State University, Milan, Italy
e-mail: umberto.solimene@unimi.it

© Springer International Publishing AG 2018

S. Masiero, U. Carraro (eds.), *Rehabilitation Medicine for Elderly Patients*, Practical Issues in Geriatrics, DOI 10.1007/978-3-319-57406-6_15

15.2 Crenotherapy

Two types of crenotherapy exist—internal and external (that includes balneotherapy).

Internal crenotherapy can be administered via hydropinotherapy (or drinking therapy), irrigations (vaginal, nasal, oral, intestinal, or rectal), and inhalations.

Hydropinotherapy is a treatment approach that uses mineral waters for drinking. The term comes from the Greek *hydro* (water) and *pino* (drink). The therapy consists in the intake of specific amounts of liquid at a given temperature and at pre-set time intervals throughout the day. Hydropinotherapy is indicated to treat urinary tract disorders, as well as bowel diseases and general gastroenteric disorders.

Thermal waters can also be used to treat chronic irritations and inflammations of the upper and lower respiratory tract. Thermal inhalation therapies can be administered in a variety of forms and approaches aimed at achieving the desired effects, classified according to a number of factors, including the chemical properties of the used mineral waters, the physical characteristics of the inhaled substances, the features of the appliances, and the dispensing mode.

Balneotherapy uses water and the mineral properties of the salts dissolved in it to treat some medical conditions, such as osteoarticular diseases. Muds, sands, and medicinal clays (also known as "fangotherapy") are also used with medical purposes. Balneotherapy is usually practiced in spas.

15.3 Hydrotherapy

Although motor disorders, connected with disabilities, are frequently observed at a later stage in life, clinical, psychological, and social conditions need to be addressed when dealing with geriatric patient rehabilitation. Such conditions add up to purely functional disorders, resulting into a complex and intricate picture for which intervention measures and procedures can hardly be identified (though this is not impossible). There is no doubt about the importance of treating elderly people despite their possible disabilities and frailties and to overlapping negative life events: the functional recovery to the level preceding the disease is a goal that can be pursued even when people get older.

Geriatric patient's rehabilitation is based on the consideration of loss events that are not confined to a specific organ or system affected, but on the entire disease that caused the disability [1].

Thermal rehabilitation could play a primary role in this respect by using water and its properties.

Hydrotherapy is a very old therapeutic approach made up of several techniques, which developed through centuries in multiple aspects. Nowadays, this approach is used to treat a variety of disorders and diseases, as well as for rehabilitation and to improve the patient's quality of life in general [2].

Hydrotherapy, in a strict sense, leverages on the properties of water, such as floating, temperature, and hydroactive pressure, regardless of the potential pharmacological properties connected with the presence of mineral salts.

A large amount of papers describe techniques including, in particular, balneotherapy to treat a variety of orthopedic, heart, and venous disorders, also involving domains like neurological physiotherapy [3] and gastroenterology, thus demonstrating the broad range of traditional indications for use of this method. The adopted methods are also simple to apply and cheap; nonetheless they require training of operators and patient's supervision, in order to ensure their implementation [1].

More recently, besides considerations deriving from the traditional use of these methods, several scientific studies were carried out and are now producing evidence on safety, effectiveness, and appropriate provision of these therapies [4]. At present, rehabilitation in water is crucial to ensure a modern and effective functional recovery of patients with orthopedic and neurological disorders [5].

The unique properties of water ensure its efficacy as a therapeutic agent. These include, most importantly, its ability to retain and release heat. Rehabilitation in water is founded on "Archimedes' principle," stating that any object, immersed in a fluid, is buoyed up by a force equal to the weight of the fluid displaced by the object, so that such object is lighter the deeper it is immersed. For example, the human body, when immersed vertically, is apparently reduced to 95% of its real weight if immersed up to the calves, to 80% when water reaches the thighs, to 50% up to waistline level, to 20% up to the armpits, to 7% at the base of the neck, and to 3% when totally immersed; this results into easier movement in water compared to the external environment when, in the event of traumas, cerebrovascular events, or orthopedic surgery (fractures, joint replacement, etc.), it would be impossible, difficult, or even harmful to load real weight on the limbs [6, 7].

Baths can be taken in plain source or in thermal water; they can contain herbs, drugs, or mineral salts. Moreover, waters can be purposefully moved and agitated, as it happens, for example, in whirlpool baths.

- Full-Immersion Hot Baths
- They are performed at a temperature of 37.7–41.1 °C, for a maximum of 20 min, and are indicated to treat musculoskeletal pain, to mitigate muscular spasms, and to stimulate perspiration [8]. In most cases they are followed by a brief cold bath; therefore, they are not indicated for very old people with organic disorders or prone to hemorrhage.
- Neutral Baths
- Neutral full-immersion baths are performed in tubs at an average 33.3–35 °C temperature. Patients should not feel warm or cold. Ideal temperature depends on the patient's conditions and reactions in water and should therefore be adjusted according to patient feelings, rather than using a thermometer. A neutral bath can last from 15 min to 4 h. The primary effect of a neutral bath is sedation, with a calming action on the nervous system. Moreover, it enhances diuresis, due to water absorption during the long-term immersion. Lastly, neutral baths tend to lower body temperature due to heat dispersion through the skin. Neutral baths are traditionally used against insomnia, pain, anxiety, irritability, and chronic tiredness [9].
- Cold Baths

- Cold baths should be performed at comfortable room temperature (water temperature should range from 15 to 18 °C). They can be repeated depending on subjective resistance. Before a cold bath, physical exercise is recommended to warm up the body, or body rubbing, or a hot footbath. After bathing, the patient will return to bed under warm covers to promote the hyperemic reaction. Cold sponge baths may follow.
- *Rehabilitation pool water* is usually kept at a 34–36 °C temperature. All authors agree that bathing at this temperature determines:
  - Amyorelaxant action, with a decrease of muscle tone ensuring smooth mobilization, due to the direct action of heat on muscle spindles, which become less sensitive to stretching, and a reduced activity of the alpha fibers with a subsequent muscle relaxation. Moreover, heat stimulates the skin thermoreceptors and indirectly reduces muscle contractures.
  - An antalgic action by raising the pain threshold, which allows to perform more aggressive exercise compared to dry mobilization [1].

Muds or peloids are natural or artificial substances that result from mixing water (thermal, sea, or lake/river water) with inorganic, organic, or mixed materials deriving from geological or biological processes. They are used for therapeutic purposes in the form of compresses or baths. Peloids include muds, loams, peats, or molds. Muds are generally indicated for rheumatic and osteoarticular diseases and for the related pain syndromes.

15.3.1 Physiological Actions

The physiological actions of hydrotherapy can be divided into thermal and mechanical. Thermal actions are produced through the application of water at temperatures higher or lower than the human body's temperature. The higher will be the change in body temperature, the stronger the effect, the other factors being equal. Mechanical actions are produced by the impact of water on the body surface (e.g., spray, shower, whirlpool bath, rubbing, etc.) [10, 11].

In order to promote healing, both local and systemic, oxygen circulation should be maximized and catabolic products should be removed; hydrotherapy is very effective for this purpose. These changes are traditionally obtained through a variety of actions on blood circulation that mainly include revulsive action, derivative action, and reflex spinal action [12].

15.3.2 Treatment

The primary goal of hydrotherapy is the same as for all therapies: treating the whole person, considering the past and present medical history, the present conditions, any regular drug intake, and any other relevant information. Once this holistic patient picture is obtained, the following steps are required:

- To use hydrotherapic treatments in a coordinated manner, integrated with any other drug treatment
- To use hydrotherapic treatments in order to fit the general and specific patient health conditions
- To explain the entire process to the patient, from the outset, before treatment, including the technique (duration, frequency, and any other relevant factors), ensuring that he will feel comfortable during execution
- To measure the patient's body temperature before starting a treatment [13]

The range of disorders and diseases for which thermal treatment is indicated has been gradually expanded in time, according to an evolution of the idea of health, which is now meant as general psychophysical well-being, rather than as the absence of a specific disease. However, preliminary medical evaluation and great care are required when applying hydrotherapy to patients with diabetes, heart disease, hypertension, kidney disorders, severe liver diseases, organ transplants, pacemaker or other medical devices, etc.

Upon implementing a hydrotherapy treatment, it is important to note that its action can take place at two separate levels: actual treatment and symptom mitigation. In fact, hydrotherapy can heal certain conditions and mitigate symptoms of others. In some cases, however, this distinction is not so sharp (e.g., in osteoarthritis, both a functional recovery and a reduced progression of the disease can be achieved), due to the fact that hydrotherapy also acts on the stimulation of the immune system; it causes a reduction of inflammation and has a hormone-modulating action. Hydrotherapy is also prescribed for many chronic and/or degenerative disorders, for which no treatment, allowing full healing, exists [14].

All hydrotherapy/crenotherapy practices should be designed according to the patient's reaction; therefore, they should start gradually and progressively adjusted. In general, elderly patients or patients with atherosclerosis, kidney disorders, or heart failure should not be submitted to cold hydrotherapy/crenotherapy, which may cause harmful hypertensive reactions; showers are contraindicated also in case of excitement [15].

Half-bust baths (up to or just above the waistline) are contraindicated in case of weakness, collapse, or risk of hemorrhage; cold baths have similar contraindications in feverish patients. Very hot baths should always be avoided, particularly in elderly patients or individuals with potential latent cardiovascular disorders.

In any case, hydrotherapic/crenotherapic treatments usually have mild side effects, even if, sometimes unexpected, that can be caused by inappropriate treatment execution or, in most cases, by individual reactions to treatment.

Common side effects of these treatments include headache (in case of intense or long-term treatment), dizziness, irritability, localized or general pain, insomnia, nausea, palpitations, weakness, and cold.

Contraindications of hydrotherapy/crenotherapy can be either relative or absolute. Relative contraindications concern a specific method or administration technique, related to patient's disease. Contraindications include, first and foremost, active neoplasms or recent surgery to remove them. Hydrotherapy/crenotherapy is also contraindicated in case of kidney failure; heart failure; severe arterial hypertension; severe organ diseases, such as cirrhosis; and immunodeficiency. Hydrotherapy/crenotherapy should not be used in case of fever or to protect other users in case of active infectious disease. Absolute contraindications discourage patients with specific diseases from submitting to any hydrotherapic approach; indeed, several studies and authors challenge this distinction, claiming that any contraindications are relative [16].

Key Points

- Crenotherapy uses the specific chemical properties of mineral waters for medical purposes.
- Hydrotherapy has physiological thermal and mechanical actions that determine local and systemic effects.
- Hydrotherapic treatments require a holistic approach.
- Hydrotherapy leverages on the properties of water and is effective in rehabilitation of many diseases, such as orthopedic and neurological disorders.
- Hydrotherapy has usually some mild effects; main contraindications are neoplasms, heart or kidney failure, severe hypertension or organ disease, fever, or infectious diseases.

References

1. Hydroglobe definition of a global framework for hydrotherapy. A FEMTEC–FORST joint project with the cooperation of ISMH and the technical support of the WHO. http://termas-world.com/documentos/hydroglobe.pdf
2. Forestier R, Erol-Forestier FB, Francon A (2016) Current role for spa therapy in rheumatology. Joint Bone Spine 84(1):9–13
3. Gabel CP, Rando N, Melloh M (2016) Slacklining and stroke: a rehabilitation case study considering balance and lower limb weakness. World J Orthop 7(8):513–518
4. Verhagen AP, Bierma-Zeinstra SM, Boers M et al (2015) Balneotherapy (or spa therapy) for rheumatoid arthritis. Cochrane Database Syst Rev 4:CD000518
5. Evcik D, Kavuncu V, Yeter A, Yıgıt I (2007) The efficacy of balneotherapy and mud-pack therapy in patients with knee osteoarthritis. Joint Bone Spine 74(1):60–65. Epub 2006 Nov 29
6. Fazaa A, Souabni L, Ben Abdelghani K et al (2014) Comparison of the clinical effectiveness of thermal cure and rehabilitation in knee osteoarthritis. A randomized therapeutic trial. Ann Phys Rehabil Med 57(9–10):561–569
7. Bidonde J, Busch AJ, Webber SC et al (2014) Aquatic exercise training for fibromyalgia. Cochrane Database Syst Rev 10:CD011336
8. Özkuk K, Gürdal H, Karagülle M et al (2016) Balneological outpatient treatment for patients with knee osteoarthritis; an effective non-drug therapy option in daily routine? Int J Biometeorol 61(4):719–728
9. Daniels J, Loades ME (2016) A novel approach to treating CFS and co-morbid health anxiety: a case study. Clin Psychol Psychother. doi:10.1002/cpp.2042

10. Wong JJ, Shearer HM, Mior S et al (2015) Are manual therapies, passive physical modalities, or acupuncture effective for the management of patients with whiplash-associated disorders or neck pain and associated disorders? An update of the bone and joint decade task force on neck pain and its associated disorders by the optima collaboration. Spine J 16(12):1598–1630
11. Sarsan A, Akkaya N, Ozgen M et al (2012) Comparing the efficacy of mature mud pack and hot pack treatments for knee osteoarthritis. J Back Musculoskelet Rehabil 25(3):193–199
12. Karagülle M, Kardeş S, Karagülle O et al (2016) Effect of spa therapy with saline balneotherapy on oxidant/antioxidant status in patients with rheumatoid arthritis: a single-blind randomized controlled trial. Int J Biometeorol 61(1):169–180
13. CJ MC, Mills PM, Pullen R et al (2004) Supplementation of a home-based exercise programme with a class-based programme for people with osteoarthritis of the knees: a randomised controlled trial and health economic analysis. Health Technol Assess 8(46):iii–iiv, 1–61
14. Langhorst J, Musial F, Klose P, Häuser W (2009) Efficacy of hydrotherapy in fibromyalgia syndrome – meta-analysis of randomized controlled clinical trials. Rheumatology (Oxford) 48(9):1155–1159
15. Yusupalieva MM (2016) The possibilities for the correction of the co-morbid anxiety and depressive disorders in the patients suffering from chronic obstructive pulmonary disease by the methods of climatic therapy. Vopr Kurortol Fizioter Lech Fiz Kult 93(3):29–33
16. Langschmidt J, Caine PL, Wearn CM et al (2014) Hydrotherapy in burn care: a survey of hydrotherapy practices in the UK and Ireland and literature review. Burns 40(5):860–864

Orthoses in Older Patients

16

S. Masiero, M. Mastrocostas, and A. Musumeci

16.1 Introduction

According to the international guidelines, orthosis is an "external applied device designed and fitted to the body to achieve structural and functional characteristics of the neuromuscular and skeletal system" [1]. Therefore, the main purpose of orthosis is the correction of an impaired function, whereas the aim of prosthesis is to substitute it. The orthoses can be used temporarily (e.g., after surgery) or permanently; they can be also static (if they do not allow movement) or dynamic. The advantages of using orthotic devices in older patients are several: ensuring postural stabilization, balance and trunk control, improving pain relief, reducing the risk of falls, correcting limb malformations, preventing progression to deformities, protecting and restraining joint mobility, and facilitating ambulation and weight-bearing. Most important features of an orthosis should be safety, practicality, functionality during all gait phases, stability, protectivity, to be appealing, and comfortable to wear. Choice of the appropriate orthotic device is crucial for an individualized rehabilitation treatment and requires knowledge of different disciplines such as anatomy, biomechanics, medical engineering, etc. In this chapter we will discuss some of the basic concepts of the spinal, upper, and lower limb orthoses and shoes that are frequently used in geriatric patients [2].

16.2 Upper Limb Orthoses

The upper-extremity orthoses are used to protect joints and to limit their movements in order to facilitate a good bone alignment. They also prevent articular deformities, compensate muscle weakness and hypotonia, and enhance postsurgical healing of bones and tendons.

S. Masiero (✉) • M. Mastrocostas • A. Musumeci
Neurorehabilitation Unit, University of Padua, Padua, Italy
e-mail: stef.masiero@unipd.it; alfredomusumeci@yahoo.com

© Springer International Publishing AG 2018

S. Masiero, U. Carraro (eds.), *Rehabilitation Medicine for Elderly Patients*, Practical Issues in Geriatrics, DOI 10.1007/978-3-319-57406-6_16

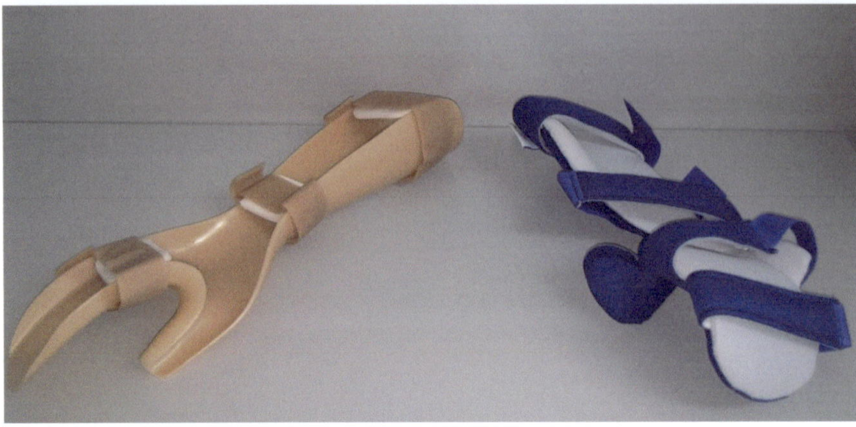

Fig. 16.1 Upper limb rigid (*right*) and semirigid static orthoses

Upper limb orthoses can be classified according to anatomical regions (shoulder, arm, elbow, wrist, hand), function, and design (nonarticular, static, serial static, static motion blocking, static progressive, dynamic, dynamic motion blocking, dynamic traction splints, tenodesis, continuous passive motion orthoses, adapted or for functional usage).

In older patients, the splints are frequently used for tendinopathies, enthesopathies, or joint sprains in order to prevent movement and reduce inflammation, facilitating thereby recovery. In rheumatoid arthritis, ulnar or radial deviation of the fingers and deformities can be treated using splints; the aim of the splint is to restore functional hand movements and to support wrist and fingers. Upper limb splint is also useful after stroke in order to control muscle hypertonia, prevent muscle and tendon retractions, and avoid physical deformities [3] (see Fig. 16.1).

16.3 Shoes and Shoe Modifications

Falls in older people are often related to footwear. Foot proprioception and plantar sensitivity worsen during age and in diabetes, peripheral neuropathies, and other medical conditions. Therapeutic shoes or shoe modifications might improve balance and reduce risk for falling; they could influence both tactile and proprioceptive mechanisms; moreover, the choice of appropriate and comfortable shoes could reduce the necessity of an orthosis [4].

Shoes should fit the shape of the foot and be one index fingerbreadth longer than the longest toe, allowing movement during standing and walking [5]. Loose or tight shoes can determine calluses, ulcers, or corns. Leather is one of the best materials to avoid this inconvenience, because it is durable and breathable, adapts itself to the patient's foot shape, and can be easily reshaped. In patients with diabetes and peripheral neuropathy, shoes should aim to decrease pressure on prominent areas through a high wide toe box. Modified or custom-made shoes are also indicated in case of ankle stiffness, edema, or joint deformity.

Foot inversion or eversion can be treated using a heel flare on either the medial or lateral heel. Distributing forces to the lateral knee compartment through lateral heel wedges may prevent valgus medial knee compartment overload in osteoarthritis.

Metatarsalgia is treated by distributing the forces to the metatarsal shafts using either a metatarsal bar or a rocker (convex) bar, positioned on the external sole in order to promote foot rollover. A metatarsal pad inside the shoe can be placed behind metatarsal heads in less severe cases. Adding an extended shank with mild rocker sole in order to decrease shoe's flexibility could treat toe pain, which occurs in arthritis and gout.

Talalgia, often caused by plantar fasciitis, calcaneal spurs, and Achilles tendon retraction, can be managed using an external calcaneal bar behind the painful site. If plantar fasciitis is associated with overpronation, a Thomas heel can help in pushing the foot toward the opposite side. Heel lifts or heel cushion relief pads can relieve Achilles tendon pain.

Leg length differences major than 10–15 mm should be treated using internal heel lifts [6].

16.4 Lower Limb Orthoses (LLO)

LLO and shoes are used to treat weakness, spasticity, pain, and joint deformities, in case of brain injury, neuropathies, arthritis, fractures, or amputation. Moreover, they improve abnormal posture or tone and can be used to correct irregular gait patterns. They should be periodically evaluated to monitor for patient's comfort, skin breakdown, and their effects on ambulation; a multidisciplinary approach is advised during patient's assessment.

According to the International Standard Organization (ISO), the classification of LLO is based on the anatomical joint, which they contain foot orthoses (FO), ankle-foot orthoses (AFO), knee orthoses (KO), knee-ankle-foot orthoses (KAFO), hip-knee-ankle-foot orthosis (HKAFO, which are used for infants in cerebral palsy), and hip orthoses (see Table 16.1).

Table 16.1 Lower limb orthoses classification

	Classifications based on design	Types
Lower limb Orthoses	Static Dynamic	Foot orthoses (FO) Ankle-foot orthoses (AFO) Knee-ankle-foot orthoses (KAFO) Knee orthoses (KO) Hip-knee-ankle-foot orthoses (HKAFO) Hip orthoses

1. Foot Orthoses (FO)

FO are useful in reducing ground reactive forces acting on lower limb joints; moreover, these devices can control pronation and supination. Three types of FO are available: soft, semirigid, and rigid. Soft foot orthoses can provide shock absorption, whereas rigid and semirigid, which are custom-made from casts of patients' feet, also support plantar arch (e.g., in case of severe foot deformities). It is fundamental, especially when using semirigid and rigid orthoses, to monitor skin looking for the presence of wounds or clinical signs of infection.

Flat and high-arched feet are managed using semirigid foot orthoses, which extend the foot and provide medial arch support. FO can also correct hyperpronation of the midfoot by acting on the longitudinal axis of the foot. The plantar buildup should be progressively increased to avoid an overcorrection of the deformities [6].

Soft soles can determine positive effect on foot pain sensation, but they may also determine plantar pressure changes with negative effects on balance; on the contrary, firm inlays may have an opposite action on the plantar surface [4].

2. Ankle-Foot Orthoses (AFO)

AFOs are the most commonly used LLO; they provide control of ankle dorsiflexion and plantar flexion and varus-valgus deviation, both static and dynamic. They also have a secondary effect on knee during ambulation: ankle plantiflexion facilitates knee extension whereas dorsiflexion helps knee flexion [2].

Static AFOs are devices made of rigid materials which keep joints in firm position; conversely, dynamic AFOs are defined using different terms with a similar meaning, such as hinged, articulating, and static progressive. AFOs are made of leather, plastic, metal, carbon composites, or a combination of these materials. Examples of static AFOs include solid ankle AFOs, ground reaction ankle-foot orthosis (GRAFO), and the patellar tendon bearing. Dynamic AFOs are posterior leaf spring, hinged (articulated) AFO, etc. [7].

The most prescribed AFOs are solid AFO, hinged AFO, and posterior leaf spring AFO. **Solid AFOs** restrict ankle motion and provide mediolateral stability of the foot; however, due to their rigidity and lack of plantar flexion, they could destabilize the knee during stance. Solid AFOs are used in the presence of ankle pain, plantar flexion spasticity, and foot drop associated with weakness of plantar flexors. **Hinged MAFOs** can be used to control ranges of motion of plantar flexion and dorsiflexion and to limit prono-supination. **Posterior leaf spring MAFOs** are flexible, they have the narrowest trimline, and the calf shell encircles less than half the circumference of calf; therefore they are not indicated in case of mediolaterally unstable ankle. They help weak ankle dorsiflexors during initial contact and swing phases of gait, preventing foot drop.

"Molded AFOs" (MAFOs) are thermoplastic and have many advantages; in fact they are lightweight, compact, easily wearable, not pliable at room temperature, and relatively inexpensive. MAFOs can be custom-made or manufactured in different sizes. Foot, ankle, and knee control depends on the anterior borders or edges at the malleolar region of the MAFOs (trimline). MAFOs consist of calf shell, calf strap, shoe insert, and, depending on the MAFO, a hinge at the malleolar level.

Metal AFOs include medial and lateral metal uprights, which are proximally attached to the limb with a calf band and distally fixed to a shoe sole by a stirrup. They are used in case of insensate skin because they have few points of contact [6].

Stroke often determines a motor impairment that mainly involves trunk, pelvis, knee, and ankle coordination both in standing position and during ambulation. Hemiparetic patients have specific gait patterns in the affected side, which is characterized by shorter step length, longer stance phase, and a shorter swing phase. They may also present an equinovarus foot, in which the weight support of the heel shifts to the lateral plantar surface, leading to imbalance, insecure gait, and, consequently, increased risk of falls. AFOs decrease the incidence of ankle contractures in patients with hemiparesis, but they should always maintain the ankle joint stiff, at the same time, in order to hold the foot in the correct position while standing and keep its clearance during swing phase [8]. However, an excessively stiff AFO will obstruct both the loading response during early phase of ground contact and the dorsiflexion during stance, causing this way instability, reduced walking speed, and a delay in recovery of ambulation [9].

AFOs have several potential disadvantages such as poor ankle hyperextension during stance and ineffective triplanar foot motion control; they also require good muscle strength and flexibility for knee control during swing. Moreover, AFOs increase bulk in the shoes and are difficult to use in case of severe spasticity [10] (Figs. 16.2 and 16.3).

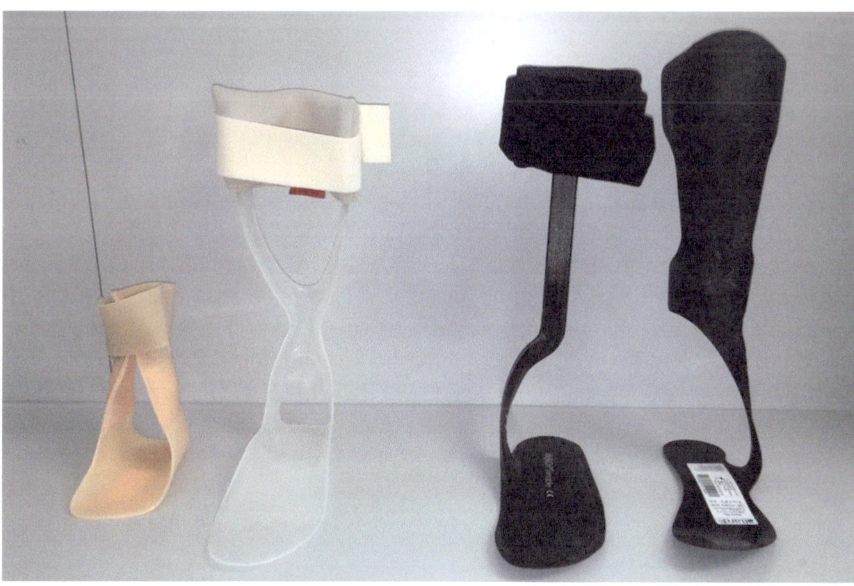

Fig. 16.2 AFOs. From *left* to *right*: AFO and posterior leaf spring AFO (in plastic material); MAFO and toe-off (in carbon composite)

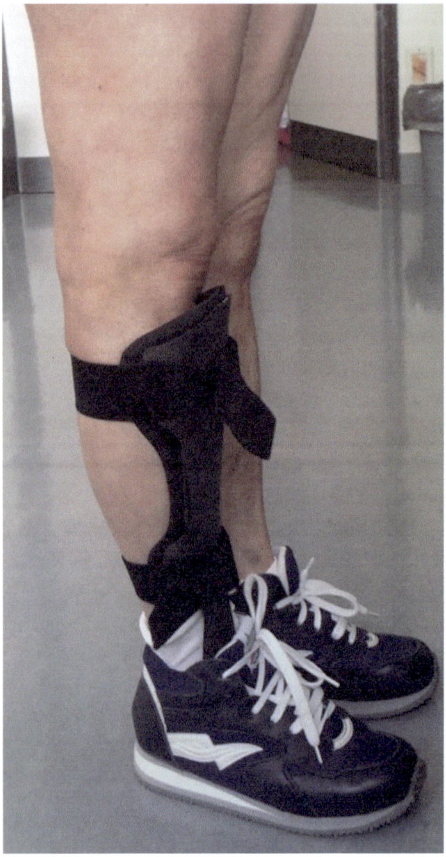

Fig. 16.3 Toe-off AFO

3. Knee-Ankle-Foot Orthoses (KAFO)

KAFOs are made of metal, leather, and plastic materials and stabilize knee, ankle, and foot, both mediolaterally and anteroposteriorly. KAFOs usually share the following components: a metal knee joint anchored to the thigh proximally and attached to an AFO distally (see Fig. 16.4). KAFOs can be classified, according to design, into passive, which do not provide any active control on knee movements; stance control (SC) KAFOs, which block the knee during the stance phase and allow free motion during the swing phase; and dynamic KAFOs, which allow knee control during both stance and swing phases. KAFOs are usually worn on both legs

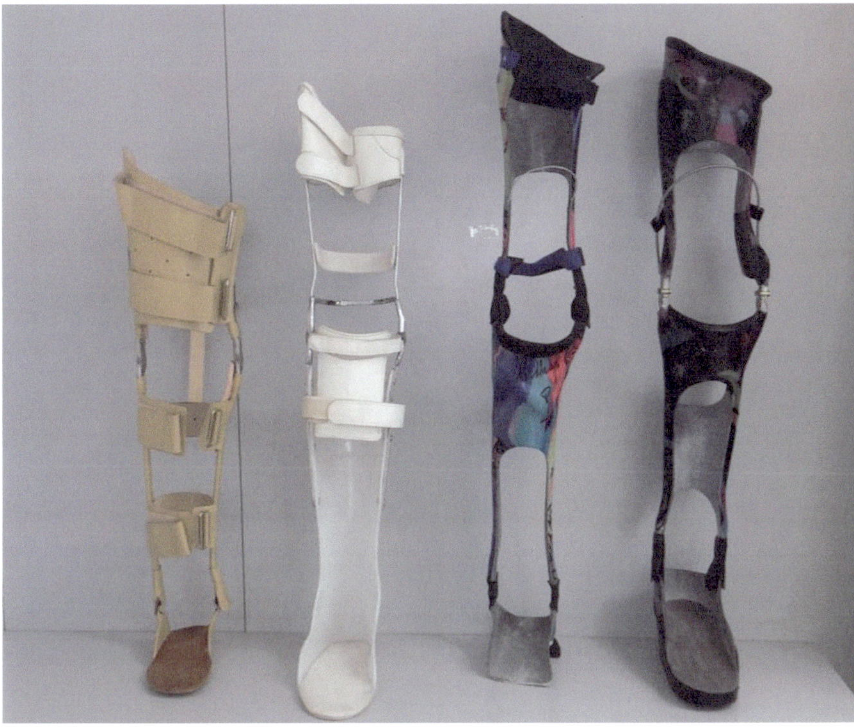

Fig. 16.4 Dynamic KAFO components: AFO, with or without plastic shell, metal uprights, knee joints, and straps

after spinal cord injuries or on one limb after poliomyelitis sequelae. KAFOs are seldom used at rest because they are difficult to don and doff [11].

4. Knee Orthoses (KO)

KO provide knee stabilization during ambulation. In osteoarthritis, these braces aim to reduce load on the knee compartments and are usually named medial or lateral. An example of an articulated KO is the Swedish knee cage, which is made of metal joint and mediolateral stays; it uses a three-point system (one above, one below, and one behind the knee) to control hyperextension during walking; in obese patients, its use can be limited (Fig. 16.5).

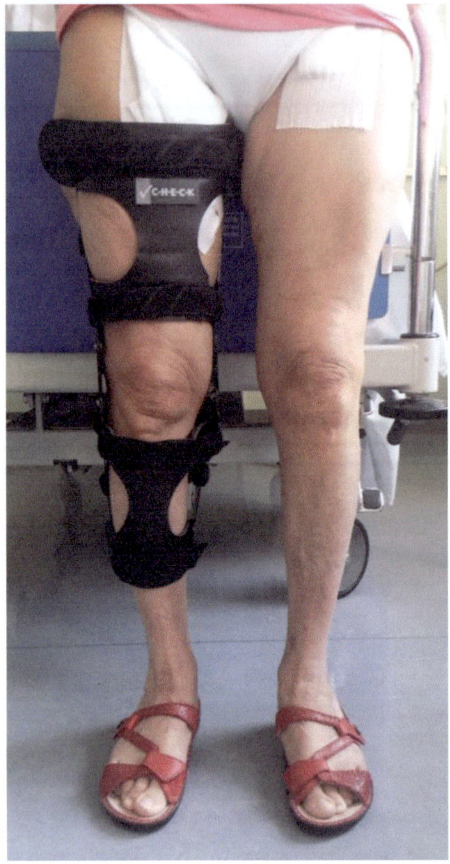

Fig. 16.5 Right knee orthosis

16.5 Spinal Orthoses (SO)

SO prevent and stabilize vertebral fractures related to osteoporosis or neoplasms, relieve back pain, and improve trunk stability in osteoarthritis, discal hernias, and paraspinal muscle insufficiency; they also correct vertebral disalignment in degenerative scoliosis and restrict range of movement after spinal surgery or trauma. SO can be flexible, rigid, or semirigid and are named according to the vertebral segments they enclose: cervical orthoses (CO), thoracolumbar orthoses (TLO), thoracolumbosacral orthoses (TLSO), and lumbosacral orthoses (LSO). Potential SO drawbacks are the difficulty to wear the brace, the risk of pressure sores, weakening of spinal muscles, osteoporosis, nerve compression damages, and restraint of thoracic cage or abdominal wall movements.

1. Cervical Orthoses (CO)

CO include cervical collars and Halo devices. Cervical collars (C-collars) can be rigid (made of plastic material) or soft (felt); they are easy to apply and very well tolerated. However, they do not completely restrict neck motion even if they give feedback to patient in order to limit excessive motions (kinesthetic reminder). CO can be used to relieve pain in the short term and may provide partial support to the cervical spine after neck injuries. C-collars are indicated in cervicalgia, spondyloarthritis, and discal hernias. Rigid CO are routinely used in the prehospital setting for trauma victims, the most frequently used are the Aspen, Malibu, Miami J collar, and Philadelphia [12, 13] (Figs. 16.6 and 16.7).

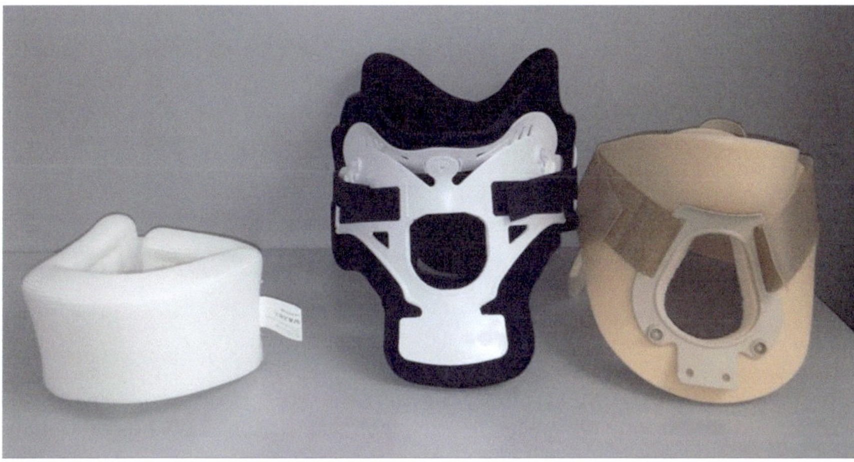

Fig. 16.6 Cervical orthoses. From *left* to *right*: soft cervical collar; Miami J collar; Philadelphia collar

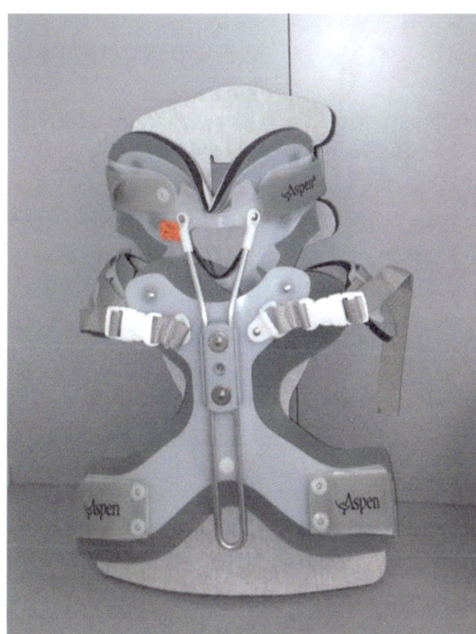

Fig. 16.7 Cervical-thoracic orthoses (CTO) provide external immobilization in the planes of flexion, extension, rotation, and lateral bending of C1–T1 levels

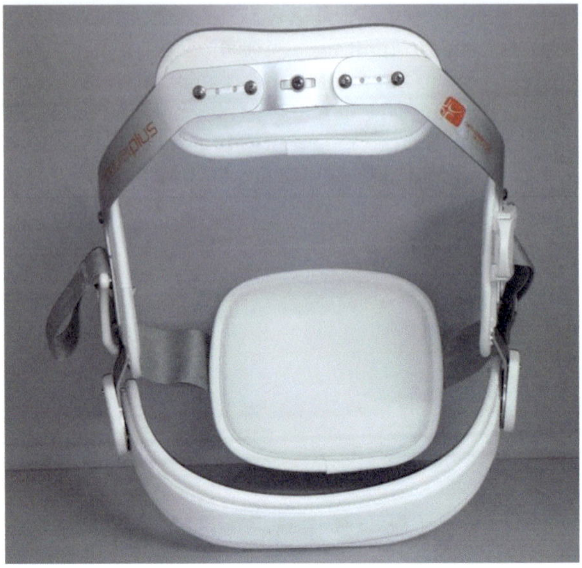

Fig. 16.8 TLSO with 3-point pressure

The Halo devices provide greater restriction in comparison to any other CO; they are made of a metal ring, which is fixed to the head by means of pins and connected to a body vest through several metal rods. Halo devices are indicated in case of cervical vertebral fractures, major cervical trauma, cervical vertebral dislocation, and neoplasms [6].

2. Thoracolumbosacral Orthoses (TLSO)

They provide spinal pain relief and fare used for primary and secondary prevention of osteoporotic fractures, especially in the inferior thoracic and upper lumbar vertebrae. In fact, TLSO restrain flexion movement, which is responsible of fragility fractures, and allow, on the contrary, extension of the thoracolumbar spine and spinal muscle strengthening. TLSO feature a 3-point pressure system to prevent flexion movements with three pads placed at the lumbar, pelvic, and sternal level, respectively (Fig. 16.8).

3. Lumbosacral Orthoses (LSO)

LSO are the most commonly prescribed SO due to their comfort and tolerability. They are made of elastic belts, provided with anterior or posterior closure. Indications for their use are mechanical lumbar pain, lumbar discal hernias, lumbar degenerative scoliosis, and lumbosacral stenosis (Fig. 16.9).

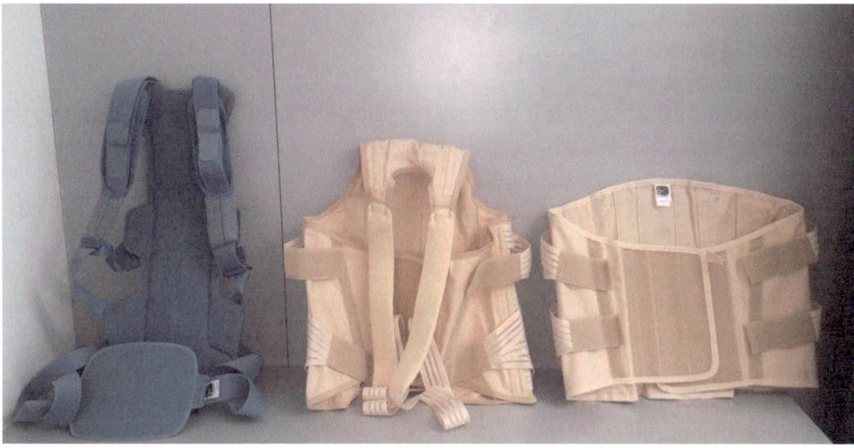

Fig. 16.9 From *left* to *right*: two semirigid thoracolumbosacral orthoses with shoulder straps and a lumbosacral corset (on the *right*)

16.6 Physical Therapy in Patients Who Use Orthotic Devices

The orthoses should be evaluated by the attending practitioner, orthotist, and physiotherapist, both before and after the prescription, in order to choose the best device with the most suitable design according to the patient's needs. It is important to design goals of treatment together with the patient and his family, taking into account the clinical situation, the individual functional assessment, the social context, and the subject's preferences [6].

Patients using orthotic devices need:

– *Education*. The program should include information on donning and doffing the orthoses and the education on skin inspection and hygiene measures of the impaired limb (e.g., patients may use compression stockings for leg edema and ulcer prevention).

Patients using orthotic devices are instructed on lower limb desensitization activities such as friction massage and tapping, in order to decrease hypersensitivity and to become more tolerant to pressure of the orthosis. Patients' family should supervise and assist relatives, notably when treatment begins.

– *Instruction on exercises to perform at home*. Range-of-motion exercises are important in elderly population in order to prevent muscle spasms and contractures. Patients may develop plantar flexion contractures due to loss of active movement, even if they use orthotic devices. Stretching exercises and an appropriate positioning of frail older patients in bed or wheelchair are, therefore, of utmost importance. Trunk and upper-extremity flexibility exercises allow more efficient performances in daily activities.

Upper-extremity strength is important for transfers in bed mobility, donning and doffing of orthotic devices, and ambulation activities. Patients using orthoses show greater energy expenditure than normal individuals; therefore, aerobic training is fundamental, provided there are no medical contraindications. Moreover, strengthening exercises of the trunk musculature improve stability, and training of the lower extremities improves gait pattern, allowing, in this way, an efficient ambulation.

It is also important to improve balance of disabled elderly in order to prevent falls and maintain independence in daily functional activities. Patients who use orthotic devices usually experience loss of balance and stability. The presence of environmental barriers, such as soft, uneven or unstable surfaces and the gait instability may increase the risk of fall injuries. Ambulation training aims to improve patient's walk on even or uneven surfaces (i.e., carpet, grass, sidewalks), from short to longer distances, using the appropriate devices. Any deviation and asymmetry in gait pattern should be promptly evaluated and corrected.

Functional training for independence in daily activities such as personal hygiene or independent transfer is part of the exercise program (e.g., from bed to wheelchair, from wheelchair to toilet, from seated to standing position, with or without the assistive devices, and vice versa).

The purpose of the stair exercises is to teach patients how to safely ascend and descend stairs using orthoses. Stair negotiation is one of the most difficult tasks for older people, and stair falls cause more than 10% of fatal fall accidents. Walking stairs requires attention, balance, and coordination. Proprioception, somatosensory, visual, and vestibular systems often deteriorate with aging; therefore, stair descent and ascent can be very difficult for older patients using orthoses [14–17]. Supervised physical therapy, mobility, and balance exercises, with or without the use of stair railings or assistive devices, can be helpful in accomplishing this very hard task [18].

From all the above, we can conclude that education and a multicomponent, progressive, personalized training program should be considered as part of the management of elderly patients who use orthotic devices.

Key Points

- The orthoses are used, usually within a rehabilitation program, to correct the impaired functions of the upper/lower limbs or of the spine.
- The correct choice of an orthotic device should be based on the clinical situation, the individual functional assessment, and the social context, focusing on patient's and caregiver's needs.
- Association of an orthotic usage with a multicomponent individualized training program improves patient's functionality.
- A periodic checkup is also necessary to control the fit of the orthosis and avoid unnecessary complications secondary to its usage.

References

1. http://www.iso.org/iso/catalogue_detail.htm?csnumber=15800
2. Cifu DX, Kaelin DL, Kowalske KJ et al (2016) Braddom's physical medicine and rehabilitation, 5th edn. Elsevier, Amsterdam, Netherlands. Chapter 12
3. Cifu DX, Kaelin DL, Kowalske KJ et al (2016) Braddom's physical medicine and rehabilitation, 5th edn. Elsevier, Amsterdam, Netherlands. Chapter 11
4. Hijmans JM, Geertzen JH, Dijkstra PU, Postema K (2007) A systematic review of the effects of shoes and other ankle or foot appliances on balance in older people and people with peripheral nervous system disorders. Gait Posture 25(2):316–323. Epub 2006 May 9
5. Xing Y, Alexander M (2002) Lower limb orthotics. EMedicine Topic 172 June
6. Pomeranz B, Adler U, Shenoy N et al (2006) Prosthetics and orthotics for the older adult with a physical disability. Clin Geriatr Med 22(2):377–394
7. Shankman GA, Manske RC (2011) Fundamental orthopedic management for the physical therapist assistant, 3rd edn. Elsevier Saunders, pp 458–462
8. Ferreira LA, Neto HP, Grecco LA et al (2013) Effect of ankle-foot orthosis on gait velocity and cadence of stroke patients: a systematic review. J Phys Ther Sci 25(11):1503–1508
9. Alam M, Choudhury IA, Bin Mamat A (2014) Mechanism and design analysis of articulated ankle foot orthoses for drop-foot. Sci World J 2014:867869
10. Bosch PR, Harris JE, Wing K (2014) American Congress of Rehabilitation Medicine (ACRM) stroke movement interventions subcommittee. Review of therapeutic electrical stimulation for dorsiflexion assist and orthotic substitution from the American Congress of Rehabilitation Medicine stroke movement interventions subcommittee. Arch Phys Med Rehabil 95(2):390–396
11. Tian F, Hefzy MS, Elahinia M (2015) State of the art review of knee-ankle-foot orthoses. Ann Biomed Eng 43(2):427–441
12. Lauweryns P (2010) Role of conservative treatment of cervical spine injuries. Eur Spine J 19(Suppl 1):S23–S26
13. Sandler AJ (1996) The effectiveness of various cervical orthoses: an in vivo comparison of the mechanical stability provided by several widely used models. Spine 21(14):1624–1629
14. Startzell JK, Owens DA, Mulfinger LM, Cavanagh PR (2000) Stair negotiation in older people: a review. J Am Geriatr Soc 48(5):567–580
15. Hamel KA, Cavanagh PR (2004) Stair performance in people aged 75 and older. J Am Geriatr Soc 52(4):563–567
16. Verghese J, Wang C, Xue X, Holtzer R (2008) Self-reported difficulty in climbing up or down stairs in nondisabled elderly. Arch Phys Med Rehabil 89(1):100–104
17. Mian OS, Thom JM, Narici MV, Baltzopoulos V (2007) Kinematics of stair descent in young and older adults and the impact of exercise training. Gait Posture 25(1):9–17
18. Cadore EL, Rodríguez-Mañas L, Sinclair A, Izquierdo M (2013) Effects of different exercise interventions on risk of falls, gait ability, and balance in physically frail older adults: a systematic review. Rejuvenation Res 16(2):105–114. doi:10.1089/rej.2012.1397

17 Taking Charge of the Lower Limb Amputee Patient: Evaluation Measures, Scales, and the Clinical Approach

Marco Traballesi, Giovanni Morone, and Stefano Brunelli

17.1 Taking Charge of the Patient

A patient-centric, interdisciplinary approach is mandatory for amputee rehabilitation. Team should integrate physicians, nurses, physical, and occupational therapists, prosthetists, psychologists, and dieticians with the objective to regain function and independence to the amputee. Patients and family members must take an active role in the process and are consulted in decisions about therapeutic and prosthetic options [1].

17.2 Clinical Evaluation

During the first evaluations, the rehabilitative team has to take into account the following aspects:

1) The cause of the amputation. In general people with an amputation due to dysvascular problems are aged and with comorbidity, while traumatic or neoplastic amputees have more phantom limb pain and psychologic disturbances [2].
2) The period of the patient's bed rest before and after the surgical treatment. The longer is this period, more severe are the complications due to hypo-mobility and muscle-tendon retraction. In particular, the shortening of the hip flexor muscles (for transfemoral and transtibial amputations) and the knee flexor muscles (for transtibial amputations). Moreover the detraining status could interfere with the conditioning exercises and the first attempts to stand up the patient [2].
3) The cognitive status and the heart/respiratory condition. Learning how to use the prosthesis, and the use itself, in particular for transfemoral amputees, needs

M. Traballesi (✉) • G. Morone • S. Brunelli
Santa Lucia Hospital, Neurorehabilitation Unit, Rome, Italy
e-mail: m.traballesi@hsantalucia.it; g.morone@hsantalucia.it; s.brunelli@hsantalucia.it

© Springer International Publishing AG 2018

S. Masiero, U. Carraro (eds.), *Rehabilitation Medicine for Elderly Patients*,
Practical Issues in Geriatrics, DOI 10.1007/978-3-319-57406-6_17

collaboration and clinical stable conditions. The energy cost of walking for a transfemoral amputee is much higher than healthy people, and this may led to breathlessness and rejection of the prosthesis usage [3].
4) The residual limb condition. Only when the surgical wound is healed and the edema is greatly reduced, it will be possible to fit the first prosthesis [2].

17.3 Pre-prosthetic Training

The first objective is to increase motor ability without the prosthesis and increase the self-awareness and the acquisition of new motor competencies.

During pre-prosthetic rehabilitation the following factors are crucial:

- Good global reconditioning
- Training of the trunk muscles and respiratory functions
- Increase of joint mobility and core stability
- Training to achieve autonomy in transferring and postural changes

Residual limb evaluation through visual inspection and palpation should highlight signs and symptoms of possible complications: skin breakdown, bone stump complications, proximal joint contractures, pain (musculoskeletal, neuromas or nerve entrapment, phantom limb), and edema. We recommend an X-ray examination of the stump with its proximal joint [1].

The objective of the pre-prosthetic phase is to prepare the residual limb and the entire body to support the locomotor abilities in the prosthesis phase. The main steps of the pre-prosthetics phase can be summarized as follows [4]:

1) Exercises to increase range of motion of proximal joint, balance competencies with growing level, proprioceptive rehabilitation with tactile, somatosensory, and pressure stimulation to achieve a new body schema
2) One leg standing inside parallel bars should be started as soon as possible. Sound limb walking training and balance training inside parallel bars. Exercises to increase coordination and resistance, possibly without hand support, to increase participation to activities of daily living
3) Training for independence during transfer from bed to wheelchair
4) Treatment of the residual limb edema with elastic bandaging
5) Tissue massage and ultrasound therapy to treat and prevent adherent scares
6) Mental/motor imagery or mirror therapy for phantom pain

17.4 Prosthetic Rehabilitation

17.4.1 The Approach to the Patient

The prosthetic rehabilitation represents the key moment of the recovery of patients affected by lower limb amputation. The choice on the kind of prosthesis (suspension system, materials, locked or unlocked knee, monoaxial or pluriassial foot, etc.)

depends on the level of mobility reached by the patients among the pre-prosthesis training: it is incorrect to prescribe prosthesis just after the surgical treatment [1, 4].

It is important to give the correct information to patients and caregivers: describe the different components of the prosthesis, identify the points of support of the socket where the patient will have to transfer the weight, describe the pain, after the first use of the prosthesis, give instruction to the patient on care and hygiene of the stump and prosthesis.

Since the ultimate goal is to give adequate movement trajectories, the task of the physiotherapist is to propose exercises that bring the patient to new appropriate motor adaptation, develop new motor skills and new coordination, transform the patient in a new unique "man-prosthesis" system.

17.4.2 Development of Balance and Coordination with the Prosthesis

The proposed exercises aim to develop a continuous coordinative tonic-postural adjustment by means of the involvement of proprioceptive mechanisms.

The first exercises involve the use of balance board which provides an unstable and sensory-stimulating surface that facilitates balance, proprioceptive training, and automatic postural reactions. These exercises take place inside the parallel bar, in the first phase with the upper limbs support and then without. The use of a mirror during the exercises is an important feedback for the patient to correct its postural changes. Anyway, it is recommended to increase the exercises difficulties as soon as possible, by blinding the patient in order to better stimulate the proprioceptive system and the balance condition [1, 4].

17.5 Return to Walking After Amputation

17.5.1 Exercises Preparatory to Walking

The first series of exercises proposed to the patient fitted with the prosthesis aims to develop the feeling with the socket through the identification and recognition of the support points and the loading areas of the stump, inside the rigid wall of the socket. These exercises gradually increase the tolerance for the load and reduce the pain. The patients become more confident with the prosthesis, and they can develop the static postural control on the frontal and sagittal planes.

Exercise progression consists in dual standby of the upper limbs, then through the use of only one support, until the patients can stand without any support. In this phase, the use of two weight machines for the visual feedback of the load on both sides is highly recommended. The patient is asked to climb up and down a step with the sound limb and then with the prosthetic limb. Upon reaching a correct load distribution, more dynamic exercises, dedicated to the rehabilitation of gait pattern, can be started [4].

17.5.2 The Rehabilitation of the Gait Pattern

At the first stage, the proposed exercises occur inside the parallel bar, with the aim to reduce the risk of postural trunk compensation during the full-step cycle in particular in the stance phase. Moreover, additional exercises are needed to develop the control of the swing phase in the sagittal and the frontal plane, paying attention to the movement patterns [4].

The progression of the walking aids use is strictly customized to the patient's ability. Usually the training steps are:

- Use of a walker with ferrules and wheels
- Two quad walker cane
- Two crutches
- One crutch or a walking stick

When the amputee has reached a good balance and safety. During the prosthetic training, the team (physician–physiotherapist–prosthetist) must constantly follow any difficulties and any progress made by the patient. The new postural adaptations and the further reduction of the residual limb edema, in fact, often requires some corrections of the proper alignment of the prosthesis in the first weeks of training.

17.5.3 The Use of a Walking Aid

In the clinical practice, generally, the rehabilitative community indicates to use the walking aid in the contralateral side to the prosthetic lower limb. Our experience leads us to prefer the use of the cane or stick in the prosthesis side for two reasons:

- Further development of the load of the prosthesis on the socket
- Developing the equilibrium condition on the prosthesis itself

If the patient uses the aid in the side contralateral to the lesion, he/she unconsciously tends to tilt the trunk to the aid; therefore, it affects the postural symmetry [1].

17.5.4 Use of Stairs

The return to using the stairs could not miss in our rehabilitation program. The patient has to go upstairs with the healthy limb and must come down the stairs with the prosthetic limb. Only transtibial amputees with a high level of mobility can safely choose which side to start.

17.6 Functional Evaluation

For a complete evaluation of people affected by lower limb amputation, we suggest the following evaluation tools:

1) For a general measure of the independency and mobility in the activities of daily living: Barthel Index [5] and Functional Independence Measures [6]. These tools are not specific for amputees but are useful in the first phase of the rehabilitation without the prosthesis and for amputees that are not able to use the prosthesis.
2) For mobility and walking evaluation: timed up and go test (TUG) [7], 2minute walking test (2minW) [8], Locomotor Capability Index-5 (LCI-5) [9], and Houghton Scale (HS) [10]. These tools are easy to administer and do not require too much time. LCI-5 and HS are specific for the prosthesis use (how, how much, in which condition, where). We suggest a routine use of these tools.
3) The Prosthetic Evaluation Questionnaire (PEQ) [11] and SATPRO [12] are two questionnaires that investigate the quality of life of the amputees and their satisfaction with the prosthesis. They are useful for research purpose.

References

1. Traballesi M, Brunelli S, Pulcini M, Pitidis A, Taggi F (2003) Trattamento riabilitativo del paziente geriatrico vasculopatico amputato di coscia: sperimentazione di un protocollo, 48 p. Rapporti ISTISAN 03/46. ISSN 1123-3117
2. Traballesi M, Brunelli S, Pratesi L, Pulcini M, Angioni C, Paolucci S (1998) Prognostic factors in rehabilitation of above knee amputees for vascular diseases. Disabil Rehabil 20:380–384
3. Waters RL, Perry J, Antonelli D, Hislop H (1976) Energy cost of walking of amputees: the influence of level of amputation. J Bone Joint Surg Am 58:42–46
4. Engstrom B, Van de Ven C (1993) Physiotherapy for amputees. The Roehampton approach. Ed. Churchill Livingstone, Edinburgh
5. Mahoney FI, Barthel D (1965) Functional evaluation: the Barthel Index. Md State Med J 14:56–61
6. Leung EC, Rush PJ, Devlin M (1996) Predicting prosthetic rehabilitation outcome in lower limb amputee patients with the functional independence measure. Arch Phys Med Rehabil 77:605–608
7. Schoppen T, Boonstra A, Groothoff JW, de Vries J, Göeken LN, Eisma WH (2003) Physical, mental, and social predictors of functional outcome in unilateral lower-limb amputees. Arch Phys Med Rehabil 84:803–811
8. Gremeaux V, Damak S, Troisgros O, Feki A, Laroche D, Perennou D, Benaim C, Casillas JM (2012) Selecting a test for the clinical assessment of balance and walking capacity at the definitive fitting state after unilateral amputation: a comparative study. Prosthetics Orthot Int 36:415–422
9. Franchignoni F, Orlandini D, Ferriero G, Moscato TA (2004) Reliability, validity, and responsiveness of the locomotor capabilities index in adults with lower-limb amputation undergoing prosthetic training. Arch Phys Med Rehabil 85:743–748
10. Devlin M, Pauley T, Head K, Garfinkel S (2004) Houghton Scale of prosthetic use in people with lower extremity amputations: reliability, validity, and responsiveness to change. Arch Phys Med Rehabil 85:1339–1344
11. Legro MW, Reiber GD, Smith DG et al (1998) Prosthesis evaluation questionnaire for persons with lower limb amputations: assessing prosthesis-related quality of life. Arch Phys Med Rehabil 79:931–938
12. Bilodeau S, Hebert R, Desrosiers J (1999) Questionnaire on the satisfaction of persons with lower-limb amputations towards their prosthesis: development and validation. Can J Occup Ther 66:23–32

Prosthetic Treatment in Elderly Population

18

Amedeo Amoresano, Gennaro Verni,
and Andrea Giovanni Cutti

The frequency of vascular diseases is constantly increasing in industrialized countries, due to the sedentary, adipogenic lifestyle and the increased life expectancy. Vascular diseases mostly affect the lower extremities, which can be subjected to very aggressive surgery, and, in about half of cases, are linked to diabetes [1].

Incidence of vascular diseases is reaching 80% of all lower-limb amputations. Amputees are, most commonly, elderly subjects over 65 years of age. Figure 18.1 reports the incidence of transfemoral amputations for the Italian population, based on NHS statistics: in 2005, this was over 88% of all amputations, in subjects over 65 years old.

Frequently, the general health condition of these amputated patients is compromised by:

- Cardiovascular failure (80% of cases)
- Respiratory diseases
- Diabetic retinopathy and/or peripheral neuropathy [2]

It follows that these patients have limited energetic resources [3] and feature low-to-average functional activity levels (K1, K2); K-levels are defined by Medicare, based on an individual's ability or potential to ambulate and navigate his/her environment; K0 patients are not eligible for prosthesis, while K4 patients have the ability or potential for prosthetic ambulation that exceeds basic ambulation skills, typical of the prosthetic

A. Amoresano (✉)
Operative Unit of Physical Medicine and Rehabilitation, Centro Protesi INAIL, Vigorso di Budrio, Bologna, Italy
e-mail: a.amoresano@inail.it

G. Verni • A.G. Cutti
Production Directorate, Centro Protesi INAIL, Vigorso di Budrio, Bologna, Italy
e-mail: g.verni@inail.it; ag.cutti@inail.it

© Springer International Publishing AG 2018

S. Masiero, U. Carraro (eds.), *Rehabilitation Medicine for Elderly Patients*, Practical Issues in Geriatrics, DOI 10.1007/978-3-319-57406-6_18

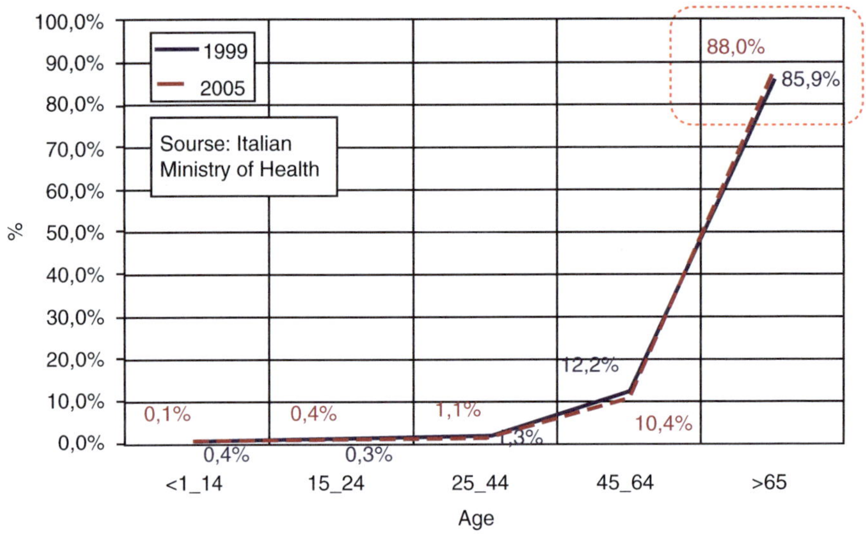

Fig. 18.1 Transfemoral amputation

demands of the child, active adult, or athlete. The high probability of successful prosthetic fitting reported among referral practices cannot be generalized to elderly individuals, but selected individuals can successfully be fitted with a prosthesis [4]. Rehabilitation efforts should best be targeted depending on needs. Rehabilitation professionals should make an educated estimate of outcomes at the beginning of rehabilitation based on the characteristics of the patients and the personal functional level on admission [5]. Considering the prosthetic application and the functional recovery that will follow, it is important to preserve as much limb as possible, with the most distal level of amputation permissible. For this reason, it is important to seriously consider:

- Foot amputations (transmetatarsal, tarsal, Syme, and Pirogoff). Transmetatarsal amputation is often used in patients with infection of the forefoot, necrosis, gangrene, and diabetic neuropathy with the aim to obtain a good functionality of the limb by preserving the midfoot. When the metatarsal bones are completely removed, the amputation level is named "Lisfranc amputation". The Chopart amputation is a disarticulation of the midfoot from the hindfoot: it is always combined with an ankle talar arthrodesis to obtain a foot with a proper support. Pirogoff level is obtained with the section of the bones of the leg over the ankle joint and with the arthrodesis of the heel's tubercle, placed in maximum talism, with the surface of section. The limb will be shortest than contralateral, suitable to sustain the weight of the body even without prosthesis. A Syme amputation is an amputation done through the ankle joint indicated for foot trauma, infection, or tumors, which allows to obtain a limb functional and painless.
- The preservation of the knee joint, if the stump achievable is longer than 4 cm, measured from the joint line [6].

- Knee disarticulation, if a full load-bearing is achievable, instead of a transfemoral amputation due to its numerous advantages from a prosthetic viewpoint.

In addition, in case of transfemoral amputation, it is always best to preserve the longest lever possible (distal stump), but with an 8–10 cm difference with respect to the contralateral knee joint line. This enables to reach two important goals:

- Reduction of the energy consumption (long lever)
- The possibility to apply the widest range of prosthetic knees and some additional components, e.g., a static rotator, avoiding an anatomical asymmetry when compared to the contralateral knee in seated position

The absence of vascular impairment of the residual limb and timely admission to the rehabilitation hospital correlated positively with effectiveness of mobility [7], but the amputation of the contralateral limb takes place within 3–4 years, in 30% of cases of amputation, based on a study of the Queen Mary's Hospital in Roehampton (UK).

Based on our experience, a bilateral transtibial amputee has a high probability to return to walk with two prostheses even in aged persons. On the contrary, for a bilateral transfemoral amputation, the probability is substantially lower and becomes null if stumps are proximal.

Elderly patients have a high probability of using a prosthesis when having an independent ambulation after transtibial amputation, without phantom pain, and they should be considered for prosthetic training [8].

All of the above stress the importance of careful clinical assessment of the patient by a multidisciplinary team: firstly, to evaluate the real potential for a prosthetic treatment and, secondly, to define a specific and customized prosthetic rehabilitation, possibly in collaboration with specialists in internal medicine, psychology [9], and cardiology.

The probability of success increases and the duration of the prosthetic-rehabilitative intervention decreases if a pre-prosthetic physio-kinesiotherapic intervention is applied. This aims to:

- Preserve the mobility of the residual joints.
- Prevent wrong postures (flexed or abducted stump) which follow after a long bed resting period or extended wheelchair use (hypokinetic syndrome) and are frequent in geriatric amputees.
- Reduce postoperative edema, thanks to an elastic-compressive monodirectional elastic bandage, or similar liners (Fig. 18.2).
- Prevent risk factors for patient falls [10].

The application of the first prosthesis should take place shortly after amputation, in the eighth–tenth week, in the absence of complications, with the aim of accelerating gait recovery and avoiding hypokinetic syndrome's effects. This goal can be obtained by means of the application of temporary endoskeletal prostheses. However, this category of prosthesis has little in common with the definitive prosthetic device, both considering the suspension system (thigh bands, harnesses, etc.) and the socket, which are little or non-customizable. These pitfalls frequently lead to prosthetic control

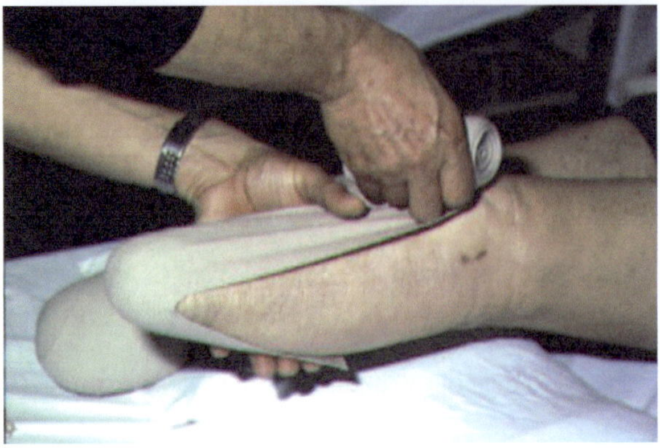

Fig. 18.2 Elastic-compressive bandage

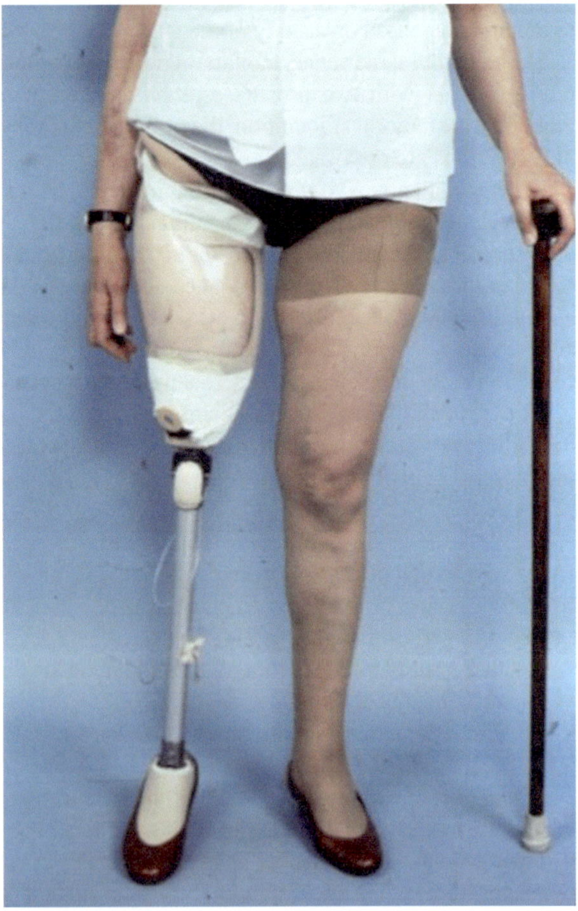

Fig. 18.3 Geriatric transfemoral prosthesis with flexible ischial containment socket and unlocking knee

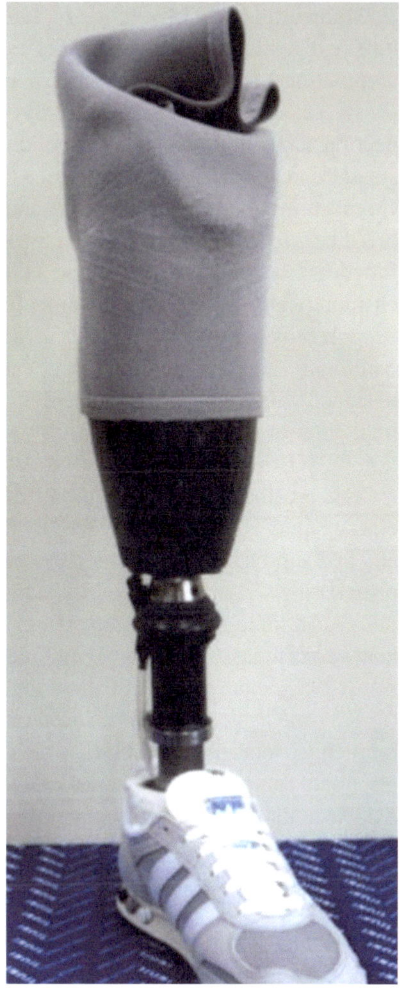

Fig. 18.4 Harmony system

issues and, consequently, to gait problems, not to mention pain, wounds, sores, and rapid muscle fatigue, which may ultimately result in depression, reject, and abandonment of the prosthesis for the majority of patients.

The application of a definitive (customized) prosthesis should also be carefully considered and followed by the renewal of the socket, after the stump stabilization.

The prostheses for geriatric patients must be designed considering technical and technological solutions that impact on three essential elements (Fig. 18.3):

- **Lightweight**, or weight containment
- **Safety**, to avoid falls
- **Comfort**

Maintaining a lightweight structure aims to limit the metabolic energy expenditure (exhaustion) during gait. This essential target is always useful after proximal amputations, due to the limited resources of high-level amputees. The weight of the prostheses can be limited, mostly through a careful choice of socket materials, connecting tubes and joints. The application of carbon fiber in the socket, instead of standard materials, enables to reduce the wall thickness and, accordingly, the weight. Connecting tubes and joints (knee and ankle), made of light alloys, titanium, or carbon fiber, reduce the weight by 25% compared to standard steel, with no effect on functionality and maximum load of the prosthesis. The choice of the solid ankle cushion heel (SACH) foot, specifically designed for geriatric amputees, can further support prosthesis weight reduction, thanks to its low weight (350 g) compared to the commonly applied prosthetic feet (about 550 g) [11]. Moreover, a geriatric foot designed with a low effective foot length improves the satisfaction and reduces proximal anterior socket pressures for poor-performing persons with transtibial amputation [12]. However, all these efforts can be vanished by the use of heavy footwear.

Safe prosthesis should avoid patient's falls, which can have dramatic effects in the elders. Safety is primarily achieved by the connection between the stump and the socket and by the prosthetic knee, if it is necessary. The safest knees feature a locking mechanism during walking, and the lock is removed only when sitting [13]. Due to their simplicity and limited functionality, compared to mono- and polyfunctional devices, these knees contribute to a further weight reduction. For instance, the lightest knee available is just 295 g and it is made of aluminum alloy. Recently, a new electronic knee, suitable for K2 patients, has been introduced on the market (Kenevo) and can be used with the joint either locked or unlocked, which is the goal of geriatric patients. Thanks to the electronic control, patients can take advantage of a highly safe articulation in potentially risky activities: uneven terrain, ramp ascending/descending, etc. However, the knee has a non-negligible weight (about 1.200 g) that must be taken into account.

The socket is equally essential for prosthesis control and safe gait. Ambulation is compromised when some room exists between the socket and the stump, even when the volume of the stump and the weight [14] of the patient are stabilized. In that case, the patient perceives the weight of the prosthesis as heavier, even when it is objectively lightweight. Possible solutions to this problem include using comfortable liners [15] (styrene, polyurethane, silicone gels, etc.) donned on the stump for transtibial and transfemoral amputees. In fact, liners ensure protection to the stump and are connected with the socket, by means of pins, straps, and magnets. Stump volume variations can be managed with one or more socks of variable thickness.

Harmony (Ottobock, D) is an alternative system specifically developed for vascular transtibial amputees (Fig. 18.4). A prerequisite for its application is the ability of the stump to tolerate the loading on its full surface. The socket, a total surface bearing (TSB) socket, is proximally sealed by a suspension sleeve. This device is essentially a pump which expels the air trapped inside the socket during socket donning. The extracted air generates a specific depression value, below the ambient pressure, and this effect enables the reactivation and maintenance of tissue perfusion, especially in the distal part of the stump, limiting volume variations. Nonetheless, the Harmony system has two disadvantages: the high cost and an increase in weight of the prosthesis (about 300 g). These inconveniences are however compensated by both the high suspension and prosthesis control level that the system ensures.

The prosthesis comfort is deeply connected to the technics and technologies that can mitigate the impacts on the stump, in particular in the areas sensitive to loads or pressures, avoiding, in this way, the occurrence of sores, wounds, and ulcerations. The skin of geriatric patients is often fragile and poorly hydrated, due to reduced vascularization, and has often a thin wrapping over bony prominences. Possible interventions to increase comfort are stump protection from stress of weight bearing (body weight) and a uniform distribution of stress over the entire surface of the stump. Stump protection can be achieved with the use of liners (styrene, polyurethane, silicone gels, etc.) combined with distal connection systems (as described above) or hypobaric [16]. Liners are always required for transtibial patients to protect the bony prominences (tibial ridge, tibial tuberosity, and head of the fibula). The presence of a distal cup with a thickness of 15–20 mm is particularly important in these liners for protecting the end of the stump.

The uniform distribution of loading is also achieved with specific shapes of the socket. In transtibial amputees, the TSB socket, which features the absence of a loading on the popliteal fossa, the loading under the patella and supracondylar walls, should be used. Suspension can be active (Harmony) or passive (one-way valve and kneepad or hypobaric system); active vacuum systems eliminate the greatest majority of the air between the liner and the socket, regulating the vacuum in a defined range. The system stabilizes the volume of the residual limb, and the high adhesion facilitates the control of the prosthesis.

An ischial containment socket with flexible walls should be adopted in transfemoral amputees with a stump in viable conditions and suitable length. This socket has the advantage to reduce ischial loadings (typical of the quadrangular socket) and to offer patients a better comfort (due to flexible materials).

It is worth remembering that the socket with flexible walls was proposed for the first time by J. Sabolich in the early 1980s, specifically for geriatric transfemoral patients, with the aim of increasing comfort in respect to rigid wall sockets and allowing small changes of volume to the stump, to some extent.

In conclusion, the prosthesis for an elderly patient should not be considered, as is usually done, unworthy of modern technologies, but an instrument for improving quality of life and the choice of components, times, and outcomes should always be carried out by a team specialized in this field of rehabilitation [17, 18].

References

1. Fleury AM, Salih SA, Peel NM (2013) Rehabilitation of the older vascular amputee: a review of the literature. Geriatr Gerontol Int 13(2):264–273. doi:10.1111/ggi.12016. Epub 2012 Dec 26
2. Eijk MS, van der Linde H, Buijck BI, Zuidema SU, Koopmans RT (2012) Geriatric rehabilitation of lower limb amputees: a multicenter study. Disabil Rehabil 34(2):145–150. doi:10.3109/09638288.2011.591888. Epub 2011 Sep 29

3. Frieden RA (2005) The geriatric amputee. Phys Med Rehabil Clin N Am 16(1):179–195
4. Fletcher DD, Andrews KL, Butters MA, Jacobsen SJ, Rowland CM, Hallett JW Jr (2001) Rehabilitation of the geriatric vascular amputee patient: a population-based study. Arch Phys Med Rehabil 82(6):776–779
5. Hershkovitz A, Dudkiewicz I, Brill S (2013) Rehabilitation outcome of post-acute lower limb geriatric amputees. Disabil Rehabil 35(3):221–227. doi:10.3109/09638288.2012.690818. Epub 2012 Jun 11
6. Adunsky A, Wershawski M, Arad M, Heruti R, Siev-Ner I, Heim M (2001) Non-traumatic lower limb older amputees: a database survey from a geriatric centre. Disabil Rehabil 23(2):80–84
7. Traballesi M, Brunelli S, Pratesi L, Pulcini M, Angioni C, Paolucci S (1998) Prognostic factors in rehabilitation of above knee amputees for vascular diseases. Disabil Rehabil 20(10):380–384
8. Van Eijk MS, van der Linde H, Buijck B, Geurts A, Zuidema S, Koopmans R (2012) Predicting prosthetic use in elderly patients after major lower limb amputation. Prosthetics Orthot Int 36(1):45–52. doi:10.1177/0309364611430885. Epub 2012 Jan 17
9. Remes L, Isoaho R, Vahlberg T, Viitanen M, Koskenvuo M, Rautava P (2010) Quality of life three years after major lower extremity amputation due to peripheral arterial disease. Aging Clin Exp Res 22(5–6):395–405. doi:10.3275/6712. Epub 2009 Dec 1
10. Vieira ER, Freund-Heritage R, da Costa BR (2011) Risk factors for geriatric patient falls in rehabilitation hospital settings: a systematic review. Clin Rehabil 25(9):788–799. doi:10.1177/0269215511400639. Epub 2011 Apr 19
11. Prince F, Winter DA, Sjonnensen G, Powell C, Wheeldon RK (1998) Mechanical efficiency during gait of adults with transtibial amputation: a pilot study comparing the SACH, Seattle, and Golden-Ankle prosthetic feet. J Rehabil Res Dev 35(2):177–185
12. Bonnet X, Adde JN, Blanchard F, Gedouin-Toquet A, Eveno D (2015) Evaluation of a new geriatric foot versus the Solid Ankle Cushion Heel foot for low-activity amputees. Prosthetics Orthot Int 39(2):112–118. doi:10.1177/0309364613515492. Epub 2014 Jan 13
13. Devlin M, Sinclair LB, Colman D, Parsons J, Nizio H, Campbell JE (2002) Patient preference and gait efficiency in a geriatric population with transfemoral amputation using a free-swinging versus a locked prosthetic knee joint. Arch Phys Med Rehabil 83(2):246–249
14. Vivanti A, Yu L, Palmer M, Dakin L, Sun J, Campbell K (2013) Short-term body weight fluctuations in older well-hydrated hospitalised patients. J Hum Nutr Diet 26(5):429–435. doi:10.1111/jhn.12034. Epub 2013 Mar 22
15. Trieb K, Lang T, Stulnig T, Kickinger W (1999) Silicone soft socket system: its effect on the rehabilitation of geriatric patients with transfemoral amputations. Arch Phys Med Rehabil 80(5):522–525
16. Samitier CB, Guirao L, Costea M, Camós JM, Pleguezuelos E (2016) The benefits of using a vacuum-assisted socket system to improve balance and gait in elderly transtibial amputees. Prosthetics Orthot Int 40(1):83–88. doi:10.1177/0309364614546927. Epub 2014 Sep 26
17. Andrews KL (1996) Rehabilitation in limb deficiency. 3. The geriatric amputee. Arch Phys Med Rehabil 77(3 Suppl):S14–S17
18. Bilodeau S, Hébert R, Desrosiers J (2000) Lower limb prosthesis utilisation by elderly amputees. Prosthetics Orthot Int 24(2):126–132

Gerontechnology, Domotics, and Robotics

19

Patrizio Sale

19.1 Introduction

Demographic studies show a continuous increase in the European population and aging: the number of people older than 50 years has exceeded 150 million. In particular, the population of the EU-28 on 1 January 2015 was estimated at 508.5 million. Older persons (aged 65 or over) had an 18.9% share (an increase of 0.4% compared with the previous year and an increase of 2.3% compared with 10 years earlier) [1]. Independent living of senior citizens is one of the main challenges linked to the aging population, due to the impact on (a) the life of the elderly people, (b) the national health systems, (c) the insurance companies, (d) the relatives, and (e) the caregivers. However, quality of life for the aging population is associated with the ability of the elderly people to live independently and with dignity without having the need to be attached to their children, grandchildren, or any other person whose help would they need for their daily life and social behavior.

Senior citizens may suffer from a number of diseases, which result in a higher risk of fall and a higher vulnerability for cardiovascular, pulmonary diseases and decline of memory function. This creates a growing interest in technologies to enable older people to remain living independently at home [2]. In particular, the physical inabilities which inevitably come with aging, together with the need of health monitoring, demand special attention which used to be possible only in healthcare structures. It is well known that the geriatrics subjects need help and/or assistance in all daily activities and in memory functions and health monitoring to remove the burden from the caregiver. The activities of daily living (ADL) for the old population in general are divided into basic ADLs and instrumental ADLs:

P. Sale, MD, PhD
IRCCS Fondazione San Camillo, Venezia, Italia

Department of Neuroscience, Rehabilitation Unit, University of Padua, Padua, Italy
e-mail: patrizio.sale@gmail.com

© Springer International Publishing AG 2018

S. Masiero, U. Carraro (eds.), *Rehabilitation Medicine for Elderly Patients*, Practical Issues in Geriatrics, DOI 10.1007/978-3-319-57406-6_19

1. Basic ADLs consist of these self-care tasks: bathing, dressing and undressing, eating, transferring from bed to chair and back into bed, voluntary control over urinary and fecal discharge, using the toilet, and walking (not bedridden).
2. Instrumental ADLs are not necessary for fundamental functioning, but enable the individual to live independently within a community (light housework, preparing meals, taking medications, shopping for groceries or clothes, using the telephone, managing money).

One of the current and future challenges in health and chronic disease management is an active participation of citizens and patients themselves in the healthcare management process. The patients' involvement in managing their own health and enhancing the awareness of their role in the framework of a collaborative and continuous care practice is very important. Currently, to reach these objectives, we can use new technologies based on monitoring system that include the connection of all required sensors to the system, under the paradigm of the Internet of Things, and sending the information to a communication layer that distributes all those signals to the corresponding system component to be properly processed.

One of the driving factors of the current electronic revolution is the vision that computing will pervade our environments. Any meaningful device or object of our everyday life will be capable of performing calculations and, at the same time, communicating transparently with any other computing device, may that be in its physical environment or remotely connected.

19.2 Gerontechnology

The gerontechnology is a new branch of assistant technologies in health and social domains combining gerontology and technology. The primary fields of application concern technological environments to health, housing, mobility, communication, leisure, and work of older people [3]. In particular, gerontechnology can help elderly people to identify and slow down the effects of the age-related modifications of the neural and musculoskeletal systems.

The management of chronicity and continuity of care can make use of innovative technologies, such as telemedicine, telehealth, and more generally information and communication technology (ICT), to ensure a networking operating mode for the total and continuous care of people with chronic disease. These new approaches are made possible thanks to recent advances in various fields such as sensor systems and smart devices that allow the analysis of data in real time. A wide range of these new technologies, including inertial sensors and video technologies at low cost, have recently been tested and in some cases combined, opening up new perspectives for relevant applications in the field of rehabilitation.

The purposes of bioengineering research in these fields are to develop new methods for the assessment of the limitations of such subjects and providing to physicians the tools to adapt and to improve interventions for motor and cognitive rehabilitation. At the same time, based on the results gathered, we could minimize if not eliminate the regular visits at home from medical personnel.

Health-enabling technologies and smart home technologies have been identified as potential measures to alleviate the consequences that demographic change will effect on societies [4]. These technologies offer support in terms of "patient empowerment," i.e., in a person's own health management [5], making more health-related data available than ever before.

19.3 Domotics

By the late 1990s, the term "domotics" was commonly used to describe any system in which informatics and telematics were combined in order to support activities at home. This word appears to be a portmanteau word formed from "domus" (Latin, meaning "house") and informatics. Therefore, it refers specifically to the application of computer and robot technologies to domestic appliances.

Smart houses (or homes) are known by a variety of names, including intelligent homes, home networking, home automation, sensor-embedded houses, and adaptive homes. Smart home technology refers to installing a home monitoring systems (sensors, actuators, and biomedical monitors) and special wiring to enable residents to program, control, and operate an assortment of appliances and other household features throughout the house. Smart homes have been defined as the integration of technology and services through home networking for a better quality of life [6]. Monitoring devices, such as sensors, are small and can be installed anywhere—inside or outside the home or worn by an individual.

A major focus of this technology, which has existed since the 1980s, has been to provide convenience, personal comfort, security, and energy conservation. While smart house technology has primarily focused on convenience and energy efficiency, this technology is increasingly targeted for use by people with disabilities and for the care of frail older adults—providing safety, security, and ease of self-management, as well as providing both on-site and remote monitoring and healthcare.

This recent increase in interest is related to:

(a) Its practicality in supporting the ability of older adults and people with disabilities to remain living independently and self-managing in their own homes for longer periods of time, supporting a major preference of all people to "age in place" in the living environment of their choice
(b) Its ability to support the significant efforts of family caregivers
(c) Its cost savings through reducing the need for expensive personal aid assistance, through reducing the need for in-person medical care, and through delaying or avoiding costly institutional care.

In particular, we can use the sensor's signals: continuous real-time measurements obtained from specific devices at different frequencies that observe the person, inertial sensors providing information about physical activity (sleep sensors, electrodermal activities, etc.), sensors measuring vital constants (arterial pressure, temperature, heart rate, sweating, body temperature, ECG signals, peripheral blood saturation, blood glucose level), environmental sensors (room humidity (dump), room

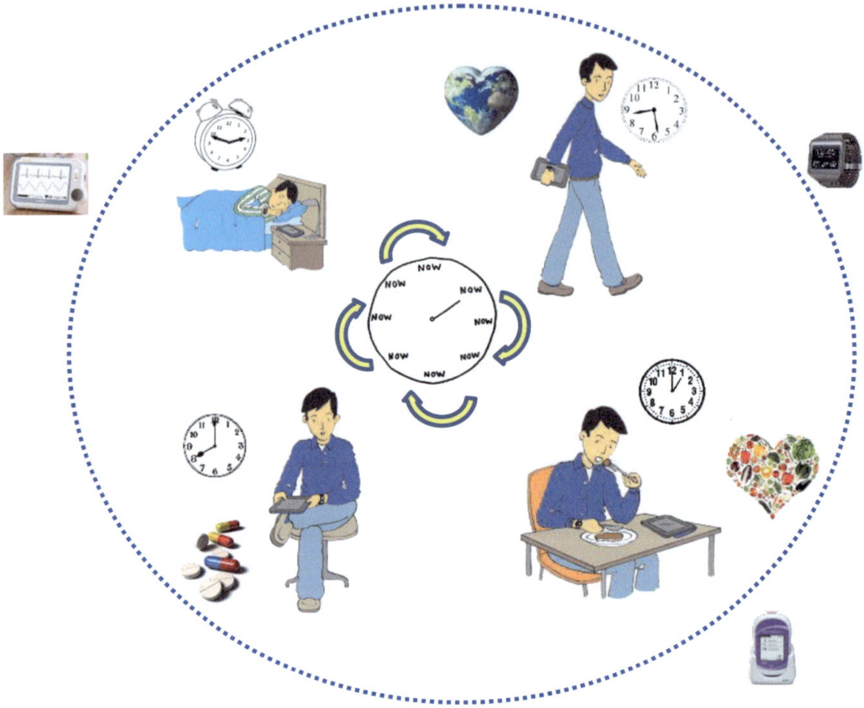

Fig. 19.1 A conceptual schema of the system and the interaction among all the subsystems included in the platfv

temperature, air quality, food sensors), Kinect sensors or video cameras (for motion capture during physical neurorehabilitation or authorized activities of daily life that will detect incorrect performances), or virtual symbolic sensors. Moreover, also the social network activity provides data for monitoring the emotional status of the person and its relationship with the community, among others (Fig. 19.1).

Smart home technology can also aid in disease prevention—for example, providing inconspicuous memory aids, such as medication reminders, or refrigerators that can evaluate an inventory of contents and provide suggestions for menus, healthy choices, and a list of groceries that need to be purchased. Vibrating bracelets or audible prompters can remind people when to eat or when to go to the bathroom, and other wrist devices monitor pulse rates and skin temperature. Sensors and wireless devices are being used in homes to monitor individuals' vital signs and whether medication has been taken, with this information sent wirelessly, through a sensor in the home or on the individual to the doctor or to family members—which is an added benefit for people who are homebound, are living in more remote rural areas, or are without immediate access to healthcare.

Several publications were identified about devices targeting:

1. Social isolation (videophonic communication, affective orthotic devices or companion-type robots, personal emergency response systems [security])

2. Autonomy loss (technologies for maintenance of autonomy in the ADL)
3. Cognitive disorders (cognitive orthotics, wandering management systems, telemonitoring) [7–10]

To analyze and to use all these data, we can use the artificial intelligence and in particular the area of decision support systems (DSS) and intelligent DSS (IDSS) to focus on developing interactive software that can analyze data including specific domain knowledge and automatic reasoning capabilities and provide answers to the relevant decisional questions from the users, thus enhancing a person or group to make better decisions [11]. Creative use of information technologies should facilitate the organization, presentation, and integration of this information to obtain individualized and systematic clinical decisions, predicated on individual patient's priorities [12]. The capability to provide a distance-based service is expected to eliminate barriers (e.g., logistical, geographical, administrative, etc.) that are currently hindering a stronger penetration of "traditional" hospitalized rehabilitation services (Fig. 19.2).

The use of ICT and domotics in general is changing the paradigm, extending with no limit the coverage area, and therefore allowing for a strong economy of scale. One of the barriers to the diffusion of e-Health is the digital divide, as the difficulty/inability of access to the network (in this case we talk about the digital divide "absolute") as well as a lack of basic knowledge enabling the use of digital technologies. The resources and satellite telecommunication services allow filling in the

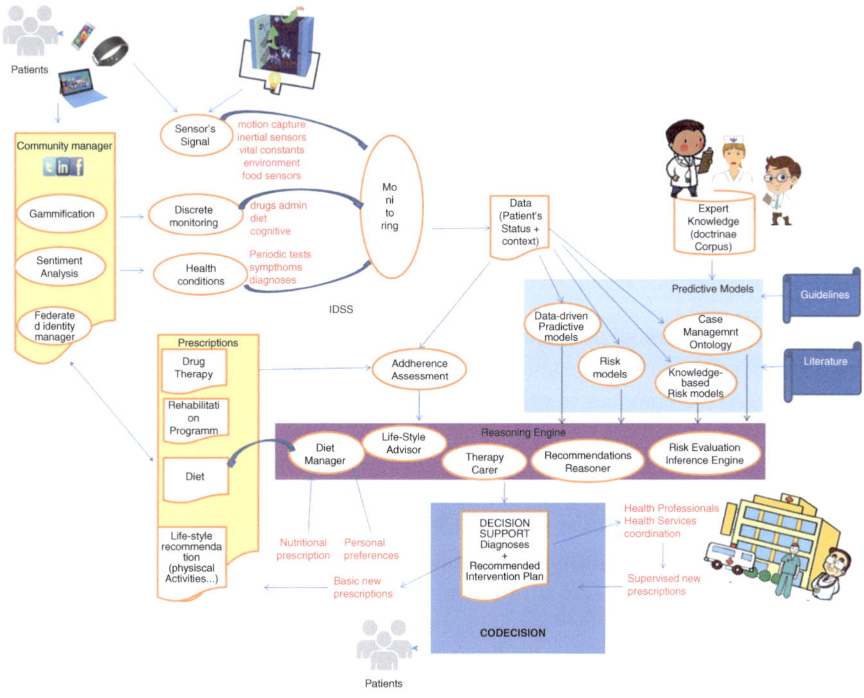

Fig. 19.2 Conceptual design of intelligent decision support system (IDSS)

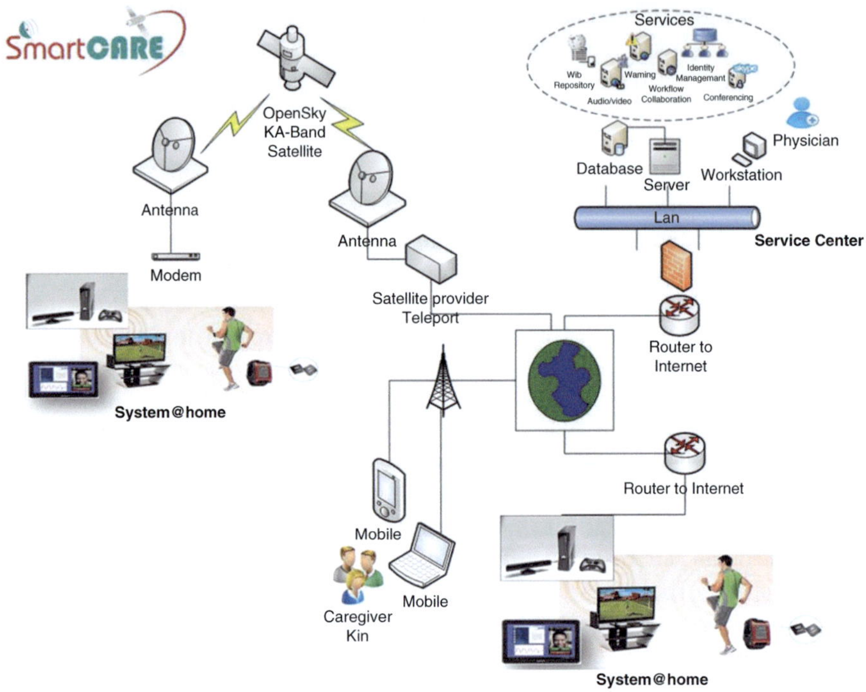

Fig. 19.3 SmartCare project architectures

gaps and delays in the spread of broadband: on the one hand, they are the only possible solution to the digital divide absolute (pure scenery satellite) and, on the other hand, they can increase the quality of telecommunications, where digital terrestrial service is already available (hybrid terrestrial and satellite scenario) [10] (Fig. 19.3).

19.4 Rehabilitation Robotics

In the field of telemedicine, robotic devices were used to help and improve the motor performance in older subjects. Rehabilitation robotics (RR) and the assistive robotics (AA) are branches of robotics, which focus on devices or machines that can help people with disability to recover and provide support in case of severe disability or physical trauma. It is unclear when this specialty was born, but the first clinical robot applications were powered human exoskeleton devices in the 1960s.

The RR and AA devices can be classified as exoskeleton, end effector, and wearable. All these robots are designed around the function and shape of the human body while the human is able to control the robotic limbs.

Numerous robotic devices for the upper and lower limb and hand function with various levels of complexity and functionality have been developed over the last 20 years. In this field, clinicians, therapists, and engineers collaborate to help the subjects with the impairments. Prominent goals in this field include developing implementable technologies that can be easily used by patients, therapists, and clinicians; enhancing the efficacy of clinician's therapies; and increasing the ease of activities in daily life.

The development of robot-aided tools for geriatric rehabilitation is a very stimulating prospective when considering their highly rehabilitative and assistive potentials. The main characteristics of all robot-aided treatment are the possibility to administer high-intensity and repetitive therapy. In fact, chronic subjects showed significant improvement in motor functions with intensive robot-assisted training, which may supplement the standard multidisciplinary rehabilitation programs, as our studies demonstrated [13, 14]. In particular, various robotic devices that assist and train upper extremity movements and hand function with various levels of complexity and functionality have been developed in the last 10 years. These devices range from simple mechanisms that support single-joint movements to more complex mechanisms with as many as 18 degrees-of-freedom (DOF) for multi-joint movements of the wrist and fingers.

The first results from clinical studies indicate that robot-assisted hand rehabilitation reduces motor impairments of the affected hand and the arm and improves the functional use of the affected hand. The different motor impairments of the hand can be viewed as resulting from problems in either motor execution or motor planning/learning. Deficits in motor execution result from weakness of wrist/finger extensors, overactive wrist/finger flexors (increased tone and spasticity), co-contraction, impaired finger independence, poor coordination between grip and load forces, inefficient scaling of grip force and peak aperture, and delayed preparation, initiation, and termination of object grip (Fig. 19.4).

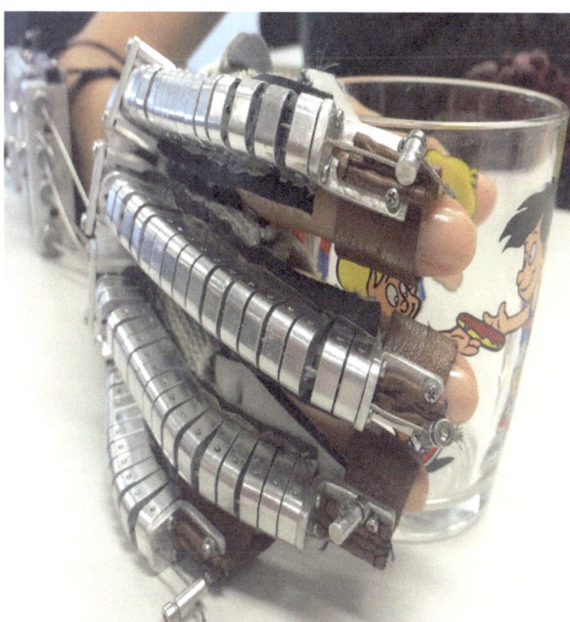

Fig. 19.4 Fingers Extending eXoskeleton (FEX) for rehabilitation and regaining mobility (Patent: PCT/IB2015/059313)

Various devices are described in literature and have been developed to train the wrist/forearm movements, individual finger movements, simultaneous finger and thumb movements (such as palmar or precision grasp), or a combination of these [15, 16].

Robotic gait training uses several devices to assist the patient move and maintain balance. Canes, crutches, walkers, and platforms are simple ambulatory-assistive devices that modify a patient's independence and functional mobility. Robot-aided walking and wearable robotic exoskeleton are considered a promising tool for gait rehabilitation in various diseases [16].

The robotic devices have been developed to relieve physical therapists from the strenuous and not ergonomic burden of manual body weight support (BWS). Furthermore, the use of robotic devices is currently advised to prevent the risk of falls and to improve gait velocity, keeping patients safe. The robotic machines can be used either as exoskeleton or end effectors, allowing practice up to 1000 steps for each session. Currently, a robotic task-specific repetitive approach, i.e., numerous practices of complex gait cycles, is regarded as the most promising to restore motor function after neurological or orthopedic diseases. Moreover, exoskeleton devices can be used to give inpatients an intensive program (in terms of many repetitions) of complex gait cycles and to allow their use in outdoor conditions [17–19].

Conclusion

Technological innovation in smart home, robotics, and ICT represents an effective solution to tackle the challenge of providing social sustainable care services for the aging population. The recent introduction of wearable technologies is opening new opportunities for the provisioning of advanced gerontechnology services based on the cooperation of a number of connected robots, smart environments, and other devices.

Key Points

- New devices were developed to help older subjects with limitation in daily activities and memory functions and for health monitoring in order to remove caregiving burden.
- Smart homes have been defined as the integration of technology and services through home networking for a better quality of life.
- The term "domotics" was commonly used to describe any system in which informatics and telematics were combined in order to support home activities. This word refers specifically to the application of computer and robot technologies to domestic appliances.
- Rehabilitation robotics (RR) and the assistive robotics (AA) are branches of robotics, which focus on devices or machines that can enhance recovery in people with disability or help them in daily activities.
- Robot-aided walking and wearable robotic exoskeleton are considered a promising tool for gait rehabilitation in various diseases.

References

1. Short analytical webnote 3/2015—Demography Report. http://ec.europa.eu/eurostat/statistics-explained/index.php/Population_structure_and_ageing#Further_Eurostat_information
2. Piau A, Campo E, Rumeau P et al (2014) Aging society and gerontechnology: a solution for an independent living? J Nutr Health Aging 18:97–112. doi:10.1007/s12603-013-0356-5
3. Micera S, Bonato P, Tamura T (2008) Gerontechnology. IEEE Eng Med Biol Mag 27(4):10. doi:10.1109/MEMB.2008.925213
4. Marschollek L (2012) Decision support at home (DS@HOME) – system architectures and requirements. BMC Med Inform Decis Mak 12:43
5. Arnrich B, Mayora O, Bardram J (2010) Pervasive or ubiquitous healthcare? Methods Inf Med 49:65–66. PubMed PMID: 20062946
6. Tiresias.org: http://www.tiresias.org/research/guidelines/smart_home.htm, quoting Smart Homes Association, i.bierhoff@smart-homes.nl, Eindhoven, The Netherlands
7. Kinsella A (1998) Home telecare in the United States. J Telemed Telecare 4:195–200
8. Ruggiero C, Sacile R, Giacomini M (1999) Home telecare. J Telemed Telecare 5:11–17
9. Bharucha AJ, Anand V, Forlizzi J et al (2009) Intelligent assistive technology applications to dementia care: current capabilities, limitations, and future challenges. Am J Geriatr Psychiatr 17:88–104. doi:10.1097/JGP.0b013e318187dde5
10. Adinolfi F, Caggianese G, Gallo L, Grosso J et al (2016) Smart care—an ICT platform in the domain of stroke pathology to manage rehabilitation treatment and telemonitoring at home. In: Proceedings of the Ninth International KES Conference on Intelligent Interactive Multimedia: Systems and Services, IIMSS 2016, Intelligent Interactive Multimedia Systems and Services, vol 55. Springer International Publishing, pp 39–49. doi:10.1007/978-3-319-39345-2_4
11. Marakas GM (1999) Decision support systems in the twenty-first century. Prentice Hall, Upper Saddle River, NJ
12. Tinetti ME, Fried T (2004) The end of the disease era. Am J Med 116:179–185
13. Sale P, Franceschini M, Mazzoleni S, Palma E et al (2014) Effects of upper limb robot-assisted therapy on motor recovery in subacute stroke patients. J Neuroeng Rehabil 11:104. doi:10.1186/1743-0003-11-104
14. Sale P, Mazzoleni S, Lombardi V, Galafate D, Massimiani MP et al (2014) Recovery of hand function with robot-assisted therapy in acute stroke patients: a randomized-controlled trial. Int J Rehabil Res 37:236–242. doi:10.1097/MRR.0000000000000059
15. Nijenhuis SM, Prange GB, Amirabdollahian F, Sale P et al (2015) Feasibility study into self-administered training at home using an arm and hand device with motivational gaming environment in chronic stroke. J Neuroeng Rehabil 12:89. doi:10.1186/s12984-015-0080-y
16. Sale P, Franceschini M, Waldner A, Hesse S (2012) Use of the robot assisted gait therapy in rehabilitation of patients with stroke and spinal cord injury. Eur J Phys Rehabil Med 48:111–121
17. Sale P, Russo EF, Russo M, Masiero S, Piccione F et al (2016) Effects on mobility training and de-adaptations in subjects with spinal cord injury due to a wearable robot: a preliminary report. BMC Neurol 16:12. doi:10.1186/s12883-016-0536-0.
18. Gwynne P (2013) Technology: mobility machines. Nature 503:S16–S17. doi:10.1038/503S16a
19. Stanford V (2002) Using pervasive computing to deliver elder care. IEEE Pervas Comput 1:10–13

Telemedicine and Physical Medicine

20

P. Rumeau

20.1 Relevance

Telemedicine is a way of practicing medicine, from a distance, with the use of information and communication technologies (ICTs).

At home, family physicians may refrain from referring to a geriatric rehabilitation specialist due to the long travel required. In institutions, residents usually have quality care (physical, occupational and speech therapists, psychologists, nursing), but physical medicine and specialized geriatric medicine are not usually available.

Geriatric rehabilitation medicine needs multidisciplinary work. But communication is difficult in practice. People available at the place of living of the patient and remote consultants cannot discuss the case together. Telemedicine is fostering collaboration; high level of academic knowledge on geriatrics, physical medicine, and care by the consultants may add to practical knowledge of the same and a better awareness of the patient's way of life by homecare professionals and family caregivers. Diagnosis and treatment can be customized to the patient's ecological needs.

20.2 Definitions

Telemedicine: The American Telemedicine Association (ATA) defines telemedicine as a clinical activity aiming at the direct improvement of the patient's condition [1].

Telehealth: It addresses the technical aspects, mostly network and organization.

P. Rumeau
Telemedicine Activity, Pôle Gériatrie du CHU de Toulouse, Toulouse, France
e-mail: rumeau.p@chu-toulouse.fr

© Springer International Publishing AG 2018

S. Masiero, U. Carraro (eds.), *Rehabilitation Medicine for Elderly Patients*, Practical Issues in Geriatrics, DOI 10.1007/978-3-319-57406-6_20

Telecare: It focuses on the place of living.

Digital medical records: These are required for telehealth but considered separately.

E-Health: For WHA "...eHealth is the cost-effective and secure use of information and communications technologies in support of health and health-related fields, including health-care services, health surveillance, health literature, and health education, knowledge and research..." [2].

Telecom: If there is no "signal" there is no telemedicine; therefore "no electricity" means "no telemedicine."

Bandwidth: It is the flow rate of information both in terms of emission (upload) or reception (download). We must be sure that the information will transfer completely and in a timely way; broadband ADSL is acceptable if access is good; otherwise warranted bandwidth is required.

Data: These include the medical information and functioning follow-up also called "**logs**" (e.g., who connected to the records, when, what they did). The medical information has to be available to both sides (applicant and consultant); each has rights to modify their part.

Server: Data servers do abide the personal data protection rules, are avoiding intrusion, and warrant safe conservation. Cloud applications are not yet eligible.

Meeting room or **point-to-point connections for videoconferencing (or audio)**: A point-to-point call, like a phone call, does not require any scheduling. Using a meeting room, each of the participants calls the same address on a server. It allows recording, access with a regular phone, technical monitoring, and support, but reservation is required.

PiP: "People in picture" is a small picture in a corner of the screen feeding back on what the other side is seeing. It is most useful to check one is seen (in the field of the camera with proper light). It gives the patient the feeling of controlling the image he is showing.

20.3 Legal and Ethical Issues

Most countries apply common medical rules to telemedicine. The 2004 legal definition in France used to put an emphasis on "perform medical acts in full respect of deontology but remotely" [3]. The main common legal aspect in telemedicine is the "medical" nature and the use of ICTs. The major consequence is that all the requirements derived from the oath of Cos in our legislations apply to telemedicine:

1. Those who practice telemedicine have to be fully qualified to perform a medical act on the remote patient where the patient stands. As an example, in the USA, only physicians from the armed forces can perform medical acts for military people all over the country, while civilian doctors can only work in the state where they are registered.

2. Telemedicine should be performed, isolated, or as part of a care process, only if the physician overseeing the act is thinking that telemedicine is for that patient, under the prevailing conditions, the most efficient or the most acceptable option.
3. The patient has the possibility to give, refuse, or withdraw his informed consent regarding the medical act itself but also the transfer and saving of his medical data.
4. The medical act has to be saved in the patient's medical records.

Regarding the use of ICTs, the physician should make sure that the technology is fit for telemedicine and covered by a guaranty by the service provider. The main issues with the technical service are the quality of the data transfer (not losing or corrupting information) and a security level sufficient to protect medical secrecy. Another issue is medicolegal responsibility: Are data saved efficiently and neutrally regarding the actors? In case of trouble, is it possible to know who did what and when, according to what information? Each participant bears full responsibility but only for what is his or hers business/responsibility.

The issue of responsibility may seem deterrent, but actually nothing is differing from consulting a patient referred by a colleague or prescribing rehabilitation. In daily practice, the legal risk is small because of better communication.

The patient's own physician is in charge of organizing care. Daily practice shows that if the patient's physician is, at least informed, at best involved, telemedicine is much more efficient.

Due to the multidisciplinary and the highly communicative nature of telemedicine, it is quite tempting to use it as a way of educating the participants. This is quite natural but ethical issues arise. The person presenting the case may wander out of the actual case for the sake of teaching and cause confusion with the care process. If real cases are used "real time," there is also a risk that a person attending might learn about the patient without his or her consent.

20.4 Telemedicine Acts in Geriatric Rehabilitation

- The patient is present and examined and/or cared during the act.
- The patient is not examined, and the diagnosis or therapeutic decisions are discussed on the medical records. The decision, regarding patient's health, may be synchronous, i.e., real-time discussion between the actors. Otherwise, it may be asynchronous: the question is sent with the records to the consulting specialist who answers without direct contact with the applicant.

See Table 20.1 for more details.

Table 20.1 Showing the different types of telemedicine relevant to geriatric rehabilitation

Applicant's side	Consultant's side	Activity	Example	Name of act
Patient ± medical ± paramedical staff	Medical staff ± paramedical staff	Examination	Stroke diagnosis	Consultation
Patient + medical or paramedical staff	Medical staff ± paramedical staff	Care or diagnosis procedure by local staff with remote guidance	Wound dressing	Medical assistance
Patient + medical or paramedical staff	Paramedical staff	Care or evaluation by local staff with remote guidance or support	Dementia diagnosis with a local psychologist	Paramedical assistance
Medical ± paramedical staff	Medical ± paramedical staff	Discussion on medical records and decision	Rehabilitation during palliative care	Synchronous expertise, staff, multidisciplinary meeting
Medical ± paramedical staff	Medical	Answer on medical records and advice	Adapting anti-thrombotic treatment in a patient already known to the consultant	Asynchronous expertise
Patient ± paramedical staff	Rehabilitation staff	Rehabilitation	Speech therapy with no speech therapist available on site	Rehabilitation
Information from a medical device "with" patient	Medical staff	Remote follow-up of a parameter or vital sign	Monitoring of weight in heart failure patient	Monitoring

20.5 The Process of a Telemedicine Act

A telemedicine act is a sequence of actions. We will describe the process that was implemented at Gérontopôle Toulouse (France) for patients from nursing home partners of the telemedicine project (Fig. 20.1).

The nursing home asks for a telemedicine appointment during the follow-up of a patient of Gérontopôle or as a first time expertise. The patient may be referred by the nursing home (i.e., by the nursing staff with the agreement of the patient's family physician and in collaboration with the coordination physician in case of chronic wounds, behavior problems, etc.) or by the patient's physician (in case of difficult diagnosis). The applicant contacts the coordination assistant (CA) by phone or secure email. The CA organizes for all the actors to be available, checks records are properly transmitted, organizes the availability of the "meeting room," and emails the date of the appointment and the directions to get connected. If advice is required on the most adequate consultant for the case, the CA will refer to the physician in charge of coordinating the telemedicine activity for proper choice.

At the said time, the actors connect. All, but only, the persons relevant to the case of the patient are present. Being in time is most important. Both sides check they can see and hear one another (PiP), everybody greets each other, patient first if present. The consultant notes all the persons attending with their profession or role. The act proper starts. This may include discussion of films, pictures, or X-rays presented during the act. When an agreement is reached by the participants on the diagnosis and treatments, the consultant writes a report on the telemedicine medical records (TMR), as an answer to the request form from the applicant. The applicant gets the report on the TMR and adds it to the patient's records.

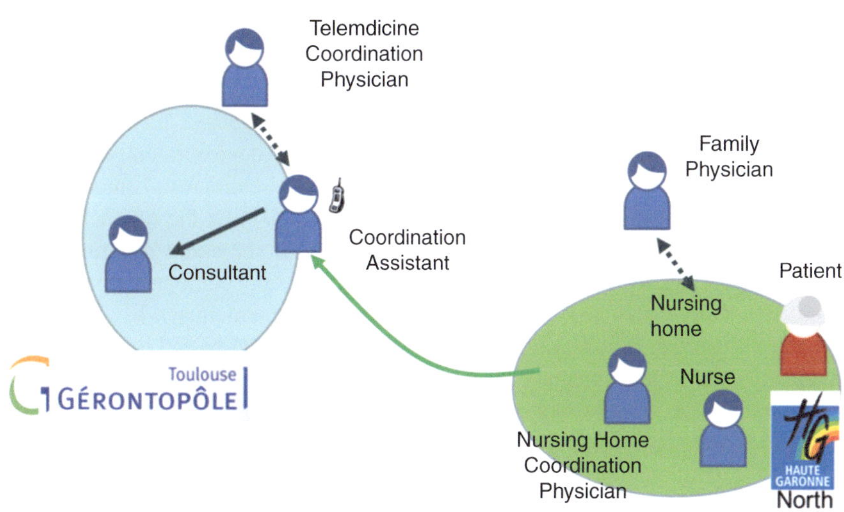

Fig. 20.1 UML diagram of actors for the provision of telemedicine for nursing homes in the north of Haute Garonne by Gérontopôle. *Full arrows* are showing compulsory participations, *dotted arrows* are showing conditional participations

20.6 Case 1: Physical Medicine in Palliative Care

Mr. B, 88 years old, has a medical history of diabetes mellitus under insulin treatment, widespread atheroma, and vascular dementia. He is referred by his GP for chronic wounds of the toes since a month and a half. A first tele-expertise is organized with the chief nurse. The pictures are provided via the TMR, and the discussion leads to a diagnosis of distal gangrene (I and II on the left, II and III on the right) and mixed pressure and ischemic, stage IV, sore (right M5 basis). Mummification of the toes and, on the fifth metatarsal, leaving the hydrogel for longer lasting wound debridement, is agreed. Morphine before dressing and adapted shoes are prescribed. One month later, the wounds have evolved as expected. The patient can stand and walk two paces without pain. However, 2 weeks later, the family says they don't want the patient to walk; this causes a major setback of patient's capabilities and the genuflexum worsens. Therefore, we agree for aided standing to lessen patient's ischemic muscle pain of lower limbs.

One month later, the physical therapist (PT) is present at the meeting, and the patient can stand by himself with no pain. The flexum, unfortunately, could not be avoided and is a limit to walk. The patient will eventually die of heart complication.

The patient would not have been able to stand repeated hospital transfers. Thanks to telemedicine, fostered by the patient's GP, he had appropriate care through global multidisciplinary management without moving from the place where he lived. This has spared him pain and has allowed him to stand and walk a bit, which he seemed to enjoy.

20.7 Case 2: Electric Wheelchair Prescription for a Patient Living at Home with a Cognitive and Motor Degeneration

Mrs. C, 75 years old, lives at home and has been diagnosed a frontotemporal degeneration with aphasia and motor control limitation (right hemiparesis) since 3 years. The patient is referred by the occupational therapist (OT) of the dementia home rehabilitation team. The patient's daughter had asked if she could benefit from an electric wheelchair for better autonomy indoors and easier social participation outdoors. Mrs. C lives in a ground floor flat; she cannot use a manual wheel chair outdoors due to fatigue. The testing by the PT shows a fair control and limited apraxia on the upper limbs and a major walk apraxia. The evaluation by the speech therapist shows an anterior aphasia with preserved work and procedural memory. Learning capabilities are also spared.

The OT, who attends the telemedicine session with the patient's daughter, provides a filmed evaluation of the test use of an electric wheelchair: home navigation, transfers, avoidance of obstacles, and observation of patient's strategy in case of double task. After discussion, the electric wheelchair is prescribed; it later proved to be a successful strategy.

Telemedicine allowed in this case a joint home evaluation by OT and physiatrist.

20.8 Case 3: Pressure Sore Healing and Beyond

Mrs. T, 90 years old, lives in a remote country nursing home; she was first referred to our day hospital because she was bedridden and had developed a sacral pressure sore. We found global lower limbs failure without spasticity, and diffuse arthrosis, dementia, and hyperthyroidism were suspected. She complained of pain, her motor scheme was greatly perturbed, and she had a major fear of walking. Her mood was bad.

Physiotherapy targeted muscle strengthening of the lower limbs and closed-chain seated work to improve proprioception while avoiding joint pain.

Two weeks later, during tele-expertise assessment, her nutritional status is improved, hyperthyroidism is confirmed, and treatment is started.

One month later, the patient can stand for a short time with some support. She is limited by shoulder and knee pain.

The next month, the PT attends the session: force is improved but there is a distal hamstring tendonitis associated to femoro-tibial osteoarthritis. This time, she receives topical anti-inflammatories on the lateral knee and is referred to day hospital.

Testing with intra-articular lidocaine confirms the intra-articular origin of pain; a lack of force (quadriceps 3−/5) is still present after analgesia. As a consequence to the day hospital, she receives viscosupplementation in a separate outpatient appointment (sodium hyaluronate 10 mg for 2 ml).

The next telemedicine session is attended by the patient herself, her PT, the coordinating physician, and head nurse of the nursing home: the patient has benefited from an increased weekly number of physiotherapy sessions, she walks over 10 m with a walker, she washes in the bathroom (instead of her bed) with some assistance, she needs some help for the transfers, and her nutritional status is improving while her hyperthyroidism is under control. Eventually, her diagnosis of dementia proved to be wrong: she had overcome her depression, and there remained no cognitive deficit. The pressure sore healed fully.

20.9 Implementation

Technology is not a problem anymore; however, telemedicine is still scarcely used: a change in medical practice is often complicated.

In this paragraph, we propose a "to-do" list, in order to help those who wish to develop a telemedicine activity:

- Contact colleagues with practical experience.
- Assess medical needs as opposed to fashion.

- Get the stakeholders involved from the early stages of the reflection (find motivated local opinion leaders) and get the required political support.
- On the one hand, do not overestimate the expected activity level. In the beginning, you will have increased work to resorb prevalence of the problem you are addressing, but then only the incidence will drive the activity.
- On the other hand, do not underestimate the impact of telemedicine: mentoring effect can spread knowledge and good practices. Another benefit is that improved care can reduce burden for the staff.
- Make sure you will get the proper workforce including support personnel and medical service provision (volunteering medical and paramedical staff with dedicated time slots).
- Get the proper procedures and agreements in order to integrate telemedicine to the rest of the healthcare system and to make the regulatory tracing easier.
- Don't forget patients' information and consent, including when the family or a legal representative is involved.
- Take into account that telemedicine requires funding before the first profits can materialize. Think about what type of indexes you are going to provide to prove your activity is worth the expense.

Conclusion

The major limit to telemedicine development is still the generally poor market model. In countries with a national health service, the issue is the funding priorities and care accessibility; in the countries where medicine is mostly private, the question is how (and how much) the patient will pay. In those countries that follow a Bismarck model, insurance companies have to make a decision according to the benefits they expect in terms of savings and confronting these benefits to the affordability of the technical infrastructures.

Telemedicine fully deserves its position within the array of medical services. It facilitates multidisciplinary teamwork, and this is relevant in care and rehabilitation of sick and handicapped elderly people who live in nursing homes or receive home services. In our experience, telemedicine, as a part of the care flow for older people, is highly beneficial and worth the effort.

To date, telemedicine research is slowly shifting from proving acceptability and feasibility to proving medical efficiency; however scientific works in this domain are still scarce. The reasons are multiple: scientific, ethical, and practical. Means are limited, and evidence-based medicine proofs are costly and require a normalized population (much unlike those we care for). Shouldn't we use, as we start, well-documented medical cases with discussion of the related literature to prove its efficacy? And then, when we will have enough activity to compare the data, could we improve the proof level using proper benchmarking with relevant selection criteria and markers?

"Take-Home Ideas"

Telemedicine is a medical activity.

Regular medical deontology and rules apply to telemedicine.

Telemedicine fosters multidisciplinary work.

A telemedicine act requires proper recording.

Physicians should only practice telemedicine with dedicated/fit technology.

Telemedicine is deployed to optimize care processes: it has to respect medical uses and customs.

Funding is a major issue.

References

1. http://www.americantelemed.org/about-telemedicine/what-is-telemedicine. Last accessed 18/07/2016
2. WHA58.28 eHealth, Ninth plenary meeting, 25 May 2005 – Committee A, seventh report, http://apps.who.int/iris/bitstream/10665/20378/1/WHA58_28-en.pdf?ua=1. Last accessed 06.09.2016
3. LOI n° 2004-810 du 13 août 2004 relative à l'assurance maladie. JORF n°190 du 17 août 2004 page 14598, texte n° 2

The Role of Nutrition in Rehabilitation of Older Adults

21

Cornel C. Sieber

21.1 Introduction

Orthogeriatric patients, one of the most frequent patient groups within geriatric rehabilitation units as well as patient post stroke—for dysphagia, see special chapter—often have nutritional problems. According to the screening and assessment methods used, the prevalence is 38–68% for the risk of malnutrition and 9–37% for overt malnutrition [1–4]. Malnutrition per se is already a risk factor for falls and fractures. Importantly, malnutrition in orthogeriatric patients is linked to a worse outcome with negative consequences both for positive rehabilitative results as well as for quality of life [1, 3, 5]. Inversely, the awareness of nutritional problems in this frail patient group in the rehabilitative setting is low.

Management of nutritional problems also includes, besides an adequate qualitative and quantitative intake of macro- and micronutrients, the patient's preferences as well as a sufficient fluid intake. As a matter of fact, older adults often show low fluid intake as thirst is usually diminishing with aging. Moreover, they often decrease their fluid intake to lower urine production and, therefore, the need for toileting (with or without help). All these factors increase the possibility of dehydration. Dehydration on the other hand is a risk factor for constipation, renal failure, falls, and also delirium.

The risk for and overt malnutrition are very frequent in this patient group of (ortho)geriatric patients. Especially in the rehabilitation setting, the patients often have not eaten enough before they were transferred to the rehabilitation center. Malnutrition is correlated with worse outcomes and even mortality in this care

C.C. Sieber
Direktor des Institut für Biomedizin des Alterns Friedrich-Alexander-Universität Erlangen-Nürnberg, Erlangen, Germany
e-mail: Cornel.sieber@fau.de

© Springer International Publishing AG 2018

S. Masiero, U. Carraro (eds.), *Rehabilitation Medicine for Elderly Patients*, Practical Issues in Geriatrics, DOI 10.1007/978-3-319-57406-6_21

setting. Patients with signs of malnutrition experience longer periods of rehabilitation to regain functional independence [6].

21.1.1 Sarcopenia, Frailty, and Cachexia

21.1.1.1 Sarcopenia

Sarcopenia is present when there is a less-than-expected muscle mass in an individual of a specified age, gender, and race [7]. Sarcopenia has emerged as a core concept to understand function and by that independence in older age. As muscle mass counts for about 40% of body mass, its decline with age is not just a part of senescence. In sarcopenia, the muscle is replaced by other tissue types, especially fat mass. After the age of 50 years, about 1–2% of muscle mass is lost every year. In addition, muscle strength decreases even faster with age, demonstrating that muscle mass is only partially responsible for strength and functionality in old age.

Even though the focus of sarcopenia research has mainly been concentrated to locomotion (e.g., gait speed, falls), muscle tissue is abundant and important in other body tissues. Loss of muscle mass in these organs also hampers functionality in affected persons. As for frailty (see below), sarcopenia may aggravate other diseases as well as their prognosis by negatively influencing their progress. Such diseases include congestive heart failure, chronic obstructive lung disease, diabetes mellitus, chronic kidney disease, diabetes mellitus, and even stroke and dementia. All these diseases are often part of the multimorbidity as seen in patients in a rehabilitation setting.

International consensus conferences have agreed on the definition of sarcopenia [8–11]. It always contains the measurements of the muscle mass (mainly by densitometry (DXA) or by bio-impedance analysis (BIA) (8.9) (Table 21.1). In addition—and this is different for example to the diagnosis of osteoporosis—a functional decline has also to be diagnosed. Here, either gait speed or handgrip strength is accepted. For more details, please see also the respective separate chapter in this book.

An upcoming clinical challenge is the fast growing overweight or obese population, which is also often seen in older adults. Even if their body mass index may be high, this does not exclude that these persons suffer in parallel of a sarcopenia, with even worse consequences for functionality. This indeed unhealthy combination is called sarcopenic obesity [12]. Even we understand more and more the pathophysiology behind sarcopenia, the diagnosis is still a matter of debate as the specific therapy [13]. This entity may even be combined with osteoporosis, now called osteosarcopenia [14].

Table 21.1 Sarcopenia according to the European Working Group on Sarcopenia [10]

Decrease muscle mass (mainly measured by DXA or BIA)
Plus
Decreased gait speed (0.8 m/s) and/or decreased handgrip strength

21.1.1.2 Frailty

Frailty may be regarded as a geriatric syndrome of decreased reserve and resistance to stressors, resulting from cumulative declines across multiple physiologic systems, causing vulnerability to adverse health outcomes including falls, hospitalization, institutionalization, and mortality. Concepts on the pathophysiological background of the frailty syndrome focus on inflammatory processes, hormonal changes, and body composition.

Nevertheless, some characteristics of frailty apply for normal aging like reduced physiologic reserve, decreased organ function and functional reserve, and loss of complexity. According to some authors, it might therefore not be possible to distinguish frailty unambiguously from advanced stages of the aging process.

The two most widely utilized approaches are the phenotypic definition of frailty developed by Fried and co-workers based on data from the Cardiovascular Health Survey [15] and the Frailty Index developed by Rockwood and co-workers [16]. The Fried definition proposes five items: weight loss, exhaustion, weakness, slow walking speed, and low levels of physical activity [15]. Frailty is diagnosed when at least three criteria are met. An individual is said to be pre-frail when one or two of these criteria are present.

A series of studies concentrated on the relationship between nutrition and frailty. It was shown that frailty is significantly associated with a daily energy intake below 21 kcal/kg body weight as well as a low protein intake [17]. The simultaneous prevalence of more than one vitamin deficiency was also significantly higher for the pre-frail and frail individuals.

Based on the results of several recent studies, the criterion weight loss may be regarded as one-dimensional. Weight loss in an obese person may have different consequences—both for morbidity and mortality—as in normal or even underweight older adults. Furthermore, the weight loss thresholds given in the Fried criteria may be too high for a European population, as shown in a study in community-dwelling older persons [18].

For the calculation of the Frailty Index by Rockwood, it is necessary to count prespecified deficits that are present in an individual [15, 18, 19]. In the most extensive study regarding this topic, Rockwood and co-workers have published yet 70 deficits that were used for the evaluation. These included active diseases, ability in the activities of daily living, and physical signs from the clinical and neurological examinations. The presence of a deficit scored 1. Theoretically, but not practically, a maximum score of 70 was possible. The Frailty Index is the score of present deficits divided by 70. The highest number of deficits the authors found in any setting was 47. Both the Fried and Rockwood Frailty criteria have recently been shown to be associated with incident disability and mortality in community-dwelling people and nursing home inhabitants.

21.1.1.3 Cachexia

Protein-energy malnutrition (PEM) has first been described as a severe clinical problem in the 1980s and 1990s with a fast increasing understanding of its pathophysiological background. Increasing research to tackle this problem came out of oncology, where cancer-associate PEM was strongly related to inflammatory processes (such as an increase in tumor necrosis factor-alpha). Even more importantly, it was and still is well known that this high inflammatory load renders nutritional treatment successes disappointing [20]. Cachexia was then defined as disease-related loss of body cell mass, not necessarily linked with concurrent weight loss. In contrast, weight loss irrespective of the effects on body composition is termed wasting disorders, and the involuntary age-associated non-disease-related—e.g., age-specific—muscle loss was called sarcopenia.

21.2 Nutrition and Fluid Demands

21.2.1 Nutritional Demands

On average, an older adult needs 25–30 kcal per kilogram body weight per day. This may be increased in catabolic states (e.g., infection, pressure sores). In hyperactive dementia patients, the caloric needs may also be significantly increased.

Protein demands are also increased in frail older adults and surpass the WHO recommendations for younger healthy adults quite a bit. So, the usual recommended 0.8 grams of protein per kilogram body weight per day have to be increased to 1.0–1.2 grams per kilogram body weight per day [21]. In the rehabilitation setting after longer catabolic periods, these demands may even go up to 1.5 proteins per kilogram body weight per day. Malnutrition in older adults after a hip fracture is indeed a bad prognostic factor "quoad"survival [22]. Older adults still have a good anabolic capacity, but the proportion of protein intake and the body protein anabolism shows a faster ceiling effect. This is why the protein intake has to be distributed over the day, at least between the main meals [23]. If this is not possible through a normal diet (even after fortification), the positive effects of oral supplements are well documented [24]. It may well be that specific oral supplements for sarcopenic patients will not only increase muscle mass but also functionality, even without an additional physical exercise program, as recently shown [25].

Micronutrient needs are usually covered when usual diet is eaten. As a rule of thumb, micronutrient deficits can be expected if a person eats less than 1200 kcal per kilogram per day over a longer period, which may be in times of a severe acute illness and then subsequently a rehabilitation period of several weeks. It is only in these cases when micronutrients need to be replaced.

21.2.2 Fluid Demands

As an overall quantity, the daily fluid intake should be between 1500 and 2000 mL. Nevertheless, many older adults—especially women—never drank this quantity during their previous adult life. So, a personal "fluid intake biography" should always be performed. As thirst tends to decrease during the normal aging process, older adults should be informed about the importance of an adequate fluid intake and be stimulated to have a drink whenever possible.

Diuretics—especially hydrochlorothizide—are not only often prescribed for both systolic hypertension and peripheral edema but are also not reevaluated if still needed in the long course. This may, besides the often induced hyponatremia, aggravate exsiccosis in times when fluid intake is especially important as in hot summer days.

The danger of exsiccosis is also frequently not seen in its consequences such as the propensity to falls. In the acute setting, fluid restriction and exsiccosis are important risk factors for delirium, especially in patients with an existing cognitive deficit.

21.3 Assessment of Malnutrition and Fluid Intake

21.3.1 Overall

As an insufficient intake of both nutrients and fluid is very frequent in the acute and rehabilitation setting in older adults, therefore, intake of both components should be documented, starting from the first day of admission in the institution. In addition, a screening for risk or overt malnutrition should be performed early during the hospitalization phase.

21.3.2 Mini Nutritional Assessment (MNA^{R}) and Nutritional Risk Screening (NRS 2002)

The Mini Nutritional Assessment (MNA^{R}) is the only screening and assessment test for malnutrition especially developed for an older person/patient group. There exists a full form as well as a short form (MNA^{R}-SF), taking around 5 min to be performed [4] (freely available under www.mna-elderly.com). Its global practicability has been well documented and has even received much more use since when body mass index (BMI) is not available; it can be replaced by calf circumference (Table 21.2). Using this screening test, the highest prevalence for risk and overt malnutrition is found in the rehabilitation setting, pointing out how important especially nutrition is in this postacute period of older adults. If this screening test is positive, one needs to add an in-depth assessment for possible treatable causes of malnutrition.

The Nutritional Risk Screening (NRS 2002) has been developed for the acute care setting and screens for those patients who will profit from a nutritional intervention during the hospital stay [26]. Is also takes only a few minutes. Whereas the MNA^{R} is more adapted for older adults, it may well be that patients are transferred from the acute care setting with a result of the NRS 2002, depending on local structures and preferences. This does not preclude that the MNA^{R} can be performed

Table 21.2 The Mini Nutritional Assessment (MNA^{R}-SF) [4]

This screening test consists of six items:

- Reduced nutritional intake within the last 3 months
- Loss of body weight within the last 3 months
- Reduced mobility within the last 3 months
- Acute disease or psychological stress within the last 3 months
- Neuropsychological problems (depression/dementia) within the last 3 months
- Actual BMI or calf circumference (CC <31 cm)

shortly after the patient is admitted to the rehabilitation center, as the test includes in its six questions one question for mobility and one for mood changes (depression and/or dementia). Indeed, when comparing the two sets in the same population, the MNA^R seems to better capture the problems in the older patient group.

When summarizing simple parameters for the screening for malnutrition in older adults, the following can be said [27]:

- An unintended weight loss of >5% of body weight within the last 3 months or >10% within the last 6 months
- A clearly reduced body mass (fat and muscle mass): body mass index (BMI) <20 kg/m^2 (please notice: the cutoff is higher in older adults than in younger ones, where the value is <18.5 kg/m^2)
- MNA^R-SF <8 points (out of 14 possible ones)

It is therefore helpful to use a checklist when searching for insufficient nutritional or fluid intake (Table 21.3).

Table 21.3 Checklist to diagnose potential insufficient food or fluid intake and malnutrition [28]

Physical limitations
• Appetite and thirst loss
• Chewing problems
• Dysphagia
• Inadequate dental status
• Eating or drinking problems due to limitations in the upper limb(s)
• Severe tiredness
• Heavily reduced vision
Psychological limitations
• Cognitive decline/dementia
• Depression
• Delirium
Diseases with impact on appetite and/or metabolism
• Diseases of the gastrointestinal tract
• Food intolerance
• Diseases with increased caloric demand (cancer, surgical intervention, pressure ulcer, dementia with hyperactivity, thyroid disease, AIDS)
Drug intake
• >5 drugs per day
• Drug with adverse side effects related to food intake (reduction of appetite, change in olfactorial and smelling capacity, nausea, dry mouth, severe tiredness, dizziness)
Additional factors
• Fear of aggravation of a preexisting existing incontinence
• Problems with toileting
• In acceptance of offered food (cultural or religious background)
• Unusual eating times
• Time pressure during meals
• Inconvenient eating situations (investigations during meal times, smell, noise)
• Insufficient food choices
• Phobia to stay slim

21.4 Interventions

21.4.1 Normal Nutritional Intake

Oral nutrition and fluid intake should be promoted in each patient both in the acute and rehabilitation setting according to his or her demands and skills [27–29]. They are summarized in Table 21.4.

Often, the patients already have a risk for malnutrition or show overt malnutrition when entering the rehabilitation center. It is crucial that during the rehabilitation phase, food and fluid intake is a cornerstone of the treatment plan besides physical activity. It is therefore important not to interrupt the meals for ward rounds or investigations. These should and can be planned during times, when not the usual meals are served. If ever possible, each patient should have the same nurse for such a long period as possible, as this nursing expert knows the skills and wishes of the patient with regard to eating and drinking, a very personal biographic part of all of us. People eat more in groups and therefore, meals should be offered to the patient in a dining room, when possible. Food intake in itself can also be well used to train tasks, sometimes with the help of an ergotherapist. As food intake can be very time-consuming and needs a lot of "hands," volunteers can be organized with proven success.

The type of provided food is also an important issue to be considered. The following tasks should be fulfilled:

- In general, a normal full diet should be offered, taking specific preferences of the patient into account ("eating biography").
- Restrictive diets should be avoided or stopped, even in overweight older adults, as they mainly loss muscle and not fat mass when dieting.
- The (temporal) need for specific diets should be considered (protein-rich, adaptive diets due to allergies, severe liver, and kidney diseases).
- Existing chewing and swallowing problems should be diagnosed, and food items with adapted food consistency be offered.

Table 21.4 This table summarizes strategies to promote fluid and energy (nutritional) intake

• Constant availability of drinks in the reach of the patient; if necessary, bottles should be opened and the fluid put in glasses adapted to the patient motoric skills
• Different types of drinks (water, soft drinks, fruit juices, tea, etc.) should be offered
• Patient has to be repetitively motivated to drink
• Patient and caregivers have to be informed about the danger of exsiccosis
• Ensure that the patient drinks in sitting position, preferentially at the table
• Patient and caregivers have to be informed about the danger of undernutrition
• Motivate the patient to eat
• Prepare the food (we also eat with our eyes! If needed, cut the food into small pieces)
• Help the patient when eating; if necessary, feed the patient
• Eating takes its time—provide enough time for the meals
• Do not disturb the patient during the meals
• Provide food between the main meals; stimulate the patient for these meals and provide help when needed

21.4.2 Postdischarge Management of Nutritional Intake

Loss of weight, body weight at admission and discharge, body mass index (or calf circumference), as well as the result of screening (MNA-SF and/or NRS 2002 or of another screening instrument) and consequently a nutritional assessment should be included in the discharge letter in a standardized fashion. In all those patients with signs of malnutrition, as well as decreased caloric and fluid intake, specific recommendations should be part of the discharge letter too. These should include recommendations to treat or compensate for problems leading to malnutrition (e.g., to see a dentist, or nutritional supplements, finger food, protein fortification, adaptation of food consistencies when swallowing problems are apparent, eating aids when motor disabilities exist).

In addition, reevaluation of the nutritional state by either the general practitioner or nursing personnel should be performed after 3 and 6 months postdischarge. As the discharge letter by the treating doctor is often not seen by the nursing staff (especially when the patient changes his living condition as, for example, from community-dwelling to nursing home), the factors mentioned above should also be part of the documentation of the nursing staff between the institutions.

Key Points

- In order to improve the pre- and post-interventional nutritional management (most often related to an orthogeriatric intervention), it is first important to search for a nutritional problem and, whenever possible, to start an adapted treatment.
- Awareness and the respective search for the risk or even an overt malnutrition and an inadequate fluid intake should be screened for early in the rehabilitation setting.
- When the screening shows a risk situation, a thorough assessment should be started in order to search for treatable causes and to look upon the specific patient demands.
- As soon a nutritional risk situation is found, an adapted intervention—often with protein-rich oral supplements—should be installed.
- Sarcopenia is often present before the acute illness—e.g., a fragility fracture—and therefore, nutritional intervention should be continued also after discharge from a rehabilitation center.

References

1. Nuotio M, Tuominen P, Luukkaala T (2016) Association of nutritional status as measured by the Mini-Nutritional Assessment Short Form with changes in mobility, institutionalization and death after hip fracture. Eur J Clin Nutr 70:393–398
2. Goisser S, Schrader E, Singler K et al (2015) Malnutrition according to Mini Nutritional Assessment (MNA) is associated with severe functional impairment in geriatric patients before and up to 6 months after hip fracture. J Am Med Dir Assoc 16:661–667

3. Drevet S, Bioteau C, Mazière S et al (2014) Prevalence of protein-energy malnutrition in hospital patients over 75 years of age admitted for hip fracture. Orthop Traumatol Surg Res 100:669–674
4. Kaiser MJ et al; MNA-International Group (2009) Validation of the Mini Nutritional Assessment short-form (MNA-SF): a practical tool for identification of nutritional status. J Nutr Health Aging 13:782–788
5. Hooper L et al (2014) Water-loss dehydration and aging. Mech Ageing Dev 136–137:50–58
6. Koren-Hakim T et al (2012) The relationship between nutritional status of hip fracture operated elderly patients and their functioning, comorbidity and outcome. Clin Nutr 31:917–921
7. Rosenberg IH (1997) Sarcopenia: origins and clinical relevance. J Nutr 127(5 Suppl):990S–991S
8. Baumgartner R, Koehler KM, Gallagher D, Romero L, Heymsfield SB, Ross RR, Garry PJ, Lindeman RD (1998) Epidemiology of sarcopenia among the elderly in New Mexico. Am J Epidemiol 147:755–763
9. Janssen I, Heymsfield SB, Robert R (2002) Low relative skeletal muscle mass (sarcopenia) in older persons is associated with functional impairment and physical disability. J Am Geriatr Soc 50:889–896
10. Cruz-Jentoft A, Baeyens JP, Bauer J et al (2010) Sarcopenia: European consensus on definition and diagnosis. Age Ageing 39:412–423
11. Muscaritoli M, Anker SD, Argiles J et al (2010) Consensus definition of sarcopenia, cachexia and pre-cachexia: joint document elaborated by Special Interest Groups (SIG) "cachexia-anorexia in chronic wasting diseases" and "nutrition in geriatrics". Clin Nutr 29:154–159
12. Zamboni M, Mazzali G, Fantin F et al (2008) Sarcopenic obesity: a new category of obesity in the elderly. Nutr Metab Cardiovasc Dis 18:388–395
13. Goisser S, Kemmler W, Porzel S et al (2015) Sarcopenic obesity and complex interventions with nutrition and exercise in community-dwelling older persons – a narrative review. Clin Interv Aging 10:1267–1282
14. Drey M, Sieber CC, Bertsch T et al (2016) Osteosarcopenia is more than sarcopenia and osteoporosis alone. Aging Clin Exp Res 28:895–899
15. Fried LP, Tangen CM, Walston J et al; Cardiovascular Health Study Collaborative Research Group (2001) J Gerontol A Biol Sci Med Sci 56:M146–M156
16. Rockwood K, Mogilner A, Mitnitski A (2004) Changes with age in the distribution of a frailty index. Mech Ageing Dev 125:517–519
17. Bartali B, Frongillo EA, Bandinelli S et al (2006) Low nutrient intake is an essential component of frailty in older persons. J Gerontol Med Sci 61A:589–593
18. Drey M, Wehr H, Wehr G et al (2011) The frailty syndrome in general practitioner care: a pilot study. Z Gerontol Ger 44:48–54
19. Rockwood K, Andrew M, Mitnitski A (2007) A comparison of two approaches to measuring frailty in elderly people. J Gerontol A Biol Sci Med Sci 62(7):738–743
20. Evans WJ, Morley JE, Argiles J et al (2008) Cachexia: a new definition. Clin Nutr 27:793–799
21. Bauer J, Biolo G, Cederholm T et al (2013) Evidence-based recommendations for optimal dietary protein intake in older people: a position paper from the PROT-AGE Study Group. J Am Med Dir Assoc 14:542–549
22. Goisser S, Schrader E, Singler K et al (2015) Low postoperative intake is associated with worse functional course in geriatric patients up to 6 months after hip fracture. Br J Nutr 113:1940–1950
23. Paddon-Jones D, Rasmussen HH (2009) Dietary protein recommendations and the prevention of sarcopenia. Curr Opin Clin Nutr Metab 12:86–90
24. Milne AC, Potter J, Vivanti A et al (2009) Protein and energy supplementation in elderly people at risk from malnutrition. Cochrane Database Syst Rev 2:CD003288
25. Bauer JM, Verlaan S, Bautmans I et al (2015) Effects of a vitamin D and leucine-enriched whey protein nutritional supplement on measures of sarcopenia in older adults, the PROVIDE study: a randomized, double-blind, placebo-controlled trial. J Am Med Dir Assoc 16:740–747

26. Kondrup J, Rasmussen HH, Hamberg O et al (2003) Nutritional risk screening (NRS 2002): a new method based on an analysis of controlled clinical trials. Clin Nutr 22:321–336
27. Cederholm T, Barazzoni R, Austin P et al (2016) ESPEN guidelines on definitions and terminology in clinical nutrition. Clin Nutr 36(1):49–64. pii: S0251-5614(16)31242-0
28. Volkert D et al (2013) Leitlinie der Deutschen Gesellschaft für Ernährungsmedizin (DGEM) in Zusammenarbeit mit der GESKES, der AKE und der DG: Klinische Ernährung in der Geriatrie. Aktuell Ernährungsmedizin 38:e1–e48
29. Huxtable S, Palmer M (2013) The efficacy of protected mealtimes in reducing mealtime interruptions and improving mealtime assistance in adult inpatients in an Australian hospital. Eur J Clin Nutr 67:904–910

22 Elderly Rehabilitation: A Clinical and Drug-Related Approach

Giulia Bellon, Marina De Rui, Nicola Veronese, Enzo Manzato, and Giuseppe Sergi

22.1 Introduction

Most of the elderly patients admitted to rehabilitation wards have undergone major orthopedic surgery due to trauma or to chronic degenerative or inflammatory conditions. Others will have neurological disorders or have experienced acute vascular events, such as ischemic or hemorrhagic stroke, or they may have had neurosurgical procedures.

All these patients will have more or less severe issues in terms of their neurological and joint functionality, which lead to impairments in their activities of daily living.

The early mobilization of elderly patients after surgery, or the remobilization of patients who have experienced long-term immobilization, can modify the unstable balance typical of aging and contain the risk of cardiovascular, respiratory, and musculoskeletal disorders.

In this context, rehabilitators need to take into account the numerous factors associated with aging and particularly elderly patients' typically high morbidity rates, use of multiple therapies, limited functional reserves, and access to social support.

G. Bellon
Department of Neuroscience, Rehabilitation Unit, University of Padua, Padua, Italy
e-mail: giulia.bellon@studenti.unipd.it

M. De Rui • N. Veronese • E. Manzato • G. Sergi (✉)
Department of Medicine, Geriatrics Division, University of Padua, Padua, Italy
e-mail: giuseppe.sergi@unipd.it

© Springer International Publishing AG 2018

S. Masiero, U. Carraro (eds.), *Rehabilitation Medicine for Elderly Patients*, Practical Issues in Geriatrics, DOI 10.1007/978-3-319-57406-6_22

22.2 Features of the Elderly Admitted to Rehabilitation Wards

Although orthopedic and neurological patients admitted to rehabilitation wards may have similar features, there is some difference between the two groups that rehabilitators should bear in mind in order to design appropriate rehabilitation programs, also considering patients' different diseases and different use of medication.

Rehabilitators must take responsibility for adapting the therapies they administer to the specific needs of the elderly. Patients arriving from neurology wards may suffer from newly diagnosed diseases that may have caused the acute event. TIA and ischemic stroke cause cerebral hypoxia, and cerebral or carotid atherosclerosis, or cardiac embolism due to arrhythmias, is the most often encountered etiology. In this setting, atrial fibrillation—with a prevalence of about 9% in individuals over 80 [1]—is the most common rhythm disorder. Such patients usually take antiplatelet (acetylsalicylic acid [ASA], clopidogrel) or anticoagulant (warfarin, new oral anticoagulants) drugs.

Hemorrhagic strokes, on the other hand, are caused by cerebral arteriovenous malformations; aneurysms; hypertensive crises associated with untreated, inadequately treated, or refractory hypertension; or an inadequate management of anticoagulant drugs. Subdural hematoma may require neurosurgery or a better control of blood pressure (with ACE inhibitors, angiotensin II receptor blockers [ARBs], beta-blockers, or calcium channel blockers).

Acute events can lead to different complications. Central hypoxic damage often impairs various functions in the hemisoma contralateral to the site of the lesion, giving rise to movement disorders (hemiparesis, hemiplegia), hypertonia, hypotonia, or impairment of somatic sensitivity. Speech disorders, balance impairments, and a disrupted coordination are other possible sequelae. Damage involving the brain stem may lead to cranial nerve disorders, with diplopia, blurred vision, bulbar weakness, dysphagia, or facial nerve damage.

The different consequences for patients with neurological issues depend on their specific clinical condition. Diaphragm or vocal cord paralysis can impair respiratory function, paving the way to a hypoxic state. Hemiplegia raises the risk of bedsores. Dysphagia may cause aspiration pneumonia.

Rehabilitators should take into account all the clinical problems that may develop in patients with neurological disorders and try to optimize their management, adapting the available therapeutic strategies to their different conditions.

Patients arriving from an orthopedic ward are characterized by the consequences of surgery and the presence of chronic diseases. In case of fractures after falls, rehabilitators should look out for trigger disorders (malnutrition, dehydration, electrolyte imbalance, osteoporosis, sarcopenia), in an effort not only to optimize a patient's management but also to prevent further acute events.

Malnutrition is an inadequate intake of macro- and micronutrients (calories, protein, vitamins, and minerals) that can be caused by functional impairments (presbyphagia) or organic disorders, but dietary or environmental factors may be involved too. Malnutrition affects 20–30% of elderly people.

Sarcopenia is characterized by a loss of muscle mass, muscle weakness, or declining physical performance. The prevalence of sarcopenia reportedly ranges from 10% to nearly 50% in individuals over 65 [2]. A gradual loss of muscle mass with aging leads to a decline in muscle strength of around 1–3% a year [2].

Bone fragility is another very important factor in the elderly that increases their risk of fractures. This condition may be caused by environmental (lack of exposure to sunlight) or dietary (inadequate intake of animal fats) factors that lead to vitamin D deficiency. The prevalence of vitamin D deficiency (<50 nmol/L) reaches as high as 100% in individuals over 70, especially among females [3].

In addition, about 45% of elderly people undergoing major surgery are found anemic on admission to the rehabilitation ward [4]. Any low hemoglobin levels that cannot be attributed to bleeding or bone marrow disorders are likely to be due to low levels of iron, folic acid, or vitamin B12.

Hyponatremia occurs in 7–10% of elderly people and is often an unrecognized contributor to their increase risk of falls [5]. Hypernatremia may also occur—albeit much less frequently, in 1% of older people [5]—and should not be overlooked because, once all potentially responsible organic diseases have been excluded, it could be due to a state of severe dehydration.

Aging coincides with profound changes in the cardiovascular system. Hypertension, type 2 diabetes mellitus, and dyslipidemia are the main risk factors for the onset of coronary artery disease, which is the first cause of death in the elderly population. For these conditions to be properly treated, elderly people often need multiple therapies. For primary prevention purposes, older people are given antihypertensive agents (ACE inhibitors, ARBs, beta-blockers, calcium channel blockers), antidiabetic drugs (oral hypoglycemic agents or insulin), and cholesterol-lowering medication (statins, phytosterols) to keep the various risk factors under control. Elderly patients with ischemic heart disease or peripheral arterial disease are also treated with antiplatelet agents and sometimes with nitrates.

Congestive heart failure affects 10% of individuals over 65 and may be caused by primary (coronary artery disease, hypertension, valve abnormalities) or secondary cardiac events (arrhythmias, anemia, hyperthyroidism). These patients are treated with beta-blockers, ACE inhibitors, anti-aldosterone agents, loop diuretics, and digoxin.

Aging also coincides with physiological changes in the respiratory system that lead to a decline in pulmonary elasticity, a reduction in alveolar surface area, and an increasing chest wall stiffness, with the onset of emphysema and a slowing expiratory flow rate. This condition gives rise to an impaired gas exchange, resulting in desaturation and hypoxia, and the situation becomes more severe in individuals who require bed rest or have limited autonomy.

Over the years, there is a gradual decline in the body's main defense systems too, and the airways are liable to organic or functional abnormalities that lead to a complex condition called *presbyphagia*, which can cause aspiration pneumonia or malnutrition.

Finally, elderly patients referred for rehabilitation may have some degree of dementia, which is treated with acetylcholinesterase (AChE) inhibitors. During their hospital stay, several factors may trigger a state of *delirium* in such patients, in which case they need treatment with antipsychotic agents.

22.3 Functional Changes in the Cardiovascular System and Energy Requirements of the Elderly Under Rehabilitation

The functional changes of different systems after surgery or immobilization and under rehabilitation are resumed in Table 22.1. The ways in which an elderly body adapts to the aerobic exercises of low to moderate intensity (VO2 25–50%) usually performed in the rehabilitation gym are much the same as those of younger people. But the elderly patient referred for rehabilitation has just suffered surgery or been bedridden for some time, with a consequent loss of the functional reserves of their body systems.

Physiologically, the cardiovascular system responds to exercise by increasing cardiac output, speeding up heart rate and left ventricular outflow, and simultaneously raising blood pressure and redistributing the blood volume in favor of the muscles involved in the physical activity underway.

Table 22.1 Physiological and clinical changes in the elderly after surgery/immobility and under rehabilitation

Systems	Physiological changes in the elderly after surgery/immobility and under rehabilitation	Clinical changes
Cardiovascular system	↓ Heart rate reached ↓ Heart's contractility ↑ Cardiac workload ↑ Blood pressure	– Orthostatic intolerance – Hypertensive crises – Tachycardia
Respiratory system	↓ Residual functional capacity ↑ Flow resistance ↓ VO2 max ↓ Maximum aerobic capacity	– ↓ Fatigue threshold
Skeletal muscle	↓ Peripheral artery vasodilation ↓ Oxygen extraction capacity ↓ Muscle work ↓ Aerobic threshold ↑ Lactate production	– Early fatigue – Muscle cramps/pain – Disclosing tendinitis, arthritis, arthrosis, bunions, or radiculitis
Metabolism	Low-intensity prolonged exercising/ moderately intense exercise (50–60% VO2 max) → metabolism of blood glucose and muscular and hepatic glycogen ↓ ↑ Consumption of glucose ↑ Muscle insulin sensitivity	– ↑ Risk of hypoglycemia
Water/electrolyte balance	↑ Body temperature ↑ Perspiration ↑ Electrolyte loss	– ↑ Dehydration – ↑ Hyponatremia/hypokalemia

During exercise, heart rate is usually lower in older people (220 minus the patient's age), while blood pressure is higher, with a consequent greater cardiac workload. Moreover, heart's contractility and peripheral artery vasodilation decline with aging [6].

Surgery and long periods of immobility determine many modifications in the cardiovascular system. For instance, orthostatic intolerance (due to recent sedation or baroreceptor-depressed sensitivity) is common. Hypovolemia (due to a loss of fluids or a reduced liquid intake) causes hypotension and tachycardia. The residual effects of sedation depress baroreceptor sensitivity, giving rise to hypotension and bradycardia. Inadequate pain control prompts tachycardia and hypertension.

In the early period of a rehabilitation program, a patient may consequently have many medical conditions. Orthostatic hypotension is frequent and identified in 50% of patients undergoing PTA, for instance [7], while hypertensive crises may occur during the rehabilitation treatment.

Although the age-related deterioration in the respiratory system is not considered a factor restricting exercise capacity, and the oxygen pressure is maintained up to maximal exercise capacity [6], an elderly patient who has just had surgery under general anesthesia or been bedridden for some time will have a lower residual functional capacity and a higher flow resistance. This means that the patient's VO2 max [6]—maximum oxygen consumption—and therefore his/her maximum aerobic capacity will be reduced and may consequently be unable to cope with the greater oxygen demand of the muscles being exercised, and this means the muscles will have a lower fatigue threshold.

When solicited by exercise, muscles divert the blood flow toward them by dilating the blood vessels (during strenuous exercise, the blood flow toward the muscles reaches 80% of the total) and increasing its oxygen extraction capacity. In the elderly, these mechanisms are less effective, as shown by the a-vO2 difference values. In addition, older people produce less muscle work for the same amount of energy resources than younger people, and this lowers the former's aerobic threshold.

For all these reasons, the lactate production threshold drops, and individuals with an impaired clearance are likely to suffer from muscle cramps, which will limit their physical activity, and the effort needed for the body to offset acidosis may increase pulmonary workload.

Complications affecting the skeletal muscle during exercise recovery are usually mild and often associated with an inadequate warm-up or over-strenuous therapeutic programs [8]. Exercise may also disclose previously existing conditions such as tendinitis, arthritis, bunions, and radiculitis or give rise to new conditions such as muscle strain.

Pain is one of the most important players that can appear during rehabilitation exercise. Its perception depends on the patient's pain threshold and may result in stopping the treatment. It can be caused by the abovementioned lactic acidosis, by an acute exacerbation of already known osteoarticular disorders, and by movements of the limb involved in the previous surgical procedure (in orthopedic patients) or affected by muscle fibrosis and tendon retraction (in cases of paresis or plegic patients) and by paresthesias or dysesthesias along root nerves damaged by orthopedic or neurological conditions (e.g., phantom limb pain in amputees).

Another crucial aspect that changes with exercise is metabolism. The basal metabolism of a person regularly engaging in physical activity increases by comparison with that of a person who is bedridden. The physical work required of a patient at a rehabilitation center is of low intensity (25–30% VO2 max) and is covered by the metabolism of fats and triglycerides in the blood or released from adipose tissue. Low-intensity prolonged training (about 1 h), or moderately intense exercise (50–60% VO2 max) determines an increase either in blood glucose consumption either in muscular and hepatic glycogen consumption.

Exercising usually coincides with an improvement in glycemic control at rest [6], both immediately due to a greater consumption of glucose in sustained aerobic activity and in the long term due to improved muscle insulin sensitivity. In this context, it is important to remember that muscle tissue metabolism can be modified by physical training, depending on the type of exercise. Patients using insulin or oral hypoglycemic agents are at greater risk of hypoglycemia when they exercise.

Patients' hydration status is also liable to change due to perspiration and the associated electrolyte loss during physical exercise, and they may become dehydrated without adequate compensation. There is an increased risk of orthostatic hypotension too in elderly people taking diuretics, antihypertensive, or hypnotic agents [8].

Electrolyte loss may lead to hypokalemia and hyponatremia, which are reflected in muscle weakness, cramps, or myalgias that interfere with the rehabilitation program.

22.4 Advice for the Physiotherapy Team

Given the frailty of most elderly patients, physiatrists and their teams have to consider not only the goals of rehabilitation but also all the aspects that can complicate its implementation (multiple therapies, comorbidities, functional reserves) in order to tailor their programs to their patients.

The complexity of elderly patients requiring rehabilitation can derive from conditions that existed prior to the acute event, which may have caused functional impairments, or from the consequences of the event itself, surgery, prolonged immobilization, and hospitalization.

The main issues to consider concern the body's principal systems. Hypertensive therapy has to be managed in order to control blood pressure appropriately during the physical exercise, but it is essential to prevent orthostatic hypotension at the same time. It may be advisable to adjust or suspend a part of the treatment, though not all antihypertensive medication can be suddenly stopped: in the case of beta-blockers and alpha-2 adrenergic agents, for instance, doing so can trigger a rebound effect. Particular attention should also be paid to patients who are diabetic or have a poor glycemic control because physical exercise is associated with an improvement in glucose tolerance.

A patient's nutritional status cannot be neglected either, because a proper diet is essential to the success of a rehabilitation program or to maintain a proportional body weight or, more importantly, to preserve from weight loss. That is why patients with a normal renal and hepatic function should ingest about 1–1.2 g/kg/day of protein as part of their daily diet [9]. Magnesium [10] and vitamin D [11] levels can also influence physical performance; therefore, their supplementation in nutrition is important.

Rehabilitation sessions, especially with orthopedic patients, also provide a good opportunity to estimate a patient's fracture risk and, where appropriate, to arrange for the secondary prevention of fractures by ensuring an adequate therapy for osteoporosis (vitamin D, calcium, antiresorptive drugs) or to refer the patient to a specialist.

Pain is a decisive factor in the outcome of rehabilitation programs and must be adequately managed. While its overtreatment can have side effects, an inadequate pain control can severely delay a patient's functional recovery and sometimes even prevent a full return to normal. Pain experienced during rehabilitation exercises is pointless and should be investigated and treated before it becomes chronic.

It is a good idea to provide patients an adequate pain relief so that they can accomplish their activities in the gym. The drugs used for inflammatory pain are usually paracetamol and NSAIDs, though attention must be paid to any presence of bleeding and to the patient's renal and liver function. If these drugs are not enough, opioids may be appropriate for some types of pain, but their use must be strictly monitored to avoid nausea, constipation, and the risk of toxicity, which is associated with their excessive dosage or the rapid conversion into morphine of some of them. Neuropathic pain can be treated with specific drugs, such as pregabalin, gabapentin, and amitriptyline.

A particular and often difficult aspect of elderly patient rehabilitation management concerns the cognitive decline and behavioral issues that can sometimes interfere with the various phases of the rehabilitation program. In this case, it may be advisable to use low-dose neuroleptics (because they have no antidopaminergic effects, apart from quetiapine) and to avoid the use of a benzodiazepines, which can cause delirium, loss of vigilance, and a muscle relaxant action that could invalidate the therapeutic success of physiotherapy.

References

1. Robert-Ebadi H, Le Gal G, Righini M (2009) Use of anticoagulants in elderly patients: practical recommendations. Clin Interv Aging 4:165–177
2. Sergi G, Trevisan C, Veronese N, Lucato P, Manzato E (2016) Imaging of sarcopenia. Eur J Radiol 85(8):1519–1524. doi:10.1016/j.ejrad.2016.04.009
3. Adami S, Romagnoli E, Carnevale V, Scillitani A, Giusti A, Rossini M, Gatti D, Nuti R, Minisola S (2011) Linee guida su prevenzione e trattamento dell'ipovitaminosi D con colecalciferolo. Reumatismo 63(3):129–147
4. Pioli G, Giusti A, Barone A (2008) Orthogeriatric care for elderly with hip fractures: where are we? Aging Clin Exp Res 20:113–122

5. Andreucci VE, Russo D, Cianciaruso B, Andreucci M (1996) Some sodium, potassium and water changes in the elderly and their treatment. Nephrol Dial Transplant 11(Suppl 9):9–17
6. Chodzko-Zajko WJ, Proctor DN, Fiatarone Singh MA, Minson CT, Nigg CR, Salem GJ, Skinner JS (2009) Exercise and physical activity for older adults. Med Sci Sports Exerc 41(7):1510–1530. doi:10.1249/MSS.0b013e3181a0c95c
7. Jans O, Bundgaard-Nielsen M, Solgaard S, Johansson PI, Kehlet H (2012) Orthostatic intolerance during early mobilization after fast-track hip arthroplasty. Br J Anaesth 108(3):436–443. doi:10.1093/bja/aer403
8. Vitulli P, Femminella GD, Ciccarelli AL, Rengo F, Lombardi A, Cellurale M, Aruta SF, Kamici K, Allocca E, De Lucia C, Rengo F (2012) Exercise training and aging. G Gerontol 60(3):172–181
9. Landi F, Calvani R, Tosato M, Martone AM, Ortolani E, Savera G, D'Angelo E, Sisto A, Marzetti E (2016) Protein intake and muscle health in old age: from biological plausibility to clinical evidence. Forum Nutr 8(5):295. http://doi.org/10.3390/nu8050295
10. Veronese N, Berton L, Carraro S, Bolzetta F, De Rui M, Perissinotto E, Toffanello ED, Bano G, Pizzato S, Miotto F, Coin A, Manzato E, Sergi G (2014) Effect of oral magnesium supplementation on physical performance in healthy elderly women involved in a weekly exercise program: a randomized controlled trial. Am J Clin Nutr 100:974–981
11. Tofanello ED, Perisinotto E, Sergi G, Zambon S, Musacchio E, Maggi S, Coin A, Sartori L, Corti MC, Baggio G, Crepaldi G, Manzato E (2012) Vitamin D and physical performance in elderly subjects: the Pro. V.A. Study. PLoS One 7(4):e34950

23 Clinical-Instrumental Evaluation of Elderly Patients During Rehabilitation

Jean-Paul Steinmetz and Elisabeth Bourkel

23.1 Introduction

Rehabilitation is a long-lasting process requiring guidance and support of the patient by a multidisciplinary rehabilitation team. A tailored intervention program which fits the patient's needs is essential to effective rehabilitation. These individualized rehabilitation programs are developed by means of constant objective, reliable, and comprehensive insights into the patient's physical, cognitive, and emotional condition. We present and discuss tools which allow mapping cognitive- and mobility-related deficits as well as the emotional state of the elderly patient. Our choice of instruments is necessarily restricted and was guided by two main criteria, which were (1) a short administration time and (2) high clinical validity and a clinical applicability of the findings. Generally, clinical-instrumental evaluation requires many different resources (e.g., time, finances) which often are not available in the clinical context due to various reasons (e.g., availability of clinicians, budget cuts, the patient's clinical condition, etc.). Given the vast amount of clinical assessment tools available in the literature, our selection of the instruments reviewed in this chapter is limited. In the mobility section, the chapter discusses physical performance batteries and screening tools like grip strength, functional independence measure, and Timed Get Up and Go Test, with a special focus on the purpose of spatial-temporal gait analyses. The second part of the chapter reviews psychometric instruments which allow analyzing the patient's cognitive capacities and emotional state.

J.-P. Steinmetz, PhD (✉) • E. Bourkel, PhD
Centre for Memory and Mobility - ZithaSenior, 13 Rue Michel Rodange, L-2430 Luxembourg City, Luxembourg

Research & Development, ZithaSenior, Luxembourg City, Luxembourg
e-mail: jean-paul.steinmetz@zitha.lu; elisabeth.bourkel@zitha.lu

© Springer International Publishing AG 2018

S. Masiero, U. Carraro (eds.), *Rehabilitation Medicine for Elderly Patients*, Practical Issues in Geriatrics, DOI 10.1007/978-3-319-57406-6_23

23.2 Evaluation of Mobility

Functional impairment is a primary geriatric condition that may remain unrecognized or may be inadequately addressed in older patients. Repeated measurements using the present instruments can be valuable in monitoring rehabilitation response and can provide prognostic information assisting the clinician to adapt the therapy.

23.2.1 Grip Strength

Grip strength is a quantitative and objective measure of isometric muscular strength of the hand as well as the forearm. The evaluation of grip strength is considered being the simplest method for assessing muscular strength; furthermore, it represents a clinical marker of poor mobility. Muscle strength assessed through grip strength has been shown to be predictive of sarcopenia and consequences associated to this syndrome (e.g., falls, low quality of life, institutionalization, mortality). Among the wide range of instruments which allow assessing grip strength, the Jamar® dynamometer has been found to provide the most accurate measure of grip strength [1]. In the rehabilitation process, the use of a standardized testing protocol is almost more important than the choice of the instrument that is used to test grip strength. A standardized testing protocol guarantees reproducibility and hence comparability between several measurements, so that the development of the patient's muscle strength throughout the rehabilitation process can be monitored. The importance of a strict adherence to a standardized testing protocol is emphasized in studies demonstrating that changes in body position result in altered grip strengths. When using a standardized protocol, grip strength measurements are found valid and useful for determining functionality, presenting very good test-retest reliabilities [2]. The administration time of a grip strength test in the clinical setting is usually under 5 min.

23.2.2 Timed Get Up and Go Test

The Timed Get Up and Go Test (TUGT) is a gait and dynamic balance screening test and assesses walking ability, balance, and fall risk in older adults. The TUGT is quick to administer (less than 5 min) and does not require any special equipment. In the TUGT, the patient sits in the chair with his/her back against the chair back. On command, the patient must stand up (without using the armrests), walk three meters at a normal pace, turn, walk back to the chair, and sit down. The TUGT has been found to be closely related with the patient's overall motor status and appears to predict everyday walking abilities [3]. The TUGT has proved to be a reliable and valid instrument, which is sensitive and specific enough to identify a risk of falling in old adults [4]. More recent research however refrains from using only the TUGT to predict falls in community-dwelling older adults, with authors making the recommendation of assessing the risk of falling in a more comprehensive manner [5].

23.2.3 Gait Analysis

The quantitative assessment of gait-related parameters enables the understanding of the mechanisms of gait disorders and the development of appropriate (rehabilitation) interventions. Quantifying spatial-temporal gait parameters by using an electronic system allows identifying subtle gait instabilities and is helpful in developing appropriate interventions and monitoring the rehabilitation process. In the present chapter, we focus on the GAITRite® system as a tool to analyze a person's gait. An advantage of the GAITRite® system is its simplicity, without the need of using functional tests to determine joint centers and axes of rotation, to determine the anthropometry of the patient and without the need of placing retroreflective markers on the skin of the patient. The GAITRite® system is composed of an electronic walkway available in lengths varying from 518 to 884 cm. The system provides the clinician with the possibility of performing a standardized and reliable analysis of a person's walking abilities in a brief amount of time. The time to analyze a patient's gait usually varies between less than 5 min and up to 20 min depending (1) on the walking protocol set up by the clinical team (one versus more walking conditions such as fast-/slow-walking trials, dual-task walking) and (2) by the overall condition or fitness of the patient. While assessing gait using the GAITRite® system, we strongly recommend applying a standardized assessment protocol. A decade ago, an important number of researchers gathered and consented on common instructions and guidelines of data collection to enhance first the reproducibility of gait measures and second to guarantee the comparability of outcomes [6]. Research has identified key domains (i.e., rhythm, phase, pace, base of support and variabilities) helping to understand and interpret gait performances from a clinical point of view [7]. More recent guides with quantitative reference values are currently being developed (Fig. 23.1).

In the clinical context, spatial-temporal gait analysis may serve to diagnose and to assess the severity of the underlying injury or the disease. Furthermore and even more important for the rehabilitation process is the continuous quantification of gait parameters allowing the evaluation of the effectiveness of the interventions. Interestingly, it is now suggested that (subclinical) gait changes can be used as a surrogate marker of future falls or disabilities and even future diseases [8].

23.2.4 Functional Independence Measure

The Functional Independence Measure (FIM) allows evaluating physical and cognitive functions among rehabilitation inpatients. Psychometric properties such as discriminative validity and internal consistency have been evaluated (see, e.g., [9]). A trained evaluator is ideally required to rate a total of 18 items (13 motor tasks and 5 cognitive tasks) on a 7-point ordinal scale ranging from complete dependence to complete independence. Generally, the FIM is used several times during a rehabilitation process to track a patient's disabilities and recoveries in detail and to determine how much assistance is required for the individual to carry out activities of

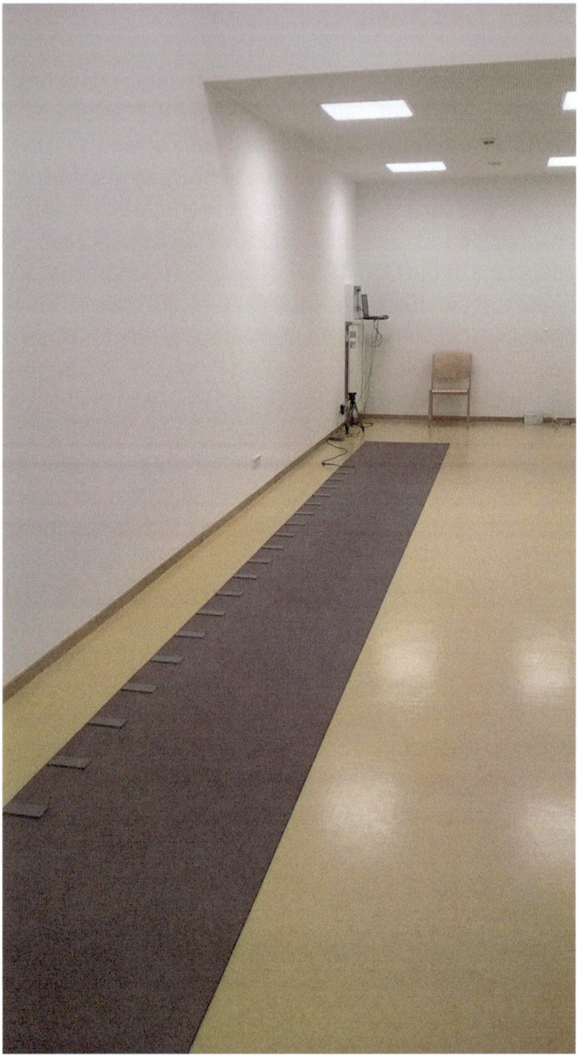

Fig. 23.1 GAITRite® platinum plus version with a 610 cm long active mat and two additional inactive extensions. Mat is connected to a portable personal computer. Room is kept neutral to reduce external influences on a patient's walking performance. *Source*: Centre for Memory and Mobility, ZithaSenior

daily living. The quality of the assessment is directly dependent of the multitude of the gathered information. Therefore, the patient's disabilities should be rated by a multidisciplinary team.

23.2.5 Short Physical Performance Battery

The Short Physical Performance Battery (SPPB) comprises different performance measures of lower extremity function. Gait, strength, balance, and endurance are measured using three short tests: (1) standing balance including tandem, semi-tandem, and side-by-side stances, (2) walking speed on an 8-foot walking course, and (3) repeated chair stances (five repetitions). The total administration time of the three tests in the clinical setting ranges from 10 to 20 min depending on the physical condition of the patient. The scale has been found to predict loss of motor function, impairments affecting the activities of daily living, mortality, and institutionalization. The SPPB has established reliabilities and validities for community-dwelling older adults. Research investigating the validity of the SPPB in acute hospitalized patients is available [10].

23.2.6 Tinetti Test

The Tinetti test or "Performance-oriented mobility assessment (POMA)" was developed by Mary E. Tinetti in 1986. The Tinetti test assesses balance (e.g., standing balance, turning 360°) and gait (e.g., step symmetry, step continuity) through a variety of different tasks. The tasks are scored and summed up, with lower scores indicating higher mobility impairments and thus a higher risk for falls. The test is well adapted to the clinical context as it does not require any special equipment. The administration time usually does not exceed 10–15 min. Different versions of the Tinetti test with a varying numbers of tasks and scoring systems are available. The majority of studies demonstrate that the different versions of the test are reliable and valid tools for assessing the mobility status of patients showing different medical conditions (e.g., Parkinson's disease; [11]). Nevertheless, when employing any version of the Tinetti test, it remains crucial that the therapist is thoroughly informed on the psychometric properties of the respective version in use.

23.3 Evaluation of Cognition and Mood Disorders

The present section reviews psychometrical instruments which allow assessing cognition and affectivity of elderly patients in an economical and valid manner. Generally, a differentiation can be made between screening tests to gain a quick and broad overview of diverse cognitive functions and function-specific neuropsychological tests assessing different cognitive functions in more detail. Older inpatients should be screened for possible cognitive deficits so that rehabilitative interventions and overall care can be adequately adapted to their cognitive status. Likewise, it is important to assess the affectivity of patients so that a possible depression can be detected and treated appropriately. Furthermore, clinical-instrumental evaluation plays an important role in the differentiation between mild states of cognitive impairments (e.g., mild cognitive impairment) and more severe cognitive impairments (e.g., dementia) and mood disorders. Symptoms of all these conditions can overlap increasing the risk of misdiagnosing. In general, the neuropsychological evaluation should be preceded by an extensive clinical interview (i.e., anamnesis), so that concerns of the patient and their acquaintances can be assessed. The knowledge about those complaints is important to guide the testing process, and accurate assessment instruments are chosen.

23.3.1 Evaluation of General Cognitive Functioning

Due to limited time resources in the clinical context, there is a need for instruments which allow a relatively quick and general overview of the cognitive deficits and capacities of a patient entering the rehabilitative process. The assessment of cognitive functions is generally a complex (and may be an intimidating) situation for people having cognitive deficits. This implies that the clinician should respond to the patient's potential anxieties and reassures the patient during the assessment. Furthermore, the purpose of the respective tests should be explained to the patient in order to promote compliance and reduce frustration. Ideally, the assessment should yield to a written report and an oral feedback to the patient [12].

The so-called screening tests allow gaining a quick and broad overview of diverse cognitive functions in a relatively short amount of time. The majority of cognitive screening instruments consist of a set of different tasks (e.g., memory tasks, word fluency tasks, etc.), whose scores are added up to determine a global score. This totalled score is (ideally) compared to representative norms or cutoff values to quantitatively determine the extent of the patient's performances or deficits.

23.3.2 Mini-Mental State (MMS)/Mini-Mental State Examination (MMSE)

One of the most commonly used screening tests for neurocognitive disorders in the medical context is the Mini-Mental State (MMS) or Mini-Mental State Examination (MMSE). The MMSE covers memory, orientation, and attention and assesses the ability to follow written and verbal commands, to name, to write a sentence, and to copy a polygon. In clinical practice, often the raw scores are interpreted, with changing recommendations concerning the cutoff scores. Perneczky and colleagues [13] concluded that the MMSE scores (maximum score is 30) are indicative of the following: 30 no dementia, 26–29 questionable dementia, 21–25 mild dementia, 11–20 moderate dementia, and 0–10 severe dementia. In general, the MMSE is easy and quick to apply and exists in different languages. In the clinical context, the correct interpretation of MMSE scores is however challenging, as the appropriate age- and education-adjusted norms should be taken into consideration. It is known that age and other factors such as psychological comorbidities may influence the results. Furthermore, ceiling effects and poor sensitivities make the detection of mild cognitive impairments in highly educated individuals difficult. Therefore, improvements were made, resulting in the MMSE-2 test [14]. Despite those supplements, it should be noted that other screening tests were developed and are available demonstrating improved sensibilities to detect milder cognitive deficits.

23.3.3 Montreal Cognitive Assessment (MoCA)

The Montreal Cognitive Assessment (MoCa) is a short screening test with high specificity and sensitivity for detecting mild cognitive deficits. It is more sensitive for discriminating mild cognitive impairment (MCI) from a healthy condition than the MMSE [15]. The MoCA can be administered in 10 min, and it includes a short-term memory recall task and contains two learning trials of five nouns and delayed recall after 5 min. Visuospatial abilities and executive functions are assessed. Furthermore, a phonemic fluency task and a two-item verbal abstraction task are included. Attention, concentration, and working memory are evaluated. Finally, language and orientation to time and place are assessed. The maximum possible score in the MoCA is 30 points. In a recent study, authors found that the MoCA cutoff for differentiating reliably a pathological sample with dementia from a sample composed of healthy controls was 23 (with a specificity of 96% and a sensitivity of 94%; [15]). A score of 19 was found to differentiate reliably between patients with MCI and patients with Alzheimer's disease, with corresponding specificities ranging from 77% [16] to 80% [15] and sensitivities ranging from 77% [15] to 87% [16].

23.3.4 DemTect

In addition to the MoCA, the DemTect (originally developed in German) is also a highly sensitive instrument to identify patients with mild cognitive impairments and patients with dementia in early stages of the disease. The DemTect is a brief test (8–10 min completion time) composed of five subtests composed of a word list, a number transcoding task, a word fluency task, a digit span reverse task, and a delayed recall of the previously learned word list. The DemTect is independent from age and education, with total scores ranging from 0 to 18. Performances ranging between 13 and 18 points are considered adequate, between 9 and 12, MCI is probable, and for performances lower than 8, further investigations are necessary as dementia is probable. A parallel version of the test (DemTect-B) has been developed demonstrating equivalent task requirements and difficulties suitable for follow-up evaluations [17].

23.3.5 Clock-Drawing Test (CDT)

Another very brief, valid test is the Clock-Drawing Test (CDT). Patients are instructed to draw a clock face with hands; afterward, the clock errors are rated to determine the score. The CDT is a marker of cognitive deficits and is useful as a screen for cognitive impairment. Associations between the CDT and executive functions, global cognitive status, visuospatial processing, and semantic knowledge have been demonstrated [18]. Sensitivities and specificities around 75% in differentiating clinically diagnosed MCI patients from healthy elderly individuals have been shown [19] (Fig. 23.2).

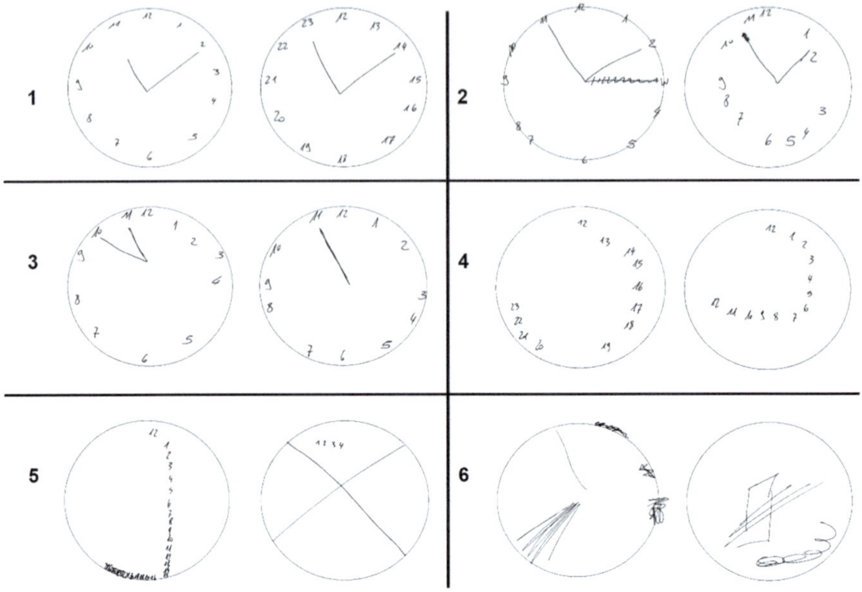

Fig. 23.2 Examples of different clock-drawing performances with corresponding ratings. *Source*: Centre for Memory and Mobility, ZithaSenior

23.3.6 Evaluation of Specific Cognitive Functions

In addition to the assessment of general cognitive functioning with screening tests, a more detailed evaluation of specific functions allows differentiating between altered cognitive functions. Assessment can focus more specifically on attention, learning and memory (e.g., Rey Auditory Verbal Learning Test or Wechsler Memory Scale, Fourth Edition), constructional praxis (e.g., Rey-Osterrieth Complex Figure Test), executive functions (e.g., Stroop test), language (e.g., Boston Naming Test), or psychomotricity (e.g., Trail Making Test).

23.3.7 Alters-Konzentrations-Test (AKT)

If attention deficits are suspected, the broad cognitive screening test can be supplemented by an (age-adapted) attention test. In the geriatric context, the nonverbal concentration test for the elderly (AKT [Alters-Konzentrations-Test]) has proven useful and valid [20]. The AKT assesses the ability of an individual to selectively allocate attention to certain stimulus characteristics and to suppress distracting characteristics. The participants' task is to identify a stimulus figure among a total of 55 two-colored (black and white) figures. Stimulus figures and distracters differ only in their colored pattern and their two-dimensional orientation. A total number of 20 figures can be correctly identified. Dependent variables are the completion time (in seconds) and the percentage of errors. The AKT has excellent psychometric properties with Spearman-Brown split-half reliabilities ranging from $r = 0.89$ to 0.99 [20]. Dependent variables are the total performance (calculated by adding the correctly identified figures and subtracting the errors), percentage of errors (percentage of distracters erroneously crossed out), and the time to complete the test (in seconds).

23.3.8 Trail Making Test (TMT)

Trail Making Test in both versions A and B is one among the most commonly used tests in clinical practice. Test form A assesses primarily visual search and psychomotor speed, whereas test form B requires attentional processing, cognitive flexibility, and working memory functions [21]. Both the time to complete each form and a normalized TMT time ((B-A)/A) to isolate the executive component of the TMT can be analyzed.

23.4 Evaluation of Depression and Neuropsychiatric Behavior

Several scales for rating depression specifically in elderly people have been developed during the last decades.

23.4.1 Geriatric Depression Scale

The Geriatric Depression Scale (GDS) is the most known and used depression rating scale for elderly people. The original version developed by Yesavage and colleagues is composed of 30 items, to be answered by yes or no (e.g., "Are you basically satisfied with your life?") leading to a maximum total score of 30. Scores ranging from 0 to 10 are considered to represent an absence of a depression-; scores of 11 or higher are indicative of a depression [22]. The GDS can be completed by the patient or in an interview with the healthcare professional. Shorter versions with fewer items are available. In the 15-item scale, a score of >/= 5 is suggestive of a depression and >/= 10 is indicative for depression. It has been demonstrated that the 15-item GDS assesses reliably the presence of depressive symptoms among older adults. An even shorter version (mini-GDS) has been developed, with a total of 4 items [23]. Importantly, shorter versions generally show lower test-retest reliabilities and are less precise in detecting illness severities. The advantage of shorter versions is however that they require less time and are easy to rate and thus better applicable in the clinical context. The GDS does not allow making a depression diagnosis but reliably indicates the emotional state of the patient. Similarly to the psychometric instruments assessing cognitive capacities described in the previous paragraphs, no diagnosis can be made by only using the GDS. It should be noted that the GDS is not recommended in patients demonstrating important cognitive deficits as self-reflection and understanding of the respective items may be compromised.

23.4.2 Cornell Depression Scale

The Cornell Scale for Depression in Dementia (CSSD) is a 19-item instrument with an administration time of approximately 20 min. The CSDD was specifically developed to assess depression in patients with dementia. As reports of patients with high cognitive deficits may be unreliable, the CSDD combines information from interviews with both the patient and the informant. The scale was found to have a high inter-rater reliability and high internal consistency (alpha coefficient of 0.84; [24]). Many of the items can be filled after observation of the patient. The ratings of the CSDD items represent the observer's impression of the patient rather than the verbal answers (of the patient or the informant) to the respective items. Each of the items is rated for severity (0 = absent, 1 = mild or intermittent, 2 = severe) with item scores being totalled. A score above 10 is associated with a probable major depression. Scores above 18 are associated with a definite major depression. Scores below 6 indicate the absence of significant depressive symptoms [24].

The CSDD and GDS both have high validity in screening for depression in the elderly; however, only the CSDD seems to be equally valid in patients with dementia and patients with no cognitive deficits. The CSDD retained its specificity and validity as a screening tool for depression of patients with dementia, while the GDS versions all decreased in validity [25].

23.4.3 Neuropsychiatric Inventory

An additional clinically useful instrument to assess neuropsychiatric disorders in patient populations is the Neuropsychiatric Inventory (NPI). The NPI is available in two versions, namely, the 10-item NPI and the 12-item NPI (see Table 23.1). Both versions can be used in the geriatric context and assess behavioral dysfunctions common in dementia. Both versions have good content validity, concurrent validity, inter-rater reliability (93.6–100% for different behaviors), and 3-week test-retest reliability (correlation, 0.79 for frequency and 0.86 for severity ratings; [26]). The NPI is administered to an informant who has detailed knowledge of the patient's

Table 23.1 Behavioral domains of the NPI

Hallucinations
Delusions
Agitation/aggression
Dysphoria/depression
Anxiety
Irritability
Disinhibition
Euphoria
Apathy
Aberrant motor behavior
Sleep and nighttime behavior change (12-item version only)
Appetite and eating change (12-item version only)

behavior. A screening question determines whether a specific behavior is present or not. If the informant indicates that the respective behavior is not present, the subquestions of the respective section are omitted. If the informant affirms the presence of the behavior, the respective subquestions are administered. The informant is then also asked to rate the severity and frequency of that behavior. In addition, the caregiver is asked to rate his or her own distress in relation to the behavior.

The Neuropsychiatric Inventory Questionnaire (NPI-Q; [27]) is a short version of the NPI to obtain information quickly. The NPI-Q is completed by the caregiver and reviewed by the clinician; it comprises only the screening question, severity rating, and caregiver distress rating of the original test. A recent study has shown that the NPI-Q is a reliable and valid tool for screening neuropsychiatric symptoms in patients with stroke and transient ischemic attack [28].

23.5 Discussion and Conclusion

The overall goal of the present chapter was to compile a set of instruments that enable the clinician to identify and to monitor cognitive deficits, emotional state, and mobility-related impairments in the rehabilitative context. We reviewed the evaluation tools which we considered to be the most significant in the rehabilitative context, while focusing both on short administration times and high clinical validities in the choice of instruments. The clinician should make a choice within the discussed instruments depending on the needs of the patient. This choice should be based on the medical history and the results of the tests which were previously administered in the rehabilitation context (e.g., the GDS should not be used to assess depression in a patient if previous test results indicate severe cognitive deficits). In order to fully match the patients' needs, the clinician should consider whether the assessment might be complemented with further tools evaluating, for example, quality of life or activities of daily living. Prior to using a clinical instrument or tool to diagnose or to monitor cognitive- or mobility-related parameters, we recommend searching for the most recent scientific developments on protocols, reliabilities, and validities of the respective tools. The respective scores should always be interpreted by using the most recent and (for the respective patient group) most representative norms available. Above all, the choice of the evaluation tools as well as their interpretation and the conclusions drawn from them should always be conducted with clinical reasoning.

References

1. Roberts HC, Denison HJ, Martin HJ, Patel HP, Syddall H, Cooper C, Sayer AA (2011) A review of the measurement of grip strength in clinical and epidemiological studies: towards a standardised approach. Age Ageing 40:423–429. doi:10.1093/ageing/afr051
2. Abizanda P, Navarro JL, García-Tomás MI, López-Jiménez E, Martínez-Sánchez E, Paterna G (2012) Validity and usefulness of hand-held dynamometry for measuring muscle strength in community-dwelling older persons. Arch Gerontol Geriatr 54:21–27. doi:10.1016/j.archger.2011.02.006

3. Podsiadlo D, Richardson S (1991) The timed "Up & Go": a test of basic functional mobility for frail elderly persons. J Am Geriatr Soc 39:142–148
4. Shumway-Cook A, Brauer S, Woollacott M (2000) Predicting the probability for falls in community-dwelling older adults using the Timed Up & Go Test. Phys Ther 80:896–903
5. Barry E, Galvin R, Keogh C, Horgan F, Fahey T (2014) Is the Timed Up and Go test a useful predictor of risk of falls in community dwelling older adults: a systematic review and meta-analysis. BMC Geriatr 14:14. doi:10.1186/1471-2318-14-14
6. Kressig RW, Beauchet O, European GAITRite Network Group (2006) Guidelines for clinical applications of spatio-temporal gait analysis in older adults. Aging Clin Exp Res 18:174–176
7. Hollman JH, McDade EM, Petersen RC (2011) Normative spatiotemporal gait parameters in older adults. Gait Posture 34:111–118. doi:10.1016/j.gaitpost.2011.03.024
8. Allali G, Annweiler C, Blumen HM, Callisaya ML, De Cock A-M, Kressig RW, Srikanth V, Steinmetz J-P, Verghese J, Beauchet O (2015) Gait phenotype from mild cognitive impairment to moderate dementia: results from the GOOD initiative. Eur J Neurol. doi:10.1111/ene.12882
9. Glenny C, Stolee P (2009) Comparing the functional independence measure and the interRAI/MDS for use in the functional assessment of older adults: a review of the literature. BMC Geriatr 9:52. doi:10.1186/1471-2318-9-52
10. Volpato S, Cavalieri M, Guerra G, Sioulis F, Ranzini M, Maraldi C, Fellin R, Guralnik JM (2008) Performance-based functional assessment in older hospitalized patients: feasibility and clinical correlates. J Gerontol A Biol Sci Med Sci 63:1393–1398
11. Kegelmeyer DA, Kloos AD, Thomas KM, Kostyk SK (2007) Reliability and validity of the Tinetti Mobility Test for individuals with Parkinson disease. Phys Ther 87:1369–1378. doi:10.2522/ptj.20070007
12. Jahn T, Werheid K (2015) Demenzen [Dementias]. Hogrefe Verlag, Göttingen
13. Perneczky R, Wagenpfeil S, Komossa K, Grimmer T, Diehl J, Kurz A (2006) Mapping scores onto stages: mini-mental state examination and clinical dementia rating. Am J Geriatr Psychiatry Off J Am Assoc Geriatr Psychiatry 14:139–144. doi:10.1097/01.JGP.0000192478.82189.a8
14. Folstein MF, Folstein SE, White T, Messer MA (2010) MMSE-2: Mini-mental state examination 2nd Edition. Psychological Assessment Resources, Inc., Lutz, FL
15. Roalf DR, Moberg PJ, Xie SX, Wolk DA, Moelter ST, Arnold SE (2013) Comparative accuracies of two common screening instruments for the classification of Alzheimer's disease, mild cognitive impairment and healthy aging. Alzheimers Dement J Alzheimers Assoc 9:529–537. doi:10.1016/j.jalz.2012.10.001
16. Trzepacz PT, Hochstetler H, Wang S, Walker B, Saykin AJ, Alzheimer's Disease Neuroimaging Initiative (2015) Relationship between the Montreal Cognitive Assessment and Mini-mental State Examination for assessment of mild cognitive impairment in older adults. BMC Geriatr 15:107. doi:10.1186/s12877-015-0103-3
17. Kessler J, Calabrese P, Kalbe E (2010) DemTect-B: ein Äquivalenztest zum kognitiven Screening DemTect-A® [DemTect-B: A parallel test version to the cognitive screening instrument DemTect-A®]. Fortschritte Neurol Psychiatr 78:532–535. doi:10.1055/s-0029-1245452
18. de JJ P, de DM M, de EN M, Malloy-Diniz LF (2013) Mapping the clockworks: what does the Clock Drawing Test assess in normal and pathological aging? Arq Neuropsiquiatr 71:763–768. doi:10.1590/0004-282X20130118
19. Yamamoto S, Mogi N, Umegaki H, Suzuki Y, Ando F, Shimokata H, Iguchi A (2004) The clock drawing test as a valid screening method for mild cognitive impairment. Dement Geriatr Cogn Disord 18:172–179. doi:10.1159/000079198
20. Gatterer G (2007) Alters-Konzentrations-Test [Test of concentration for older adults], 2nd edn. Hogrefe, Göttingen
21. Ashendorf L, Jefferson AL, O'Connor MK, Chaisson C, Green RC, Stern RA (2008) Trail Making Test errors in normal aging, mild cognitive impairment, and dementia. Arch Clin Neuropsychol 23:129–137. doi:10.1016/j.acn.2007.11.005
22. Yesavage JA, Brink TL, Rose TL, Lum O, Huang V, Adey M, Leirer VO (1983) Development and validation of a geriatric depression screening scale: a preliminary report. J Psychiatr Res 17:37–49

23. D'Ath P, Katona P, Mullan E, Evans S, Katona C (1994) Screening, detection and management of depression in elderly primary care attenders. I: the acceptability and performance of the 15 item Geriatric Depression Scale (GDS15) and the development of short versions. Fam Pract 11:260–266
24. Alexopoulos GS, Abrams RC, Young RC, Shamoian CA (1988) Cornell Scale for Depression in Dementia. Biol Psychiatry 23:271–284
25. Kørner A, Lauritzen L, Abelskov K, Gulmann N, Marie Brodersen A, Wedervang-Jensen T, Marie Kjeldgaard K (2006) The Geriatric Depression Scale and the Cornell Scale for Depression in Dementia. A validity study. Nord J Psychiatry 60:360–364. doi:10.1080/08039480600937066
26. Cummings JL, Mega M, Gray K, Rosenberg-Thompson S, Carusi DA, Gornbein J (1994) The Neuropsychiatric Inventory: comprehensive assessment of psychopathology in dementia. Neurology 44:2308–2314
27. Kaufer DI, Cummings JL, Ketchel P, Smith V, MacMillan A, Shelley T, Lopez OL, DeKosky ST (2000) Validation of the NPI-Q, a brief clinical form of the Neuropsychiatric Inventory. J Neuropsychiatry Clin Neurosci 12:233–239. doi:10.1176/jnp.12.2.233
28. Wong A, Cheng S-T, Lo ESK, Kwan PWL, Law LSN, Chan AYY, Wong LK-S, Mok V (2014) Validity and reliability of the neuropsychiatric inventory questionnaire version in patients with stroke or transient ischemic attack having cognitive impairment. J Geriatr Psychiatry Neurol 27:247–252. doi:10.1177/0891988714532017

Muscle Assessment Using 3D Modeling and Soft Tissue CT Profiling

24

Paolo Gargiulo, Kyle J. Edmunds, Iris D. Arnadottir, Ugo Carraro, and Magnus K. Gíslason

24.1 Introduction: Translational Myology and Medical Imaging

The growing field of translational myology continually seeks to define and promote the generalizability of muscle research to clinical practice via optimizing the transition of a wide variety of investigative muscle assessment modalities. Medical imaging is of particular interest in this regard, as extant literature focuses on the utilization of a wide variety of techniques to noninvasively recapitulate and quantify various internal and external tissue morphologies. In the clinical context, medical imaging remains a vital field of research for diagnostic and investigative assessment. Of the many facets of medical imaging, most current research aims to improve aspects of instrumentation design, image processing software, data acquisition methodology, and computational modeling. In particular, methods that enable the 3D visualization of internal anatomy elicit valuable information for optimizing the treatment of many pathologies, but every modality has its inherent limitations [1]. For the purposes of clinical assessment, in particular, visually simplistic imaging methods that outline noninvasive, high-resolution methodologies for assessing diseased or damaged tissues have readily been identified as a strategic priority in translational myology

P. Gargiulo (✉)
Institute for Biomedical and Neural Engineering, Reykjavík University, School of Science and Engineering, Reykjavík 101, Iceland

Landspítali, University Hospital, Reykjavík 101, Iceland
e-mail: paologar@landspitali.is

K.J. Edmunds • I.D. Arnadottir • M.K. Gíslason
Institute for Biomedical and Neural Engineering, Reykjavík University, School of Science and Engineering, Reykjavík 101, Iceland
e-mail: kyle14@ri.is; irisa10@ru.is; magnuskg@ru.is

U. Carraro
IRCCS Fondazione Ospedale San Camillo, Venezia, Italy
e-mail: ugo.carraro@unipd.it

© Springer International Publishing AG 2018

S. Masiero, U. Carraro (eds.), *Rehabilitation Medicine for Elderly Patients*, Practical Issues in Geriatrics, DOI 10.1007/978-3-319-57406-6_24

research. Although there are many extant imaging modalities that may be discussed at length in the context of translational myology, the particular methods outlined in this chapter will all be associated with X-ray computed tomography (CT).

Before delving more into the intricacies of CT, it is first important to understand a bit more about the field of translation myology. While researchers focus primarily upon diseases and comorbidities associated with natural and/or pathological changes in the muscle, muscular degeneration, in particular, has been consistently identified as a particular phenomenon of interest. Muscle degeneration is characterized by the progressive loss of muscle mass, strength, and/or function and has long been implicated as an independent risk factor for high mortality in both aging populations and individuals suffering from neuromuscular pathology or injury [2–5]. When associated with aging, this phenomenon is defined as sarcopenia—a phenomenon whose precise, quantitatively derived etiology remains debated [6–8]. When associated with a severe chronic illness, muscle degeneration, in conjunction with other forms of atrophy or weakness, is defined as cachexia. Muscle degeneration is additionally a common sequela of various types of spinal cord trauma. In general, muscle degeneration from any origin confers an increase in muscular adiposity and noncontractile tissue infiltration, which, in accordance with a loss of muscle mass, leads to an increased risk for frailty, disability, reduced mobility, and eventual hospitalization [9]. The focus of this chapter will be in the utilization of modern applications of CT imaging to better quantify muscle degeneration and the efficacy of clinical intervention.

24.2 Quantifying Sarcopenic Muscle Degeneration with Soft Tissue CT Profiling

Whether via sarcopenia, cachexia, or other trauma, muscular degeneration has been characterized by increased muscular adiposity and reduced average CT attenuation values. In this section, we discuss how distributions of these CT attenuation values can be analyzed to understand shifts in soft tissue composition as a function of age and sex.

CT images are essentially comprised of large matrices of X-ray attenuation values. These values are typically expressed in Hounsfield units (HU), where zero HU is defined by the absorptivity of water. For the purposes of clinical utility, one may consider HU values to directly represent tissue density—a notion which is very important when assessing the muscle and surrounding soft tissue. Indeed, post-processing of 3D CT images via the linear transformation of the HU image matrices allows for the segmentation of different tissue types, allowing for the clear distinction between both intra- and extra-muscular soft tissue regimes. In the simplest case, this can be applied to the distinction of fat from muscle, since HU values of fat range from −200 to −10 HU, whereas muscle HU values range from 41 to 200 HU. Disseminating tissue types between these ranges is considerably more difficult, since such voxels often represent an average of many distinct tissue elements.

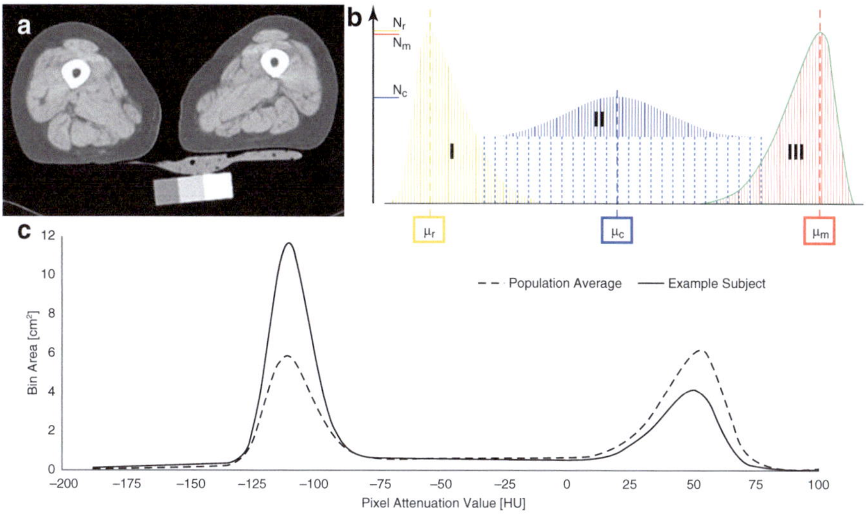

Fig. 24.1 Hounsfield distribution from a representative subject's upper leg CT slice. (**a**) Transverse CT slice of the upper legs, taken at 20 cm below the femoral head. (**b**) Representation of the tri-modal HU distribution showing (I) the fat peak, (II) the connective tissue peak, and (III) the muscle peak. Note that N represents the amplitude of these peaks, and μ represents the location of the Gaussian mean. (**c**) A representative elderly patient's HU distribution as compared to the average distribution of over 3000 elderly subjects. Note the comparatively large fat peak, the small muscle peak, and the apparent shift of the connective tissue peak toward lower-density HU values

For the purpose of quantification, the central HU regime from −10 to 41 has been defined as "loose connective or water-equivalent tissue" [10, 11].

Figure 24.1a shows an example subject's CT slice which was taken at the mid-femur, and Fig. 24.1b depicts a diagram of each of the three tissue modes of an HU distribution. Additionally, Fig. 24.1c details an example of what an average HU distribution from an elderly subject's CT scan cross section looks like, as well as one generated from over 3000 healthy elderly subjects of ages 66–86.

It is readily apparent that each of the three tissue types generates a trimodal distribution or a curve with three distinct, summed Gaussian distributions. The leftmost peak represents fat (centered around −90 HU), the rightmost peak represents muscle (centered around 65 HU), and the smaller and wider central peak represents loose connective tissue (centered around −10 HU). Each of these individual peaks can be defined by two very useful Gaussian distribution parameters: the amplitude of the curve, N, and the location of the curve's mean, μ. The amplitude of a peak simply relates to the relative volume of a tissue type, whereas the location term describes the tissue density. In general, healthy muscle is evidenced by a higher muscle peak density, whereas intramuscular fat (present from increasing adiposity of degenerating muscle) confers a less-dense fat peak. The density of the connective tissue peak may likewise change according to the degree of muscle adiposity, but this notion remains unclear [12].

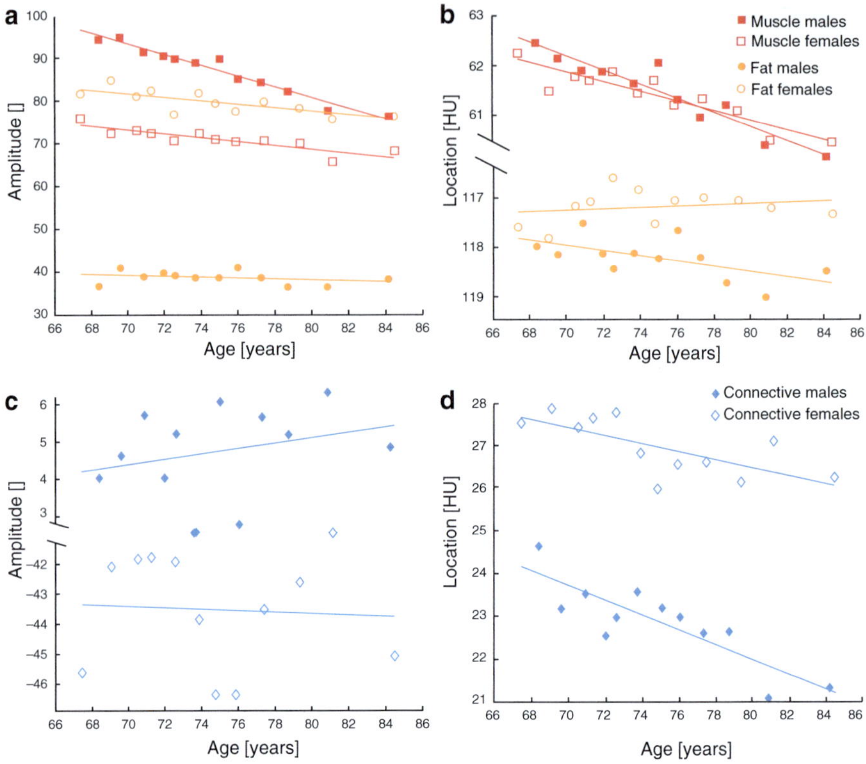

Fig. 24.2 HU distribution profiling results for over 3000 healthy elderly subjects. Linear regression was performed for (**a**) muscle and fat amplitudes, (**b**) muscle and fat locations, (**c**) connective tissue amplitudes, and (**d**) connective tissue locations

When averaged over the large elderly population and compared as a function of age and sex, clear linear trends in these peak amplitudes and locations become apparent. Figure 24.2 shows the results from this analysis.

Figure 24.2 illustrates clear differences in distribution parameters between men and women, but how these parameters vary and the degree to which they fit to linear correlation with age depends upon the tissue type. The amplitudes of both fat and muscle in both men and women decrease readily with increasing age, but men have significantly higher muscle amplitudes and lower fat amplitudes than women. Intriguingly, the locations of muscle peaks were nearly identical and decreased analogously with age in both men and women, but the women's fat peak location increased while the men's decreased. This could be interpreted as evidence that, while both sexes lose soft tissue volume similarly with age, women exhibit increased fat volume and decreased muscle volume compared to men. Furthermore, both sexes' muscle densities decrease identically with age, suggesting an analogous trend of increased adiposity in both sexes. Increasing densities for fat tissue in women could likewise be a further indicator of fatty tissue infiltration, but this conclusion is less obvious.

The degree of linear correlation in the connective tissue amplitudes and locations was much lower than fat or muscle. However, women and men exhibited marked differences with similar variance in these parameters as a function of age. Connective tissue amplitudes increased with age in men but decreased in women, while the locations decreased analogously with age for both sexes. This could suggest that lower muscle density (increased muscle adiposity) from sarcopenic degeneration could increase predictably with advanced age, but the low linear correlations in these terms give pause for any definitive conclusions.

24.3 3D Modeling: Morphological and Compositional Changes in the Muscle

As previously mentioned, many recent investigations have realized the quantitative potential of CT image analysis to quantify muscle composition and quality, and its utility for analyzing muscle degeneration in particular has been of great focus in research. As such, many investigators have assessed how changes in skeletal muscle density correlate with changes in muscular volume and function in patients suffering from a variety of conditions or diseases. We have already seen the utility of HU distribution analyses in the rigorous quantification of degenerating muscle. However, this section focuses on another utility of these CT-derived density values that has particular relevance in a clinical context: the use of density-based tissue segmentation and 3D modeling to clearly illustrate changes in muscle mass and quality.

Figure 24.3 illustrates how the *tibialis anterior* muscles of three representative subjects may be reassembled in 3D with voxel coloration that correlates to each of

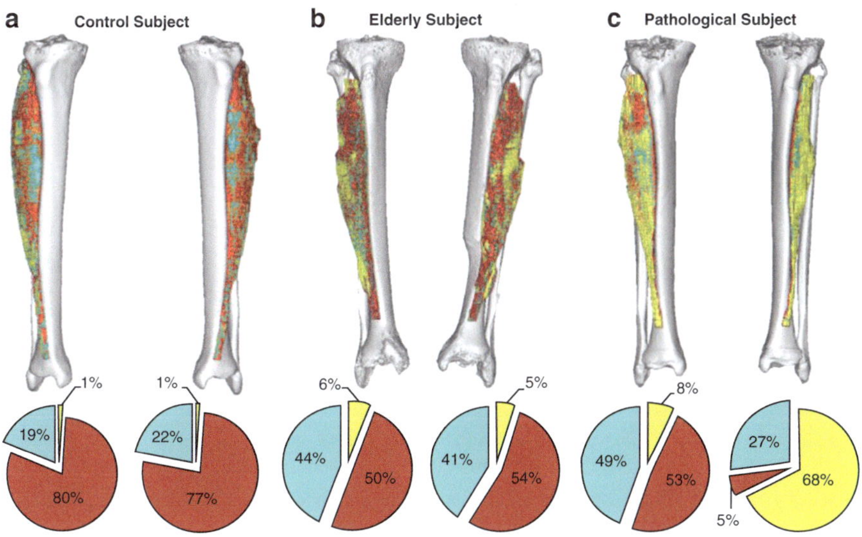

Fig. 24.3 Segmented soft tissues and compositions within the *tibialis anterior* from each subject's 3D upper leg volumes. Tissue types are as follows: fat (*yellow*), connective tissue (*cyan*), and muscle (*red*). (**a**) The control subject's composition is primarily muscle, but (**b**) the elderly subject had markedly more fat and connective tissue, to the detriment of muscle. (**c**) However, the pathological subject's healthy leg composition was analogous to those of the elderly subject, but the pathological leg comprised of nearly all fat and connective tissue

the three tissue types that were defined previously. The compositions of these tissues have likewise been calculated for each leg. As is evident from these values, the elderly subject and pathological subject (who suffered from asymmetrical lower body paralysis from a pelvic mass infiltration of the sciatic nerve) exhibited increasing amounts of fat and loose connective tissue, compared to the control subject. Likewise, the left leg of the pathological subject contains remarkably more fat than the right leg, illustrating the degeneration's severity.

The use of 3D segmentation and modeling can likewise be utilized to show changes in muscle volume and density during a targeted therapy. Figure 24.4 depicts such an example, where a patient with complete lower motor neuron denervation from a spinal cord injury underwent functional electrical stimulation (FES) treatment for 5 years, followed by 5 years of non-compliance to the therapy. It is clear that the increase in both volume and density of the *rectus femoris* muscle indicates the overall importance of the treatment—which likewise highlights the utility of the 3D segmentation process.

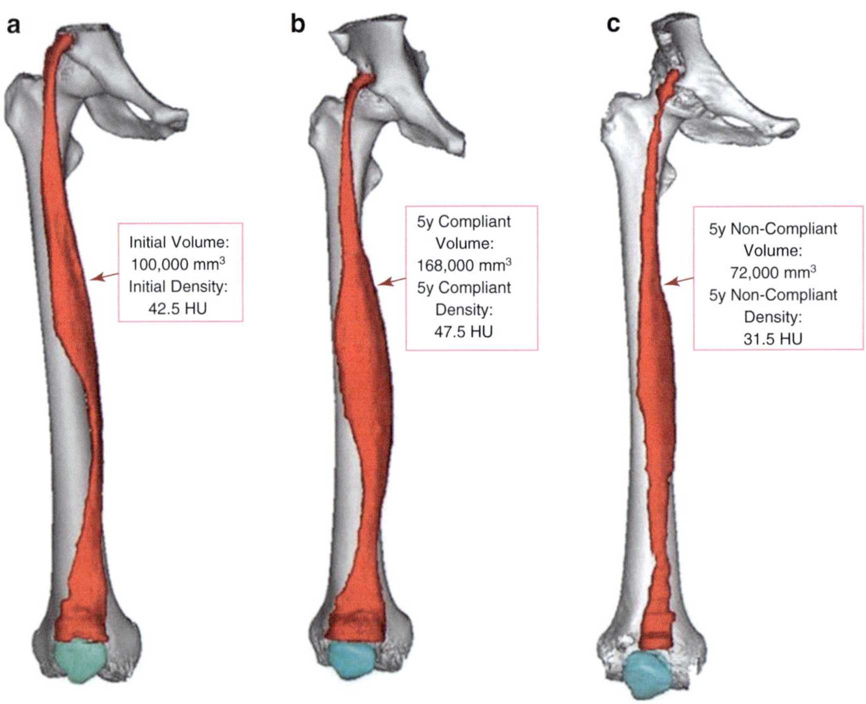

Fig. 24.4 An example of irreversible *conus and cauda equina* syndrome who underwent (**a**) an initial CT scan and segmentation before treatment, (**b**) 5 years of compliance with home-based FES treatment, and followed by (**c**) another 5 years of non-compliance to FES. As is evident above, the 3D volume and density analyses identify changes in the *rectus femoris* muscle over the timespan of the study. Figure obtained from Edmunds et al. [12]

24.4 Muscle Asymmetry and Recovery in Total Hip Arthroplasty Patients

By analyzing the muscle amplitude of patients undergoing total hip arthroplasty (THA), both pre-operation and 1-year post-operation, it is possible to determine the progression of the state of the muscle and monitor how the subject is performing over that period [13–15]. This analysis was carried out on 16 patients scheduled for primary THA, and the aforementioned trimodal muscle profiling was used to quantify any changes in muscle volume and density. The results demonstrate how, on average, patient muscle amplitudes increased in the operative leg and, to a much lesser extent, in the healthy leg.

Looking at the subject-specific progression of the muscle over the 1-year recovery period, it is evident that a majority of the patients showed an increase in muscle amplitude—many of whom likewise showed a decrease in fat amplitude, implying an improvement in muscle quality (Fig. 24.5). This demonstrates that only by analyzing the muscle in such a manner, it is possible to rigorously quantify changes in muscle volume and density before and after THA surgical intervention.

Using such an assessment technique can help to detect patients that could be considered at risk for sarcopenia and to prescribe the appropriate rehabilitation method to optimize the strengthening of their leg muscles. The success of the THA procedure depends upon the patient's ability to be mobile and create the necessary loading of their hip. This will ultimately maintain the prosthetic's strength, which will in turn lead to an increased lifespan of the implant and an increased quality of life for the patient.

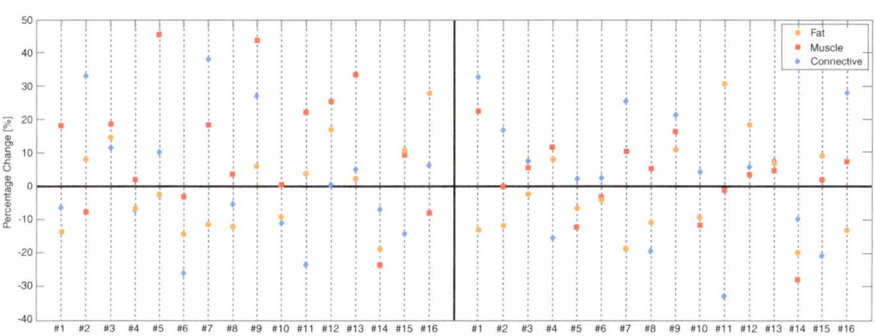

Fig. 24.5 Percentage changes in model parameters for THA patients over a 1-year recovery period. Positive values demonstrate and increase in tissue volume, and negative values indicate a decrease in tissue volume

Conclusions

In this chapter, we have shown different applications of soft tissue analysis based upon CT imaging. The analysis of fat, muscle, and loose connective tissue distributions can identify key differences between how sarcopenia may be elicited in elderly men and women. We have also shown how 3D modeling and CT image segmentation according to these three tissue types can fully describe the clinically significant extent of changes in skeletal muscle density and volume. Both the analysis of soft tissue distributions and the use of 3D modeling can likewise be useful in quantifying and characterizing patients who have undergone clinical treatments for mobility impairment, such as FES and THA. However, there is more potential in these types of mathematical analyses to correlate muscle characteristics with comorbidities.

Key Points

- Soft tissue distribution profiling from CT images can identify clear differences between how sarcopenia may affect elderly men and women.
- 3D modeling and CT image segmentation can fully describe the clinically significant extent of changes in skeletal muscle quality and volume.
- Both the analysis of soft tissue distributions and the use of 3D modeling can be useful in quantifying and characterizing patients who have undergone clinical treatments for mobility impairment.

References

1. Edmunds KJ, Gargiulo P (2015) Imaging approaches in functional assessment of implantable myogenic biomaterials and engineered muscle tissue. Eur J Transl Myol 25(2):4847. doi:10.4081/ejtm.2015.4847
2. Metter EJ, Talbot LA, Schrager M, Conwit R (2002) Skeletal muscle strength as a predictor of all-cause mortality in healthy men. J Gerontol A Biol Sci Med Sci 57(10):B359–B365
3. Rantanen T (2000) Muscle strength and body mass index as long-term predictors of mortality in initialle healthy men. J Gerontol 55A(3):168–173
4. Newman AB, Kupelian V, Visser M, Simonsick EM, Goodpaster BH, Kritchevsky SB, Harris TD (2006) Strength, but not muscle mass, is associated with mortality in the health, aging and body composition study cohort. J Gerontol A Biol Sci Med Sci 61(1):72–77
5. Goodpaster BH, Carlson CL, Visser M, Kelley DE, Scherzinger A, Harris TB, Stamm E, Newman AB (2001) Attenuation of skeletal muscle and strength in the elderly: the Health ABC Study. J Appl Physiol 90:2157–2165
6. Baumgartner RN, Koehler KM, Gallagher D, Romero L, Heymsfield SB, Ross RR, Garry PJ, Lindeman RD (1998) Epidemiology of sarcopenia among the elderly in New Mexico. Am J Epidemiol 147(8):755–763
7. Janssen I, Heymsfield SB, Ross R (2002) Low relative skeletal muscle mass (sarcopenia) in older persons is associated with functional impairment and physical disability. J Am Geriatr Soc 50(5):889–896

8. Newman AB, Kupelian V, Visser M, Simonsick E, Goodpaster B, Nevitt M, Kritchevsky SB, Tylavsky FA, Rubin SM, Harris TB (2003) Sarcopenia: alternative definitions and associations with lower extremity function. J Am Geriatr Soc 51:1602–1609. doi:10.1046/j.1532-5415.2003.51534.x
9. Janssen I, Shepard DS, Katzmarzyk PT, Roubenoff R (2004) The healthcare costs of sarcopenia in the United States. J Am Geriatr Soc. doi:10.1111/j.1532-5415.2004.52014.x
10. Helgason T, Gargiulo P, Jóhannesdóttir F, Ingvarsson P, Knútsdóttir S, Gudmundsdóttir V, Yngvason S (2005) Monitoring muscle growth and tissue changes induced by electrical stimulation of denervated degenerated muscles with CT and stereolithographic 3D modeling. Artif Organs 29:440–443. doi:10.1111/j.1525-1594.2005.29073.x
11. Carraro U, Edmunds KJ, Gargiulo P (2015) 3D false color computed tomography for diagnosis and follow-up of permanently denervated human femoral muscles submitted to functional electrical stimulation. Eur J Transl Myol 25(2):129–140
12. Edmunds KJ, Gíslason MK, Arnadottir ID, Marcante A, Piccione F, Gargiulo P (2016) Quantitative computed tomography and image analysis for advanced muscle assessment. Eur J Transl Myol 26(2):6015. doi:10.4081/ejtm.2016.6015
13. Magnússon B, Pétursson Þ, Edmunds K et al (2015) Improving planning and post-operative assessment for total hip arthroplasty. Eur J Transl Myol 25(2):4913. doi:10.4081/ejtm.2015.4913
14. Pétursson Þ, Edmunds KJ, Gíslason MK et al (2015) Bone mineral density and fracture risk assessment to optimize prosthesis selection in total hip replacement. Comput Math Methods Med 2015:162481. doi:10.1155/2015/162481
15. Gargiulo P, Péturssone T et al (2003) Assessment of total hip arthroplasty by means of computed tomography 3D models and fracture risk evaluation. Artif Organs 37(6):567–573

Part II

25 Rehabilitation of Older Patients with Rheumatic Diseases

Kerstin Mattukat, Christoph Schäfer, Inge Ehlebracht-König, and Juliane Lamprecht

25.1 Introduction

Gerontorheumatology deals with the particular features of onset, course and treatment of rheumatic diseases in patients of advanced age [1]. The initial manifestations of rheumatic diseases in elderly patients often differ from the typical findings in younger patients [2]: Non-specific general disease symptoms, e.g. non-specific complaints, a decline in physical function and/or mental confusion [2], may hinder the initial diagnosis of rheumatic diseases beyond the age of 60 [1]. The most important diseases and their management strategies are to be discussed later in the chapter. Where no guidelines for older patients are available, general guidelines are reported with respect to possible challenges in patients at an advanced age.

25.2 Rehabilitation for Older People with Rheumatic Diseases

Rheumatic medication is often the precondition to non-medical treatment in patients with rheumatic diseases. Reduction of pain and inflammation by medical treatment is essential before starting activating therapies like mobility-enhancing

K. Mattukat (✉) • J. Lamprecht
Institute of Rehabilitation Medicine, Martin Luther University Halle-Wittenberg, Halle (Saale), Germany
e-mail: kerstin.mattukat@medizin.uni-halle.de; juliane.lamprecht@medizin.uni-halle.de

C. Schäfer
Clinic for Internal Medicine II, Department of Internal Medicine, Martin Luther University Halle-Wittenberg, Halle (Saale), Germany

I. Ehlebracht-König
Center of Rehabilitation, Bad Eilsen, Germany

© Springer International Publishing AG 2018

S. Masiero, U. Carraro (eds.), *Rehabilitation Medicine for Elderly Patients*, Practical Issues in Geriatrics, DOI 10.1007/978-3-319-57406-6_25

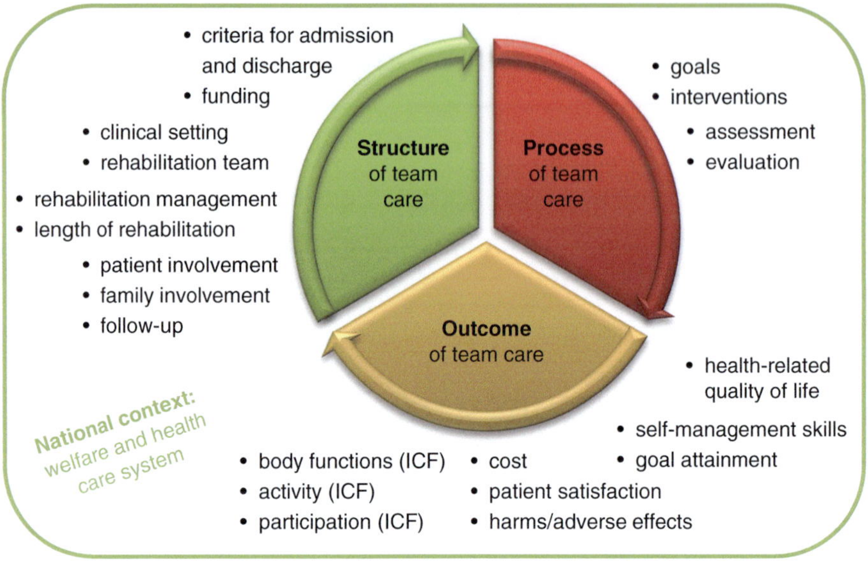

Fig. 25.1 The Scandinavian Team Arthritis Register-European Team Initiative for Care Research (STAR-ETIC) framework of arthritis rehabilitation according to Klokkerud et al. [3]

exercises. In principle, all specific disease-modifying drugs, immunosuppressant drugs and biologics can be used for the therapy of rheumatic diseases in the elderly [1]. However, careful dose selection is particularly necessary, taking into consideration age-specific limitations in organ function and metabolism [1]. Whereas the treatment goal usually comprises achievement of complete clinical remission in younger patients, the focus should shift towards reducing pain, preserving function and avoiding therapy-associated adverse effects in the elderly.

The **rehabilitation of patients with rheumatic diseases** can be described by a framework recently developed by a work group from the Netherlands [3] (see Fig. 25.1). According to the differing forms of rehabilitation services in different countries, a common framework may facilitate comparisons of rehabilitation programmes across countries and different levels of care [3].

Rehabilitation Goals Geriatric medicine aims at an *improvement of functional deficits* to *avoid disability* and *delay the need for nursing* for as long as possible [4]. Patient education and patient training are important to enhance the knowledge of the disease and its management possibilities. The goal of *remission* in the sense of "restitutio ad integrum" is illusory due to the chronic disease and frequent comorbidities of the patients as well as due to the limited future time perspective [4].

Interdisciplinary Rehabilitation Team The attending physician (e.g. the rheumatologist, the geriatrician, the orthopaedic surgeon) should *evaluate the older patient* in collaboration with the entire interdisciplinary rehabilitation team of medical specialists and non-medical professionals and *prescribe a comprehensive treatment programme* that aims to preserve and restore function [5]. Such a programme offers the geriatric patient the best opportunity to increase physical skills and function [5].

Interventions Before Surgery The elderly orthopaedic patient should be instructed to perform breathing exercises to prevent pulmonary complications and active lower limb exercises to maintain good circulation and joint mobility and to do functional exercises for mobilisation in and out of bed [5].

Interventions Postoperatively The interdisciplinary rehabilitation team has to facilitate early resumption of *active exercises* and *self-care tasks* and to discourage prolonged bed rest ("bed is bad") [4] and dependency on nursing staff and family members [5]. Physical and occupational therapy should be provided to restore mobility and self-care functions [5]. Notably, *physical therapy* (e.g. electrotherapy, hydrotherapy, thermotherapy, massages and lymphatic drainage) can help to reduce the amount of medication needed and thereby to avoid severe side effects [4]. *Occupational therapy* aims to train activities of daily living (e.g. washing, dressing and eating), including exercises to enhance fine motor skills of the fingers, strengthening exercises, sensitivity training, joint protection and the provision of aids and remedies [4]. When planning discharge, the home environment should be assessed and modifications recommended to reduce the risk of falls and to ensure independent functioning to the extent possible. As soon as the rehabilitation goals have been obtained, the patient should be discharged from the hospital, but additional therapy in terms of *rehabilitation aftercare* may be required, either at home or at an outpatient facility [5].

Place of Treatment Rehabilitation interventions are not only to be carried out in the *clinical context* (outpatient or inpatient) but also at the *patient's home* or in a *nursing home*. In recent studies, home-based rehabilitation provided the same or even higher gains regarding function, cognition, quality of life and patient satisfaction compared to inpatient rehabilitation.

Assessments The comprehensive geriatric assessment encompasses the somatic, cognitive, emotional and social resources as well as functional deficits of the patient. The *assessment of the baseline status* of an older patient with a rheumatic disease should be conducted as detailed as needed. It may include a medical examination, laboratory assessments, radiography/imaging of the joints, an inquiry of the patient's history, mobility tests, assessments of function in everyday life and well-being as well as the assessment of the socio-demographic and living background of the patient. Several assessments and patient questionnaires are available for the different matters of interests.

Pain, fatigue, daily activities, physical function, quality of life, coping, motivation, goal attainment, mental health and participation are the domains that are most central for *evaluating the effects of rehabilitation*.

Treatment Risks and Barriers *Comorbid conditions*, such as cardiovascular diseases, impaired motor and cognitive functioning, *geriatric problems*, such as sarcopenia and frailty, and the *decline of social support and income* as important resources to cope with the disease may complicate disease management strategies and limit the goals of rehabilitation programmes in elderly patients. Hence, treatment interventions have to be checked for appropriateness for people at an advanced age and must be adapted to their individual cognitive or health conditions as well as to their living background.

25.3 Rehab Interventions: State of the Art in Selected Rheumatic Diseases

The rheumatic diseases which occur most often in elderly patients include osteoarthritis, rheumatoid arthritis, polymyalgia rheumatica, giant cell arteritis (arteritis temporalis), crystalline arthropathy (gout and pseudogout), fibromyalgia, the Sjögren's syndrome [1], systemic lupus erythematosus and ankylosing spondylitis.

25.3.1 Osteoarthritis

Osteoarthritis (OA) is the most prevalent rheumatic disease with the knees being the most commonly affected joints. According to the EULAR recommendations [6], treatment of OA should be based on the localization of OA and various risk factors (age, sex, comorbidity, obesity). For the planning of interventions, the presence of inflammation, severity of structural change, level of pain and restriction of daily activities are relevant [6].

Exercise is an important non-pharmacological treatment for symptomatic OA and seems to be effective in terms of pain and function [7]. Especially aerobic and strengthening exercise as well as weight reduction improved physical function and reduced pain in patients with OA of the knee [8]. Additionally, positive effects of proprioceptive exercises and balance training have recently been shown [9]. *Manual therapy* combined with exercises is also recommended in the disease management of patients with OA. *Pharmacological interventions* encompass non-steroidal anti-inflammatory drugs (NSAIDs), COX-2 inhibitors, topical NSAIDs, topical capsaicin and chondroitin sulphate [7]. In addition to exercise and medications, *adjunctive interventions* include thermal therapies (e.g. heat, cold and ultrasound), transcutaneous electrical nerve stimulation (TENS), pulsed electromagnetic field therapy, laser therapy and electrical (galvanic) stimulation [7]. For acupuncture, TENS and low-level laser therapy, moderate-quality evidence with respect to pain reduction is reported [8]. In addition to enhancing the functional status, the improvement of psychological outcomes is also an essential factor in the treatment of OA. *Behavioural interventions*, like patient education and behavioural change techniques, lead to better psychological outcomes and a moderate pain reduction [7]. In the sense of a holistic biopsychosocial model, *walking aids* (e.g. a walking stick, walking frames), *assistive technology* and *adaptations at home* (e.g. handrails for stairs, walk-in shower, heightened chairs, beds and toilet seats) should be considered to increase the patients' independency and participation [6].

25.3.2 Gout

Today, gout patients are more clinically complex than in the past, due to various combinations of advanced age, comorbidities, drug-drug interactions and refractory tophaceous disease [10]. The disease is characterised by deposition of monosodium urate crystals in and around joints and soft tissues, resulting in painful inflammation [11]. Gout is associated with significant morbidity and mortality from both intra- and extra-articular complications and has an increased incidence in the elderly. Imaging may be helpful in making a firm diagnosis since clinical presentation in the elderly may differ from that in the younger patients.

Following evidence-based recommendations [12], specific risk factors, clinical phase and general risk factors should be considered in the treatment of gout. A comprehensive treatment of gout requires *non-pharmacological modalities* as well as *pharmacological treatments*. *Patient education* and appropriate *lifestyle counselling*, regarding weight loss in the case of overweight, low animal purine diet and reduced alcohol consumption, are core aspects of the management of gout [12]. *Dietary interventions* refer to an inclusion of skimmed milk and/or low-fat yoghurt, soy beans and vegetable sources of protein; limited intake of high-purine foods and red meat; avoidance of liver, kidneys, shellfish and yeast extracts; and an overall restriction of protein intake [13]. Patients with gout and a history of urolithiasis should be encouraged to drink more than 2 litres of water per day to avoid dehydration [13]. This is particularly important for all older persons. Herbal remedies should not be taken without medical consultation [13]. According to physical exercise, trauma to joints and intense *physical exercise* should be avoided, whereas moderate physical exercise should be encouraged [13]. Xanthine oxidase inhibitor therapy with either allopurinol or febuxostat is recommended as the first-line *pharmacologic urate-lowering therapy approach* in (chronic) gout. Medications that are commonly used in the *treatment of acute gout* include oral non-steroidal anti-inflammatory drugs (NSAIDs), colchicine, oral glucocorticoids and the injection of glucocorticoids into the affected joint [11]. In addition to the pharmacological treatment of acute gout, *ice packs* as well as *elevating and resting the affected joint* have been suggested to reduce the pain [13].

25.3.3 Rheumatoid Arthritis

Rheumatoid arthritis (RA) is a chronic inflammatory autoimmune disease characterised by joint swelling, joint tenderness and destruction of synovial joints (see Fig. 25.2), often leading to severe disability and premature mortality [14]. For people with newly diagnosed rheumatoid arthritis, treatment should follow the model

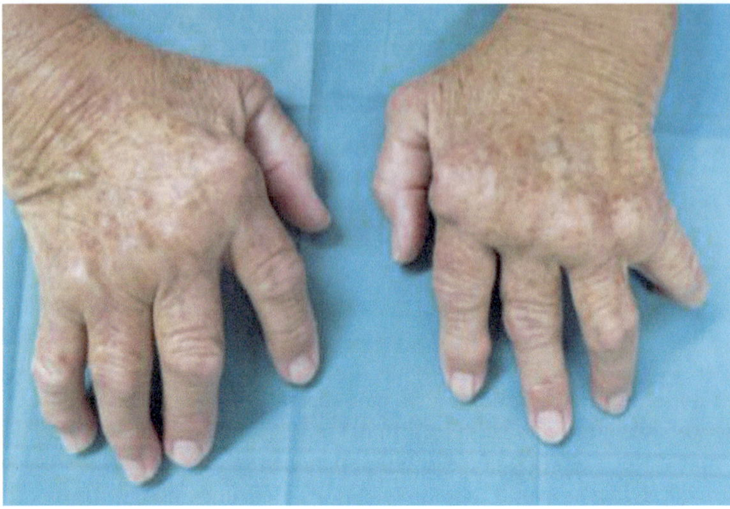

Fig. 25.2 Hands of a 70-year-old woman suffering from seropositive rheumatoid arthritis showing severe ulnar deviation in the metacarpophalangeal joints

of the patient-centred standards of care for RA in Europe [15]. This is especially true for people with late-onset rheumatoid arthritis (LORA) that first occurs in the age of 65 years and older (approx. 30% of all RA patients) [4].

The American College of Rheumatology (ACR) guideline for the treatment of RA [16] covers the use of traditional *disease-modifying antirheumatic drugs* (DMARDs), biologic agents and glucocorticoids in early (<6 months) and established (≥6 months) RA. Besides pharmacological treatment, *regular exercise* is one of the cornerstones of care in RA. Physical activity and exercise have numerous health benefits in patients with RA, e.g. improved joint health, physical function, mobility and psychological well-being as well as reduced rheumatoid cachexia and fatigue, without aggravating symptoms or inducing further joint damage. According to a recent review [17], long-term land-based aerobic exercise (e.g. bicycle ergometer, cycling or jogging) and muscle strengthening exercise (e.g. rubber expanders, circuit interval training) of moderate to high intensity reduced activity limitations and improved both cardiorespiratory fitness (i.e. oxygen uptake) and muscle strength, while short-term aerobic exercise increased cardiorespiratory fitness only. A review of the effects of rehabilitation recently stated that *physical therapy (PT)* and *occupational therapy (OT)* significantly reduce pain in RA patients. Furthermore, grip strength in various grip types (power grip, key pinch, precision pinch and tripod pinch) improved through *hand exercise therapy* (including resistance and/or active range of motion exercises) without having adverse effects on pain or disease activity [18]. With regard to the intervention content, there is some evidence in favour of a longer therapy duration and a higher therapy intensity [18]. According to a Cochrane review [19], physical activity and *psychosocial interventions* provided benefits in relation to self-reported fatigue in adults with RA.

25.3.4 Polymyalgia Rheumatica and Giant Cell Arteritis

Polymyalgia rheumatica (PMR) and giant cell arteritis (GCA) occur almost exclusively in persons aged ≥50 years [20]. GCA occurs in at least 15% of PMR patients and about 40% of GCA patients exhibit symptoms of PMR [20].The proximal pain (hip and/or shoulder) and stiffness syndrome of PMR can occur in many other rheumatologic inflammatory illnesses in older people, e.g. in late-onset RA and ankylosing spondylitis. GCA is the most common systemic vasculitis in the adult population [21]. The typical symptoms of new-onset GCA are bi-temporal headaches, jaw claudication, scalp tenderness, visual disturbances, systemic symptoms such as malaise, fever and weight loss, and polymyalgia [21].

According to the 2015 EULAR/ACR recommendations for the management of PMR [22], glucocorticoid (GC) therapy is the *pharmacological treatment* of choice—although relapses, long-term dependency and side effects (50%) are common problems. In addition, patients should have access to *education* focusing on the impact of PMR and treatment (including comorbidities and disease predictors) and to individually tailored *exercise programmes* to maintain muscle mass and function and to reduce the risk of falls (particularly in frail persons) [22]. Today, there are no studies investigating the value of further *non-pharmacological therapies* (e.g. physiotherapy, relaxation techniques, diets, etc.) in PMR, and due to insufficient clinical experience, no specific recommendation exists regarding this issue [22].

The *diagnostic assessment* of GCA comprises laboratory testing (erythrocyte sedimentation rate, C-reactive protein), imaging studies (duplex sonography, high-resolution magnetic resonance imaging, positron emission tomography) and temporal artery biopsy [21]. The standard *pharmacological treatment* is glucocorticoid therapy (adverse effects: diabetes mellitus, osteoporosis, cataract, arterial hypertension) [21]. However, treatment with high-dose steroids, especially in an elderly population with multiple pre-existing comorbidities, carries serious risks (e.g. thrombosis), resulting in high rates of GC-related adverse side effects (86% at 10 year follow-up) [23]. Therefore, immunosuppressive drugs (e.g. methotrexate) are proposed as GC-sparing therapy [23]. According to EULAR recommendations for the management of large vessel vasculitis [23], patients with GCA are at an increased risk of developing cardiovascular and cerebrovascular events and should be treated temporarily (e.g. for the first 3 months in the acute phase) with low-dose aspirin in the absence of contraindications. Fraser et al. [24] emphasised the role of *patient education* in the treatment of GCA: Patients with GCA must be informed of the risks and benefits of long-term corticosteroid use before commencing treatment, as well as the dangers of abrupt cessation of corticosteroids. They should be told that although a typical course of steroid treatment for GCA lasts 1–3 years, theirs could last longer [24]. Also, because GCA may relapse during the tapering process, patients must be advised to seek medical attention immediately whenever symptoms of GCA recur, particularly if they develop new visual blurring or blindness [24]. Almost nothing is reported in regard to *non-pharmacological treatment* of GCA (i.e. exercise, physical and occupational therapy).

25.3.5 Sjögren's Syndrome

The Sjögren's syndrome (SS) is a multisystem autoimmune disease that often affects the elderly and is characterised by hypofunction of the salivary and lacrimal glands [25]. It is often associated with other autoimmune conditions such as lupus erythematosus or rheumatoid arthritis. The diagnosis and management of SS require three areas of specialty practice: rheumatology, ophthalmology and oral medicine [25].

SS patients with dry eyes should avoid aggravating environmental factors such as low humidity (e.g. excessive air-conditioning and airline travel), limit activities that can provoke tear film instability (e.g. prolonged reading and computer use) and avoid medications that decrease tear production [26]. Multiple *artificial tear preparations* are available in the market that help alleviate the dryness by replacing the tears [26]. *Ocular ointment* as replacement therapy should be used at night due to possible visual blurring if used during the day [26]. Furthermore, topical *corticosteroid preparations* (only short term) and *cyclosporine ophthalmic emulsion* showed positive effects in past studies [26].

SS patients with chronic dry mouth should maintain a *good dental health* to prevent common dental complications (e.g. dental caries, gum disease and dental erosions) [26]. The salivary secretion can be physically stimulated by chewing *sugar-free chewing gum*, and *saliva substitutes* help to increase moisture in oral surfaces [26]. The use of pharmacological agents in elderly patients is not recommended due to missing efficacy or adverse side effects [26].

25.3.6 Ankylosing Spondylitis

Ankylosing spondylitis (AS) is a chronic, inflammatory rheumatic disease characterised by inflammatory back pain due to sacroiliitis and spondylitis and the formation of syndesmophytes leading to ankylosis (see Fig. 25.3) and is frequently associated with peripheral arthritis, enthesitis and acute anterior uveitis [27]. Approximately one-third of the patients report peripheral joint involvement, most of them in the hip, the shoulder and the knee, as well as extra-spinal manifestations affecting the bowel or the heart [28]. Furthermore, AS is often accompanied by an increased risk of cardiovascular morbidity [28]. With an estimated prevalence of 0.9% in northern European white populations, AS is a significant health burden to the community [27]. Symptoms commonly begin in late adolescence and early

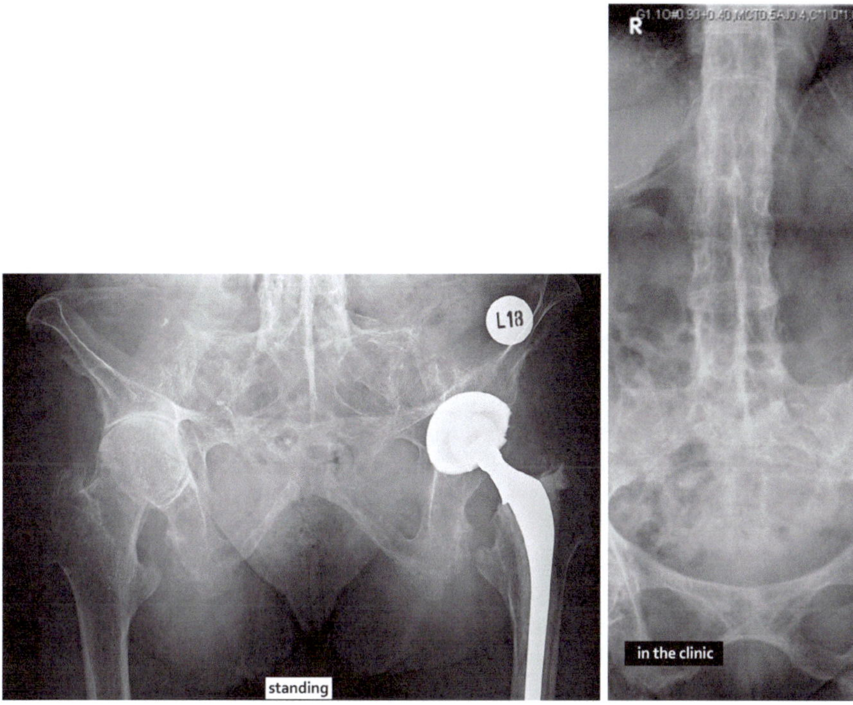

Fig. 25.3 X-rays of a 75-year-old woman suffering from ankylosing spondylitis showing complete ankylosis of sacroiliac joints and the lumbar spine, joint replacement of the *left hip* after coxitis and joint space narrowing of the *right hip*

adulthood; however, patients are able to approach an old age in relatively good health due to improved medical care.

For symptom control, exercise and non-steroidal anti-inflammatory drugs (NSAIDs) are primarily recommended by the EULAR [27]. When planning the treatment, current manifestations of the disease, the level of current symptoms, clinical findings, prognostic indicators, the general clinical status and, of course, the wishes and expectations of the patients should be taken into account [27]. *Pharmacological interventions* comprise non-steroidal anti-inflammatory drugs (NSAIDs), COX-2 inhibitors, analgesics (paracetamol, opioids) and corticosteroid injections to the local side of musculoskeletal inflammation. No evidence is reported for traditional disease-modifying antirheumatic drugs, e.g. sulfasalazine and methotrexate, regarding the treatment of axial disease [27]. Biologic agents, however, are able to reduce pain and inflammatory burden and to improve physical function in patients with axial involvement.

Exercise therapy plays a pivotal role in the treatment of AS and focuses mainly on improving and/or maintaining physical function and posture by mobility exercises, muscle strengthening, stretching of specific muscle groups and cardiorespiratory training [29]. Additionally, spa therapy and patient education have been shown to have short-term benefits regarding function in AS [27]. Exercise therapy is not able to stop the process of ankylosis, but it can avoid stiffening of the spine in an flexed position. However, in the elderly patient, this treatment goal is of lower importance, since the inflammatory course of the disease usually starts before the age of 40.

25.4 Discussion

The number of elderly patients with rheumatic diseases will continuously increase in the next few years. Therefore, it is necessary that the structures of the healthcare system for elderly patients with rheumatic diseases are prepared for this challenge [30]. Two important fields are of particular relevance: multimorbidity and the prevention of disability. These problems can be faced by structures which facilitate interdisciplinary care, e.g. institutions which provide rehabilitation for elderly patients with rheumatic diseases [30]. This can be realised in either an outpatient or an inpatient setting. Rheumatologists working in interdisciplinary fields, in outpatient practices and in specialised rheumatology hospitals have key functions in the care of elderly patients with rheumatic diseases [30] and can be supported by special, rheumatologically qualified nurses. According to concrete treatment procedures, pharmacological treatment is the mainstay in rehabilitation management of patients with rheumatic diseases, highly investigated and thus constantly improving. However, multi-medication in older multimorbid patients is difficult to handle because of incalculable cross-interactions between the single medicaments.

- **Consequently, pharmacological treatment has to be reduced as far as possible, and non-pharmacological interventions have to be increased.**

For the prevention of disability, it is necessary to activate the patients to the maximum possible. This is especially important for patients after undergoing surgery: They should be in bed as little as possible. Activation of the patients can be achieved particularly by regular physical exercise and occupational therapies. In case of acute flares and high disease activity, joints are passively moved and relaxed; physical therapies are used for pain relief. In case of low disease activity, exercise therapy helps to maintain the flexibility of the joints, to strengthen the muscles and to stabilise the patient as a whole. Last but not least, adequately adapted aids and remedies can significantly increase the patients' independence in everyday life and improve their quality of life in this way.

Key Points
- Treatment goals for older patients with rheumatic diseases are pain relief, restoration and preservation of (joint) function and maintenance of independence in everyday life.
- The pharmacological treatment should be reduced as far as possible due to possible cross-interactions and adverse side effects.
- Non-pharmacological interventions, e.g. physical, occupational and exercise therapy as well as technical aids and remedies, should be highlighted instead.
- The involvement of family members or other help providers is fundamental for the success of the rehabilitation process—especially if the older patients' self-help capacity is limited due to functional or cognitive impairment.

References

1. Wollenhaupt J (2009) Gerontorheumatology. Aspects of diagnosis, course and therapy of inflammatory rheumatic disease in advanced age. Z Rheumatol 68:397–403; quiz 404
2. Michet CJ Jr, Evans JM, Fleming KC et al (1995) Common rheumatologic diseases in elderly patients. Mayo Clin Proc 70:1205–1214
3. Klokkerud M, Hagen KB, Kjeken I et al (2012) Development of a framework identifying domains and elements of importance for arthritis rehabilitation. J Rehabil Med 44:406–413
4. Behringer W, Vogel W (2012) Geriatric treatment of rheumatic patients. Akt Rheumatol 37:52–56
5. Flanagan SR, Ragnarsson KT, Ross MK et al (1995) Rehabilitation of the geriatric orthopaedic patient. Clin Orthop Relat Res 316:80–92
6. Fernandes L, Hagen KB, Bijlsma JWJ et al (2013) EULAR recommendations for the non-pharmacological core management of hip and knee osteoarthritis. Ann Rheum Dis 72:1125–1135
7. Sarzi-Puttini P, Cimmino MA, Scarpa R et al (2005) Osteoarthritis: an overview of the disease and its treatment strategies. Semin Arthritis Rheum 35:1–10
8. Jamtvedt G, Dahm KT, Christie A et al (2008) Physical therapy interventions for patients with osteoarthritis of the knee: an overview of systematic reviews. Phys Ther 88:123–136
9. Al-Khlaifat L, Herrington LC, Tyson SF et al (2016) The effectiveness of an exercise programme on dynamic balance in patients with medial knee osteoarthritis: a pilot study. Knee 23:849–856
10. Gout TR (2009) Novel therapies for treatment of gout and hyperuricemia. Arthritis Res Ther 11:236

11. van Echteld I, Wechalekar MD, Schlesinger N et al (2014) Colchicine for acute gout. Cochrane Database Syst Rev 18(4):CD006190. doi:10.1002/14651858.CD006190.pub2: CD006190
12. Zhang W, Doherty M, Bardin T et al (2006) EULAR evidence based recommendations for gout. Part II: management. Report of a task force of the EULAR Standing Committee for International Clinical Studies Including Therapeutics (ESCISIT). Ann Rheum Dis 65:1312–1324
13. Jordan KM, Cameron JS, Snaith M et al (2007) British Society for Rheumatology and British Health Professionals in Rheumatology guideline for the management of gout. Rheumatology 46:1372–1374
14. Aletaha D, Neogi T, Silman AJ et al (2010) Rheumatoid arthritis classification criteria: an American College of Rheumatology/European League Against Rheumatism collaborative initiative. Ann Rheum Dis 69:1580–1588
15. Stoffer MA, Smolen JS, Woolf A et al (2014) Development of patient-centred standards of care for rheumatoid arthritis in Europe: the eumusc.net project. Ann Rheum Dis 73:902–905
16. Singh JA, Saag KG, Bridges SL Jr et al (2016) 2015 American College of Rheumatology guideline for the treatment of rheumatoid arthritis. Arthritis Rheumatol 68:1–26
17. Swardh E, Brodin N (2016) Effects of aerobic and muscle strengthening exercise in adults with rheumatoid arthritis: a narrative review summarising a chapter in Physical activity in the prevention and treatment of disease (FYSS 2016). Br J Sports Med 50:362–367
18. Bergstra SA, Murgia A, Te Velde AF et al (2014) A systematic review into the effectiveness of hand exercise therapy in the treatment of rheumatoid arthritis. Clin Rheumatol 33:1539–1548
19. Cramp F, Hewlett S, Almeida C et al (2013) Non-pharmacological interventions for fatigue in rheumatoid arthritis. Cochrane Database Syst Rev 23(8):CD008322. doi:10.1002/14651858.CD008322.pub2
20. Schmidt WA (2011) Polymyalgia rheumatica and giant cell arteritis in the elderly. In: Nakasato Y, Yung RL (eds) Geriatric rheumatology: a comprehensive approach. Springer, New York
21. Ness T, Bley TA, Schmidt WA et al (2013) The diagnosis and treatment of giant cell arteritis. Dtsch Arztebl Int 110:376–385; quiz 386
22. Dejaco C, Singh YP, Perel P et al (2015) 2015 recommendations for the management of polymyalgia rheumatica: a European League Against Rheumatism/American College of Rheumatology collaborative initiative. Arthritis Rheumatol 67:2569–2580
23. Mukhtyar C, Guillevin L, Cid MC et al (2009) EULAR recommendations for the management of large vessel vasculitis. Ann Rheum Dis 68:318–323
24. Fraser JA, Weyand CM, Newman NJ et al (2008) The treatment of giant cell arteritis. Rev Neurol Dis 5:140–152
25. Shiboski SC, Shiboski CH, Criswell L et al (2012) American College of Rheumatology classification criteria for Sjogren's syndrome: a data-driven, expert consensus approach in the Sjogren's International Collaborative Clinical Alliance cohort. Arthritis Care Res (Hoboken) 64:475–487
26. Yung RL, Francis S (2011) Sjögren's syndrome in the elderly. In: Nakasato Y, Yung RL (eds) Geriatric rheumatology: a comprehensive approach. Springer, New York
27. Zochling J, van der Heijde D, Burgos-Vargas R et al (2006) ASAS/EULAR recommendations for the management of ankylosing spondylitis. Ann Rheum Dis 65:442–452
28. Dagfinrud H, Halvorsen S, Vollestad NK et al (2011) Exercise programs in trials for patients with ankylosing spondylitis: do they really have the potential for effectiveness? Arthritis Care Res 63:597–603
29. Millner JR, Barron JS, Beinke KM et al (2016) Exercise for ankylosing spondylitis: an evidence-based consensus statement. Semin Arthritis Rheum 45:411–427
30. Fiehn C (2014) Which kind of structures and facilities are needed for the care of elderly patients with rheumatic diseases? Z Rheumatol 73:217–224

Cervical Pain, Lumbar Pain, and Sciatalgia

26

Andrea Furlan and Miriam Duso

26.1 Introduction

Due to the complexity of structures in the spine, determination of the cause of neck pain (NP) and low back pain (LBP) is not always possible. Age-related degenerative processes affecting the spine are found in most of the population older than 60 years and can be asymptomatic or cause NP and LBP, with or without radiculopathy. These changes can also lead to spinal stenosis and its related symptoms [1]. However, NP and LBP can be a feature of many other conditions, including serious diseases such as cancer, infections, fractures, and rheumatologic illnesses.

The elderly patient with NP and LBP has lower physical performance than their pain-free peers [2] and a lower global health as they are more frequently affected by other morbidities, especially bone and joint disorders, migraine, and cardiovascular, pulmonary, and gastric disorders [3].

A. Furlan, MD, PhD (✉)
Toronto Rehabilitation Institute - University Health Network, Toronto, ON, Canada

Department of Medicine, University of Toronto, Toronto, ON, Canada

Institute for Work and Health, Toronto, ON, Canada
e-mail: andrea.furlan@uhn.ca

M. Duso, MD
Department of Neuroscience, University of Padua, Padua, Italy
e-mail: miriam.duso@studenti.unipd.it

© Springer International Publishing AG 2018

S. Masiero, U. Carraro (eds.), *Rehabilitation Medicine for Elderly Patients*,
Practical Issues in Geriatrics, DOI 10.1007/978-3-319-57406-6_26

26.2 Neck Pain in the Elderly

26.2.1 Epidemiology

NP affects every year approximately 16–20% of the older population [2]. Many conditions can cause NP, and in the elderly population, a major cause is osteoarthritis of the cervical spine. Not all of the individuals affected by cervical osteoarthritis, however, have clinical signs or symptoms of pain. Clinicians should be aware that there are other conditions that can potentially cause neck pain, which include cervical instability, fracture, neoplastic conditions, vascular compromise, thoracic outlet syndrome, and affections of the cervical musculature such as myofascial pain syndrome, torticollis, and whiplash [4].

NP can be transitory (less than 7 days), short-duration NP (between 7 days and 3 months), and long-duration NP (>3 months) [5]. It can be classified as (a) NP without suspect of underlying serious pathology and with no or little interference with the activities of daily living (ADL), (b) NP without suspect of underlying serious pathology but with major interference with ADL, (c) NP without suspect of underlying serious pathology but with neurological deficits (motor, sensitive, weakness), and (d) NP with suspect of underlying serious pathology [5].

26.2.2 Symptoms

Localization of pain may vary: there are patients with axial pain only and patients with both axial and radiating pain. Axial pain is localized in the posterior cervical region, and it can radiate upward to the head (typically the occipital region) or to the superior trapezius or the interscapular region. If radiculopathy is present, pain radiates to the arm along the distribution of a specific nerve root, with sensory and motor symptoms such as paresthesias, dysesthesias, numbness, and weakness that follow the specific myotomal and dermatomal distribution [1]. It is important to rule out symptoms of serious underlying disease, commonly called "red flags" (see Table 26.1). For example, red flags for cervical myelopathy include gait abnormalities, resulting from sensory and motor extremity deficits (numbness, paresthesias, impaired proprioception, weakness and difficulty in fine motor tasks, hyperreflexia), neurogenic bladder, or bowel and sexual dysfunction [1].

26.2.3 Physical Exam

Physical examination of a patient who complains of NP should include evaluation of range of movement of the cervical spine (flexion, extension, rotation, and side bending), the cervical and thoracic segmental mobility test, the cranial cervical flexion test, and the neck flexor muscle endurance test. In patients with radicular symptoms, the physical examination should also include upper limb tension test, the Spurling test, the distraction test, and the Valsalva test [1]. In patients with radicular

Table 26.1 Red flags (for both neck and low back pain)

Potential cause	Red flags
Cancer	History of cancer Unexplained weight loss Progressive pain not responding to therapies Nighttime pain, pain at rest
Vertebral infection	History of infection Fever IV drug use Immunosuppression Systemic symptoms such as fever with chills, high inflammatory markers
Fracture	History of trauma Osteoporosis Steroid use Structural deformity Midline spine tenderness
Myelopathy	Pain in the extremities Weakness in the extremities Sensory deficits and/or atrophy in the extremities Hyperreflexia
Cauda equina syndrome	Bladder dysfunction Bowel incontinence Saddle anesthesia Weakness of the lower limbs Gait disturbance
Inflammatory (rheumatological) cause	Pain and stiffness worsening with rest Morning stiffness (>30 min) Altered inflammatory markers Multiple joint involvement

Adapted from Chou et al. [6], Côté et al. [7], Dagenais et al. [8], and Van Tulder et al. [9]

pain, an accurate examination helps to identify the involved nerve root: this means an accurate sensory testing, motor testing, and evaluation of deep tendon reflexes (see Table 26.2). Cervical facets can be examined by manual palpation of the spinal segments: pressure on the involved facet joints causes exacerbation of the usual symptoms. Evaluation also includes the palpation of neck muscles for tone, tenderness and contractures. Gait evaluation is important and may be abnormal if myelopathy is present. Validated scales and instruments, such as *Neck Disability Index* and *Patient-Specific Functional Scale*, allow to evaluate how pain can affect the activities of daily living (ADL). A surgeon or rheumatologist consultation may be appropriate in cases of neck pain associated with red flags [4].

26.2.4 Imaging

When imaging is necessary, a plain radiograph is the first exam to be ordered in the elderly patient with NP, eventually associated to dynamic X-rays. Advanced

Table 26.2 Cervical radicular referred pain—characteristics

Nerve root level	Sensory deficits/location of pain	Muscle weakness	Reflex
C2	Occipital, eyes		
C3	Neck, trapezius		
C4	Neck, trapezius		
C5	Shoulder, lateral arm	Deltoid, biceps	Biceps
C6	Radial forearm, first and second digits	Biceps, wrist extension	Brachioradialis, biceps
C7	Third digit	Triceps, wrist flexion	Triceps
C8	Fourth and fifth digits, ulnar forearm	Finger flexors	
T1	Ulnar arm	Hand intrinsic muscles	

Adapted from Frontera and Silver [1], Hoppenfeld [10], and Iyer [11]

imaging, such as CT, MRI, and bone scan, can be considered in case of NP, but not routinely, as there is a lack of evidence in the literature of the correlation between abnormal findings and patients' symptomatology [4]. In patients with referred arm pain, an electromyographic study can be useful to distinguish peripheral nerve entrapment syndromes from cervical radiculopathy [11].

26.2.5 Pharmacological Therapy

In transient or short-duration NP, muscle relaxants are the only pharmacological therapy suggested by current evidence. NSAIDs can be considered in order to relieve pain in patients with long-duration NP. NSAIDs must be prescribed only for short periods due to their many side effects. There is no evidence for efficacy of acetaminophen/paracetamol [4].

26.2.6 Non-pharmacological Therapies

1. Education of the patient. For patients without red flags, clinicians must educate the patients about NP, reassuring them that it is usually a condition with a good prognosis, and should advise a quick return to normal activities [4, 7].
2. Pillows seem to be beneficial in reducing pain [12] and can be recommended as part of the NP treatment.
3. Cognitive behavioral treatment might have a role in reducing pain and disability in the short term in patients affected by chronic NP, but its role is still to be demonstrated [13].
4. Exercises are used in common practice in patients with NP. Strengthening, coordination, and endurance exercises are suggested in patients with NP and neck-related headache. Stretching exercises of the scalenes, trapezius, levator scapulae, and pectoralis minor and major can also be prescribed. Centralization

exercises are not recommended [4]. Adverse effects after exercise are self-limiting and include headache; neck, shoulder, or thoracic pain; or symptom worsening [14].

5. Physical therapy modalities: Low-level laser therapy (LLLT) is recommended for chronic NP, but not for acute patients [7]. Pulsed electromagnetic fields (PEMF), repetitive magnetic stimulation, and TENS might be effective in reducing pain (low-level evidence). Galvanic current, iontophoresis, electrical muscle stimulation, and static magnetic field do not seem to be useful in reducing neck pain [15].
6. Massage can provide some relief from pain in chronic NP. It does not seem useful in acute NP [7].
7. Cervical mobilization/manipulation seems to have a role in reducing both acute and chronic NP, especially when associated with exercises [4]. Maiers et al. suggested that in elderly population, spinal manipulative therapy associated with home exercises is more effective in reducing pain and disability than exercises alone in the short term [16]. Potential risks of mobilization/manipulation are local or radiating discomfort, headache, fatigue, or more rarely dizziness and nausea (in a minority of patients); however, these symptoms are usually transitory. There is only inconclusive evidence on the association between cervical spinal manipulative therapy and cervical artery dissection [17]. Contraindications to cervical mobilization are osteoporosis, inflammatory spondylopathy, vertebral metastases, or other weakening conditions of the spine.
8. Thoracic mobilization/manipulation can reduce pain and disability [4].
9. Acupuncture seems to have a role in reducing NP [18]. Needling of myofascial trigger points, both dry needling and wet needling (using lidocaine or other local anesthetics), can be useful in relieving myofascial neck and shoulder pain; wet needling seems more effective [19].
10. Cervical collars [7], heat [7], and cervical traction are not recommended as they do not seem to provide any benefit.

26.3 Low Back Pain in the Elderly

26.3.1 Epidemiology

Prevalence of low back pain (LBP) in the elderly is approximately 25% [20]. Severe LBP seems to afflict 13% of older men and 20% of elderly women for at least 30 days every year [2].

LBP can be acute (<6 weeks), subacute (6–12 weeks), and chronic (>12 weeks). Ninety percent of patients affected by acute LBP recover within 6 weeks; however, LBP will persist more than 12 weeks in 2–7% of patients [21]. LBP can be classified in (a) mechanic or nonspecific LBP, (b) LBP associated with radicular pain, (c) LBP with an underlying serious pathology, and (d) LBP referring from a visceral disease [6, 9, 22, 27, 32].

26.3.2 Symptoms

LBP is usually defined as pain in the lower back, between the costal margin and the inferior gluteal folds [21], or the thighs; it can radiate to the legs with a radicular distribution, associated or not to sensory and motor symptoms (sciatica) [6].

26.3.3 Patient Evaluation

In limited cases, a serious disease could cause LBP. Therefore, patient evaluation must primarily aim at identifying signs, symptoms, and patient characteristics that will alert the physician ("red flags"). In particular, cancer can be suspected in a patient with LBP and a history of malignancy, nocturnal pain, symptoms at rest that do not respond to therapy, or if they are associated to weight loss. On the other hand, a history of recent trauma, osteoporosis, or recent use of steroids could be associated with a vertebral fracture, especially in the presence of an evident structural deformity of the spine. It is also important to look for symptoms of cauda equina and infection (Table 26.1).

LBP can also have visceral or non-spinal origin, such as arterial (aortic aneurysm), renal, gastrointestinal, or pelvic [22]. "Yellow flags" are emotional and behavioral factors associated with pain chronicity, such as anxiety, depression, and avoidance of normal activities resulting from fear of pain exacerbations, and should always be sought and modified with psychosocial support interventions [8].

Physical examination includes sensory testing of the lower limbs and evaluation of deep tendon reflexes and muscle strength (see Table 26.3). Special maneuvers can be helpful in distinguishing different pain sources; straight leg raising test, for example, is commonly used to detect nerve root irritation and has a high sensitivity but low specificity [6]. In case of herniated disc or bulging, disc pain radiates to the legs following a specific nerve root dermatomal irradiation (see Table 26.3), but, on the contrary, it does not have a radicular distribution when it has a myofascial origin or it is due to spinal stenosis.

Validated scales and instruments such as the Roland Morris Disability Questionnaire and Oswestry LBP Disability Scale can help the clinician in evaluating the severity of LBP and how it affects the ADL.

Table 26.3 Lumbar radicular referred pain—characteristics

Nerve root level	Sensory deficits/location of pain	Muscle weakness	Reflex	Screening test
L4	Anterior thigh, medial leg and foot	Quadriceps/tibialis anterior	Patellar	Rising from squat position
L5	Lateral thigh and leg and dorsum of foot	Extensor hallucis longus/ tibialis anterior	Hamstring	Walking on heels
S1	Posterior thigh and leg and lateral foot	Fibularis (peroneus) longus and brevis	Achilles	Walking on toes

Adapted from Hoppenfeld [10] and Manchikanti et al. [23]

26.3.4 Imaging

Imaging studies should not be routinely used in acute LBP without signs or symptoms of underlying serious disease, as their findings are not always related to symptoms. Whenever fracture is suspected, a plain radiograph is recommended. Lumbar spine plain X-ray, followed by an MRI, can be useful if cancer is suspected. MRI or CT scan should be promptly ordered in case of new-onset lumbar pain and a history of malignancy, suspected vertebral infection, spinal stenosis, cauda equina syndrome, and herniated disc [24].

26.3.5 Prevention of LBP

- Physical activity such as gardening, walking, cycling (>30 min/day), sport, or dancing should be encouraged in the aging population; moderate to high intensity physical activity, at least once a week, protects from LBP [25].

26.3.6 Pharmacological Treatment

- Paracetamol (acetaminophen) is not better than placebo for acute LBP. (Reference to Saragiotto BT, Machado GC, Ferreira ML, Pinheiro MB, Abdel Shaheed C, Maher CG. Paracetamol for low back pain. Cochrane Database Syst Rev. 2016 Jun 7;(6):CD012230). NSAIDs are more efficient than paracetamol but have more side effects. Muscle relaxants such as cyclobenzaprine or methocarbamol can also be prescribed, especially for myofascial pain syndrome. In case of more severe pain, other medications such as opioids or tramadol can be used for short periods (less than 4 weeks), but patients need to be monitored for sedation, overdose and aberrant behaviours. Tricyclic antidepressants may provide some benefit in patients with chronic LBP, especially in the presence of pain associated with neuropathic pain (such as radiculopathy), fibromyalgia or myofascial pain syndrome. Gabapentin can give some small, short-term relief in case of radicular symptoms [6].

26.3.7 Non-pharmacological Therapy

There are many conservative and interventional procedures offered in practice and described in the scientific literature; below is a list of the treatments that are most commonly used in everyday practice and those with the best current evidence.

- **Acute low back pain:**

In the absence of red flags, the patient must be reassured, and a fast return to daily activities must be encouraged. Bed rest is not recommended and should not exceed 2 days. There is no evidence in support of prescription of exercise therapy in the acute phase of LBP [9]. Spinal manipulation can be considered [6, 9], but traction does not seem to be effective [9, 30]. Physical therapy modalities such as ultrasound, TENS, or laser are not suggested [9]. Massage seems to control pain, and heat can also give some short-term relief [6, 29].

- **Chronic low back pain:**

1. Cognitive behavioral treatment seems to be moderately effective [6], and it is recommended to improve pain and function in patients suffering from chronic low back pain [26].
2. Mindfulness meditation is a technique which might have some role in improving pain acceptance [27].
3. Exercise therapy is recommended as first-line therapy in patients with chronic low back pain [26], as it seems to be effective in reducing pain and improving function. There is little evidence about which exercise modality is best in elderly patients; therefore, a practical approach is to prescribe a general exercise program that combines four types of exercises: strengthening, stretching, aerobic and relaxation ("SSAR") exercises [28].
4. Back school or group education that teaches self-management strategies can be considered to improve knowledge about pain and function in the short term [26].
5. Massage is useful to control pain and improve function, at least in the short term; but when compared to other treatments, it does not seem to have any beneficial effect on physical function [29].
6. Spinal manipulation could be useful for improving pain [26].
7. Acupuncture can be moderately effective in relieving pain [6].
8. There is limited evidence on the efficacy of physical therapies, such as interferential current, therapeutic ultrasound, laser therapy, thermotherapy, shortwave diathermy, and TENS [6, 26].
9. There is no evidence for lumbar support [26].
10. Traction is not suggested in LBP as there is no evidence supporting any type of traction (mechanical, motorized, manual, or auto-traction) [30].

Conservative interventions can be also combined. Currently, there is no recommendation about which modality is to try first; therefore, it is important to discuss the treatment with the patient and decide according to his/her preferences and availability. In any case, before considering a treatment ineffective, an adequate time of trial and observation is important.

26.4 Interventional Procedures and Surgery for NP and LBP

In those patients whose progressive symptoms do not improve with conservative treatment, invasive procedures are suggested both in NP and in LBP.

There is good evidence that cervical interlaminar epidural injections with local anesthetic, eventually associated with steroids, can be useful in NP secondary to disc herniation or radiculitis, while in discogenic pain, spinal stenosis, and postsurgical pain syndrome, evidence is fair. Efficacy of epidural lumbar injection therapy with steroids and local anesthetics has been proved with good evidence, in patients with disc herniation or radiculitis; however, there is fair evidence in case of axial or discogenic pain without herniation, spinal stenosis, facet joint pain, and postsurgery syndrome [23].

Immediate spine surgeon consultation is mandatory when suspected cauda equina and a referral to a surgeon or interventional pain specialist is recommended in patients refractory to all conservative treatments. In patients with cervical radicular pain with severe impairments, surgery may be a reasonable option. Pain relief is usually observed immediately after surgery, although it is not clear if the long-term outcome of surgery is better than conservative treatment. Currently, there is no evidence on the best surgical procedure [31]. In refractory and severely disabling LBP, the main surgical options are vertebral fusion, instrumented stabilization, and vertebral decompression. Although there is no definitive demonstration in literature of the efficacy of surgery compared to conservative treatment in the long-term pain management, surgery seems to be beneficial in degenerative spondylolisthesis and symptomatic lumbar canal stenosis [32]. A surgical treatment is a procedure that can behold many risks in the elderly and especially in patients with multiple comorbidities.

Key Points

- Neck pain and lumbar back pain are common in elderly population.
- A complete history and thorough physical examination are crucial and often the only measure needed to obtain a proper diagnosis.
- It is important to rule out red flags for serious diseases.
- Investigations such as X-ray and MRIs should be used judiciously and only when red flags are suspected or when surgery is indicated.
- Some conservative treatment may be effective in the management of neck and lumbar back pain.
- Surgery is indicated both in NP and LBP only in case of serious disease (e.g. cancer, infection) or in refractory cases to conservative treatments.

References

1. Frontera WR, Silver JK (2015) Essentials of physical medicine and rehabilitation
2. Hartvigsen J, Frederiksen H, Christensen K (2006) Back and neck pain in seniors-prevalence and impact. Eur Spine J 15(6):802–806
3. Hartvigsen J, Christensen K, Frederiksen H (2003) Back pain remains a common symptom in old age. A population-based study of 4486 Danish twins aged 70–102. Eur Spine J 12:528–534
4. Childs JD, Cleland JA, Elliott JM et al (2008) Neck pain: clinical practice guidelines linked to the International Classification of Functioning, Disability, and Health from the Orthopedic Section of the American Physical Therapy Association. J Orthop Sports Phys Ther 38(9):A1–A34. Epub 2008 Sep 1

5. Guzman J, Hurwitz EL, Carroll LJ et al (2008) A new conceptual model of neck pain: linking onset, course, and care: the bone and joint decade 2000–2010 task force on neck pain and its associated disorders. Spine (Phila Pa 1976) 33(4 Suppl):S14–S23
6. Chou R, Qaseem A, Snow V et al (2007) Diagnosis and treatment of low back pain: a joint clinical practice guideline from the American College of Physicians and the American Pain Society. Ann Intern Med 147(7):478–491
7. Côté P, Wong JJ, Sutton D et al (2016) Management of neck pain and associated disorders: a clinical practice guideline from the Ontario Protocol for Traffic Injury Management (OPTIMa) Collaboration. Eur Spine J 25(7):2000–2022. doi:10.1007/s00586-016-4467-7. Epub 2016 Mar
8. Dagenais S, Tricco AC, Haldeman S (2010) Synthesis of recommendations for the assessment and management of low back pain from recent clinical practice guidelines. Spine J 10:514–529
9. Van Tulder M, Becker A, Bekkering T et al (2006) Chapter 3. European guidelines for the management of acute nonspecific low back pain in primary care. COST B13 Working Group. Eur Spine J 15(Suppl 2):S169–S191
10. Hoppenfeld S (1976) Physical examination of the spine and extremities. Appleton Century-Crofts, East Norwalk, CT
11. Iyer S, Kim HJ (2016) Cervical radiculopathy. Curr Rev Musculoskelet Med 9(3):272–280
12. Jamal AN, Feldman BM, Pullenayegum E (2016) The use of neck support pillows and postural exercises in the management of chronic neck pain. J Rheumatol. pii: jrheum.151368. [Epub ahead of print]
13. Monticone M, Cedraschi C, Ambrosini E et al (2015) Cognitive-behavioural treatment for subacute and chronic neck pain. Cochrane Database Syst Rev 5:CD010664
14. Gross AR, Paquin JP, Dupont G et al (2016) Exercises for mechanical neck disorders: a Cochrane review update. Man Ther 24:25–45
15. Kroeling P, Gross A, Graham N et al (2013) Electrotherapy for neck pain. Cochrane Database Syst Rev (8)
16. Maiers M, Bronfort G, Evans R et al (2014) Spinal manipulative therapy and exercise for seniors with chronic neck pain. Spine J 14(9):1879–1889
17. Biller J, Sacco RL, Albuquerque FC et al (2014) Cervical arterial dissections and association with cervical manipulative therapy: a statement for healthcare professionals from the American Heart Association/American Stroke Association. Stroke 45(10):3155–3174
18. Trinh K, Graham N, Irnich D et al (2016) Cochrane acupuncture for neck disorders. Database Syst Rev 5:CD004870
19. Liu L, Huang QM, Liu QG et al (2015) Effectiveness of dry needling for myofascial trigger points associated with neck and shoulderpain: a systematic review and meta-analysis. Arch Phys Med Rehabil 96(5):944–955. doi:10.1016/j.apmr.2014.12.015. Epub 2015 Jan 7
20. Leopoldino AA, Diz JB, Martins VT et al (2016) Prevalence of low back pain in older Brazilians: a systematic review with meta-analysis. Rev Bras Reumatol (Rio J) 56(3):258–269
21. Burton AK, Balagué F, Cardon G et al (2006) Chapter 2. European guidelines for prevention in low back pain. COST B13 Working Group. 2004: 1–53. Eur Spine J 15(Suppl 2):S136–S168
22. Deyo RA, Weinstein JN (2001) Low back pain. N Engl J Med 344(5):363–370
23. Manchikanti L, Abdi S, Atluri S et al (2013) An update of comprehensive evidence-based guidelines for interventional techniques in chronic spinal pain. Part II: guidance and recommendations. Pain Physician 16:S49–S283
24. Chou R, Fu R, Carrino JA, Deyo RA (2009) Imaging strategies for low-back pain: systematic review and meta-analysis. Lancet 373(9662):463–472
25. Hartvigsen J, Christensen K (2007) Active lifestyle protects against incident low back pain in seniors: a population-based 2-year prospective study of 1387 Danish twins aged 70–100 years. Spine (Phila Pa 1976) 32(1):76–81
26. Airaksinen O, Brox JI, Cedraschi C et al (2006) Chapter 4. European guidelines for the management of chronic nonspecific low back pain. Eur Spine J 15(Suppl 2):S192–S300
27. Cramer H, Haller H, Lauche R, Dobos G (2012) Mindfulness-based stress reduction for low back pain. A systematic review. BMC Complement Altern Med 12:162

28. Henchoz Y, Kai-Lik SA et al (2008) Exercise and nonspecific low back pain: a literature review. Joint Bone Spine 75:533–539
29. Furlan AD, Giraldo M, Baskwill A et al (2015) Massage for low-back pain. Cochrane Database Syst Rev 9:CD001929
30. Wegner I, Widyahening IS, van Tulder MW et al (2013) Traction for low-back pain with or without sciatica. Cochrane Database Syst Rev 8:CD003010
31. Carragee EJ, Hurwitz EL, Cheng I et al (2008) Treatment of neck pain. Injections and surgical interventions: results of the bone and joint decade 2000–2010 task force on neck pain and its associated disorders. Spine 33(4s):S153–S169
32. Jones LD, Hemandt P, Lavy C (2014) Back pain in the elderly: a review. Maturitas 78(4):258–262

Rehabilitation of Older Patients with Osteo-metabolic Disorders

27

Giovanni Iolascon, Francesca Gimigliano, Antimo Moretti, Emanuela Covella, and Raffaele Gimigliano

27.1 Bone Physiology and Age-Related Bone Changes

27.1.1 Bone Tissue Metabolism in Older Adults

Bone tissue undergoes continuous remodeling throughout life, where resorption and formation alternatively occur. From a biomechanical point of view, the aim of bone remodeling is to repair the micro-cracks and to adapt the shape and the bone density to the mechanical load which the skeleton usually undergoes. Bone tissue also serves to store various substances, in particular calcium and phosphorus ions that can be released into the blood in order to keep steady their serum concentrations.

The 5–10% of the entire adult skeleton is replaced every year through bone remodeling [1]. Bone turnover is rigorously regulated by the coupled action of osteoblasts and osteoclasts. These two types of cells build the basic multicellular units (BMUs), whose activities are controlled by several hormones and growth factors [2].

During skeletal growth, formation exceeds resorption with a consequent increase in the total body bone mass, reaching the bone peak mass (between 20 and 25 years). Bone formation and resorption are balanced till the fourth decade of life. After this time the total bone mass will start to decrease, so that at 80 years it will be reduced to the 50% of the peak value [3]. In fact, in the elderly, bone remodeling

G. Iolascon (✉) • A. Moretti • E. Covella • R. Gimigliano
Department of Medical and Surgical Specialties and Dentistry, University of Campania "Luigi Vanvitelli", Caserta, Italy
e-mail: giovanni.iolascon@unicampania.it

F. Gimigliano
Department of Mental and Physical Health and Preventive Medicine, University of Campania "Luigi Vanvitelli", Caserta, Italy

© Springer International Publishing AG 2018

S. Masiero, U. Carraro (eds.), *Rehabilitation Medicine for Elderly Patients*, Practical Issues in Geriatrics, DOI 10.1007/978-3-319-57406-6_27

is characterized by an increase of osteoclastic resorption and a reduction of osteoblastic formation, resulting in bone mass reduction. Among the pathogenetic mechanisms involved in skeletal aging, chronic inflammation (inflammaging) has been identified as playing an important role, through the action of pro-inflammatory cytokines on bone remodeling process [4]. Several studies have shown that the levels of interleukin-6 (IL-6), tumor necrosis factor alpha (TNF-α), and IL-1, elevated in elderly [5], inhibit the production of new osteoblasts and can induce their apoptosis. Moreover, in aging, there is an alteration in growth hormone (GH) and insulin-like growth factor-1 (IGF-1) serum levels with a progressive decrease of GH secretion and consequent reduction of IGF-1 levels [6], which is further decreased by the simultaneous increase in serum IGF-binding proteins that reduces the bioavailability of IGF-1 [7]. This protein is a powerful anabolic factor that increases osteoblasts number and activity [8].

Another issue with aging is the reduction of physical activity [9]. In fact, it is well known that exercise, through the increase of the mechanical load, can positively influence bone mass [10].

Bone is a tissue that dynamically adapts its mass and architecture to the mechanical stress of daily living. Osteocytes are considered mechano-sensors that detect mechanical afferents and translate them into biochemical messages. In physiological conditions, the osteocyte network controls osteoclastogenesis and suppresses osteoblast function, thus increasing bone resorption and inhibiting bone formation. Unloading conditions promote the osteocytes production of molecules stimulating osteoclastogenesis, whereas physical activity counteracts this function by reducing both osteoclastogenesis and at the same time stimulating osteoblast function [11]. Recently it has been shown that osteocytes produce several molecules in response to mechanical stimulation: in addition to the collagen and alkaline phosphatase, these cells produce DMP1 (dentin matrix protein 1), PHEX (phosphate-regulating neutral endopeptidase on chromosome X), MEPE (matrix extracellular phosphoglycoprotein), FGF-23 (fibroblast growth factor 23), osteocalcin, osteoprotegerin, and sclerostin [12]. In particular, sclerostin is an acid glycoprotein of 190 amino acids secreted mainly by osteocytes [13]. Its function is to antagonize the Wnt signaling pathway, thus suppressing the activity of osteoblasts and downregulating bone turnover [13]. This pathway is involved in bone response to mechanical loads.

Both adequate nutrition and physical activity are necessary to achieve the genetically determined peak bone mass, which in turn is one of the most important factors that influence bone mass in old age [14].

27.1.2 Calcium, Phosphorus, and Vitamin D Metabolism in the Young Adult and in the Elderly

Bone aging is characterized by an inadequate mineralization of the osteoid tissue. It mainly depends on an impaired intestinal absorption of dietary calcium.

The trans-cellular active absorption is regulated by 1,25$(OH)_2$D that induces the synthesis of the calcium-binding protein (CBP) or calbindin, which facilitates the diffusion of calcium inside the cell toward the basolateral membrane and the extracellular fluid [15]. A variable amount of vitamin D is conducted to storage sites, mainly adipose and muscle tissues, from where it is continuously mobilized. Several studies have shown that plasma levels of both 25-OH-D3 (the vitamin D metabolite usually detected in the blood) and its biologically active form (calcitriol) decrease with aging by about 50% in both men and women. Hypovitaminosis D is an extremely common condition in the elderly because of the reduction of sun exposure, of the ability to convert vitamin D by the skin, of the vitamin D intake, of the intestinal vitamin D absorption, and of the 1-α-hydroxylase activity [16].

In the elderly, the reduced calcium availability, resulting from hypovitaminosis D, leads to an abnormal calcification of osteoid tissue, named osteomalacia. The simultaneous increase in serum PTH levels, aiming to increase the calcium levels, causes an activation of osteoclasts that leads to an excessive cortical and trabecular bone resorption resulting in osteoporosis. The coexistence of these two pathological conditions gives rise to the so-called osteoporomalacia that should be considered the typical senile bone disease.

27.1.3 Crosstalk Among Bone and Other Tissues

Bone might be considered as an endocrine organ, since it produces molecules acting not only on the bone itself but also at distance on other tissues and organs. On the other hand, bone is a target of several substances produced by other tissues. These mutual interactions play a key role in regulating relevant metabolic activities.

27.1.4 Bone and Gonads

Sex steroids affect bone and muscle growth and contribute to the maintenance of the homeostasis of these tissues during adulthood, so their deficiency can contribute to the development of osteoporosis and sarcopenia in both genders.

After menopause the major estrogen source is the adipose tissue that converts androstenedione, derived from dehydroepiandrosterone, into estrone. This latter does not exert the same trophic function on bone as estradiol; therefore, it is not able to counteract the age-dependent changes of the female skeleton. That is why the loss of bone mass, architectural integrity, and strength can be observed in female senile skeleton. In elderly men bone mass decreases with the decline of gonadal function due to the loss of Leydig cells in the testes and consequent decrease of testosterone levels [17]. However, androgens appear to be less important than estrogen in the maintenance of bone health in older men [18].

27.1.5 Bone, Muscle, and Adipose Tissue

Bone, muscle, and adipose tissues are involved in the complex energy metabolism scenario. These tissues have the same mesodermal origin and influence each other through a biochemical crosstalk producing several molecules with paracrine and endocrine activities [19]. Both osteoblasts and muscle fibers express receptors for two hormones produced by fat tissue, leptin, and adiponectin that have direct osteogenic effects [20, 21], promoting osteoblastogenesis and inhibiting osteoclastogenesis in bone marrow stromal cells as demonstrated in animal studies [22, 23]. In muscle, adiponectin increases mitochondrial number improving the oxidative tissue metabolism [24].

Another actor in bone/muscle/fat crosstalk is osteocalcin, a protein produced by osteoblasts and routinely used as a marker of bone formation. Osteocalcin stimulates the synthesis of adiponectin by adipocytes, increasing insulin sensitivity in muscles and enhancing the testosterone release in males [25].

27.1.6 Bone and Nervous System

Bone is an extremely dynamic tissue, as it continuously remodels itself, requiring a large amount of energy as well as muscle activity. Fat tissue provides the energy used to drive these complex metabolic processes. Through the mechanism of appetite regulation, the hypothalamus controls the amount of fat tissue. This anatomical region also modulates reproductive mechanisms, thus representing the link between energy metabolism and reproduction and bone metabolism, with osteocalcin as a modulator of these interactions. Hypothalamic cells present leptin receptors that stimulate the sympathetic activity, which, via osteoblastic adrenergic receptors, induces the overexpression of the gene coding for the RANKL, thus promoting bone resorption. Therefore, leptin inhibits the appetite and promotes the reproduction, energy consumption, and bone resorption.

It is likely that, within the central nervous system (CNS), there is the "control room" of the integrated management of bone-muscle-fat energy metabolism [26]. Recently, there have been identified four stages for these complex mechanisms. In the first stage, bone detects the energy requirements, and fat deposits send afferent signals to the hypothalamus. In the second stage, there is the activation of the hypothalamus and other complex neuronal network that promotes adrenergic activity in order to regulate bone metabolism (third stage), since osteoblasts express beta-adrenergic receptors. These cells modulate the synthesis of adiponectin by the adipocytes, completing the crosstalk circle between bone tissue and CNS (fourth stage). It is likely that these complex mechanisms might change with aging because of the alterations of the single components (bone, muscle, and fat) and also of the "control room" within the CNS (Fig. 27.1).

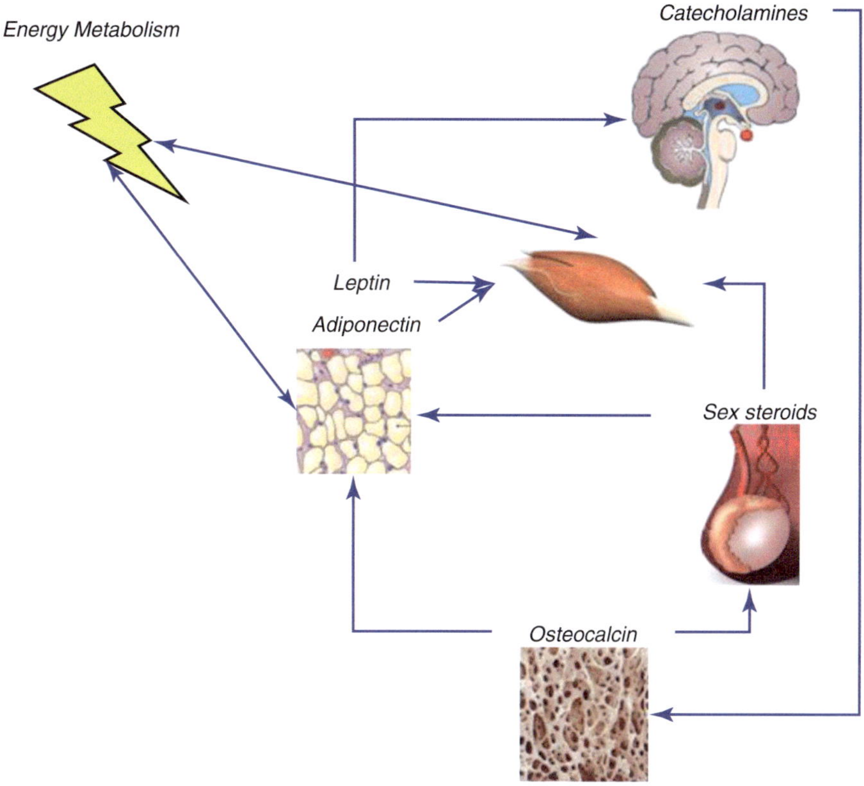

Fig. 27.1 Crosstalk among SNS, fat tissue, bone, and skeletal muscle

27.2 Osteo-metabolic Disorders in Elderly: Osteoporosis and Osteomalacia

27.2.1 Osteoporosis

27.2.1.1 Definition

Osteoporosis is a systemic skeletal disease characterized by a generalized decrease in bone density and deterioration of the microarchitecture of bone tissue that predispose to skeletal fragility resulting in increased risk of fractures [27].

From an operational point of view, the WHO defined osteoporosis when the bone mineral density (BMD) is less than 2.5 standard deviations than the mean peak bone mass of healthy young adults [27], based on a BMD measured by dual-energy X-ray absorptiometry (DXA). The normal BMD corresponds to a T-score ≥ -1;

osteopenia is defined as a T-score between -1 and -2.5; severe osteoporosis as a T-score ≤ -2.5 with a fracture.

27.2.1.2 Epidemiology

The incidence of osteoporosis increases with aging affecting most of the population over 80 years old. It is estimated that about one out of two women over the age of 50 will sustain a fragility fracture [28]. In the Italian people aged over 50, the incidence of hip fractures is more than 90,000, and vertebral fracture was detected in over 20% of people over 65 in both men and women [29].

27.2.1.3 Physiopathology

Primary or idiopathic osteoporosis includes juvenile, postmenopausal, and senile osteoporosis.

Secondary osteoporosis instead includes all clinical conditions in which the bone involvement is not the main pathologic finding, but the bone is one of the targets of primary disease or related treatments, especially those that include the use of glucocorticoids.

The main pathogenetic factor of postmenopausal osteoporosis is the estrogen depletion that worsens the age-related bone loss occurring from the age of 40 [30]. Senile osteoporosis comes from the combination of various factors: tissue aging, hormone depletion, nutritional disorders, and decrease in physical activity.

Secondary osteoporosis is caused by several diseases such as endocrine disorders and hematologic, gastrointestinal, rheumatic, and kidney diseases or by the use of medications such as glucocorticoids, anticoagulants, and other drugs [31].

Male osteoporosis can be considered primary only in 40% of cases [32], whereas most frequently it is secondary to other conditions, such as hypogonadism, alcoholism, multiple myeloma, hyperparathyroidism, malabsorption, and corticosteroid use [33], but also to androgen deprivation therapy for prostate cancer [34].

27.2.1.4 Risk of Falls and Fragility Fractures in Older Patients

Fall is the most important risk factor for fragility fractures, and the risk of falling increases exponentially with aging. The risk factors of falling can be categorized as intrinsic or extrinsic. The first ones include the physiological decline in age-related postural control mechanisms [35] and appendicular muscle strength, medications (diuretics, antiarrhythmics, antidepressants), orthostatic hypotension, and comorbidities. Neurological diseases, such as Parkinson's disease, cerebellar disorders, peripheral neuropathy, myelopathy secondary to cervical spondylosis, epilepsy, and stroke, increase the risk of falling.

Extrinsic risk factors include environmental issues, such as low or soft chairs, carpets, slippery surfaces, raised thresholds, stairs (especially the first and last step), inadequate lighting, unsuitable shoes, clutter, and wires. The reduction of the risk of falling is the main target of a non-pharmacological approach for the prevention of osteoporotic fractures [36].

Fragility fractures occur when a mechanical stress applied to the bone exceeds its strength. They result from a "low-energy" trauma due to mechanical forces equivalent to a fall from a standing height or less, which would not ordinarily cause a fracture.

27.2.1.5 Treatment of Primary and Secondary Osteoporosis

In order to reduce the risk of fragility fractures, a preventive strategy can be taken which is essentially based on exercise and lifestyle [37]. The National Osteoporosis Foundation (NOF) suggested the use of different prevention measures that include an adequate calcium and vitamin D intake, constant and regular physical activity, smoking cessation, alcoholism identification and treatment, and fall prevention. Physical activity is strongly recommended as an effective strategy to reduce the risk of osteoporosis and fracture through its beneficial effects on bone, muscle, and risk of falling [38].

The estimated risk necessary to establish the threshold of the pharmacological intervention is based on both the BMD and clinical fracture risk factors. Integrated assessment of multiple risk factors can be done through algorithms validated as the FRAX®.

The drugs commonly used for the treatment of osteoporosis and their related evidence are shown in Tables 27.1 and 27.2.

Table 27.1 Level of evidence for pharmacological treatment in postmenopausal osteoporosis

	Target of therapy			
Drugs	Hip fracture	Vertebral	Non-vertebral	BMD
Alendronate	1	1	1	1
Ibandronate		1	1	1
Risedronate	1	1	1	1
Zoledronate	1	1	1	1
Teriparatide		1	1	1
Raloxifene	1			1
Bazedoxifene	1			1
Denosumab	1	1	1	1

Table 27.2 Level of evidence for pharmacological treatment in male osteoporosis

	Target of therapy			
Drugs	Hip fracture	Vertebral	Non-vertebral	BMD
Alendronate		2		1
Risedronate		2		1
Zoledronate	2	1	2	1
Teriparatide		1		1
Denosumab		1		1

27.2.2 Osteomalacia

27.2.2.1 Definition

Osteomalacia is a metabolic bone disorder characterized by the presence of a normal bone mass, with reduced mineral content for an inadequate mineralization of the organic matrix. Patients with osteomalacia may complain of bone pain and muscle weakness and present vertebral deformity and/or pseudofractures (Looser-Milkman striae) [39].

27.2.2.2 Epidemiology

Nowadays, osteomalacia is a fairly rare disease. According to the National Institutes of Health (NIH), its incidence is less than 1/1000 [39].

27.2.2.3 Pathophysiology

Osteomalacia is linked to a reduced availability or to an altered metabolism of vitamin D or to alterations of the renal tubular reabsorption of phosphorus. The most common causes of osteomalacia are shown in Table 27.3 [40].

In the elderly osteomalacia due to vitamin D deficiency is very common [41]. Hypovitaminosis D is also very common in people with darker skin pigmentation [42], obese, and people who undergo gastrectomy or suffer from liver cirrhosis [43].

27.2.2.4 Treatment

For the treatment of osteomalacia, it is essential to identify and promptly treat the underlying cause to prevent the occurrence of fractures; furthermore it is necessary to adopt simple corrective measures regarding nutrition and sun exposure. We should encourage patients to have a higher nutritional intake (oily fish, cod liver oil, egg yolk, mushrooms, cereals, and margarine enriched of vitamin D). Early pharmacological treatment is mandatory, consisting of 50–125 μg per day of calcifediol, or 5000–10,000 IU per day of cholecalciferol for 1–2 months, with a maintenance therapy of 20 μg per day of calcifediol, or 800 IU per day of cholecalciferol.

Table 27.3 Common causes of osteomalacia

Vitamin D deficiency	• Inadequate oral intake • Inadequate exposure to sunlight • Intestinal malabsorption
Abnormal vitamin D metabolism	• Liver disease • Renal disease • Medication
Hypophosphatemia	• Low oral phosphate intake • Excess renal phosphate loss
Inhibition of mineralization	• Bisphosphonate • Aluminum • Fluoride
Hypophosphatasia	Inherited autosomal disorder

27.3 Physiatric Approach to Older Patients with Osteo-metabolic Disorders

27.3.1 Background

The global rehabilitative approach has a key role in all stages of these diseases, from prevention to functional recovery after a fragility fracture. The pivotal element of rehabilitation is the therapeutic exercise. Several studies and international guidelines suggested that this intervention is effective in increasing bone mass during skeletal growth, maintaining what has been achieved in adult life, reducing bone loss in the elderly and the risk of fractures.

In the elderly, exercise can enhance cortical thickness and strength in overloaded bone tissue. These effects might result from a diminished loss of endocortical bone and/or an increase in tissue density rather than an increase in bone size (due to periosteal apposition), even if also in elderly a progressive widening of the outer diameter occurs. These geometrical adaptations are able to increase the mechanical resistance to the compression load [44].

Two types of physical exercises are suitable for elderly: aerobic activities (walking, stair climbing, jogging, tennis, tai chi, gymnastics, dancing) and resistance exercises (where joints move against an external force given by weights, machines, or the own body weight).

The most common aerobic training in older people is walking that could be effective in maintaining BMD when combined with high-impact activities, such as jogging or stepping [45].

Therapeutic exercise could exert, through the improvement of the muscle performance, an indirect effect on bone health. However, aging is characterized by a progressive decline in aerobic exercise capacity due to the reduction in cardiovascular efficiency and skeletal muscle function caused by a decrease of mitochondrial number and activity [46]. Aerobic training stimulates the synthesis of mitochondria in the skeletal muscle with a consequent reduction of the oxidative stress and the enhancement of muscular performance [47].

Several studies suggest that the muscle strengthening produces a significant increase in femoral neck BMD [48]. Furthermore, improvement in muscle strength and performance, due to resistance exercise, might reduce the risk of falls.

At a cellular level, strengthening exercises increase the transverse diameter of type I and type II muscle fibers and of the entire lean mass, with relative increase in muscle strength [49]. Fast-velocity resistance exercises (i.e., performing a concentric phase as quickly as possible followed by an eccentric 2-second contraction phase) [50] have shown to cause a greater recruitment of motor units in type II muscle fibers counteracting atrophy in aging [51].

There is a general consensus that older people should perform moderate-intensity aerobic exercises for a minimum of 30 min 5 days a week or high-intensity aerobic activity for a minimum of 20 min 3 days per week [45]. Moderate-intensity aerobic exercise is intended, from an absolute scale, as the activity that takes place at an intensity of 3.0–5.9 times the intensity at rest or, from a relative scale based on

Table 27.4 General principles of therapeutic exercise in patients with osteoporosis

Specificity	Specific to the individual patient; specific to one or more physiological goals (bone strength, muscle strength, flexibility, cardiovascular fitness); specific to the anatomical site
Progression	Gradual increases in duration, intensity, and frequency; applied loads must remain below bone and connective tissue injury threshold, but be high enough to provide a greater than current activity stimulus to the organ system (muscle, heart, or connective tissue)
Reversibility	Positive effects of exercise will be slowly lost if the program is discontinued
Initial values	Those with initially low capacity will have the greatest functional improvement
Diminished returns	There is a biological ceiling to exercised-induced improvements in function; approaching this limit means greater effort to achieve minimal gains

individual's capacity (ranging from 0 to 10), an intensity of 5 or 6 times the intensity at rest. High-intensity aerobic exercise is the activity that takes place at an intensity of at least 6 times the intensity at rest on an absolute scale, an exercise intensity of 7 or 8 times the intensity at rest based on individual's capacity. Aerobic exercise should be performed for at least 10 consecutive minutes [52].

Bodyweight exercises or training with equipment is also useful, but should be performed slowly, with 1–3 series for each type of exercise, spacing 1–3 min of rest, for 2–3 days/week [52]. Strengthening exercises are safe, feasible, and effective to induce muscle hypertrophy and to increase strength and should be performed as soon as possible in order to prevent the progression of skeletal fragility and sarcopenia. General principles of the prescription of therapeutic exercise in osteoporotic patients have been proposed by a specific task force of the NOF [53] (Table 27.4).

27.3.1.1 Rehabilitation of Elderly Osteoporotic Patients Without Fragility Fractures and Prevention of the Risk of Falling

The rehabilitative approach to an old osteoporotic patient at risk of a fragility fracture aims to counteract the progressive osteoporomalacia and to reduce the risk of falling. The adoption of safety measures at home, the correction of modifiable intrinsic factors such as visual disturbances, pacemaker implantation in patients with sick sinus syndrome, and the gradual reduction in the consumption of psychotropic drugs are recommended according to a Cochrane review of 2012 [54].

NICE guidelines (2013) [55] support a multidisciplinary assessment and a comprehensive intervention in order to improve both physical and psychological health. It has been shown that combined programs of balance training and muscle strengthening are effective in the prevention of falls in elderly residents in the community. On the other hand, there is no scientific evidence supporting brisk walking as a preventive measure that reduces the risk of falls.

Recently, a Cochrane review underlined that the hip protectors, when correctly worn, might decrease hip fracture risk and both morbidity and mortality in elderly, especially in institutionalized individuals [56].

27.3.1.2 Rehabilitation of Elderly Patients with Fragility Fractures

The most frequent sites of osteoporotic fractures are the spine, hip, proximal humerus, and distal radius, but actually also other fractures might recognize an osteoporotic pathogenesis [29]. In many cases a surgical approach followed by a rehabilitative treatment is necessary in order to improve the functional activity and social participation and thus the quality of life of the individual. The majority of distal radius fractures is treated conservatively by closed reduction and cast/splint application for 4–6 weeks, although currently many authors prefer an internal fixation. Rehabilitation programs generally begin after cast removal and consist of range-of-motion (ROM) exercises and resistance exercise associated with occupational therapy.

Clinical vertebral fractures are commonly treated with rest and/or spinal bracing. Indications to surgery vary according to age, general clinical condition, type of fracture and spinal stability, involvement of the spinal cord, bone quality, and time from the fracture. Surgical options are frequently vertebroplasty and kyphoplasty, rarely spinal stabilization with or without fusion [57].

Rehabilitative approach begins immediately after surgery in order to recover muscle strength and spinal mobility and to enhance balance, especially during postural changes and walking. However, the strengthening of back extensor muscles is a priority [53].

Fractures of the proximal humerus are usually treated conservatively in the elderly, unless there is an unstable or displaced four-part fracture that requires surgical approach, consisting of open reduction with internal fixation or, in some cases, arthroplasty [57]. Rehabilitation starts after cast removal or surgical treatment, aiming to reduce pain and recover the ability in ADL.

Hip fracture is undoubtedly the most relevant complication of bone fragility in elderly. The main role of the physiatrist is to figure out an individual rehabilitation plan (IRP) that aims to reduce mortality and disability [58]. Hip fractures are currently treated surgically within 24–48 h from injury. Surgical intervention consists of hemiarthroplasty or total hip arthroplasty for intracapsular hip fractures, whereas osteosynthesis (screw plate or intramedullary nail) is preferred for trochanteric fractures. Considering the patient clinical condition and presence of comorbidities, rehabilitation begins immediately after surgery. Several factors should be taken into account in order to decide the timing of weight-bearing on the operated limb (Table 27.5).

Table 27.5 Factors affecting the time of total weight-bearing on the operated limb

	Early	Late
Method of fixation	Cemented prosthesis	Cementless prosthesis
Surgical approach	Mini-invasive	Traditional or trochanteric osteotomy
Bone grafting	No	Yes
Poor bone quality	No	Yes

Table 27.6 IRP and rehabilitation programs

Objectives	Rehabilitation programs
Preventing vascular complications (venous stasis, thrombosis, and pulmonary embolism)	Ankle pump exercises
Preventing pulmonary complications (atelectasis or postoperative pneumonia) especially for bedridden patients	Breathing exercises and bronchial hygiene therapy
Preventing hip dislocation of THA	Patient/caregiver education to mobility strategies in order to reduce the risk of dislocation during ADLs
Achieving functional independence before discharge	Educate patient to postural changes, transfers, and walking aids use
Maintaining an optimal level of muscle strength and endurance for the upper limb and not operated limb	Aerobic exercises and resistance training
Contrasting muscle atrophy, recovery of muscle performance in the operated limb	Progressive resistance training

The rationale for partial weight-bearing is based on the assumption that an early excessive load on the operated limb may cause micro-movements at the bone-implant interface, compromising the initial implant stability that interferes with bone healing and predispose to aseptic loosening of the implant. On the other hand, early weight-bearing after total hip arthroplasty (THA) could have potential benefits, in particular counteracting bone loss and allowing early recovery of functional activities. Patient education should be emphasized to prevent the dislocation of the prosthetic implant, through specific preventive rules. The IRP proposed by the physiatrist should include several targets that have to be addressed by rehabilitation programs as showed in Table 27.6.

Home-based programs should begin 2–3 weeks after surgery and consist of specific exercises aiming to improve muscle performance and endurance, balance, and functional ability to perform ADLs independently. Precautions to take during ADL should continue for at least 12 weeks. The rehabilitation plan proposed in outpatient setting is shown in Table 27.7.

27.3.1.3 Rehabilitation of Elderly Patients with Osteomalacia

Osteomalacia is characterized by skeletal fragility and muscle weakness that can interfere with the ADLs performance. The rehabilitative approach should be targeted to improve muscle strength and physical performance, through low-impact activities, such as gait training, avoiding high-intensity exercises that might cause microfractures or interfere with bone healing processes. In the advanced stages of osteomalacia, a significant reduction of the strength in proximal muscles of the lower limbs has been shown, thus resulting in balance impairment and consequent increased risk of falling. In this condition, resistance exercises could significantly improve muscle strength and reduce the risk of falling. Furthermore, occupational therapy can provide coping strategies in order to better perform ADLs [59].

Table 27.7 Rehabilitation plan in intermediate and advanced recovery in outpatient setting

Objectives	Rehabilitation programs
Improvement of muscle strengthening and endurance	Open chain exercises against slight resistance; bilateral exercises in closed kinetic chain against a slight resistance; unilateral exercises in closed kinetic chain like climbing stairs; muscle endurance exercises for the rest of the body
Improve cardiorespiratory endurance	Low-impact aerobic exercises, such as cycling progressive resistance training, swimming, or water gymnastics
Reduction of soft tissue retraction	Stretching techniques
Improvement of postural stability and ambulation, with progressive acquisition of the physiological gait pattern	Protected weight-bearing in the initial stages through mobility aids (e.g., crutches). Subsequently, the use of the crutches should be recommended even during long journeys in order to reduce muscle fatigue
Prepare the patient to a complete level of functional activity	Exercises for muscle strengthening, endurance, and balance training, gradually increasing the time and distance in a low-intensity walking program

References

1. Parfitt AM (1982) The coupling of bone formation to bone resorption: a critical analysis of the concept and its relevance to the pathogenesis of osteoporosis. Metab Bone Dis Relat Res 4:1–6
2. Lee CA, Einhorn TA (2001) The bone organ system: form and function. In: Marcus R, Feldman D, Kelsey J (eds) Osteoporosis, 2nd edn. Academic Press, Salt Lake City, pp 2–20
3. Duque G, Troen BR (2008) Understanding the mechanisms of senile osteoporosis: new facts for a major geriatric syndrome. J Am Geriatr Soc 56(5):935–941
4. De Martinis M, Franceschi C, Monti D et al (2005) Inflammation-ageing and lifelong antigenic load as major determinants of ageing rate and longevity. FEBS Lett 579:2035–2039
5. Nanes MSL (2003) Tumor necrosis factor-alpha: molecular and cellular mechanisms in skeletal pathology. Gene 4:1–15
6. Freemont AJ, Hoyland AJ (2007) Morphology, mechanisms and pathology of musculoskeletal ageing. J Pathol 21:252–259
7. Frystyk J (2005) Aging somatotropic axis: mechanisms and implications of insulin-like growth factor-related binding protein adaptation. Endocrinol Metab Clin North Am 34:865–876
8. Zofkova I (2003) Pathophysiological and clinical importance of insulin-like growth factor-I with respect to bone metabolism. Physiol Res 52:657–679
9. Sinaki M (1998) Musculoskeletal challenges of osteoporosis. Aging Clin Exp Res 10:249–262
10. Felsing NE, Brasel JA, Cooper DM (1992) Effect of low and high intensity exercise on circulating growth hormone in men. J Clin Endocrinol Metab 75:157–162
11. Iolascon G, Resmini G, Tarantino U (2013) Mechanobiology of bone. Aging Clin Exp Res 25(Suppl 1):S3–S7
12. Seeman E (2006) Osteocytes—martyrs for integrity of bone strength. Osteoporos Int 17: 1443–1448
13. Winkler D, Sutherland MK, Geoghegan JC, Yu C, Hayes T, Skonier JE, Shpektor D, Jonas M, Kovacevich BR, Staehling-Hampton K, Appleby M (2003) Osteocyte control of bone formation via sclerostin, a novel BMP antagonist. EMBO J 22(23):6267–6276
14. Weaver CM, Gordon CM, Janz KF, Kalkwarf HJ, Lappe JM, Lewis R, O'Karma M, Wallace TC, Zemel BS (2016) The National Osteoporosis Foundation's position statement on peak bone mass development and lifestyle factors: a systematic review and implementation recommendations. Osteoporos Int 27:1281–1386

15. Rayal-Pandya M, Porta A et al (1998) Mechanism of action of 1,25 (OH)2 D3 on intestinal calcium absorption and renal calcium transportation. In: Holick MF (ed) Vitamin D physiology, molecular biology and clinical applications. Humana Press, Totowa, pp 163–173
16. Ireland P, Fordtran JS (1973) Effect of dietary calcium and age on jejunal calcium absorption in humans studied by intestinal perfusion. J Clin Invest 52:2672–2681
17. Orwoll ES, Bilezikian JP, Vaneerschueren D (eds) (2010) Osteoporosis in men: the effects of gender on skeletal health. Elsevier, Boston
18. Manolagas SC, O'Brien CA, Almeida M (2013) The role of estrogen and androgen receptors in bone health and disease. Nat Rev Endocrinol 9:699–712
19. Reid IR (2008) Relationships between fat and bone. Osteoporos Int 19:595–606
20. Sáinz N, Rodríguez A, Catalán V, Becerril S, Ramírez B, Gómez-Ambrosi J, Frühbeck G (2009) Leptin administration favors muscle mass accretion by decreasing FoxO3a and increasing PGC-1alpha in ob/ob mice. PLoS One 4(9):e6808
21. Oshima K, Nampei A, Matsuda M, Iwaki M, Fukuhara A, Hashimoto J, Yoshikawa H, Shimomura I (2005) Adiponectin increases bone mass by suppressing osteoclast and activating osteoblast. Biochem Biophys Res Commun 331:520–526
22. Williams GA, Wang Y, Callon KE, Watson M, Lin JM, Lam JB, Costa JL, Orpe A, Broom N, Naot D, Reid IR, Cornish J (2009) In vitro and in vivo effects of adiponectin on bone. Endocrinology 150:3603–3610
23. Lee B, Shao J (2012) Adiponectin and lipid metabolism in skeletal muscle. Acta Pharm Sin B:335–434
24. Lee NK, Karsenty G (2008) Reciprocal regulation of bone and energy metabolism. Trends Endocrinol Metab 19:161–166
25. Buday B, Pach FP, Literati-Nagy B, Vitai M, Vecsei Z, Koranyi L (2013) Serum osteocalcin is associated with improved metabolic state via adiponectin in females versus testosterone in males. Gender specific nature of the bone-energy homeostasis axis. Bone 57(1):98–104
26. Gonzalez-Rozas M, Dueñas-Laita A, Perez-Castrillon JL (2015) The β-adrenergic system and bone mineral remodeling. Clin Rev Bone Miner Metab 13:114–124
27. World Health Organization Study Group (1994) Assessment of fracture risk and its application to screening for postmenopausal osteoporosis. Report of a WHO Study Group. World Health Organ Tech Rep Ser 843:1–129
28. National Osteoporosis Foundation (2013) Clinician's guide to prevention and treatment of osteoporosis. National Osteoporosis Foundation, Washington. Available at: http://nof.org/
29. Tarantino U, Capone A, Planta M, D'Arienzo M, Letizia Mauro G, Impagliazzo A, Formica A, Pallotta F, Patella V, Spinarelli A, Pazzaglia U, Zarattini G, Roselli M, Montanari G, Sessa G, Privitera M, Verdoia C, Corradini C, Feola M, Padolino A, Saturnino L, Scialdoni A, Rao C, Iolascon G, Brandi ML, Piscitelli P (2010) The incidence of hip, forearm, humeral, ankle, and vertebral fragility fractures in Italy: results from a 3-year multicenter study. Arthritis Res Ther 12(6):R226
30. Ahlborg HG, Johnell O, Turner CH, Rannevik G, Karlsson MK (2003) Bone loss and bone size after menopause. N Engl J Med 349(4):327–334
31. Riggs BL, Melton LJ 3rd (1983) Evidence for two distinct syndromes of involutional osteoporosis. Am J Med 75(6):899–901
32. Khosla S (2010) Update in male osteoporosis. J Clin Endocrinol Metab 95(1):3–10
33. Fitzpatrick LA (2002) Secondary causes of osteoporosis. Mayo Clin Proc 77:453–468
34. Adler RA, Hastings FW, Petkov VI (2010) Treatment thresholds for osteoporosis in men on androgen deprivation therapy: T-score versus FRAX. Osteoporos Int 21(4):647–653
35. Tinetti ME, Speechley M, Ginter SF (1988) Risk factors for falls among elderly persons living in the community. N Engl J Med 319:1701–1707
36. Tinetti ME, Doucette J, Claus E, Marottoli R (1995) Risk factors for serious injury during falls by older persons in the community. J Am Geriatr Soc 43:1214–1221
37. Yates CJ, Chauchard MA, Liew D, Bucknill A, Wark JD (2015) Bridging the osteoporosis treatment gap: performance and cost-effectiveness of a fracture liaison service. J Clin Densitom 18(2):150–156

38. Cosman F, de Beur SJ, LeBoff MS, Lewiecki EM, Tanner B, Randall S, Lindsay R, National Osteoporosis Foundation (2014) Clinician's guide to prevention and treatment of osteoporosis. Osteoporos Int 25(10):2359–2381
39. Whyte MP, Thakker RV (2009) Rickets and osteomalacia. Medicine 37:483–488
40. Field M, Burnett L, Sullivan D et al (2014) Clinical biochemistry and metabolism. In: Walker B, Colledge N, Raiston S et al (eds) Davidson's principles and practice of medicine, 22nd edn. Churchill Livingstone Elsevier, Edinburgh
41. Pearce S, Cheetham T (2010) Diagnosis and management of vitamin D deficiency. BMJ 340:B3664
42. Holick M (2004) Sunlight and vitamin D for bone health and prevention of autoimmune diseases, cancers, and cardiovascular disease. Am J Clin Nutr 80(6 Suppl):1678S–1688S
43. Collier J (2007) Bone disorders in chronic liver disease. Hepatology 46:1271–1278
44. Nikander R, Sievänen H, Heinonen A, Daly RM, Uusi-Rasi K, Kannus P (2010) Targeted exercise against osteoporosis: a systematic review and meta-analysis for optimising bone strength throughout life. BMC Med 8:47
45. Nelson ME, Rejeski WJ, Blair SN, Duncan PW, Judge JO, King AC, Macera CA, Castaneda-Sceppa C, American College of Sports Medicine, American Heart Association (2007) Physical activity and public health in older adults: recommendation from the American College of Sports Medicine and the American Heart Association. Circulation 116(9):1094–1105
46. Staunton L, O'Connell K, Ohlendieck K (2011) Proteomic profiling of mitochondrial enzymes during skeletal muscle aging. J Aging Res. doi:10.4061/2011/908035
47. Forbes SC, Little JP, Candow DG (2012) Exercise and nutritional interventions for improving aging muscle health. Endocrine 42:29–38
48. Howe TE, Shea B, Dawson LJ, Downie F, Murray A, Ross C, Harbour RT, Caldwell LM, Creed G (2011) Exercise for preventing and treating osteoporosis in postmenopausal women. Cochrane Database Syst Rev (7):CD000333
49. Mero AA, Hulmi JJ, Salmijärvi H, Katajavuori M, Haverinen M, Holviala J, Ridanpää T, Häkkinen K, Kovanen V, Ahtiainen JP, Selänne H (2013) Resistance training induced increase in muscle fiber size in young and older men. Eur J Appl Physiol 113(3):641–650
50. Sayers SP (2007) High-speed power training: a novel approach to resistance training in older men and women. A brief review and pilot study. J Strength Cond Res 21:518–526
51. Bottaro M, Machado SN, Nogueira W, Scales R, Veloso J (2007) Effect of high versus low-velocity resistance training on muscular fitness and functional performance in older men. Eur J Appl Physiol 99(3):257–264
52. Global recommendations on physical activity for health. World Health Organization, 2011
53. Bonner FJ Jr, Sinaki M, Grabois M, Shipp KM, Lane JM, Lindsay R, Gold DT, Cosman F, Bouxsein ML, Weinstein JN, Gallagher RM, Melton LJ III, Salcido RS, Gordon SL (2003) Health professional's guide to rehabilitation of the patient with osteoporosis. Osteoporos Int 14(Suppl 2):S1–22
54. Cameron ID, Gillespie LD, Robertson MC, Murray GR, Hill KD, Cumming RG, Kerse N (2012) Interventions for preventing falls in older people in care facilities and hospitals. Cochrane Database Syst Rev 12:12
55. NICE clinical guideline – June 2013 Falls: assessment and prevention of falls in older people
56. Santesso N, Carrasco-Labra A, Brignardello-Petersen R (2014) Hip protectors for preventing hip fractures in older people. Cochrane Database Syst Rev 3:CD001255
57. Pietri M, Lucarini S (2007) The orthopaedic treatment of fragility fractures. Clin Cases Miner Bone Metab 4(2):108–116
58. Iolascon G, Gimigliano F, Piscitelli P et al (2007) Hip fracture in Italy: analysis of DRG data. Aging Clin Exp Res 19(3 Suppl):2–4
59. Walker J (2014) Pathogenesis, diagnosis and management of osteomalacia. Nurs Older People 26(6):32–37

Rehabilitation of Older Patients with Orthopedic Diseases

28

Antonio Frizziero, Giuseppe Gasparre, Filippo Vittadini, Andrea Pignataro, Marko Bonjako, Marta Valente, Valentina Copetti, and Stefano Masiero

28.1 Tendinopathies and Metabolic Disease in Elderly

Tendon is a specialized tissue composed by collagen arranged in linear fibrils that join muscle to the bone (Figs. 28.1 and 28.2). Intrinsic mechanical properties of tendon permit to adapt and respond to loading that provide the principal mechanical stimulus for tendon cells. Tenocytes are involved in the production of collagen, matrix proteoglycans and repair proteins and result essential to maintain tendon characteristics by the capacity of remodel extracellular matrix (ECM) [1].

Several studies show that 16% of the general population and about 20% of elderly hospitals and community populations are affected by tendon pain. The most frequent symptoms that lead to tendinopathies are pain and loss of function.

Histopathologically, tendinopathies are related to unsuccessful healing response, represented by altered tenocyte proliferation, disruption and impaired organization of collagen fibers, increase in non-collagenous matrix, and neovascularization. In the chronic stage of tendinopathy, inflammation is absent or minimal; these findings may indicate that inflammation could play a role in the beginning, but not in the progression of the disease process [2].

During aging intrinsic and extrinsic factors influence biological environment and the capability of tendon to adapt itself to mechanical stimuli. Therefore, tendons show the typical macroscopic and microscopic aspects that are possible to observe in elderly in the major periarticular structure such as the shoulder, hip, knee, and foot [3].

A. Frizziero, MD, PhD (✉) • G. Gasparre • F. Vittadini • A. Pignataro • M. Bonjako
M. Valente • V. Copetti • S. Masiero
Department of Physical Medicine and Rehabilitation, University of Padua, Padua, Italy
e-mail: antonio.frizziero@unipd.it; giuseppegasaprre@hotmail.it; andreapignataro88@gmail.com; marko.bonjako@studenti.unipd.it; val.copetti@gmail.com; stef.masiero@unipd.it

© Springer International Publishing AG 2018

S. Masiero, U. Carraro (eds.), *Rehabilitation Medicine for Elderly Patients*, Practical Issues in Geriatrics, DOI 10.1007/978-3-319-57406-6_28

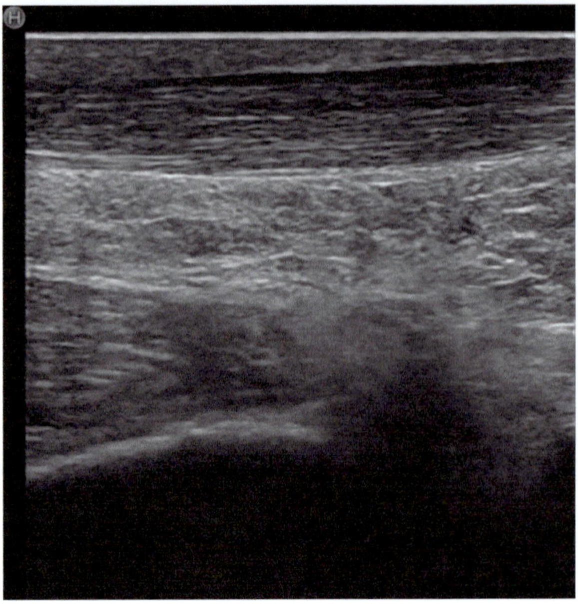

Fig. 28.1 Ultrasound image of Achilles tendon degeneration

Particularly, aging is often related to estrogen deficiency in postmenopausal women, obesity and diabetes, dysthyroidism, hypercholesterolemia, hyperuricemia, and other rare congenital metabolism disorders often involved in tendon degeneration. The presence of estrogen receptors in tenocytes has been demonstrated in human and animal trials, and these findings indicate that tenocytes are influenced by circulating estrogen level. In postmenopause, the reduction of blood estrogen is linked to the reduction in tensile strength; decrease in collagen synthesis, fiber diameter, and density; and increase degradation in tendon tissue. Hormone replacement therapy (HRT) with exogenous estrogens may improve tendon structure by preserving collagen fiber diameter. Furthermore, estrogen positively influences morphology and biomechanical properties of tendon in postmenopausal women. On the other hand, estrogen stimulation in younger women seems to have negative effects on tendons. In fact, in a study performed in young women, oral contraceptive user group was found to have lower collagen synthesis rate, compared to control women at the same age [4].

As mentioned above, a pathological condition often related to aging is diabetes mellitus type 2. Tendon alterations in diabetes are due to an excess of advanced glycation end products (AGEs) that are able to form covalent cross-link within fibers of collagen that alters their structure and consequently the capacity to respond to mechanical stimuli.

Obesity, particularly frequent in older and sedentary people, expose weight-bearing tendons to overuse due to the higher loads related to increasing adiposity. Moreover adipose tissue is an endocrine and signaling organ that can release hormones and peptides able to modify directly tendon structure. Particularly, adipokines modulate cytokines, prostanoids, and metalloproteinase production that cause a persistent low grade of inflammation that intensifies the detrimental effect of overuse on tendon.

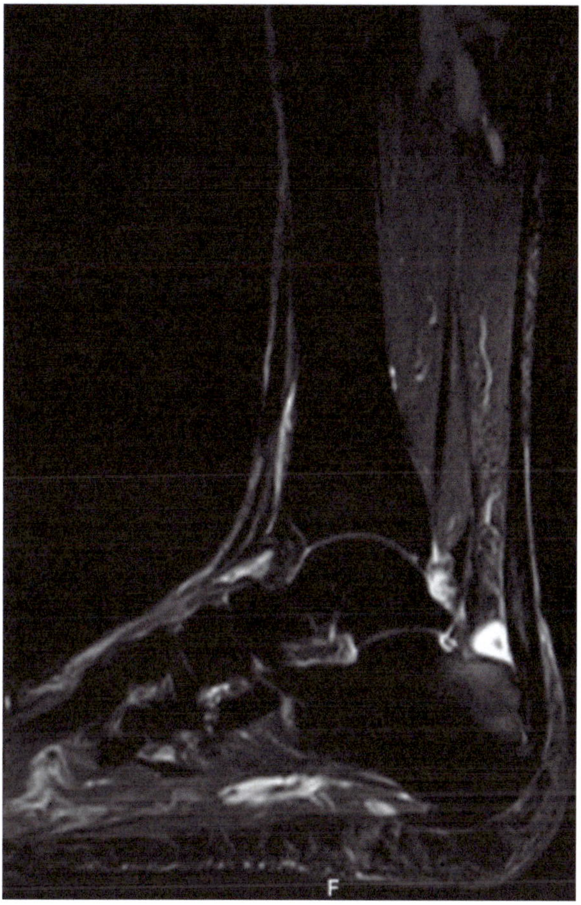

Fig. 28.2 MRI of non-insertional Achilles tendinopathy and bone marrow edema of the calcaneum

Dysregulation of thyroid hormones, another disease not rarely observed in elderly, contributes to the genesis of musculoskeletal pathologies. Hypothyroidism can be related to the onset of calcific tendinopathies due to the reduction of oxygenation with consequent metaplasia that may cause calcium deposition, especially in rotator cuff tendons [5].

Extrinsic factors such as sport activities, physical loading, occupation, and environmental conditions could affect anatomo-physiological and biological characteristics of the tendon.

Correct mechanical loading is useful to tendons to stimulate their anabolic processes and also to compensate the effects of aging. On the other hand, extreme mechanical loading, immobilization, and disuse are harmful to tendons by stimulating catabolic processes such as matrix degradation and by modifying collagen synthesis, collagen organization, cellularity, vascularity, proteoglycan content, tear density, and mechanical properties.

Preclinical and clinical studies have shown that discontinuing activity negatively influences morphology and structure of the tendon, whether there are differences in training or detraining protocols, in the study design, in the types of tendons, in subjects, or in the experimental setting involved. Therefore, the authors suggested that after a period of sudden detraining (such as after an injury) physical activity should be restarted with caution and with appropriate rehabilitation programs [6].

In people affected by tendinopathies, eccentric exercise programs are widely used in the rehabilitation of Achilles tendon midportion and patellar tendon injuries with a successful outcome. Particularly in elderly, it has been shown a general preservation of eccentric strength compared to concentric strength. High-intensity resistance training, including eccentric exercises, revealed an increase muscle mass and strength in contractions comparing to traditional training protocol [7].

Therefore it's feasible that a correct eccentric exercise protocol may be promising in the treatment and also in the prevention of tendon disorders in elderly.

28.2 Painful Shoulder in Elderly

Shoulder pain is the third most common musculoskeletal complaint in primary care physicians' offices with high prevalence among the fourth to the sixth decade.

According to population surveys, shoulder pain affects 18–26% of adults; it is the most common regional pain syndromes. Symptoms can be persistent and disabling in terms of an individual's ability to carry out daily activities both at home and in the workplace. There are also substantial economic costs involved, with increased demands on health care, impaired work performance, substantial sickness absence, and early retirement or job loss [8].

Common shoulder conditions in elderly patients include rotator cuff tendinopathy, rotator cuff tear, adhesive capsulitis ("frozen shoulder"), and glenohumeral arthritis.

Diagnosis is mainly clinical. Radiographs generally may be normal. Magnetic resonance and ultrasound are the most used diagnostic tools. Conservative treatments include rest, ice, topical analgesics, a short course of nonsteroidal anti-inflammatory drugs (NSAIDs), subacromial corticosteroid injections, and intra-articular hyaluronic acid (HA) injections [9]. HA is a component of the synovial fluid and is crucial for the lubrification and chondroprotection of joints. Several authors suggest that intra-articular injections of hyaluronic acid reduce inflammation and pain and improve joint function. Furthermore, HA stimulates type B synoviocytes producing endogenous HA with a chondroprotective effects on the whole joint [10, 11].

One of the most frequent causes of shoulder pain in elderly patients is shoulder osteoarthritis, which is a gradual, progressive, mechanical, and biochemical breakdown of the articular cartilage and other joint tissues, including bone and joint capsule. Several risk factors can lead to shoulder osteoarthritis, including aging, genetics, sex, weight, joint infection, history of shoulder dislocation, and previous injury. The loss of shoulder function can lead to depression, activity limitations, and job-performance problems.

Typical presenting symptom is progressive, activity related pain that is deep in the joint and often localized around the deltoid region and posteriorly. As the disease progresses, night pain becomes more common. Patients complain reduction of the shoulder range of movement, with the loss of the extra rotation and abduction in both active and passive mobilization [12, 13].

Therefore, rehabilitative goals are the restoration of strength and flexibility of the shoulder musculature on the upper thoracic, neck, and scapular muscle groups, including also the rotator cuff, arm, forearm, wrist, and hand. Isometric contraction exercises with normal range of motion in shoulder joint have a leading role in rehabilitation because these exercises will not only produce more strength in the stabilizers shoulder muscles groups but also help to minimize joint damage, reducing the inflammation and pain. The satisfactory outcome of flexibility exercises will be confirmed by the amplitude of mechanical bone blockade that is achieved by the size of glenohumeral deformity and osteophyte generation.

Osteoarthritis may lead to rotator cuff tendinopathy. However, rotator cuff tendinopathy may result from several factors like an alteration of tendon's structure related to overloading or underloading, hormonal and/or metabolic impairment, reduction of subacromial space, and instability of the humeral head. The entirety of rotator cuff is crucial in maintaining normal humeral head position in the glenoid during elevation, flexion, and abduction movements, producing compressive forces that stabilize the humerus against the glenoid, giving a dynamic stabilization of the glenohumeral joint. In chronic rotator cuff tendinopathy, due to pain and disuse, muscles of the rotator cuff may become weak and can fatigue earlier, leading to changes in shoulder kinematics. Weakness of the rotator cuff, especially infraspinatus, reduces this compressive force, promoting instability. This instability may lead the humeral head to an abnormal range of motion out of the glenoid center, causing impingement and tendinopathy.

Generally, pain occurs in the posterolateral and deltoid region, especially when the patient performs eccentric contractions, during sleeping on the affected side or performing overhead activities with the arm abducted more than 90°. Provocative passive movements, such as the Neer and Hawkins-Kennedy tests, increase the pain. Appropriate balance of the muscles surrounding the shoulder is fundamental for flexibility and strength. Therefore, a deficit in flexibility or strength in an agonistic muscle must be compensated for by the antagonist ones, leading to dysfunction. Consequently, the restoration of the appropriate strength and flexibility in both agonistic and antagonist muscles is very important in shoulder rehabilitation [14].

In the first phase, rehabilitation should be gentle and passive with prolonged stretchability to restore flexibility of the posterior capsule, muscle balance, and scapulothoracic and glenohumeral muscular control and stability. Patients should be well educated to prevent incorrect postures and movements to avoid the occurrence of any exacerbating activities. Pendulum exercises, wall walking, or towel exercises are very effective in improving range of motion and in facilitating optimal motor pattern. Capsular stretching, pectoralis minor stretching as well as reducing upper trapezius activation are recommended to improve soft tissue tightness because it can cause anterior and superior humeral head migration, resulting in impingement. Very important in this early stage is the restoration of shoulder kinematics using wall push-ups and biofeedback exercises because an altered motion may lead to glenohumeral joint instability.

The next phase of treatment is the muscle strengthening. This phase should be performed in a pain-free range of motion. Therefore, before beginning a strengthening program, it is important to identify tight or short muscles and if flexibility was restored. Strengthening should begin with the muscles that support the shoulder. We can use shoulder shrugs, rowing, and push-ups for strengthening both agonistic and antagonist muscles, because only a proper balance in strength of these two groups helps return range of motion and the normal kinematics between the scapula and the glenohumeral joint.

Specific strengthening exercises of the serratus anterior, typically including supine protractions and wall push-up exercises, should be used in the early stages of rehabilitation, while dynamic hugs and push-up varieties are commonly utilized in later stages of rehabilitation. Strength exercises for rotator cuff tendinopathy should be initiated with low-load activities and progressing as patient comfort permits [15, 16]. An effective treatment strategy that leads to a tendon strengthening is also the eccentric training [17].

The last phase is the proprioceptive training. The most important result of this phase is the restoration of neuromuscular coordination of the muscles that provides a synergistic activation of muscles. The proprioceptive phase should begin with closed kinetic chain exercises.

Usually, shoulder pain in elderly people is associated also with an adhesive capsulitis of the shoulder, which is a common condition characterized by spontaneous onset of pain, progressive restriction of movement of the shoulder, and disability that restricts activities of daily living, work, and leisure. The disease is characterized by three stages including the painful phase, the freezing or adhesive phase, and the healing phase. This condition is more frequent in women after the age of 50 years and involves the nondominant shoulder too. The primary etiology is still unknown, but it is associated with different secondary causes, like immobilization, diabetes, hypothyroidism, autoimmune diseases, and treatment of breast cancer.

Contraction and fibrosis of the capsule lead to pain and stiffness of the joint when the capsule is stretched during typical shoulder range of motion [18].

Generally, the treatment goals are focused to decrease pain and inflammation and increase shoulder range of motion. Rehabilitation protocol is based on stretching, strengthening, pendulum, pulley, and shoulder wheel and wall-climbing exercises, overhead stretches, and crossed adduction of the affected arm. It is mandatory to start rehabilitation exercises as soon as possible because it helps to reduce pain, to improve the pain-free range of motion, and to prevent further joint capsule contraction. The next step of the treatment is a graduated exercise program that leads to rotator cuff muscles and periscapular stabilizers strengthening. To maintain an adequate range of motions and to prevent recurrence, every patient should continue the exercise program at home [19, 20].

Also an excessive thoracic kyphosis is considered a predisposing factor for shoulder pain, but, to date, the relationship between these two conditions is uncertainty. It has been demonstrated that older adults with a large thoracic kyphosis had reduced arm elevation, but further researches are needed to investigate the nature of the link between shoulder pain and thoracic spine posture and to examine the specific value of thoracic postural rehabilitation in populations with painful shoulders.

28.3 Osteoarthritis

Osteoarthritis (OA) is a chronic disease that causes pain and substantial disability. It primarily affects the hip, knee, and hands (but also the shoulder and spine). This condition limits severely the daily activities and quality of life for many individuals in industrialized countries [21]. It affects at least 20 million Americans, a number that is expected to double over the next two decades [22]. Hip and knee osteoarthritis (OA) are the main causes of the poor health of older people worldwide [23] and are considered to be the most serious musculoskeletal disorders [24, 25].

Therefore, the effective management of hip and knee OA is a priority of the World Health Organization.

Osteoarthritis is a disorder of the whole joint and affects the cartilage, synovial tissue, subchondral bone, ligaments, and muscles. The critical occurrence in OA is the damage of cartilage, caused mainly by the degradation of type II collagen [26]. This process, at the cellular level, is mediated by releasing and responding to inflammatory mediators. OA often requires decades to develop and has a range of associated risk factors that it is possible to divide in general and local ones. General risk factors enclose older age, female gender, obesity (particularly in knee and hip OA), genetics, and muscle weakness. Local risk factors include an altered distribution of loads on the articular surfaces (e.g., the varus-valgus knee, evolution of congenital hip dysplasia, impingement hip syndrome, etc.), previous joint injuries, and articular alterations produced by inflammatory or septic arthritis.

Clinically patients complain about joint pain related to activity, stiffness [27], and, in severe OA, joint deformity.

Idiopathic osteoarthritis recognizes a genetic predisposition and it is typical for elderly. However, OA can also affect young people secondary to trauma, malformations, metabolic and rheumatic diseases, repetitive works (using vibrating tools, repetitive operations under load, or no physiological positions), etc.

Diagnosis is based on clinical and instrumental evaluation. To date, the most commonly used classification of hip and knee OA is the Kellgren and Lawrence grade [28] (Figs. 28.3 and 28.4), although it has several criticisms and radiographic signs of osteoarthritis not always are closely associated with pain [29]. However, in addition to correct clinical staging, it is also important to assess the functional level and the quality of life of patients affected by osteoarthritis. The American College of Rheumatology recommends to administer several scales to better stage the pathology such as Harris Hip Score, Oxford Hip Score, WOMAC, Hip disability and Osteoarthritis Outcome Score (HOOS), and Knee injury and Osteoarthritis Outcome Score (KOOS).

The management of osteoarthritis is still heterogeneous [30].

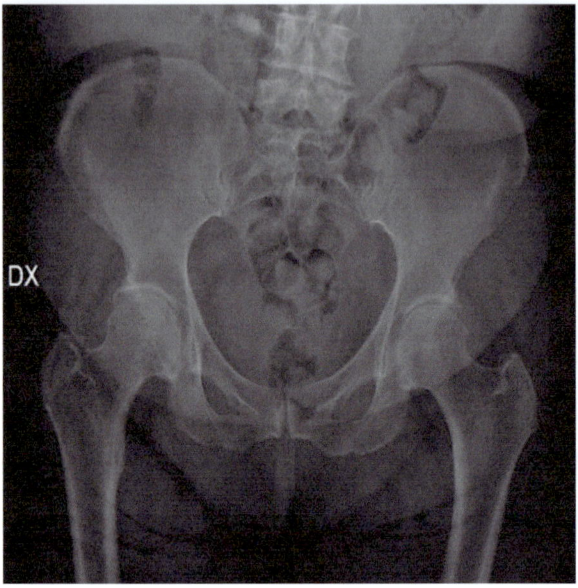

Fig. 28.3 Standard radiographic anteroposterior pelvis projection showing bilateral reduction of the hip joint space with subchondral sclerosis and initial deformities of the femoral head

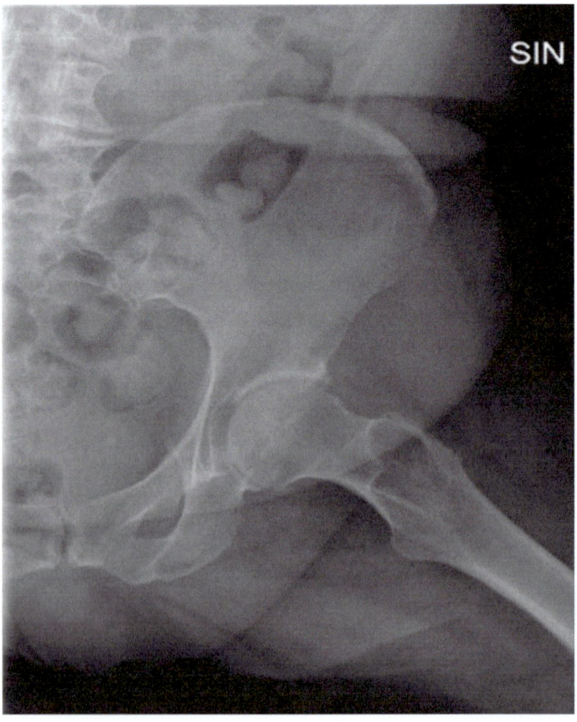

Fig. 28.4 Standard radiographic lateral view of the left hip joint showing signs of osteoarthritis

The treatment's options for osteoarthritis include conservative and surgical interventions. Conservative treatments aim to prevent progression and reduce symptoms such as joint pain and impairment of functions. Pharmacologic therapies and non-pharmacologic modalities are commonly used for the initial treatment of OA. Pharmacologic therapies include acetaminophen and topical and oral nonsteroidal anti-inflammatory drugs (NSAIDs). Although NSAIDs are effective in relieving pain and improving function, they should only be used in short term because of side effects [31]. Topical and systemic corticosteroids, opioids, and intra-articular drug injection may be useful. The effects of intra-articular injections of corticosteroids, as regards decreasing joint pain, are less effective over time than the hyaluronic acid injections. To date, evidences about the effectiveness of intra-articular injections of PRP are increased.

Non-pharmacologic modalities can include weight loss, aerobic exercise, muscle-strengthening exercises, neuromuscular education, dietary supplements, walking aid, bracing, and physical modalities.

In older people affected by knee or hip OA, a first approach should be weight reduction associated to perform a regular aerobic activity and joint protection brace, aimed to decrease the load on the joints of the lower limbs. The main advice should be to avoid prolonged postures and activities that overload the joint. Walking aids such as a cane or walker can decrease load on affected joints, and a simple walking stick reduces hip loading by 20–30%.

Clinical guidelines recommend that people with hip and knee osteoarthritis wear appropriate footwear, although there is no evidence supporting their use. Heel raises can be used to achieve pelvic obliquity and improve joint congruence in the setting of a functional leg-length discrepancy. In patients with knee OA and mild/moderate varus or valgus instability, a knee brace can reduce pain and improve stability and the risk of falling [32].

Exercises are a very important tool of conservative management for OA and are universally recommended by clinical guidelines [33]. Exercises should be prescribed in the early stages of OA or as preventive treatment. There is a growing evidence that the pathologic processes of OA may lead to a dysfunction of the joint surrounding muscles rather than within the cartilage. Moreover, preoperative neuromuscular exercises may constitute a viable adjunct therapy to hip or knee arthroplasty. In fact, several studies have shown that a preoperative neuromuscular exercise program leads to an earlier onset of postoperative recovery in self-reported ADL. In literature exercise programs have proven more effective in the knee OA than hip OA. There is no evidence that certain types of exercises have a better outcome than others. Generally, muscle strengthening, aerobic reconditioning, joint mobility, muscular stretching, and coordination and proprioception exercises are prescribed. Recommendations for dosage and progression of exercise in older people and people with chronic disease are aerobic moderate-intensity training for at least 30 min/day or up to 60 min and progressive strength training involving the major muscle groups for at least 2 days/week at a level of moderate to vigorous intensity. But people with chronic disease who do not reach the recommended level should perform exercises as their abilities and condition allow.

Unfortunately, physicians do not recommend physiotherapy or a program of exercises to every patient. Moreover, patients, especially elderly, often may be uncompliant to the physical work, and it is related to the increased risk of inactivity and morbidity.

Aquatic exercises have been recommended as an option for people with hip osteoarthritis because in water the percentage of body weight supported by the lower limbs is lower. Although there is strong evidence on their effectiveness compared to exercises performed on the ground, aquatic exercises are very useful for patients with obesity or neuro-musculoskeletal disorders.

The use of physical modalities such as ultrasound, electromagnetic fields, and low-level laser therapy in clinical practice is controversial and varies between countries. However, the American College of Rheumatology Clinical Guidelines recommends to instruct patients in the use of thermal agents.

Surgery should be considered only in the case of unsatisfactory results obtained with conservative treatments.

We cannot close off this section without discussing hand OA because of it high prevalence in the population, more than knee/hip OA. Because of the important functional significance of the thumb, trapeziometacarpal (TM) OA is more significant in fact of disability than osteoarthritis of other fingers.

Generally, TM OA is more frequent in women than men, but the prevalence strongly increases with aging in both genders.

Patients with TM OA reported persistent pain at the thumb base which limits their hand functions, reducing both thumb mobility and hand strength, affecting their daily activities (holding objects, preparing meals, writing), and causing a considerable reduction in quality of life, particularly in older people. While the results of surgical procedures have been well studied, gaps remain in research about the effectiveness of conservative treatments. Management of TM OA includes joint protection, education, assistive devices, hand exercises, pharmacological therapy, corticosteroid/hyaluronic acid injections, orthoses, and physical modalities.

To date, several studies have shown that hyaluronic acid injections induce a decrease of pain and an improvement in function that are also preserved in the medium to long term. Therefore, hyaluronic acid may be a safety and valid therapeutic option, which should be considered when other conservative therapies (like NSAIDs) were ineffective or contraindicated, before surgery [10].

28.4 Total Joint Replacement

According to national and international guidelines and the 2014 Osteoarthritis Research Society International (OARSI) recommendations, rehabilitation is considered the core treatment of OA and is widely indicated in primary care settings. Joint replacement is recommended if conservative treatment failed in reducing pain and improving quality of life or in patients with end-stage OA. About 119 per 100 thousand persons per year undergo total hip arthroplasty (THA) and a slightly lower number in total knee arthroplasty (TKA) worldwide.

28.4.1 Rehabilitation After Total Knee Arthroplasty (TKA)

TKA is considered as one of the useful medical interventions in terms of pain relief, improvement in function, and consequently in quality of life for patients suffering from end-stage OA. These patients show a modified gait pattern due to pain, with reduced gait speed and step length and increased time in double limb stand.

Outcomes following TKA depend on surgical technique and implant longevity; preoperative levels of knee pain, strength, flexibility, and functional ability; and, of course, on the adequacy of rehabilitation following surgery [34].

In the last decade, several authors began to argue on preoperative physiotherapy and exercise programs (called "pre-rehabilitation") for its capability to potentially improve early postoperative pain and function and consequently reduce recovery time and hospitalization in patients undergoing joint replacement. Pre-rehabilitation programs typically include warm-up, lower limb stretching and strengthening, aerobic training, and, in some protocol, step training. Proprioceptive and balance training or home exercises have also been proposed in some studies [35]. Villadsen et al. in their review underline the importance of a neuromuscular rehabilitation protocol as a viable treatment, combined to other preoperative exercise, to optimize and accelerate postoperative recovery until 3 months after TKA [36].

However, to date, the knowledge of the role of pre-rehabilitation remains debatable due to the limited number of studies in literature with small sample size, heterogeneous protocol, and conflicting results. Standard rehabilitation after TKA focused on decrease swelling, recovery of knee range of motion (KROM), enhancement of muscle control and strength in the involved lower limb, and improvement of patients' independence in daily life.

There are several rehabilitative approaches for recovery of strength and range of motion after TKA, with a focus on exercise therapy, balance training, aquatic therapy, continuous passive motion, cold therapy and compression, neuromuscular electrical stimulation, and transcutaneous electrical nerve stimulation.

Dedication and commitment to rehabilitation may help patients attain and exceed their preoperative activity levels [34]. It has been shown that early mobilization, achieved within 24 h after knee joint replacement surgery, can result in a reduced length of hospital stay and consequently limited onset of complications [37].

Rehabilitation after total joint replacement differs in where, how, and when it is delivered. After discharge from an acute care hospital, people who have had a primary total knee replacement may receive inpatient or outpatient physiotherapy. Inpatient physiotherapy is delivered in a rehabilitation hospital or specialized hospital unit. Outpatient physiotherapy is done either in an outpatient clinic (clinic-based) or at home (home-based). Rehabilitation protocol may be administered immediately after surgery (within the first 5 days) and in the early recovery period (within the first 3 months) after discharge [38].

Rehabilitation program often includes bed mobility and transfers with the least amount of assistance while maintaining appropriate weight-bearing (WB) precautions, ambulation with the use of an assistive device for 8–30 m, and climbing the stairs to allow for independence with household activities while maintaining appropriate WB. In the first days, the patient may regain at least 80° of passive and active range of motion of the knee to perform sit-to-stand transfers with minimal compensatory activity. Next step, the patient may consider to improve knee active range of motion (AROM) from 0 to 110° of flexion and gain knee extension less than or equal to −10°. Patient may also independently perform straight leg raise (SLR) exercise and keep in mind recommendations/precautions that include the use of proper positioning of the lower extremity, range of motion, and strengthening exercises of the entire lower limb with emphasis on knee extensor and flexor muscle groups.

The use of a *continuous passive motion* (CPM) machine *may* be indicated according to surgeon preference or in cases where postoperative knee range of motion (ROM) is severely restricted due to revision or reconstructive surgery, severe postoperative pain, limb's girth and/or edema, or impaired ability to participate in ROM exercises.

It is necessary to exclude any sign of deep vein thrombosis (DVT): increased swelling, flushing, and calf pain.

It is important to assess patients' pain using the visual analogue scale and administer, if required, analgesic or anti-inflammatory drugs 30–60 min prior to treatment. Cryotherapy is recommended following physical therapy treatment to reduce pain, discomfort, and swelling in the knee joint.

Neuromuscular electrical stimulation (NMES) for quadriceps can be prescribed in case of important decreased of muscular tone and mass.

The last step of rehabilitation protocol includes gait training on flat surfaces and on stairs and proprioceptive training to improve spatial awareness of the lower limb and whole body in functional activities. Patients are encouraged to wean from crutches approximately at the end of the second week from surgery. The American College of Sports Medicine Guidelines suggest aerobic training, muscle strengthening exercises, and flexibility exercises to improve overall elderly's health.

28.4.2 Rehabilitation After Total Hip Arthroplasty (THA)

Due to aging and the increase in life expectancy, the demand for joint replacement surgery to improve elderly's quality of life is growing.

Clinical pathways tend to reduce the hospitalization in acute care after surgery. Therefore, the preoperative rehabilitation of patients has become a topic of great scientific interest [39].

Before surgery, an educational program and a physical preparation may represent a useful adjunct, with low risk of adverse effects, particularly in subject with depression, anxiety, or unrealistic expectations, who may respond well to preoperative education that is stratified according to their physical, psychological, and social need [40].

Further, surgical approach (posterior, anterior lateral, or lateral incision) addresses the therapist in postoperative rehabilitation management.

For 3 months after THA (Fig. 28.5), patients should avoid hip flexion over 90°; avoid internal rotation of the lower extremity, not crossing the midline of the body; avoid sitting on low and soft surfaces; and use a raised toilet seat.

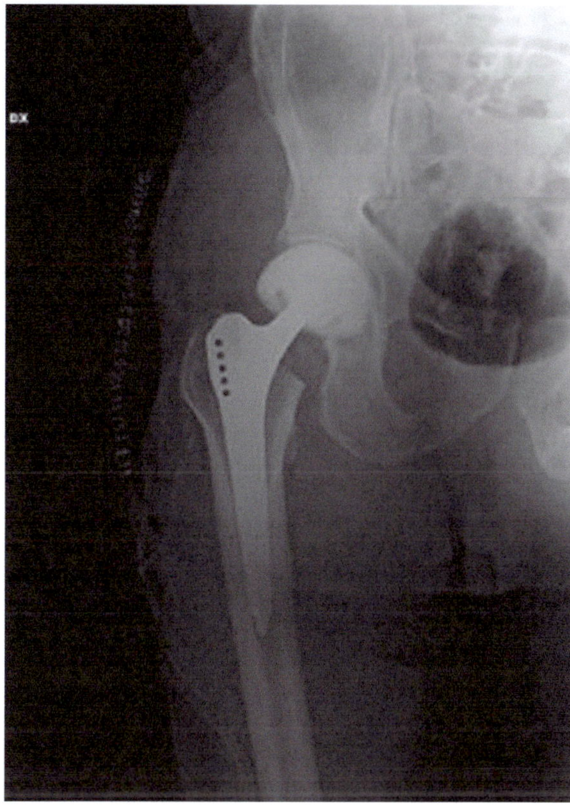

Fig. 28.5 Standard radiographic anteroposterior view of the right hip joint after total hip replacement

Postoperative rehabilitation is essential after total joint replacement in order to ensure pain-free function of the joint and improve the patient's quality of life [41].

The rehabilitative protocols will include passive and active flexion, extension, and abduction of the hip and strength training with focus on isometric and functional hip flexor and quadriceps control, hamstrings, as well as hip abductors, adductors, and gluteal muscles. In addition, cardiopulmonary exercises that include deep breathing, coughing, and ankle pump are recommended. Closed chain exercises can be started when the patient shows good pain control, muscle strength, and balance. Resistive exercises for the quadriceps and hamstrings are generally not used in the acute phase of rehabilitation but are commonly initiated within 2 months postoperatively.

Gait training on even surfaces, stair training, balance and coordination activities, and postural exercises are also recommended.

Neuromuscular exercise can be used as an adjuvant therapy in patients with osteoarthritis for both preoperative rehabilitation and to achieve an earlier onset in postoperative recovery [42].

Patients may also benefit from a home-based rehabilitation program supervised by a physiotherapist, if there were no pre- or postoperative reasons for prolonging the hospitalization [40].

However, to date, it is not possible to build up a detailed evidence-based exercise protocol after THA due to the lack of evidence in literature.

28.5 Rehabilitation After Hip Fractures

Hip fracture refers to a fracture occurring in the area between the edge of the femoral head and 5 cm below the lesser trochanter. They can be subdivided into intracapsular and extracapsular fractures (Fig. 28.6). Most of the hip fractures occur in older people with an average age of around 80 years, females predominate over males by about four to one. There are various risk factors: increasing age, osteoporosis, osteomalacia, metastatic disease, falls, and minor traumas (secondary to instability, lack of core strength, gait disturbance, sensory impairment) [43]. Clinically subjects with hip fractures complain about pain; leg flexion, adduction, and extra-rotation; and inability to load.

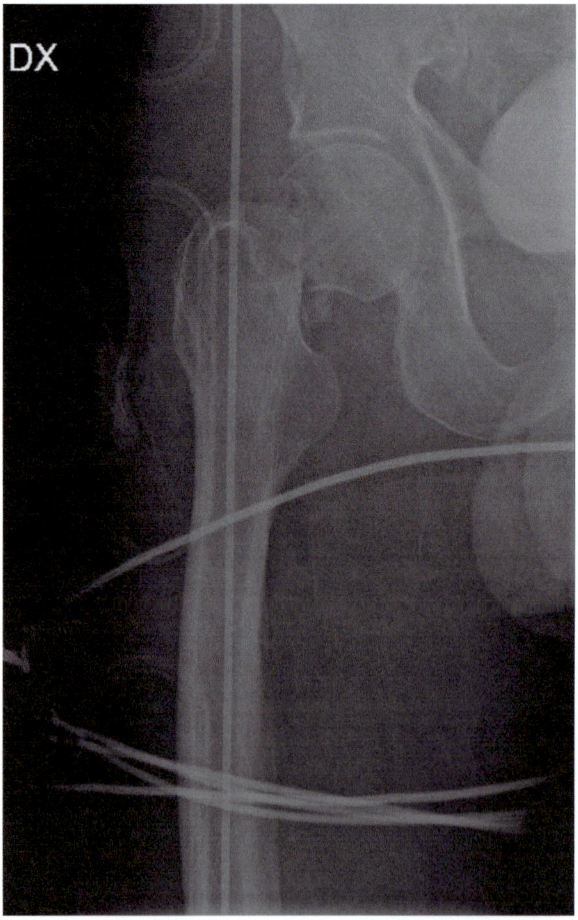

Fig. 28.6 Standard radiographic anteroposterior view of the right hip showing femoral neck hip fracture

Diagnosis is made with imaging: hip X-rays, MRI, or CT. Intracapsular fractures include sub-capital and transcervical fractures, undisplaced or displaced (Garden's classification). Extracapsular fractures include per-, inter- and subtrochanteric, best subdivided by their degree of comminution. Surgery is the best treatment and allows early mobilization of the patient. Undisplaced intracapsular fractures should be treated by internal fixation; in displaced intracapsular, one internal fixation and arthroplasty produce similar final outcomes, but the first one has a marginally lower mortality at the expense of an increased reoperation rate. Different types of arthroplasty exist for the hip: hemiarthroplasty and total hip replacement (THR). Results of hemiarthroplasty are initially better, but if the patient survives more than 3–5 years, then function deteriorates; total hip replacement may be better than hemiarthroplasty after 3 years but has higher incidence of early dislocation. Therefore many factors besides the type of fracture must be considered when deciding a surgical approach and type of implant: age, previous physical mobility, previous mental agility, and condition of the bone and joints. Primary arthroplasty is better than internal fixation for displaced intracapsular hip fractures. There is an increasing body of evidence to support THR over hemiarthroplasty in selected patients: patients with preexisting joint disease, medium/high activity levels, and a reasonable life expectancy (active patients aged less than 75–80 years) should have THR rather than hemiarthroplasty as primary treatment. THR, however, is unsuitable for patients with dementia due to their higher dislocation rate [44–46]. Complications from internal fixation depend on the quality of the reduction (20–36% after internal fixation, 6–18% after hemiarthroplasty). The common surgical approaches for hemiarthroplasty for intracapsular hip fractures are anterolateral or posterior. The operative treatment of extracapsular fractures includes reduction and internal fixation (extramedullary sliding screw and plate or intramedullary gamma nail). Mortality following hip fractures is high: about 10% died within 1 month and one third within 12 months. Complication rates are higher in elderly patients and could be divided into early complications (neurovascular damage, blood loss, compartment syndrome, infections) and later complications (fat embolism, deep vein thrombosis, pulmonary embolism, infections, shortening, angulation, malalignment, avascular necrosis, delayed union and nonunion, higher reoperation rates in older and female patients). Rehabilitation's aim is to improve dexterity, ability, strength, endurance, and ROM, return to a pre-fracture functional level, and empower the patient in activities of daily living (ADL). Purposes for a correct rehabilitative program are pain's pharmacological control; venous thromboembolism prevention with anticoagulant, vitamin D, and calcium supplementation in patients found to be deficient on laboratory evaluation; early mobilization and ROM (range of motion) and muscle strength recovery of all districts; training of hip extensors, abductors, knee extensors, and plantar flexors with key role in ambulation and transfers; and proprioceptive exercises to recover the balance (tracking and stretching, Freeman tablets, stabilometric platform) [47–49]. Gait recovery asks chosen aids use, like crutches or other assistive device to reduce risk and fear of falls and speed up patient's moving autonomy [50]. A variety of postoperative care programs following surgery for hip fractures have been employed: early stages include bed rest and restricted weight bearing. Rehabilitation begun as soon as possible after surgery, often within a day with initial goals to help people retain the level of strength they had before the fracture and to prevent immobilization's problems. As soon as possible, patients are encouraged to sit in a chair to reduce pressure sores and blood clots' risk and facilitate the transition to standing. They are taught to do daily exercises to strengthen the trunk and arm. Deambulation exercises with therapist are started after 4–8 days, when patient can bear full weight on the injured leg. Stair-climbing exercises are started soon after walking is resumed. Exercise, training, and muscle stimulation minimize impairments (reduced strength) and improve the physical performance of walking. The aim of a multidisciplinary care programs is to enhance activities of daily living and extend exercise program with a positive impact on physical function [51]. Patient are taught not to lift or push heavy objects or sit in a chair for long periods of time; not to stoop over 90°, reach, or jump when sitting; and not to cross their legs, and occupational therapists teach how to do daily activities safely while their hip is healing, using long-handled devices (reaches and long-handled shoe horns) in order not to bend [52–54].

In conclusion, rehabilitation after femoral fracture is important to lead the patient, throw various program stages, to his pre-fractural situation. Multidisciplinary care includes different figures that can help patients in their recovery. It's mandatory to begin mobilization as soon as possible after surgery, to prevent complication and to speed up healing.

28.5.1 Lumbar Spinal Stenosis

Because of aging, diseases of the vertebral column are becoming very frequent. Degeneration processes of the intervertebral disks, vertebral bodies, and adjoining structures usually cause them. One common consequence of these processes is the narrowing of vertebral canal, spinal stenosis (SS).

SS may be caused by a wide variety of conditions, as spine arthritis, herniated disks, spinal tumors, Paget's disease, and spinal injuries. The constriction of the spinal canal usually occurs in the cervical or lumbar tract. Lumbar spinal stenosis has [55] an estimated prevalence of 19% in the general population and up to 47% in people over age 60 [56]. It is the most common reason for spine surgery in patients over 65.3 [57]. Degenerative LSS anatomically can involve the central canal, lateral recess, or foramina. Anatomic narrowing of the spinal canal or foramen is a central component of LSS, but not sufficient to produce symptoms. In fact, studies in asymptomatic populations have found that up to 20% of subjects had imaging findings of spinal stenosis [58]. Indeed, to cause symptoms, the spinal narrowing resulting from the degenerative changes must induce vascular involvement of the vessels supplying the cauda equina or increase pressure on the nerve root complex.

At today, the natural history of spinal stenosis remains largely unknown [59]. The most common symptom in LSS is neurogenic claudication, also known as pseudoclaudication. Neurogenic claudication refers to a set of symptoms involving the groin, buttock, anterior thigh, and posterior part of the leg and feet. Leg symptoms may include pain, fatigue, weakness, paraesthesia, and nocturnal leg cramps.

Symptoms can be unilateral or more commonly bilateral. Low back pain often accompanies the other symptoms. Moreover, neurogenic bladder dysfunctions can be reported.

Features of neurogenic claudication are:

1. Pain is increased by lumbar extension and decreased by lumbar flexion.
2. Symptoms are exacerbated by standing or walking and are relieved by sitting; instead nonspecific low back pain, which is commonly exacerbated by prolonged sitting.
3. Lying on the side (permitting lumbar flexion) is more comfortable for patients.
4. The distance that can be walked before symptoms occur is increased by forward bending of the spine.
5. Patients tend to adopt a position with hip and knee lightly flexed.
6. Walking uphill is better tolerated than downhill walking.
7. In contrast to those with vascular claudication, sitting but not standing relieves symptoms.

There are still no widely accepted diagnostic or classification criteria for the diagnosis of LSS. Diagnosis of spinal stenosis is complex and usually begins with a medical history and physical examination. X-ray and MRI scans are used to determine the extent and location of SS. MRI has become the test of choice for diagnosing spinal stenosis SS. CT is a useful noninvasive study in patients who have contraindications to MRI.

Electrodiagnostic studies may be helpful when there is concern about additional neurologic compromise, such as peripheral polyneuropathy.

A correct treatment must be based on pain and disability rather than on the severity of the stenosis.

Conservative therapies are appropriate for first-line management of symptomatic patients, and they include drugs, lifestyle modification, physiotherapy, and spinal injections.

Analgesics, NSAIDs, muscle relaxants, and opioids are frequently used in patients with LSS. There is little evidence that intranasal calcitonin, intramuscular calcitonin, methylcobalamin, or intravenous lipoprostaglandin E(1) provides long-term benefit [60].

Some works demonstrated that people with LSS are likely more sedentary and inactive than healthy subjects, with many implications for overall health and risk for inactivity diseases. So, an important target of intervention should increase physical activity in daily life and weight loss, which helps to prevent diseases of inactivity, but it is also effective for improving pain and function. Increasing time spent in light-intensity activity is appropriate as initial goal. Aerobic activity such as bicycling or swimming should be recommended. The use of a lumbosacral corset can increase walking distance and decrease pain, even if there is no evidence that results are sustained once the brace is removed [60].

Stretching and strengthening exercises for the lumbar spine and hip region have been supported for patients with LSS, despite few randomized studies have evaluated them. Traction, electrical stimulation, or TENS has poor evidences of efficacy in the treatment of lumbar spinal stenosis.

Epidural corticosteroids injections for LSS, radiologically guided or not, may result in short-term (2–3 weeks) symptoms relief, sometimes permanent.

Patients with LSS who do not improve after nonsurgical treatments are usually treated with surgery.

28.5.2 Facet Joint Syndrome

Face joint syndrome (FJS) is a syndrome in which back pain is due to the facet joints. Although its existence had long been questioned, facet syndrome is now an accepted clinical entity.

The reported prevalence rate varies widely in different studies depending on the diagnostic criteria used. Furthermore, several studies have estimated that 5–15% of chronic low back pain is caused by the intervertebral joints [61].

FJS is thought to be the result of repetitive stress and cumulative microtrauma in vertebral joints. This leads to inflammatory state, which can lead to the filling of the facet joint with fluid, stretching the joint capsule, and generating subsequent pain. Inflammatory changes around the facet joint can also irritate the spinal nerve by foraminal narrowing. However, the precise mechanism that produces pain remains unknown. Predisposing factors for FJS pain include spondylolisthesis, degenerative disc disease, and advanced age.

Facet syndrome is diagnosed by clinical characteristics and by excluding other causes of lower back pain. Other possible causes of back pain in the differential diagnosis include discogenic pain, sacroiliac joint pathology, ligamentous injury, and myofascial pain.

There are no physical examination findings pathognomonic for diagnosis. Affected persons usually feel dull pain in the cervical or lumbar spine that can radiate into the buttocks and legs. Symptoms primarily manifest in the lumbar spine, due to the overlying body weight and the strong mobility. Pain is worsened by stress on the facet joints, as lateral flexion, prolonged standing, or walking.

X-rays are used to determine if there are abnormalities in the spine. CT scan shows more detail about facet joint surfaces. Diagnostic blocks of medial nerve branch with local anesthetic joint injections are gold standard to determinate if the facet joints are a source of pain [62].

Furthermore, facet joint injections are also commonly administered to alleviate back pain. Because each facet joint receives dual innervation from adjacent levels, several levels usually need to be treated. Injections are usually administered under fluoroscopy (FS), computed tomography (CT) scanning, or US guidance.

US guidance is a rapid, safe, and more easy to perform than the other two, which expose patient to ionizing radiation and can only be performed in specially equipped pain clinics. US-guided injections are a good treatment choice for facet syndrome of the low lumbar spine [63]. Thermocoagulation of dorsal rami branches is another technique used for the treatment of facet syndrome.

Key Points

- A correct eccentric exercise protocol may be promising in the treatment and also in the prevention of tendon disorders in elderly.
- Shoulder's rehabilitation protocol is based on stretching, strengthening, pendulum, pulley, and shoulder wheel and wall-climbing exercises, overhead stretches, and crossed adduction of the affected arm.
- Exercises are a very important tool of conservative management for OA and are universally recommended by clinical guidelines. Exercises should be prescribed in the early stages of OA or as preventive treatment.
- Preoperative physiotherapy called "pre-rehabilitation" is a valid tool for its capability to potentially improve early postoperative pain and function and consequently reduce recovery time and hospitalization in patients undergoing joint replacement.
- Postoperative rehabilitation is essential after total joint replacement in order to ensure pain-free function of the joint and improve the patient's quality of life.
- Rehabilitation after femoral fracture is important to lead the patient to his pre-fractural situation. It's mandatory to begin mobilization as soon as possible after surgery, to prevent complication and to speed up healing.

References

1. Abate M, Schiavone C, Salini V et al (2013) Occurrence of tendon pathologies in metabolic disorders. Rheumatology (Oxford) 52:599–608
2. Narici MV, Maffulli N, Maganaris CN (2008) Ageing of human muscles and tendons. Disabil Rehabil 30(20–22):1548–1554. doi:10.1080/09638280701831058
3. Frizziero A, Vittadini F, Gasparre G, Masiero S (2014) Impact of oestrogen deficiency and aging on tendon: concise review. Muscles Ligaments Tendons J 4:324–328. doi:10.11138/mltj/2014.4.3.324
4. Burgess KE, Pearson SJ, Onambèlè GL (2010) Patellar tendon properties with fluctuating menstrual cycle hormones. J Strength Cond Res 24(8):2088–2095
5. Kubo K, Ikebukuro T, Maki A, Yata H, Tsunoda N (2012) Time course of changes in the human Achilles tendon properties and metabolism during training and detraining in vivo. Eur J Appl Physiol 112:2679–2691. doi:10.1007/s00421-011-2248-x
6. Frizziero A, Salamanna F, Della Bella E, Vittadini F, Gasparre G, Nicoli Aldini N, Masiero S, Fini M (2016) The role of detraining in tendon mechanobiology. Front Aging Neurosci 8:43. doi:10.3389/fnagi.2016.00043. eCollection 2016. Review
7. Frizziero A, Trainito S, Oliva F, Nicoli Aldini N, Masiero S, Maffulli N (2014) The role of eccentric exercise in sport injuries. Rehabilitation. Br Med Bull 110(1):47–75
8. Mitchell C, Adebajo A, Hay E, Carr A (2005) Shoulder pain: diagnosis and management in primary care. BMJ 331:1124
9. Holmes RE, Barfield WR, Woolf SK (2015) Clinical evaluation of nonarthritic shoulder pain: diagnosis and treatment. Phys Sportsmed 43(3):262–268
10. Frizziero A, Maffulli N, Masiero S, Frizziero L (2014) Six-months pain relief and functional recovery after intra-articular injections with hyaluronic acid (mw 500–730 kDa) in trapeziometacarpal osteoarthritis. Muscles Ligaments Tendons J 4(2):256–261

11. Porcellini G, Merolla G, Giordan N et al (2015) Intra-articular glenohumeral injections of HYADD®4-G for the treatment of painful shoulder osteoarthritis: a prospective multicenter, open-label trial. Joints 3(3):116–121. doi:10.11138/jts/2015.3.3.116
12. Guo J, Wu K, Guan H, Zhang L, Ji C, Yang H, Tang T (2016) Three-year follow-up of conservative treatments of shoulder osteoarthritis in older patients. Orthopedics 39:e634–e641
13. Millett PJ, Gobezie R, Boykin RE (2008) Shoulder osteoarthritis: diagnosis and management. Am Fam Physician 78(5):605–611
14. Osborne JD, Gowda AL, Wiater B, Wiater JM (2016) Rotator cuff rehabilitation: current theories and practice. Phys Sportsmed 44(1):85–92
15. Littlewood C, Ashton J, Chance-Larsen K, May S, Sturrock B (2012) Exercise for rotator cuff tendinopathy: a systematic review. Physiotherapy 98:101–109
16. Page MJ, Green S, McBain B, Surace SJ, Deitch J, Lyttle N, Mrocki MA, Buchbinder R (2016) Manual therapy and exercise for rotator cuff disease. Cochrane Database Syst Rev
17. Camargo PR, Alburquerque-Sendín F, Salvini TF (2014) Eccentric training as a new approach for rotator cuff tendinopathy: review and perspectives. World J Orthoped 5(5):634–644
18. Seah KTM, Chee YH, Hindle P, Murray IR, Robinson CM (2012) Frozen shoulder. Bone Joint J 94-B(1):1–9
19. Escamilla RF, Hooks TR, Wilk KE (2014) Optimal management of shoulder impingement syndrome. Open Access J Sports Med 5:13–24
20. Page MJ, Green S, Kramer S, Johnston RV, McBain B, Chau M, Buchbinder R (2014) Manual therapy and exercise for adhesive capsulitis (frozen shoulder). Cochrane Database Syst Rev (8)
21. A National Public Health Agenda for Osteoarthritis 2010. Centers for Disease Control and Prevention. www.cdc.gov/arthritis/docs/OAagenda.pdf. Accessed 24 Aug 2012
22. United States Senate Committee on Health, Education, Labor and Pensions, Subcommittee on Aging (2004) Center for Disease Control's role in combating the burden of arthritis. Department of Health and Human Services, Washington
23. WHO (2003) The burden of musculoskeletal conditions at the start of the new millennium. World Health Organ Tech Rep Ser 919:i–x, 1–218
24. Bijlsma JWJ, Knahr K (2007) Strategies for the prevention and management of osteoarthritis of the hip and knee. Best Pract Res Clin Rheumatol 21:59–76
25. Dawson J, Linsell L, Zondervan K et al (2004) Epidemiology of hip and knee pain and its impact on overall health status in older adults. Rheumatology 43:497–504
26. Goldring MB, Otero M (2011) Inflammation in osteoarthritis. Curr Opin Rheumatol 23:471–478
27. Bijlsma JW, Berenbaum F, Lafeber FP (2011) Osteoarthritis: an update with relevance for clinical practice. Lancet 377:2115–2126
28. Reijman M, Hazes JM, Koes BW, Verhagen AP, Bierma-Zeinstra SM (2004) Validity, reliability, and applicability of seven definitions of hip osteoarthritis used in epidemiological studies: a systematic appraisal. Ann Rheum Dis 63:226–232
29. Nieuwenhuijse MJ, Nelissen RG (2015) Hip pain and radiographic signs of osteoarthritis. BMJ 351:h6262
30. van den Ende CHM, Bierma-Zeinstra SMA, Vliet Vlieland TPM, Swierstra BA, Voorn en Joost Dekker TB (2010) Conservatieve behandeling van heup- en knieartrose. Ned tijdschr geneeskd 154:a1574
31. Pencharz JN, Grigoriadis E, Jansz GF et al (2002) A critical appraisal of clinical practice guidelines for the treatment of lower-limb osteoarthritis. Arthritis Res 4(1):36–44
32. Zhang W, Moskowitz RW, Nuki G et al (2013) OARSI recommendations for the management of hip and knee osteoarthritis, Part II: OARSI evidence-based, expert consensus guidelines. Ann Rheum Dis 72(7):1125–1135
33. Fernandes L, Hagen KB, Bijlsma JW, Andreassen O, Christensen P, Conaghan PG et al (2013) EULAR recommendations for the non-pharmacological core management of hip and knee osteoarthritis. Ann Rheum Dis 72:1125–1135
34. Mistry JB, Elmallah RD, Bhave A, Chughtai M, Cherian JJ, McGinn T, Harwin SF, Mont MA (2016) Rehabilitative guidelines after total knee arthroplasty: a review. J Knee Surg

35. Wang L, Lee M, Zhang Z, Moodie J, Cheng D, Martin J (2016) Does preoperative rehabilitation for patients planning to undergo joint replacement surgery improve outcomes? A systematic review and meta-analysis of randomised controlled trials. BMJ Open
36. Villadsen A (2016) Neuromuscular exercise prior to joint arthroplasty in patients with osteoarthritis of the hip or knee. Dan Med J
37. Guerra ML, Singh PJ, Taylor NF (2015) Early mobilization of patients who have had a hip or knee joint replacement reduces length of stay in hospital: a systematic review. Clin Rehabil 29
38. Health Quality Ontario (2005) Physiotherapy rehabilitation after total knee or hip replacement: an evidence-based analysis. Ont Health Technol Assess Ser 5
39. Khan F, Ng L, Gonzalez S, Hale T, Turner-Stokes L Multidisciplinary rehabilitation programmes following joint replacement at the hip and knee in chronic arthropathy (Review). Cochrane Database Syst Rev
40. Jansen E, Brienza S, Gierasimowicz-Fontana A, Matos C, Reynders-Frederix-Dobre C, HateM SM (2015) Rehabilitation after total knee arthroplasty of hip and knee. Rev Med Brux
41. McDonald S, Page MJ, Beringer K, Wasiak J, Sprowson A (2014) Preoperative education for hip or knee replacement. Cochrane Database Syst Rev
42. Di Monaco M, Castiglioni C (2013) Which type of exercise therapy is effective after hip arthroplasty? A systematic review of randomized controlled trials. Eur J Phys Rehabil Med
43. NICE Guidelines, Clinical guideline, Hip fracture: management, 2011
44. Parker MJ, Gurusamy KS, Azegami S (2010) Arthroplasties (with and without bone cement) for proximal femoral fractures in adults. Cochrane Database Syst Rev (6). Art. No.: CD001706. doi:10.1002/14651858.CD001706.pub4
45. Marya SKS, Thukral R, Singh C (2008) Prosthetic replacement in femoral neck fracture in the elderly: results and review of the literature. Indian J Orthop 42(1):61–67
46. Hopley C, Stengel D, Ekkernkamp A, Wich M (2010) Primary total hip arthroplasty versus hemiarthroplasty for displaced intracapsular hip fractures in older patients: systematic review. BMJ 340:c2332
47. Mendelsohn ME, Overend TJ, Petrella RJ (2004) Effect of rehabilitation on hip and knee proprioception in older adults after hip fracture: a pilot study. Am J Phys Med Rehabil 83(8):624–632
48. Martimbianco A, Polachini L, Chamlian TR, Masiero D (2008) Effects of proprioception in the rehabilitation process of hip fractures. Acta Ortop Bras 16:2
49. Ishii Y, Terajima K, Terashima S, Matsueda M Joint proprioception in the elderly with and without hip fracture. J Orthop Trauma 14(8):542–545
50. Ferrarese N, Romeo A et al (2008) Surgical rehabilitation of femur fractures. literature review and therapeutic rationale. Scienza riabilitativa 10(2):19–27
51. Auais M, Eilayyan O, Mayo N (2012) Extended exercise rehabilitation after hip fracture improves patients' physical function: a systematic review and meta-analysis. Am Phys Ther Assoc 92(11):1437–1451
52. Moroz A Rehabilitation after a hip fracture; Merck manual
53. Maxey L, Magnusson J (2007) Rehabilitation for the postsurgical orthopedic patient, 2nd edn. Mosby
54. Handoll HHG, Sherrington C, Mak JC (2011) Interventions for improving mobility after hip fracture surgery in adults. Cochrane Database Syst Rev (3):CD001704. doi:10.1002/14651858.CD001704.pub4
55. Conway J, Tomkins CC, Haig AJ (2011) Walking assessment in people with lumbar spinal stenosis: capacity, performance, and self-report measures. Spine J 11:816–823
56. Kalichman L, Cole R, Kim DH, Li L, Suri P, Guermazi A et al (2009) Spinal stenosis prevalence and association with symptoms: the Framingham Study. Spine J 9:545–550
57. Deyo RA, Gray DT, Kreuter W, Mirza S, Martin BI (2005) United States trends in lumbar fusion surgery for degenerative conditions. Spine 30:1441–1445-1447
58. Jarvik JG, Deyo RA (2002) Diagnostic evaluation of low back pain with emphasis on imaging. Ann Intern Med 137(7):586–597
59. Johnsson KE, Rosen I, Uden A (1992) The natural course of lumbar spinal stenosis. Clin Orthop Relat Res (279):82–86

60. Watters WC 3rd, Baisden J, Gilbert TJ, Kreiner S et al (2008) Degenerative lumbar spinal stenosis: an evidence-based clinical guideline for the diagnosis and treatment of degenerative lumbar spinal stenosis. Spine J 8(2):305–310. Epub 2007 Dec 21
61. Manchikanti L, Pampati V, Fellows B, Bakhit CE (1999) Prevalence of lumbar facet joint pain in chronic low back pain. Pain Physician 2:59–64
62. Datta S, Lee M, Falco FJ, Bryce DA, Hayek SM (2009) Systematic assessment of diagnostic accuracy and therapeutic utility of lumbar facet joint interventions. Pain Physician 12:437–460
63. Dong Hwan Yun MD, Hee-Sang Kim MD, Seung Don Yoo MD et al (2012) Efficacy of ultrasonography-guided injections in patients with facet syndrome of the low lumbar spine. Ann Rehabil Med 36:66–71

Rehabilitation for Older Patients with Musculoskeletal Oncologic Disease

29

G. Trovarelli and P. Ruggieri

29.1 Introduction

If rehabilitation program of patients with orthopedic pathology collaboration between physicians (orthopedic surgeon, physiatrist, physiotherapist, and rehabilitation nurse) is important, the multidisciplinary team is essential in patients with orthopedic oncology pathology. The rehabilitation process in oncologic patient should be placed inside the oncologic treatments (chemotherapy and radiotherapy) and the follow-up check visits. Moreover, despite the progresses in treatment of cancer patients, considering the psychological implications in these patients, in their relatives, and in healthcare professionals is fundamental.

29.2 Malignant Bone Tumors

Metastasis, myeloma, and chondrosarcoma are the most frequent malignant bone lesions in older patients (>50 years old) [1].

The skeleton is the third site for metastases after the lung and liver, and the first cause of bone metastasis is due to visceral carcinomas as breast, lung, prostate, and kidney, followed by cancer of the digestive system, bladder, thyroid, and uterus [1–6]. About 15–20% of all carcinomas clinically manifests bone metastasis, whose incidence is increased in the last decades due to rise of cancer patients in relation with early diagnosis and with improvement of the surgical and medical treatments resulting in higher survival of patients. The most frequent sites for skeletal metastasis are the spine, pelvis, proximal femur, and proximal humerus, even if any bone can be affected [1–7].

Myeloma is a hematologic malignant bone marrow tumor, originating from B-lymphoid cells and differentiating in plasma cells that produce specific monoclonal proteins [1].

G. Trovarelli • P. Ruggieri (✉)
Department of Orthopedics and Orthopedic Oncology, University of Padua, Padua, Italy
e-mail: pietro.ruggieri@unipd.it

© Springer International Publishing AG 2018

S. Masiero, U. Carraro (eds.), *Rehabilitation Medicine for Elderly Patients*,
Practical Issues in Geriatrics, DOI 10.1007/978-3-319-57406-6_29

Myeloma can be multiple or solitary (plasmacytoma) and usually affects patients older than 60 years old. It involves especially the spine, skull, ribs, and the meta-epiphyses of appendicular long bones, particularly proximal femur and proximal humerus.

Chondrosarcoma is the most frequent primary malignant bone tumor in adult patients with a pick age of incidence between 40 and 70 years [1]. It is predominant in limb girdles and in the knee, involving usually diaphysis or metaphysis of the long bone as proximal femur, proximal humerus, distal femur, and proximal tibia.

Surgical and rehabilitation treatments are similar in patients with metastasis and myeloma, while patients with chondrosarcoma require different strategy due to more higher chances to heal.

Surgical treatment consists especially in resection of affected bone and reconstruction with modular prosthesis that allows repairing any bone defect [2–26]. Cemented stem is used in case of bone metastasis or myeloma or if the bone is osteoporotic [2–6], while press-fit stem is used in case of primary bone tumor [11, 24, 26]. Nowadays, custom-made 3D-printed prostheses are also available to reconstruct pelvic defect in order to ensure a more anatomic reconstruction [8]; modular total reverse shoulder prostheses could be used after proximal humerus resection (if to save the deltoid muscle with its innervation is feasible) in order to obtain better functional results [13–20].

29.3 Rehabilitation After Resection and Reconstruction for Bone Tumor

The rehabilitation program aims to shorten recovery time in patients with metastasis and myeloma; while it should get stable long-term results in patients with chondrosarcoma, given that these patients have about 90% of chance to heal.

29.3.1 Rehabilitation Program After Proximal Humerus Resection and Reconstruction with Standard Modular Prosthesis [4, 13, 14, 19]

Standard modular shoulder prostheses are spacers that allow to preserve movements of the elbow, hand, and wrist; shoulder range of motion is limited at only few degrees of anteposition. The patient has to wear a Velpeau brace for 4 weeks in order to permit the remaining soft tissue healing avoiding dislocation of prosthesis. An immediate mobilization of the elbow, hand, and wrist is indicated.

29.3.2 Rehabilitation Program After Proximal Humerus Resection and Reconstruction with Modular Total Reverse Shoulder Prosthesis [13, 15–20]

The patient has to wear a shoulder brace at 30–45° of abduction for 4 weeks. Immediate progressive mobilization is indicated, and it consists in passive circumduction and pendulum movements limited to 30° for 4 weeks, then full range of movement exercises, and later exercises against resistance. Shoulder immobilization for 4–6 weeks (encouraging to exercise with the elbow, hand, and wrist) is indicated in patients with deltoid reinsertion.

29.3.3 Rehabilitation Program After Acetabular or Proximal Femur Resection and Reconstruction with Modular Prosthesis [2, 3, 5–8, 10, 12, 21]

The patient has to wear a pelvic-thigh brace locked in extension and slightly abducted for 4 weeks and then unlocked up to 90° for 4 more weeks in order to permit the remaining soft tissue healing avoiding dislocation of prosthesis. In distal femur reconstruction, deambulation with a walker or crutches is allowed after the second postoperative day: progressing up to full weight-bearing is permitted after 1 week in cases of cemented stem and after 3 weeks in case of press-fit stem.

29.3.4 Rehabilitation Program After Distal Femur Resection and Reconstruction with Modular Prosthesis [11, 22–26]

Mobilization with a walker or crutches is allowed after the second postoperative day: progressing up to full weight-bearing is permitted after 1 week in cases of cemented stem and after 3 weeks in case of press-fit stem. Initiation of ROM is permitted the second postoperative day encouraging the patient to reach 90° of knee flexion before hospital discharge.

29.3.5 Rehabilitation Program After Proximal Tibia Resection and Reconstruction with Modular Prosthesis [11, 12, 22, 26]

In proximal tibia reconstructions, the extensor mechanism and wound coverage are usually performed with rotation of the gastrocnemius muscle flap eventually associated with augmentation with artificial ligament. Mobilization with a walker or crutches is allowed after the second postoperative day: progressing up to full weight-bearing is permitted after 1 week in cases of cemented stem and after 3 weeks in case of press-fit stem. Patient has to wear a straight-leg brace for 6 weeks before initiation of ROM, in order to permit the healing of extensor mechanism.

Key Points

- Multidisciplinary care team is fundamental in patients suffering from bone malignancies.
- Most common malignant bone lesions in older patients are metastasis, myeloma, and chondrosarcoma.
- The rehabilitation program aims to reduce recovery time in patients with metastasis and myeloma and to obtain long-term functional results in more stable patients with chondrosarcoma, after surgery.

References

1. Campanacci M (1999) Bone and soft tissue tumors: clinical features, imaging, pathology and treatment. Springer, New York
2. G G (2016) Results of the treatment of bone metastases with modular prosthetic replacement—analysis of 67 patients. J Orthop Surg Res 11:20
3. Henrichs MP, Krebs J, Gosheger G, Streitbuerger A et al (2014) Modular tumor endoprostheses in surgical palliation of long-bone metastases: a reduction in tumor burden and a durable reconstruction. World J Surg Oncol 12:330
4. Wedin R, Hansen BH, Laitinen M, Trovik C et al (2012) Complications and survival after surgical treatment of 214 metastatic lesions of the humerus. J Shoulder Elb Surg 21(8):1049–1055
5. Guzik G (2016) Treatment of metastatic lesions localized in the acetabulum. J Orthop Surg Res 11(1):54
6. Calabró T, Van Rooyen R, Piraino I, Pala E et al (2016) Reconstruction of the proximal femur with a modular resection prosthesis. Eur J Orthop Surg Traumatol 26(4):415–421
7. Guzik G (2015) The use of LUMIC prosthesis for the treatment of periacetabular metastases. Ortop Traumatol Rehabil 17(6):593–602
8. Chen X, Xu L, Wang Y, Hao Y, Wang L (2016) Image-guided installation of 3D-printed patient-specific implant and its application in pelvic tumor resection and reconstruction surgery. Comput Methods Prog Biomed 125:66–78
9. Angelini A, Drago G, Trovarelli G, Calabrò T, Ruggieri P (2014) Infection after surgical resection for pelvic bone tumors: an analysis of 270 patients from one institution. Clin Orthop Relat Res 472(1):349–359
10. Angelini A, Calabrò T, Pala E, Trovarelli G et al (2015) Resection and reconstruction of pelvic bone tumors. Orthopedics 38(2):87–93
11. Pala E, Trovarelli G, Calabrò T, Angelini A et al (2015) Survival of modern knee tumor megaprostheses: failures, functional results, and a comparative statistical analysis. Clin Orthop Relat Res 473(3):891–899
12. Grimer RJ, Aydin BK, Wafa H, Carter SR et al (2016) Very long-term outcomes after endoprosthetic replacement for malignant tumours of bone. Bone Joint J 98-B(6):857–864
13. Dieckmann R, Liem D, Gosheger G, Henrichs MP et al (2013) Evaluation of a reconstruction reverse shoulder for tumour surgery and tribological comparision with an anatomical shoulder arthroplasty. Int Orthop 37(3):451–456
14. Griffiths D, Gikas PD, Jowett C, Bayliss L et al (2011) Proximal humeral replacement using a fixed-fulcrum endoprosthesis. J Bone Joint Surg Br 93(3):399–403
15. Streitbuerger A, Henrichs M, Gosheger G, Ahrens H et al (2015) Improvement of the shoulder function after large segment resection of the proximal humerus with the use of an inverse tumour prosthesis. Int Orthop 39(2):355–361
16. Guven MF, Aslan L, Botanlioglu H, Kaynak G et al (2016) Functional outcome of reverse shoulder tumor prosthesis in the treatment of proximal humerus tumors. J Shoulder Elb Surg 25(1):e1–e6
17. Kapur RA, McCann PA, Sarangi PP (2014) Reverse geometry shoulder replacement for proximal humeral metastases. Ann R Coll Surg Engl 96(7):e32–e35
18. Bonnevialle N, Mansat P, Lebon J, Laffosse JM, Bonnevialle P (2015) Reverse shoulder arthroplasty for malignant tumors of proximal humerus. J Shoulder Elb Surg 24(1):36–44
19. Teunis T, Nota SP, Hornicek FJ, Schwab JH et al (2014) Outcome after reconstruction of the proximal humerus for tumor resection: a systematic review. Clin Orthop Relat Res 472(7):2245–2253
20. Kaa AK, Jørgensen PH, Søjbjerg JO, Johannsen HV (2013) Reverse shoulder replacement after resection of the proximal humerus for bone tumours. Bone Joint J 95-B(11):1551–1555
21. Hobusch GM, Bollmann J, Puchner SE, Lang NW et al (2016) What sport activity levels are achieved in patients after resection and endoprosthetic reconstruction for a proximal femur bone sarcoma? Clin Orthop Relat Res Mar 28. [Epub ahead of print]

22. Bus MP, van de Sande MA, Fiocco M, Schaap GR et al (2015) What are the long-term results of MUTARS® modular endoprostheses for reconstruction of tumor resection of the distal femur and proximal tibia? Clin Orthop Relat Res Dec 9. [Epub ahead of print]
23. Zimel MN, Farfalli GL, Zindman AM, Riedel ER et al (2016) Revision distal femoral arthroplasty with the compress(®) prosthesis has a low rate of mechanical failure at 10 years. Clin Orthop Relat Res 474(2):528–536
24. Pala E, Trovarelli G, Angelini A, Ruggieri P (2016) Distal femur reconstruction with modular tumour prostheses: a single institution analysis of implant survival comparing fixed versus rotating hinge knee prostheses. Int Orthop 40(10):2171–2180
25. Capanna R, Ruggieri P, Biagini R, Ferraro A et al (1991) The effect of quadriceps excision on functional results after distal femoral resection and prosthetic replacement of bone tumors. Clin Orthop Relat Res (267):186–196
26. Mittermayer F, Krepler P, Dominkus M, Schwameis E et al (2001) Long-term followup of uncemented tumor endoprostheses for the lower extremity. Clin Orthop Relat Res 388:167–177

Age-Related Macular Degeneration: Prevention of Blindness and Low-Vision Rehabilitation

30

Edoardo Midena, Elisabetta Pilotto, and Enrica Convento

30.1 Introduction

Age-related macular degeneration (AMD) is a common cause of vision impairment and blindness affecting approximately 9% of the global population. The World Health Organization (WHO) has recognized blindness as one of the handicaps that mostly affects individuals, families, and society. Visual impairment has a serious impact on older adults' ability to perform daily activities, dramatically interfering with their ability to live independently [1]. The loss of that ability can greatly reduce a person's sense of independence and well-being. Visual impairment has also been associated with reduced survival in a population-based survey. Foremost, the loss of vision has been and remains one of the most feared chronic disabilities.

In 1973, the WHO established that elimination of avoidable blindness was justified not only from a humanitarian point of view but also from a social and economic perspective. It has been estimated that the annual worldwide productivity cost of blindness was US 168 billion dollars based on 1993 data for prevalence rates, gross domestic products, and populations [2]. These costs will increase dramatically in the future as population aging is also increasing [3]. Decreased vision not only can lead to changes in occupation and missed time from work but also increased need for patient caregivers (e.g., family, friends, hired help).

Approximately 0.4% of the general population has late or advanced AMD with the prevalence of advanced AMD rising to 8% among those 75 years of age and

E. Midena, MD, PhD (✉)
Department of Ophthalmology, University of Padua, via Giustiniani 2, 35128 Padua, Italy

Fondazione GB Bietti per l'Oftalmologia, IRCCS, Roma, Italy
e-mail: edoardo.midena@unipd.it

E. Pilotto, MD • E. Convento, MSc
Department of Ophthalmology, University of Padua, via Giustiniani 2, 35128 Padua, Italy
e-mail: elisabetta.pilotto@unipd.it; enrica.convento@unipd.it

© Springer International Publishing AG 2018

S. Masiero, U. Carraro (eds.), *Rehabilitation Medicine for Elderly Patients*,
Practical Issues in Geriatrics, DOI 10.1007/978-3-319-57406-6_30

older [4]. While the prevalence of all types of AMD has somewhat declined over the past decade, due to enhanced medical prevention and treatment options, the number of people with all types of AMD is expected to increase due to the rapid and consistent growth of the aging population. Recent projections estimate that worldwide the number of individuals with AMD will reach 196 million in 2020 and 288 million in 2040 [5].

In this chapter, we describe signs and symptoms of AMD, the functional visual impairment due to the development of a central dense scotoma, and the low-vision rehabilitation strategies to improve visual performance of patients affected by late AMD.

30.2 Age-Related Macular Degeneration

Symptoms of AMD are mainly due to a loss of central vision, which is required for activities such as reading, driving, and recognizing faces. Moreover, a common negative consequence of the vision impairment caused by AMD is increased functional disability, which put AMD patients at increased risk for mental health problems such as high level of clinical depression and anxiety. Among older adults with visual impairment, those with AMD seem to be particularly at risk for depression compared to other eye diseases [6].

AMD is clinically divided into two different clinical forms: the dry form and the exudative form. Subretinal deposits (drusen) and areas of hyperpigmentation and/or hypopigmentation of the retinal pigment epithelium (RPE) are the earlier clinical manifestations of dry AMD, with consequent thinning of the retina. This structural retinal change leads to decreased visual function, not necessarily associated to visual acuity reduction. Retinal sensitivity impairment develops much earlier than visual acuity changes, and it happens in a short time [7].

The atrophic late-stage manifestation of dry AMD is represented by geographic atrophy (GA). GA, which is commonly bilateral, is characterized by the development of areas of retina atrophy, which slowly progresses over time. Areas of GA are functionally characterized by a dense scotoma, whose extension corresponds to the atrophic area [8]. Therefore, the progression of GA is associated with progressive loss of visual function. However, atrophic areas initially spare the central part of the macula, the fovea, and patients are unaware of their functional condition. As long as the fovea remains unaffected, retinal fixation maintains central and stable. This means that even a small residual area of retinal sensitivity is useful for fixation in patients with progressive atrophic lesions due to AMD, with consequently good visual acuity. When GA progresses, involving the central foveal area, fixation migrates. Therefore, an extrafoveal preferential fixation location (known as *preferred retinal locus* (PRL)) develops, usually located at the edge of the area of atrophy, in a location closer to the foveal region, thus providing the best functional result [9].

The exudative (or neovascular or wet) form accounts for nearly 90% of all severe visual loss from AMD. Its main characteristic is the development of choroidal neovascularization (CNV), which exudates and bleeds, and evolves toward a macular scar, with loss of the central vision. Visual impairment in eyes with CNV is associated with early progressive deterioration not only of visual acuity but also of retinal fixation and macular sensitivity. This functional deterioration manifests as decreased fixation stability, loss of central fixation, and impaired retinal sensitivity with the development of a dense scotoma. In eyes with progressive deterioration, the inability to maintain a PRL within the fovea progresses until complete absence of foveal visual perception is established and the PRL becomes totally eccentric. Eccentric fixation develops early in exudative AMD, a functional difference from GA, in which, as long as a 2° central area of the fovea is spared by the atrophy, the fixation area remains central and stable [10].

Current treatment for AMD consists of medical treatment (intraocular injections of anti-vascular endothelium growth factor (anti-VEGF) for neovascular or exudative AMD) and vitamin therapy (for the early form of AMD). However, for many patients, medical treatment is either not indicated (e.g., anti-VEGF treatment is not effective for dry AMD), or when it is, many patients may continue to experience psychological distress or reduction of their visual function. Low-vision rehabilitation aims to reduce vision-related disability by maximizing residual vision through training in the use of optical and assistive devices, orientation and mobility skills, and general compensatory strategies. Moreover, some studies have shown improvement in depression following low-vision treatment [6].

30.3 Low-Vision Rehabilitation

In 1986, the American Foundation for the Blind sponsored the first international conference in low-vision rehabilitation (LVR). For the first time, researchers in most of the disciplines involved in LVR shared their clinical, research, and practical experiences with visually impaired people. Modern LVR was defined as a multidisciplinary professional service which provides methods and means for optimal use of residual visual function, training of residual vision-related skills, and reintegration in society. This definition was subsequently endorsed in 2007 from others associations and groups representing the visually impaired people [11].

The reduced visual acuity in patients with late-stage AMD leads to loss of reading ability. Therefore, reading ability restoration is one of the main objectives in low-vision rehabilitation. Adaptive strategies to reduce the impact of disabilities due to vision loss develop naturally and quite early. One of such strategy in AMD patients is an attempt to reduce the impact of scotoma on central fields of vision, developing scotoma awareness and displacement abilities. To perform it, incoming images land on eccentric PRL, which possess superior visual capabilities and assume the functions of the lost macula area.

One of the basic tenets of modern LVR is the concept of PRL assuming "macular function" after central vision loss. However, in about 25% of cases, the PRL develops onto an "unfavorable" retinal area and hence is useless [12]. In addition

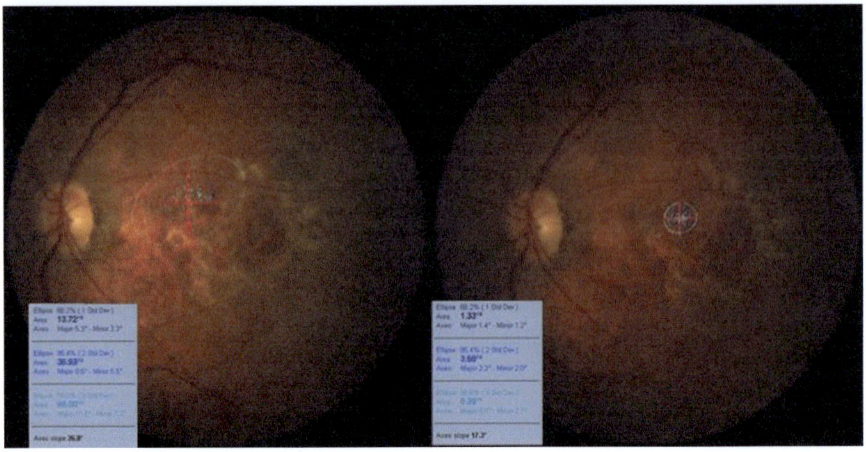

Fig. 30.1 Microperimetry fixation evaluation in the left eye of a patient with late form of exudative age-related macular, before (*left*) and after (*right*) biofeedback training using MP1. After rehabilitation, the macular area used to fixate becomes smaller. Therefore, being fixation more stable, visual performances improve

to traditional low-vision aids and reading rehabilitation training, a new method for PRL rehabilitation is the biofeedback training using an instrument, commonly known as microperimeter. The biofeedback techniques available with the microperimeter MP-1 (Nidek Technologies, Padua, Italy) provide an effective method for PRL rehabilitation, by training fixation accuracy and stability, and refixation precision skills.

Microperimetry is the diagnostic technique which not only allows to exactly correlate, in real time, the sensitivity threshold of any individual point of the retina with its clinical appearance, but it also documents the location and stability of fixation. Therefore, microperimetry allows investigating site and characteristics of the PRL. It was observed that in AMD eyes, PRL and highest retinal sensitivity loci, identified by mean of microperimetry, are two separate entities with no identical physical location. The aim of low-vision rehabilitation interventions should be relocation of PRL to loci with highest retinal sensitivity, identified by means of microperimetry, because reading speed improves if a new PRL is established in an area that is more favorable for reading (Fig. 30.1).

Moreover, microperimetry is useful to assess the site and characteristic of PRL before and after rehabilitation. Greater fixation stability with better PRL at the end of vision rehabilitation explains the improvement of visual efficiency.

Previous studies demonstrated that the use of the MP-1 microperimeter acoustic biofeedback techniques in patients with macular diseases makes it possible to improve their visual performance, such as distant and near visual acuity, reading speed, reading comprehension, stabilizing fixation behavior or relocating the PRL, or both. Moreover, MP1-microperimeter offers a different biofeedback strategy, which uses a structured light stimulus (flickering pattern) plus acoustic biofeedback. Both methods seem to improve visual function. However, flickering pattern biofeedback training seems more useful in the rehabilitation of patients with low vision at the late stage of AMD, allowing to increase not only fixation stability and reading speed but retinal sensitivity and visual acuity, too [13].

Conclusion

New therapeutic strategies for exudative AMD have reduced the incidence of visual acuity reduction, preventing or slowing the development of a macular scotoma. However, due to the aging population, AMD is still one of the major causes of legal blindness among older people. Therefore, low vision treatment has an important role in the rehabilitation of the patients with central scotoma due to late AMD. The modern low-vision treatment, assessing components of residual visual function, such as retinal sensitivity, and functional vision, such as PRL and fixation stability, aims to adequately train residual area of the retina to fixate to improve visual performance.

Key Points

- Age-related macular degeneration is one of the major causes of legal blindness among older people.
- Loss of visual function reduces a person's sense of independence and well-being.
- Low-vision rehabilitation is a multidisciplinary professional service which provides methods and means for optimal use of residual visual function, training of residual vision-related skills, and reintegration in society.

References

1. Rubin GS, Roche KB, Prasada-Rao P et al (1994) Visual impairment and disability in older adults. Optom Vis Sci 71:750–760
2. Smith AF, Smith JG (1996) The economic burden of global blindness: a price too high. Br J Ophthalmol 80:276–277
3. Meads C, Hyde C (2003) What is the cost of blindness? Br J Ophthalmol 87:1201–1204
4. Klein R, Peto T, Bird A et al (2004) The epidemiology of age-related macular degeneration. Am J Ophthalmol 137:486–495
5. Wong WL, Su X, Li X et al (2014) Global prevalence of age-related macular degeneration and disease burden projection for 2020 and 2040: a systematic review and meta-analysis. Lancet Glob Health 2(2):e106–e116
6. Horowitz A, Reinhardt JP, Boerner K (2005) The effect of rehabilitation on depression among visually disabled older adults. Aging Ment Health 9(6):563–570
7. Midena E, Vujosevic S, Convento E, Manfrè A, Cavarzeran F, Pilotto E (2007) Microperimetry and fundus autofluorescence in patients with early age-related macular degeneration. Br J Ophthalmol 91:499–503

8. Pilotto E, Convento E, Guidolin F, Abalsamo CK, Longhin E, Parrozzani R et al (2016) Microperimetry features of geographic atrophy identified with en face optical coherence tomography. JAMA Ophthalmol 134:873. doi:10.1001/jamaophthalmol.2016.1535
9. Sunness JS, Applegate CA, Haselwood D, Rubin GS (1996) Fixation patterns and reading rates in eyes with central scotomas from advanced atrophic age-related macular degeneration and stargardt disease. Ophthalmology 103:1458–1466
10. Midena E, Radin PP, Pilotto E et al (2004) Fixation pattern and macular sensitivity in eyes with subfoveal choroidal neovascularization secondary to age-related macular degeneration. A microperimetry study. Semin Ophthalmol 19:55–61
11. Markowitz SN (2016) State-of-the art: low vision rehabilitation. Can J Ophthalmol 51:59–66
12. Mandelcom MS, Podbielski DW, Mandelcorn ED (2013) Fixation stability as a goal in the treatment of macular disease. Can J Ophthalmol 48:364–367
13. Amore FM, Paliotta S, Silvestri V et al (2013) Biofeedback stimulation in patients with age-related macular degeneration: comparison between 2 different methods. Can J Ophthalmol 48:431–437

Rehabilitation in Diseases of the Sense Organs in Older Adults: Hearing and Balance

31

Roberto Bovo, Alessandro Castiglione, and Alessandro Martini

31.1 Introduction

31.1.1 Hearing Impairment

More than 40% of the population beyond the age of 65 years suffers from hearing impairment. On the other hand, the prevalence of dementia exceeds 10% at this age, thus leading to correlational studies between hearing loss and cognitive decline. In fact, as widely reported in the literature, there is strong evidence that hearing loss in older adults is associated with both cognitive impairment and aging [1]. For example, a severe hearing loss can increase the risk of developing dementia in the next years of approximately fivefolds. Consequently, the auditory rehabilitation of the elderly should not be limited to restore hearing function and should take into careful consideration the effects, causes, and consequences of the sensorial deprivation on central processes in terms of speech perception and quality of life.

To date, the most appropriate testing is represented by otoscopy, tonal and speech audiometries, dichotic test, and speech audiometry in noise (open or closed set) with or without adaptive study. Good outcomes of proper clinical practice have been accompanied by the continuously expanding clinical indications for digital hearing aids [2]. Moreover, even very old people can benefit from procedures that were previously recommended for younger patients, such as cochlear implantation [3].

It is thought that auditory rehabilitation can reduce the cognitive "load" (the neural activity needed to achieve a task, in particular understanding/recognizing the spoken word), social isolation, anxiety, and depression. Recent research suggests to us that the geriatric patient response is influenced by the spiral ganglion cells (number, efficiency, synapses, connections, and synchrony), by central plasticity

R. Bovo • A. Castiglione • A. Martini (✉)
Neuroscience Department, Operative Unit of Otolaryngology, Padua University, Padua, Italy
e-mail: roberto.bovo@sanita.padova.it; alessandro.castiglione@unipd.it; alessandromartini@unipd.it

© Springer International Publishing AG 2018

S. Masiero, U. Carraro (eds.), *Rehabilitation Medicine for Elderly Patients*, Practical Issues in Geriatrics, DOI 10.1007/978-3-319-57406-6_31

(positive versus negative or adaptive versus "maladaptive"), by central auditory processing disorders, and by diseases of the nervous system, including neurodegenerative conditions. The effects of the auditory training on short-term memory have been previously reported, and nonetheless it is surprising to notice that a significant improvement does not necessarily require a training period, or, in other words, hearing aid users can experience a reduction in cognitive performances without hearing aids. In addition, working memory has a crucial role in understanding spoken words in noisy environments; consequently, short-term memory assessment could be a predictive factor for rehabilitative outcomes [1].

31.1.2 Auditory Rehabilitation with Hearing Aids

Historically, hearing aid ownership and regular use of hearing aids have been found to be low. In fact, it is estimated that only one out of five people who could benefit from a hearing aid actually wears one. The reasons given included trouble handling the aid and little opportunity to converse with others, difficulty inserting the earmold, difficulty coping with signals in noise, lack of recognition of hearing loss, advanced age and poor health, and less than ideal matching of the aid to the loss of hearing [2, 5]. Digital hearing aids now offer a number of advantages over analogue hearing aids including improved sound quality, increased comfort, digital feedback reduction, digital noise reduction, digital speech enhancement, automatically switching listening programs for different listening environments, directional microphones, remote controls, smaller size and open fit design, and flexibility in manipulation of the frequency, compression, and gain. When feasible, a bilateral/binaural rehabilitation through digital devices is desirable. Unfortunately, a pejorative course after this practice is also possible, and in these patients, it should be avoided. Unfortunately, despite all these improvements in hearing aids, the underuse among older adults is still of significant concern. Identifying factors that affect hearing aid usage are necessary for devising appropriate rehabilitation strategies to ensure greater use of hearing aids. In current practice, a strategy exclusively aimed to compensate for the peripheral loss is not enough, because of persisting sensations of "inability to understand words, even hearing them." Very common is also the difficulty to understand speech in noise despite adequate amplification. Further research is needed to enable/ensure sufficient and efficient communication skills in all possible situations.

31.1.3 Auditory Rehabilitation with Cochlear Implant

Approximately 1% of the population above 65 years has a severe to profound loss, which cannot benefit from hearing aids. This percentage is estimated to rise to 16% in the over 80 years old age group, and it will probably grow by more than twofold in the next 40 years. Cochlear implantation (CI) is a safe and effective procedure even in the most elderly patients [3]. In fact, the risk of anesthetic and surgical complications remains low provided that a thorough multidisciplinary evaluation is performed before the procedure. Moreover, the cost-effectiveness still remains acceptable, including patients over 70 years of age, because, even if healthcare costs are high, the savings in terms of indirect costs and quality of life (QoL) are important. Cochlear implantation dramatically improves auditory function and speech perception and has an outstanding impact on the social life, activities, and self-esteem of the old patient. Health-related quality of life questionnaires show a statistically significant benefit when the preoperative health status is compared with the postoperative health status. Moreover, several authors observed that when compared to younger adult patients, cochlear implant recipients older than 65 years showed similar benefit in most measures. Finally, among patients with pre-implant severe tinnitus, a partial or total tinnitus reduction was observed in approximately 70% of cases.

31.1.4 Dizziness

Dizziness represents largely a problem in the elderly, being the most common reason patients over the age of 75 years seek medical attention. The term dizziness is often misused, as patients include many sensations as vertigo, disequilibrium, and light-headedness. Different causes for such sensations are reported. Cardiovascular, neurological, or locomotor disease, deterioration in sensory organs, vestibular dysfunction, and adverse drug effects are the most common. For the vestibular system, aging is associated with degeneration of the main receptor structures, which in the elderly patient may overlap to neurodegenerative processes. The clinical relevance of the problem is high if one considers that persons who simultaneously had balance, vision, and hearing difficulty had an over eightfold higher risk for fear of falling compared to persons who did not have any of these three sensory difficulties [4].

31.1.5 Rehabilitation of Dizziness, Vertigo, and Unsteadiness

Patients with a prevalent dysfunction of the vestibular system can be treated effectively with vestibular rehabilitation (VR), which includes both a "generic" type and more specific protocols. In generic VR, patients are provided with a series of tasks to perform that require them to use their eyes, while their head is moving and possibly when their body is also moving. On the other hand, specific protocols have been initially proposed by Cawthorne and Cooksey [6], followed by many others in subsequent decades [7, 8]. A frequently used protocol is reported in Table 31.1. It is important to begin with simpler exercises and progress to harder ones. Also, the exercises need to be moderately challenging, but safe enough, so patients do not fall while doing them.

VR has been shown to promote significant improvements in several aspects of balance, including vestibulo-visual interaction during head movements, static and dynamic postural stability in conditions of conflicting sensory information, and

Table 31.1 A protocol of exercises to be done daily for at least 60 min over split sessions

Focus on an object while moving the head side to side, up and down (20 times each)
In standing position, shrug shoulder and rotate
In sitting position, bend forward and place an object on the ground (20 times)
Focus on object moving from arm's length to about 6 in. away from the face
Sitting to standing with eyes open, than eyes shut
Throw ball from hand to hand above eye level (20 times), than under the knee (10 times each knee)
Stand on one foot with eyes open (3 times for 10 s each foot), with eyes shut (3 times for 10 s each foot)
Change from sitting to standing and turn around in between (10 times)
Walk a straight line from heel to toe (5 times for 10 paces)

diminished individual sensitivity to head movements [7]. Avocational activities can also be excellent for vestibular rehabilitation, provided that they involve using the eyes while the head and body are in motion. Of course, many avocational activities require this—dancing, yoga, tai chi, golf, and tennis are probably the most adequate for the elderly. Nevertheless, just walking around the block looking from side to side may be a useful activity. Older subjects should find one that is fun, safe, and somewhat stimulating. Most studies on VR are carried out with patients suffering from bilateral vestibular loss (BVL), although an increasing number of data is available regarding people with symptomatic unilateral vestibular loss (UVL). Unfortunately, the data on rehabilitation outcomes of these patients are still not conclusive. In a recent study on BVL, roughly 80% of patients do not improve independently of age, gender, time course of manifestation, and severity: thus, the prognosis seems less favorable than assumed previously [8]. These patients have a "visual dependence," so they should avoid walking in the dark or without corrective lenses if they have refraction disorders, especially in open spaces. On the opposite, there is a moderate to strong evidence that VR is an effective management for UVL patients and in the studies with a follow-up assessment (3–12 months), positive effects were maintained.

Benign paroxysmal positional vertigo (BPPV) is the most frequent type of peripheral vertigo in the elderly and is still an under-recognized entity. Even on specific questioning, positional vertigo is often not reported by patients suffering from BPPV. Instead, they complain of dizziness, light-headedness, or unsteadiness. This might be due to unconscious limitation and avoidance of movements and positions that evoke vertigo. Thus, a diagnostic positioning test (Hallpike or Semont) should be carried in the elderly complaining of dizziness or vertigo, with the only exception of patients with spinal contraindication, as disc herniation or other severe pathologies of the vertebral column. Unfortunately, most studies on BPPV reveal a low success rate in the treatment of this entity and a higher frequency of recurrences in elderly patients compared to the general population [9]. In a recent Cochrane meta-analysis [10], it was concluded that although there is evidence that the Epley maneuver is an effective treatment for posterior canal BPPV (based on the results of controlled trials with relatively short follow-up), there is no good evidence that this treatment provides a long-term resolution of symptoms. In treated old patients, the estimated recurrence rate of BPPV is 30–50% [10, 11], and the natural resolution of untreated cases is around 20–30% [11]. The maneuver involves sequential movement of the head into four positions, staying in each position for roughly 30 s, with the aim to remove debris or "ear rocks" out of the sensitive part of the ear (posterior canal) to a less sensitive location.

Cochlear implant (CI) may have a double opposite effect on dizziness and risk of falling. On one hand, CI may improve physical activities and auditory scene analyses and reduce cognitive load, thus improving balance and reducing the risk of falling. On the other hand, damage of the vestibular system due to postoperative labyrinthitis and subsequent fibrosis has been observed in around 3–4% for the semicircular canals and 31% for the saccule. Thus, in a CI candidate undergoing implantation of an "only balancing ear," the risk to the labyrinth should be considered and discussed with the patient: when all other factors are equal, the "worse balancing ear" should be implanted.

In conclusion, a multifactorial approach could be the best solution for a number of elderly people, who generally suffer from multiple deficiencies. Intervention needs to be tailored to each patient to obtain the maximum effect, designing different exercises for individuals with different kinds of deficiency [6–9]. Avocational activities may also have a role in improving the patient's equilibrium. Unfortunately, several studies have demonstrated that the results achieved can soon be lost if seniors revert to their previous sedentary lifestyle and limited activity. One way to avoid this is to continue the training at home whenever feasible, possibly prescribing more straightforward exercises to help patients maintain a minimal but continuous practice routine [11].

Key Points

- Hearing loss in older adults is associated with both cognitive impairment and aging. Auditory rehabilitation can reduce the cognitive "load," social isolation, anxiety, and depression.
- Dizzy elderly people generally suffer from multiple deficiencies. A multifactorial approach could be the best solution. Intervention needs to be tailored to each patient to obtain the maximum effect, designing different exercises for individuals with different kinds of deficiency.

References

1. Martini A, Castiglione A, Bovo R, Vallesi A, Gabelli C (2014) Aging, cognitive load, dementia and hearing loss. Audiol Neurootol 19(Suppl 1):2–5
2. Perez E, Edmonds BA (2012) A systematic review of studies measuring and reporting hearing aid usage in older adults since 1999: a descriptive summary of measurement tools. PLoS One 7(3):e31831
3. Orabi AA, Mawman D, Al-Zoubi F, Saeed SR, Ramsden RT (2006) Cochlear implant outcomes and quality of life in the elderly: Manchester experience over 13 years. Clin Otolaryngol 31:116–122

4. Bovo R, Faccioli C, Martini A (2014) Dizziness in the elderly. Hearing Balance Commun 12:54–65
5. Jenstad L, Moon J (2011) Systematic review of barriers and facilitators to hearing-aid uptake in older adults. Audiol Res 1:91–96
6. Cooksey FS (1946) Rehabilitation in vestibular injuries. Proc R Soc Med 39:273–275
7. Hall CD, Herdman SJ, Whitney SL, Cass SP, Clendaniel RA, Fife TD, Furman JM, Getchius TS et al (2016) Vestibular rehabilitation for peripheral vestibular hypofunction: an evidence-based clinical practice guideline. J Neurol Phys Ther 40:124–155
8. Zingler VC, Weintz E, Jahn K, Mike A, Huppert D, Rettinger N et al (2008) Follow-up of vestibular function in bilateral vestibulopathy. J Neurol Neurosurg Psychiatry 79:284–288
9. Batuecas-Caletrio A, Trinidad-Ruiz G, Zschaeck C, Del Pozo de Dios JC, de Toro GL, Martin-Sanchez V et al (2013) Benign paroxysmal positional vertigo in the elderly. Gerontology 15:408–412
10. Hilton MP, Pinder DK (2004) The Epley (canalith repositioning) maneuver for benign paroxysmal positional vertigo. Cochrane Database Syst Rev 2:CD003162
11. Brandt T, Huppert T, Hüfner K, Zingler VC, Dieterich M, Strupp M (2010) Long-term course and relapses of vestibular and balance disorders. Restor Neurol Neurosci 28:69–82

Rehabilitation of Ageing People with Neurological Disorders

32

Alessandra Del Felice, Leonora Castiglia, Elena Demertzis, Laura Bernardi, Marie Ursin, Håkon Ihle-Hansen, Guri Hagberg, Ragnhild Munthe-Kaas, and Hege Ihle-Hansen

32.1 Epidemiology of Neurological Disorders in the Elderly

Neurological conditions are a common cause of severe disability in the elderly and constitute a heavy burden on healthcare and social services.

According to the World Health Organization (WHO), 15 million people suffer stroke worldwide each year. Of these, nearly 6 million die and another 5 million are permanently disabled. In Europe, stroke was responsible for around 470,000 deaths in 2015 (http://ghdx.healthdata.org/gbd-results-tool).

In many developed countries, the incidence of stroke is declining, even if the overall rate of stroke remains high because of the aging of population. In the developing world, however, the incidence of stroke is increasing. Stroke is the second leading cause of disability after dementia and globally the second leading cause of death above the age of 60 years (http://ghdx.healthdata.org/gbd-results-tool).

Traumatic brain injury (TBI) is a major cause of long-term disability in industrialized and developing countries. An estimated 10 million people are affected

A. Del Felice, MD, PhD (✉) • L. Bernardi, MD • L. Castiglia, MD • E. Demertzis, MD
Department of Neuroscience, Section of Rehabilitation, University of Padua,
Via Giustiniani, 3, 35128 Padua, Italy
e-mail: alessandra.delfelice@unipd.it

M. Ursin, PhD • H. Ihle-Hansen, MD • G. Hagberg, MD • R. Munthe-Kaas, MD
H. Ihle-Hansen, MD, PhD
Department of Research, Vestre Viken Hospital Trust, Bærum Hospital,
3004 Drammen, Norway

© Springer International Publishing AG 2018

S. Masiero, U. Carraro (eds.), *Rehabilitation Medicine for Elderly Patients*,
Practical Issues in Geriatrics, DOI 10.1007/978-3-319-57406-6_32

annually by TBI, and it will surpass many diseases as the major cause of death and disability by the year 2020 [1].

The burden of TBI is evident worldwide and is especially prominent in low- and middle-income countries, which face a higher proportion of risk factors for TBI and have health systems ill-equipped to address the consequent disability. Latin America and sub-Saharan Africa show the highest TBI-related incidence rate, varying from 150 to 170 per 100,000 compared to a global rate of 106 per 100,000 [1]. The age-related distribution sees two peaks, one in the young, mainly related to road accidents, and a second, which is gaining impact in western countries, in the elderly generally related to accidental falls [2].

About 2.5 million people around the worldwide are affected by multiple sclerosis (MS). MS is typically diagnosed in the second or third decade of life. Due to better medical and nursing care, an increasing number of people with MS are entering or have reached senescence [3]. In addition, there is another group of elderly subjects with MS, which are those with late-onset MS. Recent estimates calculated the percentage of people with MS older than 65 years to be between 9% and 14% [3].

Peripheral neuropathies are another common cause of disability in older people. In 2009, the prevalence of peripheral neuropathy worldwide has been estimated to range from 2% to 8% of the population [4]. Small fiber neuropathy is the most common type of neuropathy in people over the age of 50 years [5]. Guillain–Barré syndrome, the most common form of acute inflammatory neuropathy, represents 11% of causes of neuropathies in people aged 65 years [6].

Parkinson's disease has a prevalence of around 0.3% of the general population and of 1% in people over 60 years of age [7] in industrialized countries, with a clear-cut age- and sex-related trend (i.e., higher prevalence in the older and in men) [8, 9]. Environmental exposure to toxics, such occupational ones (e.g., pesticides and heavy metals) [10], and genetic factors [11] have been recognized as potential etiological factors. Disease progression can lead to subcortical dementia. Dysphagia, frequently occurring during later stages, increases risk of aspiration and pulmonary complications. Parkinson negatively affects quality of life with advancing of disease, with an increased risk of falls, reduced autonomy in activities of daily life (ADL), and lastly social avoidance.

In 2015, the WHO ranked neurological disorders fifth among all causes of years of life lost to disability (YLDs) in people over 70 years of age, after other non-communicable diseases, musculoskeletal disorders, diabetes/urogynecological/hematological/endocrinological, and cardiovascular diseases.

From 1990 to 2015, there was an increase of YLDs related to neurological conditions, with a higher prevalence of Alzheimer's disease and multiple sclerosis in women, and of Parkinson's disease, epilepsy, and motor neuron disease in men (Table. 32.1 for neurological conditions, Figs. 32.1 for cerebrovascular disease).

Table 32.1 YLDs (years lived with disability) and DALYs (disability-adjusted life years) associated with neurological disorders (cerebrovascular disease not included) in people aged 70 years and over for both sexes in 2015. Source: https://vizhub.healthdata.org/gbd-compare/

YLDs	Percentage of total YLDs	YLDs (100000 population)	DALYs	Percentage of total DALYs	DALYs (100000 population)
8,170,557.87	8.51 %	2,052.34	23,817,243.48	6.62%	5,982.59

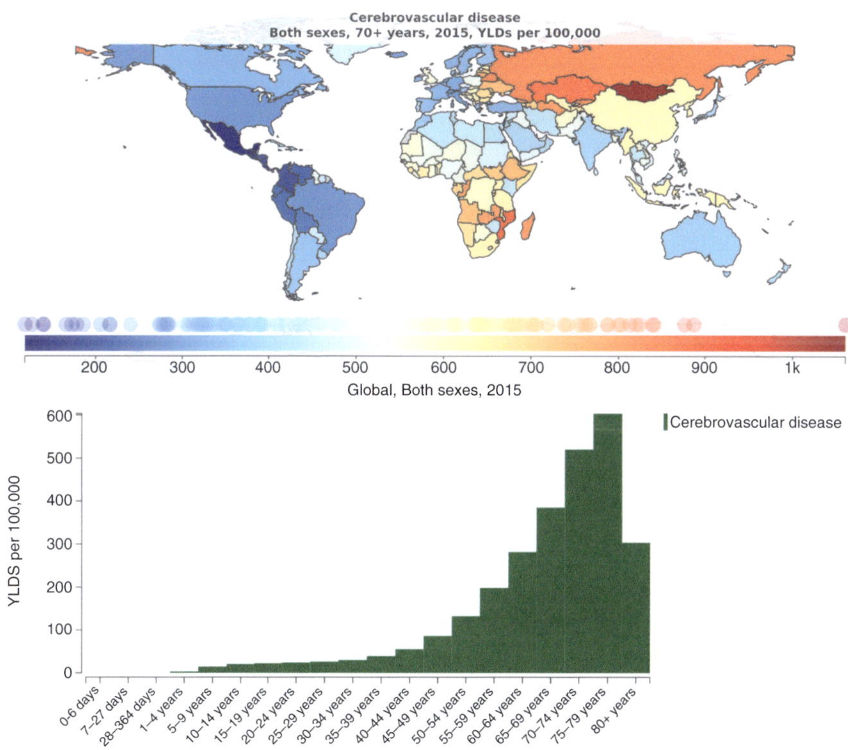

Fig. 32.1 YLDs (years lived with disability) related to cerebrovascular disease in elderly people in the world and YLDs per 100,000 persons related to neurological condition based on age. Source: https://vizhub.healthdata.org/gbd-compare/

32.2 Brain Reserve and Neuroplasticity

Brain reserve is the brain's resilience to pathological damage or changes. The greater the brain reserve, the less likely an individual will demonstrate disturbance associated with a central nervous system (CNS) lesion. The majority of studies focused on the concept of cognitive brain reserve, confirming that the level of education and cognitive skills in general (i.e., bilingualism, multiple hobbies, etc.) retard the onset of dementia or cognitive impairment [12, 13]. An emerging concept is motor brain reserve, in which neurophysiological/neuroimaging or structural markers are searched to predict who will recover better from a motor perspective after a CNS insult.

Motor reserve has been linked to the strength or modularity of cerebral motor networks: the better cortical areas involved in motor behavior are interconnected and maintain communication after the insult, the better the motor recovery will be. These assessments, conducted either with high-density EEG or with functional resonance imaging (fMRI), are time-consuming and require highly skilled teams. An alternative surrogate has been suggested to be cortical thickness of motor areas, or the extent of the cortex covered by the hand knob: both parameters require a simple structural MRI and can be determined by ad hoc software [14].

The issue of brain reserve parallels that of neuroplasticity, in that a higher functioning brain is likely to have higher potential for neuroplasticity. Neuroplasticity is the potential of the brain to rearrange and rewire; it can be part of a physiological process, i.e., during growth, or a reaction to a damage to the CNS. It affects microscopic level, e.g., by modifying neurotransmitters release or modulating synaptic expression, mesoscopic level with modifications of neuronal ensembles interactions, and macroscopic level when the cortex rearranges and modifies its structure.

We refer the reader to Chap. 2 (the ageing brain) for a more detailed discussion of neuroplasticity in the elderly.

32.3 Rehabilitation of Functional Impairments

According the World Health Organization (WHO), the aim of rehabilitation is to maximize function and minimize limitation of activity and restriction of participation resulting from an underlying impairment or disease, promoting an innovative paradigm in rehabilitation. WHO's International Classification of Functioning, Disability, and Health (ICF) includes medical, biological, and social aspects of disability, and can be used as a framework to collate all elements and goals in rehabilitation.

Rehabilitation should boost residual functions, and not focus on lost capacities. It might not be possible to return to motor baseline performance, but personal and psychological resources and remaining functions shall be the basis for a sound rehabilitation.

Table 32.2 Four steps in the rehabilitation process

1	Assessment	To identify and quantify the person's needs
2	Goal setting	To define realistic and attainable goals for improvement
3	Intervention	To assist in the achievement of goals
4	Reassessment	To assess progress against agreed goals

Adapted form Langhorne et al. [15]

Rehabilitation typically entails a cyclical process [15], involving four steps as detailed in Table 32.2.

Healthcare professionals working in neurological rehabilitation need to explore the social, psychological, and cultural background of the person to be rehabilitated, to identify expectations and values, and agree upon goals with each individual during the entire rehabilitation process. An increasing literature is highlighting the advantages provided by self-management programs [16], which include, among other interventions, involving people in decision making, emphasizing problem solving, promoting healthy lifestyle, and educating people on how to self-manage. Setting agreed-upon plans and following up on the extent to which goals are achieved have been reported the most effective intervention [17] in these programs, stressing the need for appropriate goal setting paradigms [18].

Given the complexity of impairments of elderly people with neurological dysfunctions, the need for multidisciplinary teams has been advocated. The integrated competences of neurologists, geriatricians, physical medicine doctors, physical and occupational therapists, neuropsychologists, speech and language therapists, and social workers are highly recommended.

32.3.1 Clinical Presentation and Functional Impairments in Stroke, Traumatic Brain Injury, and Multiple Sclerosis

32.3.1.1 Stroke

Stroke is the consequence of impaired oxygen supply to a brain region. It can be ischemic if the defective supply depends on either a vessel occlusion by an embolus or a thickening of the arterial wall or reduced perfusion, or hemorrhagic if a ruptured vessel impairs cerebral blood flow. In the latter case, the detrimental effects of hypoxia are coupled with the irritative effects of hemoglobin derivatives on brain tissue. Clinical presentation is heterogeneous, according to the lesioned brain area or to the disrupted cerebral network. Motor and language impairment are frequent signs following a middle cerebral artery occlusion, but symptoms range from sensory and visual disturbances to full-blown neuropsychological deficits. Due to the phenomenon of *diaschisis* (Greek for disconnection), some deficits regress spontaneously during the first days post-stroke, as the neural connections between distant areas are restored or alternative ones created.

Stroke treatment has advanced significantly over the recent years. The concept of ischemic penumbra, i.e., the tissue surrounding the ischemic core and still viable, which could be rescued if an adequate blood flow can be reinstated, has provided the conceptual basis for a paradigm shift in stroke therapy. Evidence of the benefits of thrombolysis and intra-arterial interventions, effectiveness of the multidisciplinary stroke unit [19], as well as the focus on rapid transfer of people with stroke to hospital has transformed the treatment. This change saves lives and improves outcome. However, only a small proportion of the stroke population will benefit from thrombolysis or mechanical clot retrieval. Stroke survivors will mostly still be in need of rehabilitation provided by the multidisciplinary team starting from the stroke unit up to the community level.

Many stroke survivors are left with significant residual disabilities, with 22% unable to walk again and between 24% and 53% requiring assistance with activities of daily living [20–22]. Functional outcome has been related to clinical signs [trunk control and lower-limb (LL) strength i] [23], integrity of corticospinal tracts [24, 25], and neuronal reorganization and cortical connectivity [26–28].

32.3.1.2 Traumatic Brain Injury

Traumatic brain injury (TBI) refers to damage to the brain caused by an external physical force. The leading cause of brain injury in the elderly is falls [2]. Older age, comorbidity, and medications including blood thinners are all risk factors for increased severity. CT scans in the acute setting and after a few months from the event to exclude subdural hematomas are recommended as part of the diagnostic process. Injuries that require admission to a neuro-intensive care unit usually undergo the same functional assessment as stroke patients.

In a closed head injury, damage occurs because of a blow to the person's head or having the head stop suddenly after moving at high speed. This causes the brain to move forward and back or from side to side, such that it colliding with bony structures that surrond it. This jarring movement bruises brain tissue, damages axons, and tears blood vessels. Edema often ensues, increasing intracranial pressure, which can cause further damage to the brain by preventing blood flow to the tissue. Therefore, after a closed head injury, damage can occur in specific brain areas (localized injury) or throughout the brain (diffuse axonal injury). Instrumental investigations assessing damage severity include neurophysiological recordings [electroencephalogram (EEG); somatosensory evoked potentials (SSEPs)], neuroimaging with diffusion tensor imaging (DTI) and diffusion weighted imaging (DWI), and measurements of increased intracranial pressure.

The goal of the acute treatment is to prevent any further, or secondary, injury to the brain. Decreasing and controlling intracranial pressure is a major target of medical treatment in the early phase after trauma. According to the severity of TBI and the residual damage, the issues posed to the rehabilitation physician vary. More mild cases can present with little or no motor impairment, but present a variety of cognitive impairments, for which cognitive and vocational, if the person is still in working age, rehabilitation are advised. More severe cases usually present with motor and sensory deficits and spasticity, the degree of which is often important and requires drastic medical therapies, and cognitive disturbances that can include persistent alterations of consciousness. A comprehensive approach to patient and family is required in these cases, offering an adequate psychological support to family members.

32.3.1.3 Multiple Sclerosis

Multiple sclerosis (MS) is an inflammatory disease of the central nervous system. Typically, MS is diagnosed between age 20 and 50. Its course varies widely, with a relatively benign relapsing–remitting form with a restitution *ad integrum* in between attacks, to aggressive primary progressive forms which cause severe disability early on in the course of the disease. Life expectancy is only slightly reduced due to MS (6–7 years reduction in a large French cohort) [29]. Older people with MS will undergo normal age-related changes in function as well as those associated with MS progression. Involvement of any site in CNS is possible; this implies a variety of sign and symptom, which range to motor and sensory impairments, cerebellar dysfunctions, sphynteric problems, dysphagia. Cognitive deficits develop later in the course of the disease. Functional impairments thus vary according to the neurological signs and the severity of disease progression. There is a disability progression with disease duration, with the percentage of subjects in need of walking aids increasing from 15% to 76% after an average 45 years of disease, and a 63% of subjects independent in activities of daily living at disease onset compared with a mere 8% in older age [30]. Progression rates have been substantially lowered after the advent of disease-modifying therapies [31].

32.3.2 Rehabilitative Approaches to Impairments Due to Lesions of Central Nervous System

Neurological rehabilitation foundation rests on the concepts of restoration and compensation.

In the very early phases after an acute event, restoration is more likely to happen [32]. Restoration is based on the potential of brain tissue adjacent and/or distant from a lesion to undergo plastic changes that include axonal sprouting, rewiring of previously unconnected brain areas, and modulation of cerebral excitation/inhibition to promote behavior. These changes can be facilitated, in motor deficits, by repetitive task-specific training, with high numbers of repetitions providing the strongest stimulus for neuronal rearrangement. Excessive or non-correctly directed training can indeed have detrimental effects on plasticity, possibly facilitating the so-called maladaptive plasticity—i.e., changes in brain function that foster dysfunctional interactions of cortical areas that translate in defective behavior.

Conversely, compensation is based on the incorporation of residual competencies into functional motor schemes, in order to provide the subject with the means of performing a task in alternative ways—may it be using a different motor strategy or a device.

32.3.2.1 Stroke

After discharge from the acute stroke unit, standardized pathways guide the rehabilitation process, stressing the need for multidisciplinary care, optimizing length of stay in intensive neurorehabilitation units, and providing a framework for early supported discharge. Early supported discharge is an approach that promotes discharge from hospital to community-based rehabilitation as soon as possible once appropriate support is in place for both patient and carer.

Evidence is building up that it is quantity of rehabilitation to impact on outcome [33, 34], with task oriented training particularly effective [35]. One study was able to provide up to 300 h of therapy over 5 weeks [33] compared to the standard-of-care 75 h over the same period: the authors reported an increase of the Fugl-Meyer score between 8 and 11 points.

Short and frequent early rehabilitation sessions have been demonstrated to improve the odds of favorable motor outcome after 3 months from the event [36, 37]. Involvement of family members in an early stage can partially replace resources and help for rehabilitation needs.

Interventions seek to restore motor control in gait and transfer, to improve upper limb activities, to assist in coping with activities of daily living (ADL), and to enhance participation. Advice and instructions are provided to the subject, family, and other members of the interdisciplinary stroke team regarding treatment and prevention of complications such as shoulder pain, venous thrombosis, and falls.

The optimal time window for physical activity after stroke, the intensity, type of activity, and duration for best brain repair processes are not yet fully elucidated; indeed, we know that a neuro-restorative window closes after 3 months from the event [32] and that excessive physical strain in the very early phases of recovery can be counterproductive [38]. However, moderate forced exercise seems to reduce lesion volume and protect perilesional tissue against further oxidative damage and inflammation at least for the short term (4 weeks) in post-stroke patients [39].

Different treatment approaches have been tested to improve function.

A recent Cochrane review [40] reported moderate-quality evidence of a beneficial effect for upper limb functional recovery of constraint-induced movement therapy (CIMT), mental practice, mirror therapy, interventions for sensory impairments, virtual reality, and a relatively high dose of repetitive task practice, suggesting that these may be effective interventions. Moderate-quality evidence also suggested that unilateral arm training may be more effective than bilateral arm training. The same authors provide additional guidance on fields still to explore, such as non-invasive brain stimulations, hands-on therapy, music therapy, pharmacological interventions; they also provide updated reviews on the efficacy of biofeedback, Bobath therapy, electrical stimulation, reach-to-grasp exercise, repetitive task training, strength training, and stretching and positioning.

For upper limb rehabilitation, constraint-induced movement therapy (CIMT), possibly associated with robotics and mental practice with motor imagery, was shown to be beneficial in improving arm function. CIMT consists in the forced non-use of the healthy arm, on which a mitten is worn, in order to force the use of the affected side. Subjects who benefit more from CIMT are those with active wrist and finger extension on the affected side. However, open questions remain on the applicability of CIMT, ranging from the number of hours needed per day, that in the majority of studies is very high, to its long-term effects, to the detrimental psychological consequences in severely impaired subjects that end up frustrated by the little functional use of the affected hand whilst having the healthy one blocked.

Mirror therapy builds on the concept of mirror neurons, i.e., neuronal ensembles that fire when a person observes an individual of a similar species performing a motor task [41]. In clinical practice this has been translated in exercises performed with the healthy limb using a box with inbuilt mirrors in which the affected arm is positioned: the final effect is that the subject observes his/her healthy limb moving in the mirror, as if observing the affected arm instead, thus promoting the functioning of mirror neurons and the rearrangement of sensory motor areas (SM). Motor imagery rests on the same neurophysiological principle: Rearrangement of SM by motor imagery is supported by neurophysiology and neuroimaging, which provides evidence of an overlapping activation of sensorimotor cortices with active, passive, or imagined movements [42–44]. Mentally rehearsing a movement thus promotes the same mechanism as active movement, and is indeed a technique used also by professional musicians and sport players.

Interventions for sensory impairment vary widely—e.g., stimulation with different surfaces, modulation of limb positioning in space, etc.,—and are all based on the recovery of the proprioceptive incoming information on which movement is tuned or the recovery of afferent inputs to central sensory areas.

Robotic devices are getting momentum in rehabilitation, given the chance to provide high-intensity, repetitive, task-specific, interactive treatment of the impaired limb (passive and/or active-assisted exercises). In addition, they allow monitoring subjects' motor recovery, measuring changes in forces and movement kinematics. These robotic devices demonstrate improvement of motor function and, in few studies, also of strength of the upper limb, but generally not of performances in ADLs, raising the question of the generalizability of this training. For the moment being, no guidelines on UL robotic training exist; a recent revision [45] shows that robotic treatment cannot be considered a stand-alone approach, but needs to be integrated with conventional therapy. In addition, often elederly subjcets are less familiar with such devices and thus less likely to benefit of this training.

Simultaneous bilateral training may be no more effective than other upper limb interventions to improve performance in activities of daily living (ADL) or motor functional outcome of the upper limb, but the methodological quality of studies focusing on this topic may be questioned. Other authors reported better functional outcome after bilateral training based on the differential functional lateralization of upper limb [46].

Physiotherapy is effective in the recovery of lower-limb motor function, postural control, and walking ability especially in the early phase after stroke. The association of electromechanical assisted training for walking has been shown to improve the odds of independent over-ground walking, although only people in the acute stage who are not ambulant seem to show improvement [47].

Interventions to facilitate sitting and standing balance include repetitive task-specific training and biofeedback with a moving platform. Task-specific training might improve sit-to-stand function and standing balance, while biofeedback with a force plate or a moving platform showed improvement in stand symmetry alone. Unequivocal indication on the best approach to facilitate the recovery of balance following stroke is still missing.

Cardiorespiratory physical fitness training is the only interventions with a robust evidence for a benefit on walking ability measured in terms of gait speed [48]; improvements have been obtained also with high-intensity physiotherapy, repetitive task training, and electromechanical gait training with exoskeleton robots or robotic end-effectors. Treadmill walking with body weight support also seems to achieve a better and earlier walking independence after stroke.

The use of virtual reality, a relatively recent approach that simulates the practice of functional tasks, is not yet commonplace in clinical rehabilitation settings, but seems to be effective if coupled with standard therapy [49].

Ankle-foot orthoses might also improve gait performance and reduce energy expenditure of gait in patients who have persistent foot drop.

The aforementioned interventions are generally possible if the subject has a preserved range of motion (ROM), whereas strength is not a prerequisite. The main cause for ROMs reduction is spasticity, a velocity dependent increase of muscle tone that can lead in the long term to rheological modifications and contractures of soft tissues. Pharmacological interventions include oral antispastic agents (baclofen, benzodiazepines, dantrolene, $\alpha 2$ receptor agonists) and injections of botulinum toxin in affected muscles in cases of focal spasticity, or nerve blocks. The use of splinting after treatment is usually recommended.

32.3.2.2 Traumatic Brain Injury

The rehabilitation of subjects with traumatic brain injury is normally distinguished into two phases, the acute and the post-acute phase.

Individuals with TBI are typically admitted to the intensive care unit for close observation and medical interventions.

Some preventive rehabilitation procedures may be initiated in the intensive care unit such as body positioning and early mobilization to prevent secondary damage such as pneumonia, contractures, or pressure decubitus ulcers.

As early as possible, individuals with brain injuries will begin intensive rehabilitation.

The focus is on retraining activities of daily living, pain management, cognitive and behavioral therapies, pharmacological management of medical issues or of spasticity, with the option of administration of intrathecal baclofen via an implantable pump, assistive technology (e.g., prescription of wheelchairs and gait aids), environmental manipulation (e.g., installation of lifts, ramps and rails, and bathroom adaptations), as well as family education and counselling.

Community rehabilitation follows discharge from an inpatient rehabilitation service. Helping a person with TBI return to maximum independence and participation in the community is an extremely difficult task. Family support, education, and counselling are vital and likely to be needed for a prolonged period.

32.3.2.3 Multiple Sclerosis

Although rehabilitation has no direct influence on disease progression, it has been shown to ease the symptoms of MS by enhancing self-performance and independence. Whatever premorbid status, an adapted early mobilization is important to avoid further loss of function. The setup of community services is of uttermost importance in this disease, given the long-term disability it entails.

Physical therapy for MS might includes a physical exercise program, motor and sensory balance training, gait training and training in the use of mobility aids (canes, crutches, wheelchairs), and other assistive devices. Aerobic training can help to enhance aerobic capacity and isometric strength, and possibly ease psychological disturbances (anxiety and depression) and fatigue. Respiratory training can be effective for improving respiratory functions and cough reflex. Physical therapy can also include pelvic floor training which may help address urinary/bladder symptoms (incontinence, urgency, and frequency).

Spasticity can initially be managed with changes in daily activities or physiotherapy. If these approaches are unsuccessful, pharmacological treatments can be beneficial in the management of spasticity. Pharmacological management should always be accompanied by physiotherapy.

Training in swallowing with triggering of reflexes, training of the swallowing process, compensatory measures, and appropriate consistency of food and liquids can help to improve the process of swallowing and reduce the risk of aspiration.

Occupational therapy provides training in energy conservation techniques and the use of adaptive tools and devices to simplify tasks at home and at work. Strategic modifications to the home and workplace are recommended to ensure accessibility.

32.3.3 Clinical Presentation and Functional Impairments in Neuropathies

Neuropathy is a disorder of peripheral nerves, characterized by a damage to the myelin sheet or the axon, which causes altered conduction in sensory or motor nerves. Typical symptoms can be pain, paresthesia, dysesthesia, and/or hypostenia. More severe forms include vegetative symptoms and/or trophic changes. More than 100 forms have been described [50]. Frequent forms in the older are chronic demyleinating neuropathies, often associated with hematological alterations. Motor and sensory symptoms can both be present. Some forms are paraneoplastic (i.e., caused by a likely cross-reaction with tumor antigens) and are expected to progress in parallel with the underlying disease. Small fibers neuropathies are also common in older age and cause burning pain and unpleasant temperature sensation.

Among the most disabling neuropathies are the acute inflammatory forms, which are clinically and pathophysiologically heterogeneous group. Guillain–Barré syndrome (GBS) is an acute polyneuropathy consisting of different subtypes. In as many as two-thirds of GBS patients, the onset of weakness occurs 1–3 weeks following an upper respiratory illness, gastrointestinal infection, or vaccination. Incidence is 1.1 cases per 100,000 people per year in the northern hemisphere [51]. Therapy includes plasma exchange and intravenous immunoglobulin. The typical clinical picture is one of diffuse, progressive weakness, which can in the most severe cases involve also respiratory muscle. Sensory involvement is exceptional.

GBS and other inflammatory polyneuropathies are a group of disorders that is often associated with significant long-term disability. In addition to motor or respiratory deficits, affected people develop psychosocial problems resulting in complex disability, which may require treatment in a specialist rehabilitation service. However, in comparison to other long-term neurological conditions (such as brain injury, stroke, or multiple sclerosis) there are relatively few published studies of rehabilitative treatments and outcome. Further research is needed to define treatments to prevent 20% of subjects from being left with persistent and significant disability. Guillain–Barré syndrome is thought to be amendable to multidisciplinary care, but the evidence base for its effectiveness is unclear [52].

32.3.3.1 Rehabilitative Approach to Hypostenia of Peripheral Origin

The prolonged immobility experienced by many patients with hypostnia puts them at significant risk for position-related nerve compression, skin ulceration, and contractures. Subjects that are intubated/sedated and those with significant sensory loss may not notice the symptoms that typically occur with these injuries. Careful body positioning, appropriate bracing, pressure point padding, and frequent position changes are all warranted. People with incomplete eye closure from facial weakness are also at risk for exposure keratitis. Good corneal hygiene with artificial tears, lubricants, careful lid-taping, or protective eye domes is essential [53].

Physical therapy should be initiated as soon as possible. In severely affected people, passive range-of-motion exercises prevent contractures. As subjects improve, other modalities and functional exercise programs are recommended. Despite scarce evidence-based data, physical therapy for GBS as an inpatient and continuing upon discharge is associated with better outcomes and recommended for all but the mildest cases. Physical therapeutic modalities involve a progressive mobility program, encompassing maintenance of posture, alignment, and joint range of motion, provision of orthotics, endurance exercises, muscle strengthening, and gradual gait training using gait aids. Care should be paid not to overwork muscle groups; exercise programs should initially be non-fatiguing and targeting antigravity muscles; progressively, more aggressive strengthening exercise can be prescribed. Overworking muscles in people with peripheral nerve involvement can lead to paradoxical weakening. Stretching program can prevent the onset of muscle contractures.

Muscle weakness, paralysis, balance impairment, and fatigue may result in need of assistive devices. The option for mobility devices varies from ankle-foot orthoses, canes, crutches, walkers, and wheelchairs. People with prolonged residual weakness of calf, and most commonly anterior compartment musculature, benefit from ankle-foot orthosis and shoes with good stabilization around the ankle joint.

32.3.3.2 Rehabilitative Approach to Hypoesthesia, Pain, and Proprioceptive Deficits of Peripheral Origin

Hypoesthesia rehabilitation after a peripheral nerve lesion is based on plastic reorganization of the somatosensory cortex: training aims at eliciting function of the residual sensory nerve fibers, whichever type they may be, and associate the re-learned sensation. Programs include touch exercise, in which the subject touches different objects/surfaces comparing them with the unaffected limb with a growing level of complexity, transcutaneous vibratory stimulation and global complex activities in which motor and sensory tasks are combined.

Pain is a common but often overlooked feature of neuropathies, occurring in more than half of the patients subjcets. It often precedes the development of weakness due to the higher vulnerability of sensory nerve fibers and persists long after recovery [53]. Transcutaneous electrical nerve stimulation (TENS) may be effective in reducing pain, but there are diversities in published research regarding its effectiveness and results are not conclusive. Pharmacological therapy can be an option.

Chronic demyelinating polyneuropathies have recently [54] shown to be sensitive to proprioceptive perturbation despite sensory impairment, encouraging a rehabilitation aimed at promoting the recovery of proprioceptive information rather than the compensation by visual information.

Altered sensation and proprioception, coupled with muscle weakness, is often cause of distal deformities; prescription of insoles or adapted shoes plus ergonomic adjustments is recommended.

32.3.4 Clinical Presentation and Functional Impairments in Parkinson's Disease

32.3.4.1 Etiopathogenesis

Parkinson's disease is a progressive neurodegenerative disorder caused by loss of neurons in the substantia nigra pars compacta and the locus coeruleus in the midbrain. The cell loss leads to striatal dopamine depletion and to a consequent dysfunction of the basal ganglia-thalamo-cortical pathways. The disease generally affects the elderly.

32.3.4.2 Clinical Picture

The main features of Parkinson's disease are resting tremor, rigidity, bradykinesia, and postural disturbances.

Resting tremor may be an early sign in approximately 70% of subjects and usually starts unilaterally; it has a frequency of 3–7 Hz. Bradykinesia refers to slowness of movement and typically starts distally, presenting as impaired manual dexterity and short-stepped shuffling gait. Gait freezing and festination occur when the disease progresses. Freezing of gait is reported in up to 50% of PD individuals and normally occurs when attempting to initiate gait or turning around, stepping through a doorway or approaching a terminal object; it is associated with higher disease severity and longer disease progression. Rigidity is an increase in resistance to passive movement and develops in 90% of people with Parkinson's disease. Postural instability is a common motor feature in PD and increases the risk of falls [55].

Other motor features of Parkinson's disease include hypomimia, eyelid apraxia, hypophonia, micrographia, dysphagia. Non-motor symptoms include cognitive dysfunction, mood disorders, psychosis, sleep disturbance, olfactory dysfunction, pain, sensory disturbance, and autonomic dysfunction.

32.3.4.3 Management of PD

The treatment of Parkinson's disease can be divided into pharmacological, non-pharmacological, and surgical. Available pharmacological treatments are symptomatic. Levodopa is the most effective drug for the treatment of the akinetic symptoms of Parkinson's disease.

Non-pharmacological therapy includes education, support group services, nutrition and physical, occupational, and speech therapy.

Surgical management such as deep brain stimulation (DBS), thalamotomy, and pallidotomy are reserved for people with advanced Parkinson's disease with motor fluctuations despite of pharmacological therapy.

32.3.4.4 Exercises and Neuroplasticity

It has been shown that exercise is beneficial to physical functioning, health related QoL, strength, balance, and gait speed [56]. Current rehabilitation approaches often use compensatory strategies as the basis of therapeutic management. There is a growing body of evidence on the benefits of exercise in terms of neuroplasticity and ability of the brain to self-repair. It has been demonstrated [57] that exercise protects against the onset of symptoms in PD, stimulates dopamine synthesis in the surviving dopaminergic cells, and reduces symptoms. In particular, goal-based exercises and aerobic exercises increase synaptic strength (increasing neurotransmission, receptor density, and dendritic spine formation) and increase trophic factors, blood flow, immune system, neurogenesis, and metabolism. Therefore, circuitry of basal ganglia, cortex, thalamus, cerebellum, and brainstem strengthen, improving motor and cognitive behavior, mood, and motivation.

It has been suggested [58] that there are five key principles of exercise that enhance neuroplasticity in PD: (1) intensive physical activity maximizes synaptic plasticity; (2) complex activities promote greater structural adaptation; (3) activities that are rewarding increase dopamine levels and therefore promote learning/relearning; (4) dopaminergic neurons are highly responsive to exercise and inactivity; and (5) if exercise is introduced at an early stage of the disease, progression can be slowed. The clinical effect depends not only on a correct goal-based exercise, but also on the motor and cognitive residual capacity of the subject (Fig. 32.2).

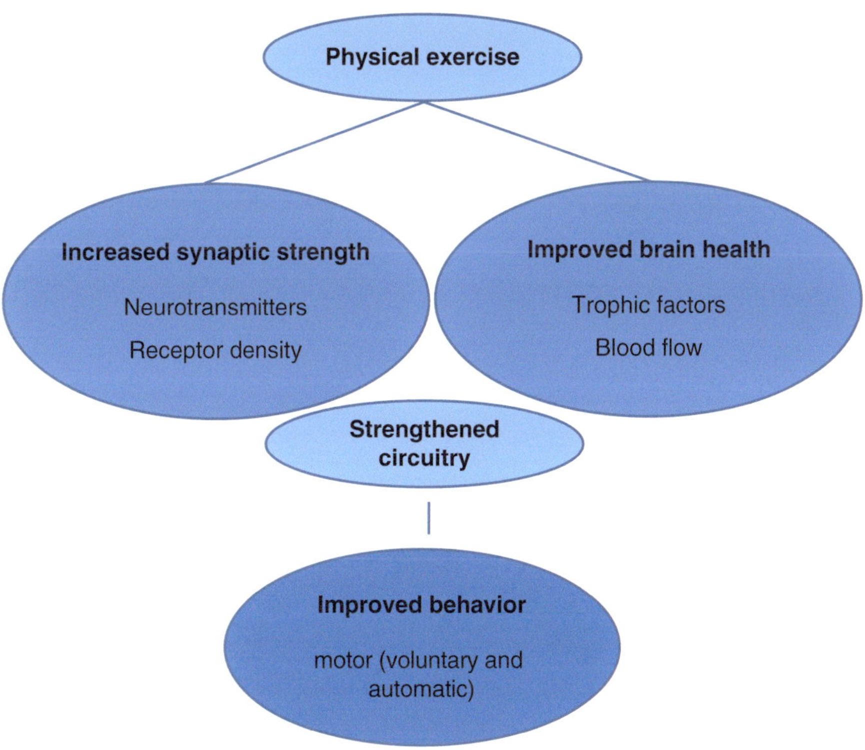

Fig. 32.2 Exercise and neuroplasticity

32.3.4.5 Rehabilitation of Postural, Gait, and Balance Disturbances in Parkinson's Disease

Current PD guidelines recognize the potential role of some rehabilitation interventions as a mean to improve subjects' functionality and help them and their families to cope with disability and functional limitations due to PD [59, 60] (Table 32.3 and Table 32.4).

Table 32.3 Rehabilitative goals and therapeutic interventions in Parkinson's disease

Stages of PD	Goals	Therapeutic interventions
Early stage	• Prevention of inactivity • Promoting physical capacity • Decreasing fear of falling	• Promoting active lifestyle • Education about preventing inactivity and increasing physical capacity • Active exercises (training group) to improve balance, strength, joint mobility, aerobic capacity • Partner/caregiver participation
Intermediate stage	• Prevention of falls • Decrease limitation in transfer, posture, dexterity, balance, gait, dysphagia	• Active exercises (also at home) and functional activity through: – General strategies – Specific strategies: Cognitive movement strategies, external (visual, spatial, step length, auditory, rhythmical, step frequency) and internal cueing (attention) • Multitasking • Botulinum toxin injections (camptocormia, Pisa syndrome)
Advanced stage	• Maintenance of vital functions • Prevention of decubitus lesions • Prevention of contracture and ankylosis	• Postural adaptation for bed or wheelchair • Active-assisted mobilization • Education for prevention of decubitus lesions and contracture/ankylosis

Table 32.4 Motor issues in PD and rehabilitation techniques

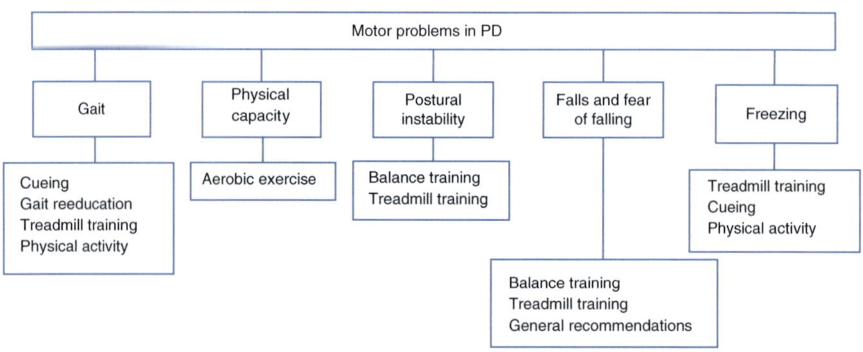

Gait disorders have a negative impact on quality of life (QoL). This related to immobility (causing loss of independence) and increased risk of falling. Most of the rehabilitation studies in Parkinson's disease have focused on treatment of balance and gait disorders. Physiotherapy is the most commonly used procedure as an adjunct to drug therapy to treat PD movement disorders. At the moment, there is no uniformity of approaches for physiotherapy in PD. Rehabilitation for PD covers a number of different treatment techniques, largely centered on active exercises and re-education of mobility [61], aimed at maximizing functional ability and minimizing secondary complications within a context of education and support for the person [56].

Different approaches can be identified: exercises aimed at improving sensorimotor integration; balance training; a combination of strengthening and balance exercises; balance training with stepping; treadmill training; training for reducing falls.

The balance training allows the subject to improve postural control and the ability to plan an appropriate postural strategy. An example of balance exercises is that in which the subject is required to maintain balance while standing on foam support bases of different consistency, on moveable platforms with different degrees of stability, or while the therapist is applying sternal or dorsal pulling. Other exercises emphasize coordination between leg and arm movement during walking as well as locomotor dexterity while stepping over an obstacle. These types of exercises require continuous feedback and feedforward postural adjustment.

Using several sensory cueing strategies may be a valuable approach in order to improve gait performance in people with PD. Visual cues can be helpful in alleviating freezing episodes. For example, carrying an inverted walking stick, so that the handle acts as a horizontal cue at foot level, was able to decrease the number of freezing episodes in participants.

32.4 Non-Invasive Brain Stimulation in Neurorehabilitation

32.4.1 Introduction

The goal of neurorehabilitation is to minimize functional disability and maximize patients' function, ideally by using surviving nervous tissue. Adjunct interventions that can optimize the response of the nervous system to the rehabilitative training might be useful to enhance recovery.

Non-invasive brain stimulation (NIBS), such as transcranial magnetic stimulation (TMS) and transcranial direct current stimulation (tDCS), appears to be a promising therapeutic option as an add-on intervention to conventional rehabilitative strategies. The use of NIBS therapy led to the neologism of "electroceuticals," which stresses the use of currents as a treatment.

They target brain areas to facilitate or inhibit cortical activity to guide neural plasticity during recovery. TMS can also measure neuronal output and interactions between different neuronal assemblies to evaluate progress during rehabilitation.

32.4.2 Types of NIBS

TMS applies a magnetic field to induce an electrical current in the underlying cortical tissue; the magnetic field is generated by a stimulating coil positioned on the scalp that overlies the targeted cortical area.

tDCS is a technique that elicits constant weak electric currents applied directly to the scalp via two surface electrodes (anode and cathode); it does not cause depolarization as TMS does, but modifies electrical properties of the extracellular medium.

Compared to invasive stimulation, NIBS techniques have several advantages that render it attractive for clinical use, such as having relatively scarce adverse effects, being safe, and with relatively few contraindications. Moreover, given that tDCS is easy to use, relatively inexpensive, portable, and suitable for at-home-use, it has the potential to become an adjunct to current neurorehabilitation strategies.

32.4.3 Basic Mechanisms of Action of NIBS

Neuroplastic changes of brain connectivity are the basis of various cognitive, motor, and behavioral processes. During the last years it became increasingly clear that pathological alterations of connections between neurons are involved in many alterations of brain function and after a brain lesion. Therefore, modification of such pathological plasticity or enhancing beneficial plasticity manipulating cortical excitability may be an interesting new therapeutic approach to enhance recovery.

TMS can be applied with different paradigms. To modulate plasticity, repetitive transcranial magnetic stimulation (rTMS) is mainly used, based on its potential to induce long-lasting changes via synaptic associative plasticity. Stimulation frequencies of ≤1 Hz inhibit cortical excitability, while frequencies ≥5 Hz are facilitatory.

tDCS induces plasticity via a sub-threshold polarity-dependent stimulation that modifies neuronal resting membrane potentials and spontaneous discharge rates (without direct neuronal depolarization); this results in enhanced/reduced cortical excitability, with the neuronal firing rates increased by anodal and decreased by cathodal stimulation (Fig. 32.3).

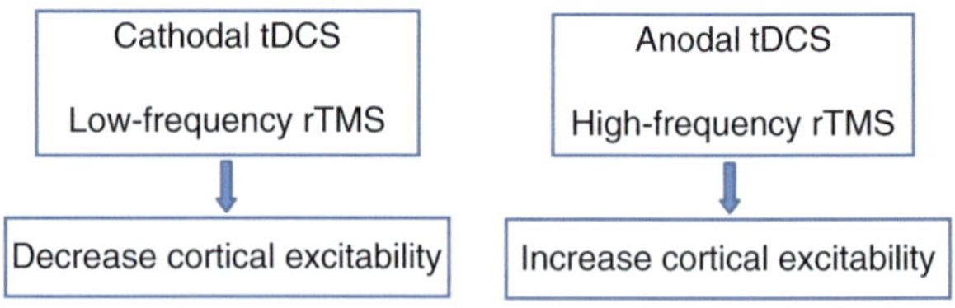

Fig. 32.3 Effects of NIBS on cortical excitability

32.5 Potential Therapeutic Application of NIBS in Neurorehabilitation

A large body of studies has emphasized the potential of non-invasive brain stimulation to complement rehabilitation effects enhancing neuroplasticity in the elderly and in subjects with neurological diseases. First studies looked at post-stroke motor rehabilitation, but were soon followed by studies on people with neurodegenerative disease, movement disorders, epilepsy, post-stroke language, attentional, or executive deficits.

rTMS and tDCS have demonstrated facilitation of cognitive and motor processing. Promising results have been reported in post-stroke motor rehabilitation. On the basis of the inter-hemispheric imbalance hypothesis, NIBS is used to restore equilibrium between two homologous brain areas, modulating excitability of the affected perilesional cortex and the intact contralesional hemisphere [62].

It has been suggested that upregulation of the lesioned hemisphere and/or downregulation of the non-lesioned hemisphere with tDCS enhances the outcomes of rehabilitation in stroke individuals [63]. Repeated sessions and long-term stimulation with tDCS over several days or weeks in conjunction with physical/occupational rehabilitation might have additive and enhanced recovery effects [64]. These effects may last for days or weeks beyond the end of the stimulation period and have been attributed to a persistent modification of post-synaptic connections, similar to long-term potentiation (LTP) and long-term depression (LTD).

High frequency rTMS administered to the affected hemisphere and low-frequency rTMS to suppress the controlesional overactivity were also shown to promote motor recovery in stroke patients [65]. A recent review has found that rTMS could decrease spasticity measured by Modified Ashworth Scale in multiple sclerosis, spinal cord injury, and stroke, while TDCS can modulate spasticity with a variable effect depending on severity and/or undelying neurological disorder [66, 67].

tDCS as adjunct to physical therapy could be an optional approach to enhance the neurophysiological mechanisms that compensate impairments in Parkinson's disease. Recent studies confirmed that tDCS applied to the motor cortex had significant results on motor function in subjects with Parkinson's disease [38]. A possible beneficial effect of tDCS stimulation specific for PD could be the induction of dopamine release in the caudate nucleus via the glutamatergic corticostriatal pathways [68]. TDCS may also have a neuroprotective role in PD by reducing the oxidative damage of dopaminergic neurons [68]. As in motor learning, tDCS appears to influence cognitive networks in PD by altering cortical excitability in key cognitive regions which are implicated in executive function impairment such as the dorsolateral prefrontal cortex [38].

A major drawback of tDCS is the lack of a significant effect once results are pooled together in meta-analysis (for a review see [69] on cognitive outcomes), or the variability in stimulation paradigms which hampers the definition of effective intervention.

These findings suggest nonetheless that transcranial magnetic stimulation and transcranial direct current stimulation could be develop into useful adjuvant strategies in neurorehabilitation. TDCS has a high potential to be routinely administered in parallel to intensive cognitive or motor training in neurological diseases. However, NIBS has to be further assessed in large multicenter randomized-controlled trials to examine not only function, but also activities and participation, and define adequate protocols. Issues related to its application in the elderly, such as best targets and parameters, shall be more throughly studied: they can often differ from those udes in younger populations, and thus impact on outcomes [70]

32.6 Aerobic Exercise and Neuroprotection

32.6.1 Introduction

Acute and chronic neurodegenerative diseases are characterized by progressive loss of structure or dysfunction of neurons. The processes of neurodegeneration have several etiological factors, either genetically determined or externally driven (such as excitotoxicity, ischemia, and oxidative stress).

Neurons are metabolically active cells, which depend on mitochondrial ATP production to satisfy their energetic needs. In contrast with other cell types, neurons are susceptible to impairment of ATP production and consequently at risk for cellular dysfunction when this production is compromised. It becomes clear that mitochondrial failure (with contribution of neurotoxicity) is critical in induction of neuronal death or dysfunction in ischemia/reperfusion injury as well as in chronic forms of neurodegeneration (i.e., Alzheimer's disease, Parkinson's disease, amyotrophic lateral sclerosis).

32.6.2 Mechanisms of Neuronal Injury: Excitotoxicity and Mitochondrial Dysfunction

Neuronal degeneration may be mediated by concomitant causal mechanisms. Excitotoxicity plays an important role and is initiated and mediated by an overload of glutamate, which results in increased intracellular calcium levels and mitochondrial dysfunction. Mitochondria deficits are responsible in turn of a failure in energy supply and production of high concentrations of oxidants, which all contribute to necrosis and apoptosis. A consequence of ATP deficiency is a dysfunction of energy-dependent membrane ion pumps. This allows a massive influx of Ca2+ into the cell, leading to cytotoxic edema. The energy depletion causes a failure of the energy-dependent presynaptic reuptake of glutamate increasing the accumulation of this neurotransmitter in the extracellular space and thereby excitotoxic neuronal damage. Hyperactivation of N-methyl-D-aspartate (NMDA), alpha-amino-3-hydroxy-5-methyl-isoxazole-4-propionic acid (AMPA) and metabotropic glutamate receptors increases further intracellular Ca2+ concentrations which trigger the activation of degradative enzymes (e.g. proteases and phospholipases) that degrade cytoskeletal proteins and extracellular matrix proteins or hydrolyse membrane phospholipid. Excessive glutamate also increases nitric oxide, which forms oxidant compounds responsible for increased mitochondrial membrane permeability and eventually failure. An additional mechanism of neuronal cell death is endoplasmic reticulum failure triggered by oxidative compounds and accumulation of misfolded proteins. Lastly, brain insults activate the release of cellular mediators including pro-inflammatory cytokines (tumor necrosis factor, interleukin-1 and interleukin-6), prostaglandins and complement with induction of chemokines and adhesion molecules and mobilization of immune cells, causing a progression of tissue damage.

32.6.3 Neuroprotection Options in Rehabilitation

Neuroprotection aims at preventing or slowing disease progression by halting or at least slowing loss of neurons. Neuroprotective treatments usually target oxidative stress and excitotoxicity, with the ultimate goal of preserving neuronal membrane function and energy production.

There is emerging evidence suggesting that aerobic exercise is neuroprotective, preventing age-related brain atrophy and enhancing performance in healthy populations [71, 72] and in populations with neurodegenerative diseases [73]. Moderate forced exercise reduces lesion volume and protects perilesional tissue against oxidative damage and inflammation at least for the short term (4 weeks) in post-stroke survivors [39]. Indeed, optimal parameters (day post-stroke, intensity, mode, and duration) to influence brain repair processes are not yet defined.

A growing field in neuroprotection is pharmacological intervention, which aims at modulating excitotoxicity and cortical excitability in the early phases after an acute CNS insult. In stroke, fluoxetine [74] administered early after the event facilitates motor outcome at 3 months. Citicoline, essential for the biosynthesis of membrane phospholipids, has also provided benefits in humans in reduction of stroke consequences, in particular in less severe and older subjects [75]. Other compounds have been trialled with positive results in animal models on the basis of interactions with the neurotoxic mechanism. Taurin is reported to protect against oxidative stress and restore endogenous antioxidant levels by inhibiting calcium influx [76]. N-methyl-D-aspartate receptor (NMDA receptor) partial antagonists appear promising compounds, with S-Methyl-N, N-diethyldithiocarbamate sulfoxide (DETC-MeSO) and memantine effective in reducing stroke consequences in rodent models [77, 78]. Memantine is currently licencesed in USA and Europe for treatment of Alzheimer disease. Neuroprotection is indeed a promising approach and likely to transform apprach in neurorehabilitation in the coming years.

Key Points

- Neurological diseases are a common cause of severe disability in the elderly and are more frequent with increasing age.
- The rehabilitation process consists of four main steps: assessment, goal setting, interventions, and reassessment, and aims to optimize a person's overall function and participation in the society and to reduce the limitations.
- People with neurological diseases, both acute and chronic, require a structured and organized support system. Rehabilitation begins immediately after the hospitalization or diagnosis in order to improve older subject's potential for recovery.
- Promising option for the improvement of neurorehabilitation outcomes are emerging: they include robotic treatment, virtual reality training, noninvasive brain stimulation, and pharmacological neuroprotection. Application of these techniques needs to be tailored to the elderly, with ad hoc protocols and targets.

References

1. Hyder AA, Wunderlich CA, Puvanachandra P, Gururaj G, Kobusingye OC (2007) The impact of traumatic brain injuries: a global perspective. Neuro Rehabilitation 22(5):341–353
2. Peeters W, van den Brande R, Polinder S, Brazinova A, Steyerberg EW, Lingsma HF, Maas AI (2015) Epidemiology of traumatic brain injury in Europe. Acta Neurochir 157(10):1683–1696. doi:10.1007/s00701-015-2512-7. Epub 2015 Aug 14
3. Awad A, Stuve O (2010) Multiple sclerosis in the elderly patient. Drugs Aging 27(4):283–294
4. Medifocus Guidebook on Peripheral Neuropathy (2009) A comprehensive patient guide to symptoms, treatment, research, and support
5. Strait S, Medcalf P (2012) Peripheral neuropathy in older people. GM J
6. Le Forestier N, Bouche P (2006) Peripheral neuropathy in the elderly. [Neuropathies du sujet age: etiologies et conduite pratique]. Psychologie Neuropsychiatrie Du Vieillissement 4(2):109–119
7. Nussbaum RL, Ellis CE (2003) Alzheimer's disease and Parkinson's disease. N Engl J Med 348:1356–1364
8. Fall PA, Axelson O, Fredriksson M et al (1996) Age-standardized incidence and prevalence of Parkinson's disease in a Swedish community. J Clin Epidemiol 49;637–641
9. Mayeux R, Marder K, Cote LJ et al (1995) The frequency of idiopathic Parkinson's disease by age, ethnic group, and sex in northern Manhattan, 1988–1993. Am J Epidemiol 142:820–827
10. de Lau LM, Breteler MM (2006) Epidemiology of Parkinson's disease. Lancet Neurol 5(6):525–535
11. Przedborski S (2017) The two-century journey of Parkinson disease research. Nat Rev Neurosci 18(4):251–259
12. Ott A, Breteler MM, van Harskamp F, Claus JJ, van der Cammen TJ, Grobbee DE et al (1995) Prevalence of Alzheimer's disease and vascular dementia: association with education. The Rotterdam study. BMJ 310(6985):970–973. PubMed PMID: 7728032. Pubmed Central PMCID: PMC2549358
13. Cobb JL, Wolf PA, Au R, White R, D'Agostino RB (1995) The effect of education on the incidence of dementia and Alzheimer's disease in the Framingham study. Neurology 45(9): 1707–1712. PubMed PMID: 7675231

14. Jouvent E, Sun ZY, De Guio F, Duchesnay E, Duering M, Ropele S, Dichgans M, Mangin JF, Chabriat H (2016) Shape of the central sulcus and disability after subcortical stroke: a motor reserve hypothesis. Stroke 47(4):1023–1029. doi:10.1161/STROKEAHA.115.012562
15. Langhorne P, Bernhardt J, Kwakkel G (2011) Stroke rehabilitation. Lancet 377(9778):1693–1702
16. De Silva D. Helping people help themselves. A review of the evidence considering whether it is worthwhile to support self-management. 2011
17. Warner G, Packer T, Villeneuve M, Audulv A, Versnel J (2015) A systematic review of the effectiveness of stroke self-management programs for improving function and participation outcomes: self-management programs for stroke survivors. Disabil Rehabil 37(23):2141–2163
18. Playford ED, Siegert R, Levack W, Freeman J (2009) Areas of consensus and controversy about goal setting in rehabilitation: a conference report. Clin Rehabil 23(4):334–344
19. Stroke Unit Trialists' Collaboration (2007) Organised inpatient (stroke unit) care for stroke. Cochrane Database Syst Rev 4:CD000197. PubMed PMID: 17943737
20. Irish Heart Foundation (2000) Council on Stroke: Towards Excellence in Stroke Care, Dublin
21. Irish Heart Foundation, in association with the Department of Health and Children, National Audit of Stroke Care, Dublin, Ireland, April 2008
22. AHA Impact of Stroke (Stroke statistics), accessed 19 December 2016
23. Manganotti P, Patuzzo S, Cortese F et al (2002) Motor disinhibition in affected and unaffected hemisphere in the early period of recovery after stroke. Clin Neurophysiol 113:936
24. Veerbeek JM, Van Wegen EE, Harmeling-van der Wel BC, Kwakkel G (2011) EPOS investigators. Is accurate prediction of gait in nonambulatory stroke patients possible within 72 hours poststroke? The EPOS study. Neurorehabil Neural Repair 25(3):268–274
25. Jones PS, Pomeroy VM, Wang J, Schlaug G, Tulasi Marrapu S, Geva S, Rowe PJ, Chandler E, Kerr A, Baron JC (2016) SWIFT-cast investigators. Does stroke location predict walk speed response to gait rehabilitation? Hum Brain Mapp 37(2):689–703
26. Ward NS (2015) Does neuroimaging help to deliver better recovery of movement after stroke? Curr Opin Neurol 28:323
27. Ward NS, Brown MM, Thompson AJ et al (2003) Neural correlates of motor recovery after stroke: a longitudinal fMRI study. Brain 126:2476
28. Burke Quinlan E, Dodakian L, See J et al (2015) Neural function, injury, and stroke subtype predict treatment gains after stroke. Ann Neurol 77:132
29. Leray E, Moreau T, Fromont A, Edan G (2016) Epidemiology of multiple sclerosis. Rev Neurol (Paris) 172(1):3–13
30. Kister I, Chamot E, Salter AR, Cutter GR, Bacon TE, Herbert J (2013) Disability in multiple sclerosis: a reference for patients and clinicians. Neurology 80(11):1018–1024
31. University of California, San Francisco MS-EPIC Team, Cree BA, Gourraud PA, Oksenberg JR, Bevan C, Crabtree-Hartman E, Gelfand JM, Goodin DS, Graves J, Green AJ, Mowry E, Okuda DT, Pelletier D, von Büdingen HC, Zamvil SS, Agrawal A, Caillier S, Ciocca C, Gomez R, Kanner R, Lincoln R, Lizee A, Qualley P, Santaniello A, Suleiman L, Bucci M, Panara V, Papinutto N, Stern WA, Zhu AH, Cutter GR, Baranzini S, Henry RG, Hauser SL (2016) Long-term evolution of multiple sclerosis disability in the treatment era. Ann Neurol 80(4):499–510
32. Zeiler SR, Krakauer JW (2013) The interaction between training and plasticity in the post-stroke brain. Curr Opin Neurol 26(6):609–616
33. McCabe J, Monkiewicz M, Holcomb J, Pundik S, Daly JJ (2015) Comparison of robotics functional electrical stimulation, and motor learning methods for treatment of presistent upper extremity dysfunction after stroke: a randomized controlled trial. Arch Phys Med Rehabil 96(6):981–990
34. Kwakkel G, Winters C, van Wegen EE, Nijland RH, van Kuijk AA, Visser-Meily A, de Groot J, de Vlugt E, Arendzen JH, Geurts AC, Meskers CG, EXPLICIT-stroke consortium (2016) Effects of unilateral upper limb training in two distinct prognostic groups early after stroke: the EXPLICIT- stroke randomized clinical trial. Neurorehabil Neural Repair 30(9):804–816
35. Veerbeek JM, van Wegen E, van Peppen R, van der Wees PJ, Hendriks E, Rietberg M, Kwakkel G (2014) What is the evidence for physical theraphy poststroke? A systematic review and meta-analysis. PLoS One 9(2):e87987
36. Bernhardt J, Churilov L, Ellery F et al (2016) Prespecified dose-response analysis for a very early rehabilitation trial (AVERT). Neurology 86(23):2138–2145

37. AVERT Trial Collaboration Group, Bernhardt J, Langhorne P et al (2015) Efficacy and safety of very early mobilisation within 24 h of stroke onset (AVERT): a randomised controlled trial. Lancet 386(9988):46–55
38. Broeder S, Nackaerts E, Heremans E, Vervoort G, Meesen R, Verheyden G, Nieuwboer A (2015) Transcranial direct current stimulation in Parkinson's disease: neurophysiological mechanisms and behavioral effects. Neurosci Biobehav Rev 57:105–117
39. Austin MW, Ploughman M, Glynn L, Corbett D (2014) Aerobic exercise effects on neuroprotection and brain repair following stroke: a systematic review and perspective. Neurosci Res 87:8–15
40. Pollock A, Farmer SE, Brady MC, Langhorne P, Mead GE, Mehrholz J, van Wijck F. Interventions for improving upper limb function after stroke. Cochrane Database Syst Rev. 2014:12;(11):CD010820. doi: 10.1002/14651858.CD010820.pub2.
41. Rizzolatti G, Sinigaglia C (2016) The mirror mechanism: a basic principle of brain function. Nat Rev Neurosci 17(12):757–765
42. Pfurtscheller G, Aranibar A (1979) Evaluation of event-related desynchronization (ERD) preceding and following voluntary self-paced movement. Electroencephalogr Clin Neurophysiol 46:138–146
43. Formaggio E, Storti SF, Cerini R, Fiaschi A, Manganotti P (2010 Dec) Brain oscillatory activity during motor imagery in EEG-fMRI coregistration. Magn Reson Imaging 28(10):1403–1412
44. Formaggio E, Masiero S, Bosco A, Izzi F, Piccione F, Del Felice A (2016) Quantitative EEG evaluation during robot-assisted foot movement. IEEE Trans Neural Syst Rehabil Eng
45. Veerbeek JM, Langbroek-Amersfoort AC, van Wegen EE, Meskers CG, Kwakkel G (2017) Effects of robot-assisted therapy for the upper limb after stroke. Neurorehabil Neural Repair 31(2):107–121
46. Mani S, Przybyla A, Good DC, Haaland KY, Sainburg RL (2014) Contralesional Arm Preference Depends on Hemisphere of Damage and Target Location in Unilateral Stroke Patients. Neurorehabil Neural Repair 28(6):584–93. doi: 10.1177/1545968314520720
47. Mehrholz J, Thomas S, Werner C, Kugler J, Pohl M, Elsner B (2017) Electromechanical-assisted training for walking after stroke. Cochrane Database Syst Rev 5:CD006185
48. Saunders DH, Sanderson M, Hayes S, Kilrane M, Greig CA, Brazzelli M, Mead GE (2016) Physical fitness training for stroke patients. Cochrane Database Syst Rev 3:CD003316
49. Laver KE, George S, Thomas S, Deutsch JE, Crotty M (2015) Virtual reality for stroke rehabilitation. Cochrane Database Syst Rev 2:CD008349. doi:10.1002/14651858.CD008349.pub3
50. National Institute of Neurological Disorders and Stroke Peripheral neuropathy fact sheet. (2012). Available from: http://www.ninds.nih.gov/disorders/peripheralneuropathy
51. Sejvar JJ, Baughman AL, Wise M, Morgan OW (2011) Population incidence of Guillain-Barré syndrome: a systematic review and meta-analysis. Neuroepidemiology 36:123–133
52. Khan F, Ng L, Amatya B, Brand C, Turner-Stokes L (2010) Multidisciplinary care for Guillain-Barre syndrome. Cochrane Database Syst Rev 06(10):CD008505. PubMed PMID: 20927774
53. Harms M (2011) Inpatient management of guillain-barré syndrome. Neurohospitalist 1(2):78–84
54. Provost C, Piccinini G, Tasseel-Ponche S, Lozeron P, Arnulf B, Yelnik A (2016) Sensory information treatment during disturbed standing posture in chronic acquired demyelinating polyneuropathies (CADP). Ann Phys Rehabil Med 59S:e123. PubMed PMID: 27676757
55. Postuma RB, Berg D, Stern M, Poewe W, Olanow CW, Oertel W, Obeso J, Marek K, Litvan I, Lang AE, Halliday G, Goetz CG, Gasser T, Dubois B, Chan P, Bloem BR, Adler CH, Deuschl G (2015) MDS clinical diagnostic criteria for Parkinson's disease. Mov Disord 30(12):1591–1601
56. Smania N, Picelli A, Geroin C, Ianes P, La Marchina E, Zenorini A, Gandolfi M (2011) Balance and gait rehabilitation in patients with Parkinson's disease. In: Rana AQ (ed) Diagnosis and treatment of Parkinson's disease. ISBN 978-953-307-465-8
57. Sutoo D, Akiyama K (2003) Regulation of brain function by exercise. Neurobiol Dis 13:1–14
58. Fox CM, Ramig LO, Ciucci MR, Sapir S, McFarland DH, Farley BG (2006) The science and practice of LSVT/LOUD: neural plasticity-principled approach to treating individuals with Parkinson's disease and other neurological disorders. Semin Speech Lang 27:283–299
59. Keus SJH, Munneke M, Graziano M et al (2014) European Physiotherapy Guidelines for Parkinsons Disease. KNGF/ ParkinsonNet, The Netherlands.

60. Oertel WH, Berardelli A, Bloem BR et al (2011) Late (complicated) Parkinson's disease. In: BaB G (ed) European handbook of neurological management, 2nd edn. Blackwell Publishing, Hoboken, NJ, pp 237–255
61. Morris ME (2000) Movement disorders in people with Parkinson disease: a model for physical therapy. Phys Ther 80(6):578–597
62. Hummel FC, Cohen LG (2006) Non-invasive brain stimulation: a new strategy to improve neurorehabilitation after stroke? Lancet Neurol 5(8):708–712
63. Madhavan S, Shah B (2012) Enhancing motor skill learning with transcranial direct current stimulation - a concise review with applications to stroke. Front Psych 3:66
64. Schlaug G, Renga V, Nair D (2008) Transcranial direct current stimulation in stroke recovery. Arch Neurol 65(12):1571–1576
65. Schulz R, Gerloff C, Hummel FC (2013) Non-invasive brain stimulation in neurological diseases. Neuropharmacology 64:579–587
66. Gunduz A, Kumru H, Pascual-Leone A. Outcomes in spasticity after repetitive transcranial magnetic and transcranial direct current stimulations. Neural Regen Res. 2014;9(7):712–8. doi: 10.4103/1673-5374.131574.
67. Del Felice A, Daloli V, Masiero S, Manganotti P. Contralesional Cathodal versus Dual Transcranial Direct Current Stimulation for Decreasing Upper Limb Spasticity in Chronic Stroke Individuals: A Clinical and Neurophysiological Study. J Stroke Cerebrovasc Dis. 2016;25(12):2932–2941. doi: 10.1016/j.jstrokecerebrovasdis.2016.08.008.
68. Lu C, Wei Y, Hu R, Wang Y, Li K, Li X (2015) Transcranial direct current stimulation ameliorates behavioral deficits and reduces oxidative stress in 1-methyl-4-phenyl-1,2,3,6-Tetrahydropyridine-induced mouse model of Parkinson's disease. Neuromodulation 18(6):442–446. discussion 447
69. Horvath JC, Forte JD, Carter O (2015) Quantitative review finds no evidence of cognitive effects in healthy populations from single-session transcranial direct current stimulation (tDCS). Brain Stimul 8(3):535–550
70. Tatti E, Rossi S, Innocenti I, Rossi A, Santarnecchi E (2016) Non-invasive brain stimulation of the aging brain: State of the art and future perspectives. Ageing Res Rev 29:66–89. doi:10.1016/j.arr.2016.05.006
71. Cotman CW, Berchtold NC (2002) Exercise: a behavioral intervention to enhance brain health and plasticity. Trends Neurosci 25(6):295–301
72. Kramer AF, Erickson KI, Colcombe SJ (2006) Exercise, cognition, and the aging brain. J Appl Physiol (1985) 101(4):1237–1242
73. Ahlskog JE, Geda YE, Graff-Radford NR, Petersen RC (2011) Physical exercise as a preventive or disease-modifying treatment of dementia and brain aging. Mayo Clin Proc 86(9):876–884
74. Chollet F, Tardy J, Albucher JF, Thalamas C, Berard E, Lamy C, Bejot Y, Deltour S, Jaillard A, Niclot P, Guillon B, Moulin T, Marque P, Pariente J, Arnaud C, Loubinoux I (2011) Fluoxetine for motor recovery after acute ischaemic stroke (FLAME): a randomised placebo-controlled trial. Lancet Neurol 10(2):123–130
75. Secades JJ, Alvarez-Sabín J, Castillo J, Díez-Tejedor E, Martínez-Vila E, Ríos J, Oudovenko N (2016) Citicoline for acute ischemic stroke: a systematic review and formal meta-analysis of randomized, double-blind, and placebo-controlled trials. J Stroke Cerebrovasc Dis 25(8):1984–1996
76. Menzie J, Pan C, Prentice H, Wu J.-Y. (2014) Taurine and central nervous system disorders. Amino Acids 46(1):31–46. doi:10.1007/s00726-012-1382-z
77. Mohammad-Gharibani P, Modi J, Menzie J et al (2014) Mode of action of S-methyl-N, N-diethylthiocarbamate sulfoxide (DETC-MeSO) as a novel therapy for stroke in a rat model. Molecular Neurobiology 50(2):655–672. doi: 10.1007/s12035-014-8658-0
78. Chen HSV, Wang YF, Rayudu PV et al (1998) Neuroprotective concentrations of the N-methyl-D-aspartate open-channel blocker memantine are effective without cytoplasmic vacuolation following post-ischemic administration and do not block maze learning or long-term potentiation. Neuroscience 86(4):1121–1132. doi: 10.1016/S0306-4522(98)00163-8

Cognitive Rehabilitation in Healthy Aging

33

Clara Casco

33.1 Introduction

Neurocognitive frailty is currently considered as the biggest risk to successful aging. Cross-sectional aging data show an age-related decline in almost all cognitive functions—speed of processing, inhibitory functions, working memory, and long-term memory—except world knowledge, which may even show some improvement [1–3]. One influential view is that age-related cognitive decline is a problem of brain plasticity which manifests itself in a change in neural communication. Cognitive decline in aging is associated with a reduced coordination between brain regions mediating high-level cognitive functions and by an increase in functional brain activity, particularly in the frontal cortex [3, 4]. These functional imaging studies reveal a more widespread activation pattern in older adults [5, 6] and an increase in frontal bilaterality [4], reflecting increased difficulty in recruiting specialized neural mechanisms. Based on this evidence, a scaffolding theory of aging has been proposed, according to which compensations due to neuroplasticity (scaffolding) are critical factors in understanding the aging mind [3]. The need for these compensatory mechanisms may be reduced when the task involves repetition of stimulus processing. For example, a task involving semantic judgment is associated with left hemisphere prefrontal cortex activation in younger and bilateral activation in older adults. Repeated semantic associations lead to similar response time benefit (repetition priming) in younger and older adults. However, whereas repetition priming leads to reduction of left lateralized activation in both younger and older adults, older adults also show reduction of right prefrontal activation [7]. The evidence of reduced asymmetry of prefrontal

C. Casco
Department of General Psychology, University of Padua, Padua, Italy
e-mail: clara.casco@unipd.it

© Springer International Publishing AG 2018

S. Masiero, U. Carraro (eds.), *Rehabilitation Medicine for Elderly Patients*,
Practical Issues in Geriatrics, DOI 10.1007/978-3-319-57406-6_33

activation in the elderly suggest reduced compensatory recruitment of right prefrontal regions. These results are relevant for showing that it is possible to induce restorative plasticity in the older brain. Indeed, the ability to change synaptic weights by long-term potentiation (LTP) or long-term depression (LTD) persists throughout adult life into senescence, and so rewiring may also take place in the mature brain [8].

This suggests that the role of neuroplasticity may be bidirectional: if it contributes to age-related cognitive decline, it could also potentially result in the restoration of sensory, cognitive, and motor systems in the aging brain.

Plasticity-based restoration requires cognitive rehabilitation imparted with neurobehavioral training methods. Mental training may have the potential of either *differentiating preservation* (Fig. 33.1, left), by which high levels of mental stimulation lead to less negative (or more positive) relations between age and level of cognitive performance, or *preserving differentiation* (Fig. 33.1, right) by which differences in performances are preserved during adulthood [9]. However, mental training by itself is not enough to produce restorative plasticity. To do so, the training task has to be devoted to improve performance of the specific low-level neural mechanisms that needs to be restored. For example, training a low-level mechanism involved in memory should produce significant effects on memory performance, while other cognitive outcome measures should show no effect. Furthermore, the training effect should transfer to untrained memory tasks relying on the low-level trained memory mechanism. Moreover, the effect of training should endure at follow-up and possibly increase.

Based on these premises, in the next section, we will briefly review three neurobehavioral approaches typically used to improve cognitive functioning in normal aging, namely, strategy training, processing training, and multitasking training, focusing on what extent they are appropriate to induce neuroplasticity with positive consequences in the aged brain.

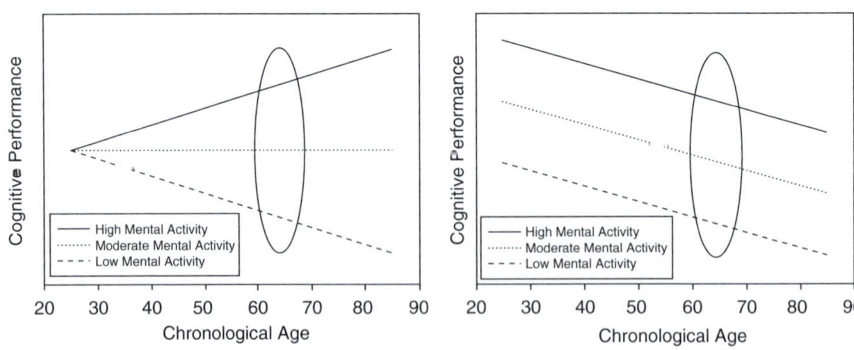

Fig. 33.1 The differential preservation hypothesis of cognitive performance across ages (*left*)—by which the level of cognitive performance late in life depends on the level of cognitive performance during adulthood—and preserved differentiation hypothesis (*right*), by which difference in performance during adulthood is preserved (From Salthouse [9])

33.2 Neurobehavioral Training Methods

33.2.1 Strategy Training

To increase performance in tasks that older adults perform inefficiently, strategy training methods are typically used. Strategy methods have been used to improve memory, reasoning, and executive functions, a set of cognitive processes that are necessary for the cognitive control of behavior (for a review [10]).

Strategy training is typically used to improve memory functions. The protocol involves instructions relative to one or more internal mnemonic strategies to be employed in the recall task. These involve mentally visualizing landmarks along a well-known route (method of loci), organizing information into meaningful categories, forming visual images and mental associations between the item to remember and faces, numbers, or objects (pegword). A seminal meta-analysis [11] revealed a positive effect of mnemonic strategies that ranged between small Cohen's *d* effect sizes (mean difference between the training and control group divided by the pooled standard deviation) for imagery ($d = 0.14$), moderate for pegword ($d = 0.5$), and larger ($d \geq 0.8$) for the method of loci, the name-face, and the organization strategies. A following large-scale study involving 2832 participants aged 65–94 years [12] confirmed that strategy-based and speed of processing training resulted in reliable cognitive improvement; in addition, the effects of cognitive training were maintained after 2 years and transferred to cognitive demanding everyday functioning. The general outcome from these studies [13, 14] is that the benefit of training with laboratory-based memory tasks is significant, although task specific.

Strategy training methods have also been used for improving reasoning or executive functions in elderly. Boron et al. [15] used inductive reasoning training tasks in which participants were required to recognize novel pattern rules and to use them to solve similar problems. A control group was trained with a spatial orientation task, regarding the ability to mentally rotate figures. The reasoning training group showed significantly greater gain in accuracy with respect to the spatial orientation group, independently of the speed of responding. Furthermore, Levine et al. [16] trained goal management strategies involving the identification of high-risk situations, stopping "automatic pilot" behavior, and breaking down goals into sub-goals and found an improvement mainly regarding subjective reports.

Overall, these "strategy training" protocols are instrumental for the improvement in specific and laboratory-based tasks, but they do not appear successful in generally improving memory, reasoning, and executive functions. Furthermore, the requirements of specificity and endurance to infer neuroplasticity are met, but that of transfer to untrained cognitive domains is not.

33.2.2 Processing Training

These protocols involve training on tasks mediated by a particular process and assessment of post-training improved efficiency on untrained stimuli and tasks engaging the same process. The goal of processing training is to obtain transfer of training to different tasks that individuals perform outside the laboratory setting. Indeed, while task-specific improvement in laboratory tasks has been well documented, the clinically relevant question of whether laboratory training improvement can transfer to tasks that older adults perform outside the laboratory has been less researched.

One goal of processing training is to reduce the age-dependent deficit in intracortical inhibition, possibly associated to alterations in GABA-mediated inhibition [17]. Wilkinson and Yang [18] addressed the issue of whether "inhibition training" had positive consequences on inhibitory behavior. They examined the inhibition retest learning in older adults using a color-word Stroop retest training paradigm and showed that training reduced the interference effects. Most importantly, the improvement was not item specific although it did not transfer to other tasks. These results suggest that the well-reported age-dependent inhibitory deficits are reversible and can be modified in older age.

Another aspect of sensory and cognitive processing that may have a broad effect on cognitive functions is speed of processing. Both human and animal studies reveal that age-dependent reduction in processing speed results from inefficient neuromodulation. In particular the reduction in dopamine receptors has been shown to have a key role in slowing down speed of processing [5]. In humans, aging-related reduction of dopamine receptors D2 [19] has been shown to result in decline of processing speed in word and face recognition. The relationship between speed of processing and cognitive efficiency is well described by Salthouse [20], according to whom the reduction of speed of processing with age may affect the speed with which many cognitive operations can be executed and this cause can be primary with respect to other relevant causes such as working memory [21]. Evidence for transfer effects of training in perceptual speed tasks comes from Salthouse and Tucker-Drob [22], indicating that test-retest effects in perceptual speed remained substantially equivalent between tasks using different items with respect to tasks using similar items. Considering the strong connection between the cognitive processing speed abilities and everyday performance (driving, mobility, gait, functional reach, risk for falling), training speed of processing may have the potential to improve everyday life among older adults.

In addition to inhibitory and speed processing, other basic processes have been trained with positive outcomes on transfer tasks. For example, training-dependent improvement in single and dual tasks of attention, working memory, and manual control, which involve relatively low-level cognitive processes, is predictive of improvement in unrelated tasks, such as driving in older adults [23]. These results are particularly important when considering that the trained tasks, in particular attention and motor ones, are significant factors (together with those involving perceptual, executive functions) in accounting for driving performance [23]. From these results, it can be suggested that transfer of training-dependent improvement from a laboratory setting to real-world task performance relies on the improved capability of distributing attention among concurrently performed skills.

Even the improved capability of shifting processing priorities seems relevant in inducing transfer. For example, effects of transfer in training executive functions, as probed by improvement in the capability of task switching, have been found: practicing in a variety of dual-task switching tasks improved the ability to switch between unpracticed pairs of near tasks in older age [24]. This result is important because daily life, such as reading newspaper or cooking a meal, often demands mental flexibility in shifting between different tasks.

Despite the evidence that processing training has good generalization potential, more often strong specificity has been reported. One potential problem of these training paradigms, which may prevent generalization to tasks normally performed in day-to-day life, is that they focus on single-task training.

33.2.3 Multitasking Training

A promising alternative in the field of training regimes to improve cognitive abilities is provided by multitasking training. Multitasking, which involves cognitive control, i.e., the capability of developing different action control and/or filtering out interference from irrelevant tasks, is reduced by aging. One measure of multitasking ability is to involve participants in performing two tasks in isolation and together [25]. It has been suggested that a less controlled multitasking training protocol, with a custom-designed 3-D video game (NeuroRacer), may lead to reduced multitasking costs in older adults [26]. After training, the older group performance improved to, and beyond, the level of the untrained younger group. The improvement was retained at 6 months follow-up. Most importantly the effect of training transferred to untrained cognitive control abilities (enhanced sustained attention and working memory), suggesting that these training protocols may enhance the ability to learn new tasks. Both the trained and the transfer behavioral effects of training were associated to a modulation of the neural mechanism underlying cognitive control, i.e., increased in midline frontal theta power, as assessed by electrophysiology. These results highlight the vigorous plasticity of the prefrontal cognitive system in the aging brain. However, how exactly neural responses to constituent tasks adapt with training remains to be characterized. One speculative hypothesis is that multitasking learning allows task representations to become more distinct after training.

33.3 New Directions in the Field of Plasticity in Aging

Phenomena of plasticity in the aging brain representing flexible recruitment of brain areas and reflecting structural and functional changes (either substitutive or in response to restorative learning and experience) have been highlighted by functional magnetic resonance imaging (fMRI).

Modulation of neural activity is necessary in order to show a causative relation between neural activation and plasticity. There are two safe and noninvasive methods to manipulate neural activity: repetitive transcranial magnetic stimulation (rTMS) and transcranial direct current stimulation (tDCS). rTMS is obtained by applying brief electrical pulses via a coil to a specific brain region; depending on the pulse arrangement, rTMS activates or inhibits neural activity under the coil and may also enhance or inhibit regions whose activity interferes with task performance. tDCS operates by applying a small amount of current through two electrodes attached to the scalp. TMS and tDCS modulation of specific brain regions may increase speed and accuracy in activities based on attention, perception, and memory [27]. Indeed, one week of object location learning with anodal tDCS applied over the temporoparietal cortex led to a large increased of memory performance compared to the sham control group that learned without anodal tDCS [28]. Moreover, older adults' performance in complex motor skill tasks was enhanced by tDCS applied to the motor cortex [29]. Importantly, anodal tDCS over right but not left dorsolateral prefrontal cortex increased the proportion of performance errors that were consciously detected, indicating that this area is involved in error awareness and that tDCS may restore the weakness that older adults present in this function. Meinzer et al. [30] used fMRI to investigate neurofunctional correlates of a tDCS-induced modulation of performance in a semantic word generation task. tDCS significantly improved performance in older adults up to the level of younger controls and significantly reduced task-related hyperactivity in bilateral prefrontal cortices, the anterior cingulate gyrus, and the precuneus.

Although these results are relevant in pinpointing the tDCS-induced task-related changes in the activity of specific brain regions, the suggestion that neurostimulation may result in a promising cognitive enhancer in aging is still speculative. Data on the time course and duration of the effects are needed in order to propose that neurostimulation methods may have an impact in day-to-day life.

33.4 Open Questions

The studies reviewed above show a considerable progress toward the goal of restoring sensory, cognitive, and motor systems in the aging brain. Box 33.1 summarizes the extent to which the various training protocols meet the essential requirements to produce significant benefits in cognitive rehabilitation. However, beside the efficacy, it should also be considered that training programs involve strong commitment and compliance on part of participants. Moreover, to provide positive outcomes in clinical setting, there are open issues to be addressed. One crucial question regards the degree to which motivation systematically influences cognitive performance in the elderly. Another issue regards the non-satisfactory transfer effects in everyday life activities. However, training-related changes in brain functions and structure are promising indicators of the fact that training may provide substantial changes in the neural mechanisms underlying cognitive performance.

Box 33.1 Each neurobehavioral training method (Strategy, Inhibitory processing, Processing speed, Low-level cognition and Multitasking) whether it fulfills the essential requirements to produce significant benefits in cognitive rehabilitation

General considerations on the training effects	Strategy training	Inhibitory processing training	Processing speed training	Low-level cognition: attention, w. memory	Multitasking training
Do the training effects last?	Yes	Possibly	Possibly	Possibly	Yes
Does the training transfer to untrained items?	Unlikely	Yes	Yes	Yes	Yes
Do the training effects generalize to real-world tasks?	No	Possibly	Possibly	Yes	Yes
Is the training successful without compliance/ motivation?	No	No	No	No	No
Is the training protocol useful for several cognitive functions?	Unlikely	Yes	Yes	Yes	Yes

Key Points

- Neurocognitive frailty is currently considered as the biggest risk to successful aging.
- Cognitive rehabilitation aims at modulating brain activation, consequent reduction of compensatory recruitment, and increase in restoration-based plasticity.
- Strategy training, processing training, and multitasking training methods are used to increase performance in tasks that older adults perform inefficiently.
- New neurostimulation techniques (repetitive transcranial magnetic stimulation (rTMS) and transcranial direct current stimulation (tDCS)) are safe and noninvasive methods used to manipulate neural activity.

References

1. Cansino S, Guzzon D, Martinelli M, Barollo M, Casco C (2011) Effects of aging on interference control in selective attention and working memory. Mem Cognit 39(8):1409–1422
2. Cansino S, Guzzon D, Casco C (2013) Effects of interference control on visuospatial working memory. J Cogn Psychol 25(1):51–63

3. Park DC, Reuter-Lorenz P (2009) The adaptive brain: aging and neurocognitive scaffolding. Annu Rev Psychol 60:173
4. Cabeza R (2002) Hemispheric asymmetry reduction in older adults: the HAROLD model. Psychol Aging 17(1):85
5. Li SC, Lindenberger U, Sikström S (2001) Aging cognition: from neuromodulation to representation. Trends Cogn Sci 5(11):479–486
6. Logan JM, Sanders AL, Snyder AZ, Morris JC, Buckner RL (2002) Under-recruitment and nonselective recruitment: dissociable neural mechanisms associated with aging. Neuron 33(5):827–840
7. Bergerbest D, Gabrieli JD, Whitfield-Gabrieli S, Kim H, Stebbins GT, Bennett DA, Fleischman DA (2009) Age-associated reduction of asymmetry in prefrontal function and preservation of conceptual repetition priming. Neuroimage 45(1):237–246
8. Das A, Huxlin KR (2010) New approaches to visual rehabilitation for cortical blindness: outcomes and putative mechanisms. Neuroscientist 16(4):374–387
9. Salthouse TA (2006) Mental exercise and mental aging evaluating the validity of the "use it or lose it" hypothesis. Perspect Psychol Sci 1(1):68–87
10. Cabeza R, Nyberg L, Park D (2004) Cognitive neuroscience of aging: linking cognitive and cerebral aging. Oxford University Press, Oxford
11. Verhaeghen P, Marcoen A, Goossens L (1992) Improving memory performance in the aged through mnemonic training: a meta-analytic study. Psychol Aging 7(2):242
12. Ball K, Berch DB, Helmers KF, Jobe JB, Leveck MD, Marsiske M, Unverzagt FW (2002) Effects of cognitive training interventions with older adults: a randomized controlled trial. Jama 288(18):2271–2281
13. Rebok GW, Carlson MC, Langbaum JB (2007) Training and maintaining memory abilities in healthy older adults: traditional and novel approaches. J Gerontol B Psychol Sci Soc Sci 62(Special Issue 1):53–61
14. Lustig C, Shah P, Seidler R, Reuter-Lorenz PA (2009) Aging, training, and the brain: a review and future directions. Neuropsychol Rev 19(4):504–522
15. Boron JB, Turiano NA, Willis SL, Schaie KW (2007) Effects of cognitive training on change in accuracy in inductive reasoning ability. J Gerontol B Psychol Sci Soc Sci 62(3):P179–P186
16. Levine B, Stuss DT, Winocur G, Binns MA, Fahy L, Mandic M, Bridges K, Robertson IH (2007) Cognitive rehabilitation in the elderly: effects on strategic behavior in relation to goal management. J Int Neuropsychol Soc 13(01):143–152
17. Heise KF, Zimerman M, Hoppe J, Gerloff C, Wegscheider K, Hummel FC (2013) The aging motor system as a model for plastic changes of GABA-mediated intracortical inhibition and their behavioral relevance. J Neurosci 33(21):9039–9049
18. Wilkinson AJ, Yang L (2012) Plasticity of inhibition in older adults: retest practice and transfer effects. Psychol Aging 27(3):606
19. Bäckman L, Ginovart N, Dixon RA, Wahlin TBR, Wahlin Å, Halldin C, Farde L (2000) Age-related cognitive deficits mediated by changes in the striatal dopamine system. Am J Psychiatry 157(4):635–637
20. Salthouse TA (1996) The processing-speed theory of adult age differences in cognition. Psychol Rev 103(3):403
21. DeLuca J, Chelune GJ, Tulsky DS, Lengenfelder J, Chiaravalloti ND (2004) Is speed of processing or working memory the primary information processing deficit in multiple sclerosis? J Clin Exp Neuropsychol 26(4):550–562
22. Salthouse TA, Tucker-Drob EM (2008) Implications of short-term retest effects for the interpretation of longitudinal change. Neuropsychology 22(6):800
23. Cassavaugh ND, Kramer AF (2009) Transfer of computer-based training to simulated driving in older adults. Appl Ergon 40(5):943–952
24. Karbach J, Kray J (2009) How useful is executive control training? Age differences in near and far transfer of task-switching training. Dev Sci 12(6):978–990

25. Garner KG, Dux PE (2015) Training conquers multitasking costs by dividing task representations in the frontoparietal-subcortical system. Proc Natl Acad Sci 112(46):14372–14377
26. Anguera JA, Boccanfuso J, Rintoul JL, Al-Hashimi O, Faraji F, Janowich J, Kong E, Larraburo Y, Rolle C, Johnston E, Gazzaley A (2013) Video game training enhances cognitive control in older adults. Nature 501(7465):97–101
27. Gutchess A (2014) Plasticity of the aging brain: new directions in cognitive neuroscience. Science 346(6209):579–582
28. Flöel A, Suttorp W, Kohl O, Kürten J, Lohmann H, Breitenstein C, Knecht S (2012) Non-invasive brain stimulation improves object-location learning in the elderly. Neurobiol Aging 33(8):1682–1689
29. Zimerman M, Nitsch M, Giraux P, Gerloff C, Cohen LG, Hummel FC (2013) Neuroenhancement of the aging brain: restoring skill acquisition in old subjects. Ann Neurol 73(1):10–15
30. Meinzer M, Lindenberg R, Antonenko D, Flaisch T, Flöel A (2013) Anodal transcranial direct current stimulation temporarily reverses age-associated cognitive decline and functional brain activity changes. J Neurosci 33(30):12470–12478

Cognitive Rehabilitation Therapy for Neurologic Diseases

34

Patrizio Sale and Giovanni Gentile

Cognitive rehabilitation therapy (CRT) is the multisensory goal-oriented programme of relearning or compensating for cognitive skills and abilities that have been altered or lost after brain damage. In particular, CRT is focused on improving cognitive functions (memory, attention and concentration) and daily living skills (i.e. using the telephone, managing medication and handling money). Cognitive impairments can indeed strongly interfere with safety, productivity, independence and personal relationships and, more generally, with the human global functioning.

Cognitive rehabilitation was born in the twentieth century and developed by physicians, scientists and health professionals to manage the acquired disability of thousands of head-injured veterans coming back from the world wars [1]. In the last decades, the high long-term impact of acquired brain injury (ABI), particularly traumatic brain injury (TBI), has been recognized, and CRT programmes have become more and more accurate.

If at the beginning the CRT seemed to be focused exclusively on training the cognitive skills and processes, nowadays the emphasis shifted on producing and obtaining functional changes.

34.1 Principles of Cognitive Rehabilitation Therapy

The main principle of CRT is *brain plasticity* which refers to a peculiar capacity of the brain of changing its neural network organization and functioning, producing new synapses (sprouting) or removing (pruning) the older ones. Indeed, acting on

P. Sale (✉)
Rehabilitation Unit, Department of Neuroscience, University of Padua, Padua, Italy
e-mail: patrizio.sale@gmail.com

G. Gentile
I.R.C.C.S. San Camillo Hospital, Venice, Italy

© Springer International Publishing AG 2018

S. Masiero, U. Carraro (eds.), *Rehabilitation Medicine for Elderly Patients*, Practical Issues in Geriatrics, DOI 10.1007/978-3-319-57406-6_34

brain plasticity with a structured environmental experience will definitively change the brain functionality and reorganization as well as the subject behaviour [2]. This consideration should be joined to the assumption of *modularity of the cognitive processes*, according to which the brain is organized into subcomponents relatively independent specialized to perform specific functions. If a damaged cognitive module retains part of the neural substrate, then it is possible, through appropriate stimulation, to obtain the reacquisition of the cognitive process. Otherwise, cognitive rehabilitation should help the patient to develop compensatory mechanisms, taking advantage of the brain's ability to perform complex tasks using alternative cognitive processes [3].

Overall, the approach of CRT is focused on reducing disability. It aims to enhance functioning and independence in patients with cognitive deficits due to a neurological condition aiming to lessen impairments, to restore the lost cognitive functions and to reduce the disabling impact of such cognitive deficits [4]. The rehabilitation programme is developed according to each subject's specific need. CRT follows a process of identifying areas of impairment, facilitating compensatory mechanisms to rapidly improve some functions and challenging the brain to restore them.

34.2 Hierarchy of Cognitive Processes

A stimulation of a cognitive function can also lead to a dysfunctional plasticity. Sturm et al. (1997) have shown that subjects receiving a stimulation of basic attentional function compared to those who received higher attentional processes training had a better outcome; moreover the second ones showed a decline of their cognitive skills [5].

Cognitive functions are modular and hierarchically organized, and basic processes serve higher functions allowing the brain to complete complex tasks. Treating each function as independent could cause huge mistakes.

Since the aim of CRT is to reduce the disability derived from cognitive impairments, the rehabilitation programme should be designed to take into account such issues. It is fundamental to provide rehabilitation tasks sticking to a hierarchical framework of cognitive functions, whereby lower-level cognitive skills (e.g. sustained attention) are involved and stabilized before proceeding with treatment of higher level cognitive domains (e.g. executive functions).

34.3 Bottom-Up and Top-Down Processes in CRT

Among the techniques and the approaches of CRT, a distinction has been proposed by Robertson and Murre [6] who describe two ways of how a CRT programme could be designed: the "bottom-up" versus "top-down" approaches.

The bottom-up process can be described as "retraining the brain from the bottom up". This approach is based on providing the injured network with strong external perceptual, motor or sensory stimuli which produce a readaptation of perceptive processes influencing the recovery of the impaired cognitive function.

Examples of this kind of approach can be found in those treatments focused on motor recovery, where the high number of repetitions of specific movements (e.g. fine movements of the fingers) produces a significant improvement of the targeted area motor function. The repetition induces plasticity and adaptation, by means of synaptic growth, of neurons around the damaged area of the brain.

This approach is also commonly adopted for rehabilitation of spatial neglect with prism adaptation stimulation technique. It consists of displacing the visual field of the subject rightward using specific prismatic lenses, and then the subject is asked to perform a repetitive motor task (reaching an object in front of him). In order to compensate this shift, the subject has to perform the movement toward the opposite side (left), resulting in a leftward displacement of sensorimotor coordinates.

On the other hand, top-down processing refers to how our brain use information coming from the environment through one or more sensory systems. This approach is based on the fact that the higher brain regions can regulate and select the sensory information that have to be processed. These regions have been identified in the frontal lobe and the thalamus. Such areas enhance attention, expectancy and motivation resulting in a higher improvement of the performance in a rehabilitation context.

This kind of approach is widely used in CRT and is determined by the direct intervention of the cognitive processes of the subject, allowing a cognitive function improvement or the development of compensatory strategies through metacognitive processes. According to point of view, the recovery appears as strongly related to the cohesion of frontal attentional networks. Having said that, subject awareness and executive function level should be strongly taken into account within the design and development of a CRT programme. It will lead the rehabilitation strategy, giving priority to the recovery of more basic processes.

34.4 The Neuropsychological Assessment

The responsible professional for the comprehensive assessment of the cognitive level is the neuropsychologist who performs a set of tests and investigations in order to develop an accurate picture of the subject's levels of cognitive, emotional and interpersonal functioning, including areas of spared ability or compensatory strength and the subject's ability of carrying out everyday functional activities.

The neuropsychological behavioural assessment investigates cognitive skills as planning, problem-solving, attentional capacity, learning efficiency and memory, emotional regulation and interpersonal effectiveness.

Cognitive domains are usually measured through a psychometric/quantitative approach which uses tests and specifically designed to best assess different cognitive functions and their subcomponents; moreover functionality and mood are assessed as well. An accurate assessment is necessary in order to inform the designing of a CRT: it gives the opportunity to the rehabilitation therapist to get a detailed analysis of strengths and weaknesses of subject's skills and abilities so that it is possible to find the proper route for the recovery of lost functions.

34.5 Outcome and Efficacy

Even if the literature body dealing with CRT has strongly increased in the last decade, methodological problems still affect the measurement of efficacy and the evaluation of CRT outcomes. The main issue is given by the high heterogeneity of subjects, each one necessitating different and specific treatment and settings; moreover often there's a huge gap between the mandates of rehabilitation facilities which are more prone to have a clinical approach instead of a research approach. There is a consensus on the validity of the efficacy of CRT; however most of the results are lacking of strength since the majority of the treatments often relies on single-case or small-group studies which easily result affected by methodological biases and contribute to giving a fuzziness to the whole CRT picture. Controlled studies with large numbers of subjects that either compare different treatments or use a non-treatment control group are still quite limited.

The efficacy of a CRT intervention could be also measured with specific scales such as the Functional Independence Measure (Granger and Hamilton 1987), the Disability Rating Scale for Severe Head Trauma (Rappaport et al. 1982) and the Glasgow Outcome Scale (Jennett and Bond 1975) or other scales that assess the autonomy and the functionality of the subject [7–9].

A final consideration concerns the difference between evaluating the *efficacy* intended as "treatments that are beneficial for patients or clients in well-controlled treatment studies" and *effectiveness* which refers to the ability of treatment in being transferred "from the research clinic to community and private practice settings". For instance, an effective result after an attention-based training is that the subject is able to come back to work.

34.6 Techniques and Areas of Intervention

There are different strategies and techniques that can be used to assist people with cognitive impairments in optimizing management of their daily lives and activities. These strategies have been incorporated into goal-oriented cognitive rehabilitation interventions that aim to (1) draw on retained strengths to support adaptive behaviour and (2) achieve optimum levels of well-being by targeting performance on personally relevant goals.

Several techniques, such as auditory and/or visual attention tasks and memory training, can help the subjects to achieve the goals of the treatment. Due to the individual response to treatment, it is preferable to try different strategies to determine what works best for each individual; two approaches are usually adopted: the restorative (remedial) approach or the compensatory approach. The main fields of treatment in cognitive rehabilitation concerned attention, the visuospatial and/or praxic functions, language and/or communication, memory and executive functions.

34.7 Factors Affecting Cognitive Rehabilitation

Many different factors influence recovery from damage to the brain. Some of these, such as demographic factors, are fixed and not subject to manipulation. We can, however, use information about such factors to make informed predictions about a client's natural course of recovery. Factors related to the injury itself are also not typically under the control of rehabilitation specialists, though medical science is certainly making inroads in decreasing the secondary damage caused by stroke and trauma, primarily through innovative pharmacological interventions.

34.8 CRT in Stroke Population

The terms *stroke* and *cerebrovascular accident* (CVA) are both used to describe brain damage or dysfunction that occurs as a result of some disruption in the vascular supply to or of the brain. Stroke is one of the three major neurological causes of death and disability, together with TBI and dementia. Both cerebral haemorrhage and cerebral infarction (thrombosis, ischaemia) can cause a widespread set of cognitive deficits, and more in general damages are related to the brain area/network by the CVA.

34.8.1 CVA Involving the Middle Cerebral Artery

Common cognitive impairments associated with left middle cerebral artery CVA include aphasia, oral and limb apraxia and verbal learning impairments, whereas the most common deficits following right middle cerebral artery CVA include visuospatial impairments, nonverbal learning impairments, impaired awareness of deficits, impairments in the pragmatic aspects of communication and impaired attention. Aphasic syndromes have been reported following lesions involving many structures, including the internal capsule, the lenticulostriate area, the thalamus and the basal ganglia.

34.8.2 CVA Involving the Anterior Communicating Artery

The anterior communicating artery is a common site for *aneurysms:* bleeds involving aneurysms in this territory commonly result in a syndrome characterized by confabulation, disinhibition, unconcern, severe anterograde and retrograde amnesia, executive function impairments and limited awareness.

Rehabilitation programme for each typology described above is addressed by the cognitive functions damaged by the CVA; moreover it takes into account priorities related to basic cognitive functions/skills that necessitate to be recovered.

34.9 CRT in Patient with Dementia

Nowadays cognitive rehabilitation is strongly indicated for people with an acquired brain injury like stroke or traumatic brain injuries, who often show memory, language and attention deficits. For those cases, many structured programmes have been developed and showed their efficacy and effectiveness in treating such impairments. However little is known about neurodegenerative disease like Alzheimer, Parkinson and other dementias. Recent literature reviews have shown that multimodal approaches of cognitive stimulation combined with physical activity and occupational therapy can produce a significant effect in treating subjects with mild cognitive impairment [10]. Other studies suggest that such interventions could improve symptoms, if the intervention is performed early or in the premorbid stage of disease. Therefore, a comprehensive neuropsychological assessment and monitoring would be crucial to identify in time people at risk of developing cognitive decline in order to provide, where possible, a cognitive stimulation intervention.

Conclusions

Although our understanding of brain plasticity and of the mechanisms underlying it is still quite primitive, what is emerging provides substantial evidence for more plasticity in the adult brain than was previously believed. At the same time, these new discoveries highlight the complexity of the overall challenge of rehabilitation. Implications for best clinical practice are confusing at times, but this reflects where the field is in the process of assimilating and applying new information. Although a greater understanding of the biological underpinnings of recovery is exciting and vital to the field, it is important to keep in mind many of the principles of rehabilitation practice that we know facilitate the recovery process. Consider, for example, the important role that mood and motivation play in rehabilitation and the importance of building a therapeutic relationship that will maximize a patient's engagement in the rehabilitative process.

Key Points

- Cognitive rehabilitation is a goal-oriented programme that aims to improve cognitive functions (memory, attention and concentration) and daily living skills (i.e. using the telephone, managing medication and handling money).
- The rehabilitation programme is developed according to each subject's specific needs.
- The goal is to improve performance in tasks that are important to the subjects.
- Two approaches are usually adopted: the restorative (or remedial) approach or the compensatory approach.

References

1. Wilson BA (2002) Cognitive rehabilitation in the 21st century. Neurorehabil Neural Repair 16(2):207–210
2. Kolb B, Gibb R (2014) Special section: review. Searching for the principles of brain plasticity and behavior. Cortex 58:251–260
3. Fodor J (1985) Precis of the modularity of mind. Behav Brain Sci 8(1):1–42
4. Sohlberg MM, Mateer C (1989) Introduction to cognitive rehabilitation: theory and practice. Guilford Press, New York
5. Sturm W, Willmes K, Orgass B, Hartje W (1997) Do specific attention deficits need specific training?. Neuropsychological Rehabilitation 7(2):81–103.
6. Robertson IH, Murre JM (1999) Rehabilitation of brain damage: brain plasticity and principles of guided recovery. Psychol Bull 125(5):544
7. Keith RA, Granger CV, Hamilton BB, Sherwin FS (1987) The functional independence measure: a new tool for rehabilitation. Adv Clin Rehabil 1:6–18. PubMed PMID: 3503663.
8. Rappaport M, Hall KM, Hopkins K, Belleza T, Cope DN (1982) Disability rating scale for severe head trauma: coma to community. Arch Phys Med Rehabil 63(3):118–23. PubMed PMID: 7073452
9. Jennett B, Bond M (1975) Assessment of outcome after severe brain damage. Lancet 1(7905):480–4. PubMed PMID: 46957
10. Bredesen DE et al (2016) Reversal of cognitive decline in Alzheimer's disease. Aging 8(6):1250–1258. Available at: http://www.ncbi.nlm.nih.gov/pubmed/27294343. Accessed 4 Jan 2017

Neurobehavioral Rehabilitation of Visual Deficits in Older Patients

35

Clara Casco

35.1 Neuroplasticity in Aging

Aging is associated with a progressive slowing down of information processing and with a diminished capacity in encoding, representing, and maintaining information, as well as in selecting relevant information and discarding irrelevant one. These changes are associated, at neurobiological level, with a neuromodulatory decline. A correlation has been suggested between cognitive decline and the decrease in cholinergic markers, although the role of Ach in modulating learning and memory may not be specific [1]. The level of acetylcholine (Ach) affects neural spatial integration and may be related to the states of arousal and attention [2]. In the aged human cortex, genes involved in GABA-mediated inhibitory neurotransmission are downregulated [3], thus affecting low-level cortical balance between excitation and inhibition in sensory tasks [4–8]. Specifically, reduced strength of surround suppression in the central visual system, a visual function essential for isolating object contours and region boundaries in crowded natural scenes, may result from age-related reduced efficiency of GABAergic inhibitory mechanisms in the visual cortex [9]. Moreover, age-dependent reduction in the ability to signal visual sensory stimuli above background activity (signal-to-noise ratio) is likely to have deficient dopaminergic modulation as a neurochemical correlate [10].

Cerebral metabolic decline is associated with inefficient interneuronal communication with consequent reduced efficacy of interconnections among neurons in brain areas involved not only in cognitive but also in sensory processing. Indeed, MRI (Magnetic Resonance Imaging) data reveal a significant age-associated reduction of the size of visual cortical areas V1, V2, and to lesser extent V3, possibly associated with a decreased number of cortical connections [11].

C. Casco
Department of General Psychology, University of Padua, Padua, Italy
e-mail: clara.casco@unipd.it

© Springer International Publishing AG 2018

S. Masiero, U. Carraro (eds.), *Rehabilitation Medicine for Elderly Patients*, Practical Issues in Geriatrics, DOI 10.1007/978-3-319-57406-6_35

Changes in synaptic connections affect cortical plasticity in the aged brain as assessed by the measurement of age-dependent threshold variation for long-lasting modulation in synaptic signal transmission (long-term potentiation and depression, LTP and LTD) [12].

In addition to changes in brain activation, neuromodulatory-dependent impairment of cortical and subcortical representations of sensory inputs determines a self-reinforcing downward spiral of reduced interaction with challenging environments, which significantly contributes to cognitive decline. Not only does alteration of neural information processing lead to less distinct neural representations and memory traces, but it also results in a more simplified behavior. In adapting to this reduced complexity, the brain simplifies even more the representations supporting perception and action. Age-related cognitive decline is therefore a problem of brain plasticity with negative consequences.

A large and growing body of human studies have documented that plasticity with negative consequences in the older brain can be reversed. The therapeutic target is to induce plasticity with positive consequences in the older brain by modulating the balance between excitatory and inhibitory networks. Extensive basic research focused on the role of endogenous neuromodulator release such as norepinephrine, acetylcholine, serotonin, or dopamine in regulating positively excitation-inhibition balance [13]. A different approach, either independent or combined with regulation of endogenous neuromodulation, is to induce neuroplasticity neurobehaviorally. This is achieved through perceptual learning (PL), a long-term sensitivity improvement with some basic sensory tasks as a result of active training on that task. Through PL, physical and functional decline can be slowed down, arrested, and inverted [14]. Neurobehavioral training resulting in PL strengthens neuromodulatory control, enhances LTP, restores neural connections, increases signal-to-noise ratio, and improves the specificity of cortical representations [15].

Neural plasticity induced neurobehaviorally by PL reduces sensory deficits by improving neural representations which become narrowly tuned along physical dimensions. Moreover, because low- and high-level brain mechanisms work together to process incoming information at increasing levels of complexity, it may be expected that neurobehavioral training resulting in PL in low-level task would transfer to higher-level functions. Decades of cumulative research have provided evidence that PL mediates cortical plasticity, thus engaging competitive brain networks so as to refine the selective representation of sensory input and transfer these improvements to interacting systems.

35.2 Improvement of Visual Functions in Healthy Aging

PL has been shown to improve a variety of visual functions. One recent study revealed a PL improvement of contrast sensitivity in older adults. After 7 days of training using a forced-choice orientation discrimination task, older adult's performance was as good as that of younger adults prior to training. The effects of PL were independent of retinal illuminance changes and transferred to untrained orientations but not to visual acuity [16]. Orientation discrimination was found to improve in older adults during training, in particular when the orientation discrimination task was difficult and the orientation to be discriminated was embedded in additive visual noise [17]. Training to discriminate the direction of motion of sine wave gratings (an image where the luminance varies as a sign wave) embedded in visual noise reduced contrast threshold in the elderly and the effect of PL transferred to other motion tasks, suggesting higher tolerance to external noise rather than reduction of additive internal noise [18]. Importantly, PL of motion tasks involving low-level central visual mechanisms transfers to higher-level visual functions [19]. Berry and coworkers [19] trained older participants in discriminating the expansion/contraction of a sine wave grating presented within a 2D Gaussian window and found, 10 h later, better performance in the older group that was trained during the 10-h interval relative to the untrained control group. Training transferred to an untrained task consisting in discriminating whether two consecutive directions of coherently moving dots were the same or different, both when the task was purely perceptual and, most importantly, when working memory was involved by interposing a delay between the two stimuli. Moreover, the electrophysiological response to the stimulus (event-related brain potentials, ERPs) was recorded. The comparison of ERPs measured at two intervals showed a training-dependent modulation of the deflection of a negative voltage component with a latency of 120–220 ms (N1). The amplitude of this component was significantly decreased at the second interval for the trained, but not for the control group. Moreover, PL has been shown in tasks approximating real-world demands of dividing attention simultaneously among multiple stimuli and tasks. For example, Richards et al. [20] involved younger and older observers in PL of a useful field of view task (UFOV), in which participants performed the localization of peripheral targets. Performance in this task was impaired by engaging simultaneously attention to a central letter which observers had to identify. However, in both groups, the impairment due to divided attention was reduced, and, when older subjects were provided with enough practice, their attentional costs did not differ from those of the younger group.

In addition to the evidence of PL-dependent improvement in aging, several studies provide evidence that PL is associated with brain plasticity. Chang et al. [11] involved observers in three training sessions. They found a 28% reduction of temporal threshold, defined as the interval between texture and mask to reach 80% accuracy in a texture discrimination task (TDT). Before, PL thresholds in TDT were uncorrelated with areal size of V1, V2, or V3 for all groups. For the older group only, individual improvement due to PL was significantly correlated with areal size of V3. Importantly, for the older group, the correlation between PL effects and areal size was found in V3, whereas in younger adults, PL is associated with a specific modulation of functional activation in the trained location of V1 [21–24]. Note that V3 shows the smallest age-associated size reduction. This could explain why it compensates for the age-dependent reduced functional plasticity of V1. Indeed, assuming that reduced areal size reflects a reduction in the number of facilitatory and inhibitory connections whose strength is modulated by PL [25], this would affect negatively the potentiality of PL in areas of reduced size such as V1, whereas

PL would be preserved in larger areas with a larger number of neural connections, such as V3.

In addition to changes in areal size, it has been shown [26] that PL leads to a change in cortical connectivity in the older brain. The study was based on the hypothesis that PL potentiates signal transmission as indexed by fractional anisotropy (FA) that reflects neural properties such myelin thickness and axonal diameter. Younger and older observers were involved in PL of TDT, and FA values associated with PL were obtained using two MRI techniques: diffusion tensor imaging, a MRI technique that can measure macroscopic axonal organization in nervous system, and functional MRI BOLD signals elicited during the task. Results showed that the older but not the younger group showed significant changes in FA, suggesting a different PL mechanism in the two groups: only in older observer PL is associated with a reorganization of white matter.

Altogether, neurobehavioral and MRI findings suggest that sensory plasticity is preserved for training in older adults.

35.3 Rehabilitation of Visual Diseases in Elderly

In the present session, we review evidence of positive outcomes resulting from the rehabilitation of sensory diseases in older patients. We focus on presbyopia, optic neuropathy, and age-related macular degeneration.

Presbyopia Presbyopia is a common type of refractive error associated with the experience of blurred vision which causes limitation in daily activities such as reading, sewing, or working at the computer and goes together with a reduction of near visual acuity, contrast sensitivity, and processing speed. The consequence of blurred input to the cortex may be a reduced neural activation and a sluggish neural response. Based on the hypothesis that blurred vision results in less efficient spatiotemporal neural coding, Polat et al. [27] involved presbyopic observes in a neurovisual training protocol, consisting in detecting a low-contrast target presented with high-contrast collinear and iso-oriented flankers. They showed that PL resulted in improved visual acuity and contrast sensitivity. Most importantly, reading speed improved by 17 words/min following training.

Optic Neuropathy Reduced vision following prechiasmatic damage had been considered irreversible until recently. However, recent studies [28, 29] used alternating weak current (repetitive transorbital alternating current stimulation, rtACS) delivered by stimulation electrodes applied transorbitally with the eye closed to patients with optic nerve damage aged 52–62 years. Results showed that the application of rACS resulted in a significant recovery of visual functions. Restorative effects were revealed by objective measures of visual acuity, visual field size with static and dynamic perimetry, and electrophysiological responses in V1 (e.g., the P100 positive component, peaking at 100 ms). Moreover, rtACS reduced limitations in vision-related activities in daily life and in vision-specific quality of life.

AMD Age-related macular degeneration (AMD) is a prominent cause of vision loss typically occurring in older people. It reduces visual acuity and contrast sensitivity, and it also affects reading, driving, or other important activities of daily living. AMD patients frequently develop an eccentric area of fixation. It is therefore of great clinical relevance to evaluate effectiveness of a PL technique for improving eccentric vision in these patients. Several studies have investigated the potential of PL in enhancing reading speed using either trigram letter recognition [30, 31] or rapid serial visual presentation (RSVP) tasks [32, 33]. The general result is that the speed of word recognition can be enhanced by PL across a range of ages. However, it is not clear whether the improvement simply depended on changes in the retinal locus chosen for fixation or on fixation stability.

Various studies suggest that the improvements in peripheral PL are likely to represent genuine plasticity of the visual system despite the older age of the observers.

To address the issue of plasticity, Maniglia et al. [34] investigated the effect of PL on contrast detection for a target flanked by high-contrast collinear elements. PL was enduring and transferred to visual acuity and contrast sensitivity; most important of all, PL reduced inhibition by the flankers at short distances in the younger group and improved facilitation by the flankers at medium distanced in the AMD group. This indicates that PL reduced inhibitory lateral interactions in the trained younger group and increased facilitatory ones in AMD patients, suggesting different mechanisms of plasticity. Rosengarth et al. [35] found that improvements obtained in oculomotor and/or reading training by AMD observers (average age 73 years) resulted in short-term functional and structural brain changes. Furthermore, Plank et al. [37] reported that PL enhances eccentric vision with central vision loss. Most importantly, the PL-dependent improvement was associated with a modest alteration in BOLD response in the early visual cortex.

The results show that PL has strong, noninvasive, and long-lasting rehabilitative potential for one of the main causes of visual disability in Western countries.

Conclusion

In summary, although interconnections among neurons become less efficient as a result of metabolic decline and subregulation of neural communication, neurobehavioral and imaging findings suggest that sensory plasticity is preserved for training in adults with age-related visual decline. The key points of modulation of sensory plasticity by PL are noninvasivity, enduring improvement in visual functions as assessed up to 1-year follow-up, and better quality of life.

Key Points

- The efficiency of interconnections among sensory neurons is reduced in the aged brain.
- Cortical plasticity decline can be reversed through neurobehavioral restorative training.

References

1. Blokland A (1995) Acetylcholine: a neurotransmitter for learning and memory? Brain Res Rev 21(3):285–300
2. Roberts MJ, Zinke W, Guo K, Robertson R, McDonald JS, Thiele A (2005) Acetylcholine dynamically controls spatial integration in marmoset primary visual cortex. J Neurophysiol 93(4):2062–2072
3. Loerch PM, Lu T, Dakin KA, Vann JM, Isaacs A, Geula C, Wang J, Pan Y, Gabuzda DH, Li C, Prolla TA (2008) Evolution of the aging brain transcriptome and synaptic regulation. PLoS One 3(10):e3329
4. Betts LR, Taylor CP, Sekuler AB, Bennett PJ (2005) Aging reduces center-surround antagonism in visual motion processing. Neuron 45(3):361–366
5. Casco C, Guzzon D, Moise M, Vecchies A, Testa T, Pavan A (2014) Specificity and generalization of perceptual learning in low myopia. Restor Neurol Neurosci 32(5):639–653
6. Casco C, Robol V, Barollo M, Cansino S (2011) Effects of aging on visual contour integration and segmentation. Invest Ophthalmol Vis Sci 52(7):3955–3961
7. Casco C, DiStefani E, Pinello L, Sato G, Battaglini L (2015) Hyper-vision of mirror symmetry in patients with macular degeneration reflects parafoveal cortical reorganization. Restor Neurol Neurosci 34(1):67–77
8. Leventhal AG, Wang Y, Pu M, Zhou Y, Ma Y (2003) GABA and its agonists improved visual cortical function in senescent monkeys. Science 300(5620):812–815
9. Peters MA, Thompson B, Merabet LB, Wu AD, Shams L (2013) Anodal tDCS to V1 blocks visual perceptual learning consolidation. Neuropsychologia 51(7):1234–1239
10. Li SC, Lindenberger U, Sikström S (2001) Aging cognition: from neuromodulation to representation. Trends Cogn Sci 5(11):479–486
11. Chang LH, Yotsumoto Y, Salat DH, Andersen GJ, Watanabe T, Sasaki Y (2015) Reduction in the retinotopic early visual cortex with normal aging and magnitude of perceptual learning. Neurobiol Aging 36(1):315–322
12. Burke SN, Barnes CA (2006) Neural plasticity in the ageing brain. Nat Rev Neurosci 7(1):30–40
13. Bavelier D et al (2010) Removing brakes on adult brain plasticity: from molecular to behavioral interventions. J Neurosci 30(45):14964–14971
14. Mahncke HW, Bronstone A, Merzenich MM (2006) Brain plasticity and functional losses in the aged: scientific bases for a novel intervention. Prog Brain Res 157:81–109
15. Van Praag H, Kempermann G, Gage FH (2000) Neural consequences of environmental enrichment. Nat Rev Neurosci 1(3):191–198
16. DeLoss DJ, Watanabe T, Andersen GJ (2015) Improving vision among older adults behavioral training to improve sight. Psychol Sci 26(4):456–466
17. DeLoss DJ, Watanabe T, Andersen GJ (2014) Optimization of perceptual learning: effects of task difficulty and external noise in older adults. Vision Res 99:37–45
18. Bower JD, Andersen GJ (2012) Aging, perceptual learning, and changes in efficiency of motion processing. Vision Res 61:144–156
19. Berry AS, Zanto TP, Clapp WC, Hardy JL, Delahunt PB, Mahncke HW, Gazzaley A (2010) The influence of perceptual training on working memory in older adults. PLoS One 5(7):e11537
20. Richards E, Bennett PJ, Sekuler AB (2006) Age related differences in learning with the useful field of view. Vision research 46(25):4217–4231
21. Furmanski CS, Schluppeck D, Engel SA (2004) Learning strengthens the response of primary visual cortex to simple patterns. Curr Biol 14(7):573–578
22. Schwartz S, Maquet P, Frith C (2002) Neural correlates of perceptual learning: a functional MRI study of visual texture discrimination. Proc Natl Acad Sci 99(26):17137–17142
23. Walker MP, Stickgold R, Jolesz FA, Yoo SS (2005) The functional anatomy of sleep-dependent visual skill learning. Cereb Cortex 15(11):1666–1675

24. Yotsumoto Y, Watanabe T, Sasaki Y (2008) Different dynamics of performance and brain activation in the time course of perceptual learning. Neuron 57(6):827–833
25. Piëch V, Li W, Reeke GN, Gilbert CD (2013) Network model of top-down influences on local gain and contextual interactions in visual cortex. Proc Natl Acad Sci 110(43):E4108–E4117
26. Yotsumoto Y, Chang LH, Ni R, Pierce R, Andersen GJ, Watanabe T, Sasaki Y (2014) White matter in the older brain is more plastic than in the younger brain. Nat Commun 5
27. Polat U, Schor C, Tong JL, Zomet A, Lev M, Yehezkel O, Sterkin A, Levi DM (2012) Training the brain to overcome the effect of aging on the human eye. Sci Rep 2
28. Sabel BA, Fedorov AB, Naue N, Borrmann A, Herrmann C, Gall C (2011) Non-invasive alternating current stimulation improves vision in optic neuropathy. Restor Neurol Neurosci 29(6):493–505
29. Gall C, Sgorzaly S, Schmidt S, Brandt S, Fedorov A, Sabel BA (2011) Noninvasive transorbital alternating current stimulation improves subjective visual functioning and vision-related quality of life in optic neuropathy. Brain Stimul 4(4):175–188
30. Yu D, Cheung SH, Legge GE, Chung ST (2010) Reading speed in the peripheral visual field of older adults: does it benefit from perceptual learning? Vision Res 50(9):860–869
31. Astle AT, Blighe AJ, Webb BS, McGraw PV (2015) The effect of normal aging and age-related macular degeneration on perceptual learning. J Vis 15(10):16–16
32. Chung ST (2011) Improving reading speed for people with central vision loss through perceptual learning. Invest Ophthalmol Vis Sci 52(2):1164–1170
33. Tarita-Nistor L, Lam D, Brent MH, Steinbach MJ, González EG (2013) Courier: a better font for reading with age-related macular degeneration. Can J Ophthalmol 48(1):56–62
34. Maniglia M, Pavan A, Sato G, Contemori G, Montemurro S, Battaglini L, Casco C (2016) Perceptual learning leads to long lasting visual improvement in patients with central vision loss. Restorative Neurology and Neuroscience 34(5):697–720
35. Rosengarth K, Keck I, Brandl-Rühle S, Frolo J, Hufendiek K, Greenlee MW, Plank T (2013) Functional and structural brain modifications induced by oculomotor training in patients with age-related macular degeneration. Front Psychol 4:428
36. Plank T, Rosengarth K, Schmalhofer C, Goldhacker M, Brandl-Rühle S, Greenlee MW (2014) Perceptual learning in patients with macular degeneration. Front Psychol 5:1189
37. Casco C, Barollo M, Contemori G, Battaglini L (2017) The Effects of Aging on Orientation Discrimination. Frontiers in aging neuroscience 9

Rehabilitation of Communicative-Pragmatic Ability and Ageing

36

Alberto Parola and Francesca M. Bosco

36.1 Introduction

The ability to communicate effectively in a social context may decrease as a consequence of the normal ageing process and may be caused by physiological and neurological changes as well as changes in the personal environment, such as a reduction in the number of social contacts and changes to the social role, as in the case of retirement, which usually characterise old age. Older adults frequently show a generalised cognitive decline [1], caused by a reduction in the cortical connectivity of the frontal lobe [2], which primarily affects high-order cognitive functions such as executive functions, i.e. planning, working memory and inhibition, and is accompanied by an alteration in hearing and speech processes. These modifications may affect the ability to use language, resulting in difficulty with name retrieval and recalling, circumlocution, reduction of the syntactic complexity of sentences and prosodic alterations, which may be accompanied by a defective emotion recognition [3]. In addition to a possible generalised cognitive decline during the normal ageing process, many neurological disorders occur in late adulthood; the most prevalent diseases that often impair communicative ability in old age are stroke, traumatic brain injury, dementia (in particular, Alzheimer's disease) and Parkinson's disease. Individuals with Parkinson's disease present prosodic difficulties, such as reduced speech stress, monotonic pitch and inappropriate pauses, as well as reduced information content of a discourse, and pragmatic deficits [4]. Individuals with dementia exhibit deficits in word retrieval, circumlocution, production of irrelevant utterances, lack of coherence and rapidly shifting topics [5]. The communicative disorders reported in people with brain damage are heterogeneous in nature and vary according to the size and origin (vascular or traumatic) of the lesion, but the most

A. Parola (✉) • F.M. Bosco
Department of Psychology, University of Turin, Turin, Italy
e-mail: a.parola@unito.it; francesca.bosco@unito.it

© Springer International Publishing AG 2018

S. Masiero, U. Carraro (eds.), *Rehabilitation Medicine for Elderly Patients*,
Practical Issues in Geriatrics, DOI 10.1007/978-3-319-57406-6_36

prevalent disturbances include aphasic symptoms; difficulties in modulation and recognition of the tone of voice; verbosity; tangentiality; social inappropriateness; pragmatic and inferential deficits, especially in understanding the most complex forms of language (irony, metaphor, idioms); and narrative disorders [6–8].

In patients, communicative disorders are an obstacle to a full recovery from injury and the return to previous daily activities. Language and communicative rehabilitation is thus extremely important in order to limit the social consequences of communicative disorders in old age.

36.2 Rehabilitation of Communicative Disorders in Brain-Injured Patients

We will now focus on the rehabilitation of communicative disorders in older people with brain damage (BD). The first aim of communicative rehabilitation is to identify the specific profile of communicative impairment, in order to provide a rehabilitative programme focused on the patient's difficulty. Traditionally, rehabilitative approaches have focused on the recovery of linguistic ability, but the recovery of linguistic function does not necessarily correspond to an actual improvement in the ability to communicate in a real-life context. Moreover, even if patients with BD frequently exhibit deficits that also affect non-verbal, i.e. gestural, communication, the majority of treatments focused on the verbal modality do not address the remediation of non-verbal forms of communication [9]. To overcome these limits, some authors have proposed the pragmatic approach (see [10]), such as the functional communication treatment [11], where aphasic patients are trained to implement non-verbal strategies to solve everyday communicative tasks, or the Promoting Aphasics' Communication Effectiveness [12], in which an examiner requires patients to describe a card, with the help of the therapist, that gives him feedback and suggests compensatory strategies in order to improve the efficacy of his communicative performance. A distinctive feature of the pragmatic approach is the presence of the group, which recreates the cognitive demands set by a real-life communicative setting, such as rapid and overlapping turn-taking and promoting generalisation of the skills acquired in the training. The group also favours the creation of new social relationships, extending the social and supportive network of the participants.

Patients with BD often show behavioural disturbances, referred to as 'personality changes' and attributable to brain damage, that limit their communicative skills, making them over-talkative, socially inappropriate, aggressive and perseverative. To overcome difficulties in communication, social skills training has also been proposed [e.g. [13]]. This training includes a wide range of techniques such as modelling, role play, feedback, self-monitoring and group discussion, with the aim of fostering prosocial and adaptive communicative behaviour. The role played by the patient's caregiver(s) is another important aspect of communicative rehabilitation. The therapist provides useful advice to the patient's caregiver(s), helping them to know the cause and to manage the consequences of the disorders and suggesting how to reinforce the compensatory strategies proposed during rehabilitation.

Other important issues, such as the level of awareness of deficits and the general cognitive profile of the patients, have to be addressed in rehabilitation with older adults with BD. Indeed, the cognitive decline, as in executive functioning and theory of mind, i.e. the ability to attribute mental states to oneself and to other people, or a scarce awareness of these deficits, could dramatically limit the treatment efficacy. Recently, Gabbatore et al. [14] proposed the cognitive pragmatic treatment (CPT), an articulated training programme created to improve the communicative ability of patients with BD. The CPT consists of 24 group rehabilitation sessions, each focused on a different aspect of communication. The treatment takes into account the linguistic, non-verbal and paralinguistic expressive means, encouraging patients to use all the communicative modalities and preserved abilities to reach the communicative goals set by a specific task. The techniques used include role play, the viewing of video clips showing communicative exchanges followed by group discussion, and exercises using audio and printed material. The efficacy of the CPT has been demonstrated in a sample of patients with traumatic brain injuries, who reported better communicative performance that remained stable 3 months after the end of the treatment.

36.3 Rehabilitation Programme in Healthy Seniors

In normal ageing, the psychosocial consequences of communicative difficulties in daily activities may be serious. Older adults often experience a reduction in social contacts, and communicative difficulties can further weaken their social network. In addition, older adults frequently have the need for assistance services, and "the ability to communicate successfully, including speaking, listening, reading, and writing, is a critical factor in obtaining health care" [15]. The benefits of the approaches aimed at assessing and enhancing communicative ability are therefore not limited to patients but could be extended to adults who are experiencing communicative difficulties connected with the normal process of ageing. Communicative treatments aimed at improving and enhancing communicative skills could help them to prevent their cognitive decline and preserve their communicative abilities. A key consequence of communicative improvement is the maintenance and reinforcement of the social and supportive network, which positively reflects on the quality of life. Finally, some critical issues should be considered when older adults are included in rehabilitative treatment: the rhythm and timing of the activity should be carefully tailored to the needs of older adults. Cognitive decline and physical fatigue can indeed reduce their attention and their responsiveness during the treatment, and the role of the experimenter is to constantly monitor and prevent possible treatment withdrawal.

Conclusion

To date few studies have focused on the assessment (and rehabilitation) of communicative difficulties in healthy and non-healthy elderly subjects, despite the actual existence of such difficulties and the serious social consequences of these disorders. Further research is needed in order to better delineate the origin and the profile of these disorders and their consequences in real life. A better understanding of these communicative impairments and of the efficacy of the rehabilitation programmes addressing this issue is also necessary.

Key Points
- Communicative disorders and ageing: origin and consequences
- Rehabilitation of communicative disorders in older people with brain damage
- Rehabilitation programme in healthy older adults

References

1. Glisky EL (2007) Changes in cognitive function in human aging. In: Brain aging: models, methods, and mechanisms. David R. Riddle, CRC Press, Taylor & Francis, NY/USA pp 3–20
2. Hess TM (2005) Memory and aging in context. Psychol Bull 131(3):383.3
3. Burdon P, Dipper L, Cocks N (2016) Exploration of older and younger British adults' performance on The Awareness of Social Inference Test (TASIT). Int J Lang Commun Disord 51(5):589–593
4. Berg E, Björnram C, Hartelius L, Laakso K, Johnels BO (2003) High-level language difficulties in Parkinson's disease. Clin Linguist Phon 17(1):63–80
5. Bayles KA, Tomoeda CK, Cruz RF, Mahendra N (2000) Communication abilities of individuals with late-stage Alzheimer disease. Alzheimer Dis Assoc Disord 14(3):176–181
6. Orange JB (2009) Language and communication disorders in older adults: selected considerations for clinical audiology. Hear Care Adults:87–102
7. Bosco FM, Angeleri R, Sacco K, Bara BG (2015) Explaining pragmatic performance in traumatic brain injury: a process perspective on communicative errors. Int J Lang Commun Disord 50(1):63–83
8. Parola A, Gabbatore I, Bosco FM, Cossa FM, Gindri P, Sacco K (2016) Linguistic, extralinguistic and paralinguistic abilities in patients with right hemisphere damage (RHD). Journal of Neurolinguistics 39:10–25
9. Angeleri R, Bosco FM, Zettin M, Sacco K, Colle L, Bara BG (2008) Communicative impairment in traumatic brain injury: a complete pragmatic assessment. Brain Lang 107(3):229–245
10. Carlomagno S, Blasi V, Labruna L, Santoro A (2000) The role of communication models in assessment and therapy of language disorders in aphasic adults. Neuropsychol Rehabil 10(3):337–363
11. Aten JL, Caligiuri MP, Holland AL (1982) The efficacy of functional communication therapy for chronic aphasic patients. J Speech Hear Disord 47(1):93–96
12. Davis GA, Wilcox MJ (1985) Adult aphasia rehabilitation: applied pragmatics. College-Hill Press, Worthing, England
13. Ylvisaker M, Turkstra LS, Coelho C (2005) Behavioral and social interventions for individuals with traumatic brain injury: a summary of the research with clinical implications. Semin Speech Lang 26(4):256–267
14. Gabbatore I, Sacco K, Angeleri R, Zettin M, Bara BG, Bosco FM (2015) Cognitive pragmatic treatment: a rehabilitative program for traumatic brain injury individuals. J Head Trauma Rehabil 30(5):E14–E28
15. Yorkston KM, Bourgeois MS, Baylor CR (2010) Communication and aging. Phys Med Rehabil Clin N Am 21(2):309–319

Neuropsychological Aspects of Language in Older Adults

37

Andrea Marini

37.1 Introduction

Language relies on the integrated organization of a within-utterance or microlinguistic dimension, which is required for intrasentential functions, and a between-utterance or macrolinguistic dimension, necessary for intersentential functions [1]. The microlinguistic dimension organizes phonemes into morphemes and words (lexical processing). It also determines the syntactic context required by a word in order to generate well-formed sentences (syntactic processing) and the literal meaning expressed by single words (lexical semantics) and entire sentences (phrasal semantics). The macrolinguistic dimension determines the contextually appropriate meaning of a word or sentence (pragmatic processing) and connects sentences or utterances by means of cohesive and coherent links in order to formulate the main theme of narrative discourse and integrate its linguistic and conceptual features (discourse processing). This complex cognitive function declines gradually in the elderly [2], as a consequence of the complex interplay between the intrinsic deterioration of the linguistic system and the cognitive decline [3]. This brief chapter focuses on some of the alterations induced by healthy aging on language production skills.

37.2 Age-Related Effects on Microlinguistic Processing

Even if the mental lexicon keeps growing during the lifespan and older adults usually have larger vocabularies than younger individuals [2, 4] at least until they enter in their 80s and 90s [5], studies assessing naming skills and tip of the tongue states

A. Marini
University of Udine, Udine, Italy

Claudiana - Landesfachhochschule für Gesundheitsberufe, Lorenz-Böhler-Straße 13, Bozen 39100, Italy
e-mail: andrea.marini@uniud.it

© Springer International Publishing AG 2018

S. Masiero, U. Carraro (eds.), *Rehabilitation Medicine for Elderly Patients*, Practical Issues in Geriatrics, DOI 10.1007/978-3-319-57406-6_37

in healthy aging show that the ability to retrieve words from memory weakens already after the age of 50 [6] but significantly deteriorates in people in their 70s [7]. Similarly, also grammatical skills gradually decline with age: older individuals produce fewer complex sentences [8] and have more difficulties in the retrieval of function words [9]. The possibility of an age-induced grammatical weakening is supported also by the results from studies using different techniques. For example [10], older participants produced narrative descriptions with more morphological errors and fewer complete sentences than younger groups of individuals aged from 20 to 60 years. It has been suggested that this grammatical weakening is at least partly related to the decline in verbal working memory which is frequently observed in the elderly [11].

Overall, the studies focusing on microlinguistic production skills in the elderly suggest that both lexical and grammatical skills deteriorate with aging. Even if most of the existing reports have focused on the traditional assessment of lexical and grammatical skills (e.g., naming tasks and sentence generation tasks), in order to have a more detailed picture of lexical and grammatical production skills in the elderly, there is a need for more studies employing tasks that allow speakers to produce samples of narrative discourse [12].

37.3 Age-Related Effects on Macrolinguistic Processing

The process of aging affects also macrolinguistic abilities. The narratives produced by older individuals are typically characterized by augmented verbosity [13] and reduced cohesive and coherent organization. For example, Kemper and Sumner [11] showed that the narrative discourse produced by persons in their 70s and 80s contained more errors of both local (i.e., missing or ambiguous referents and topic shifts) and global (i.e., tangential utterances and semantically erroneous formulations) coherence than that of adults in their 20s and 30s. The absence of a significant difference between the oldest group's performance and that of the middle-aged suggests that the production of local coherence errors is a gradual side effect of aging, which is likely to start already when people enter in their 50s. Aging weakens also global coherence, i.e., the ability to semantically relate remote utterances within a given discourse. When older adults are involved in spontaneous conversation, they produce more off-topic speech than younger individuals (e.g., [14]). This is why the narrative discourse of older people is often perceived as vague and incoherent. The narrative weaknesses observed in the elderly might not entirely depend on a linguistic disturbance per se [3]. According to the *inhibition deficit hypothesis* [15], in the elderly, the ability to suppress irrelevant pieces of information and focus on the main stream of a narrative might be weakened because of a declined ability to monitor the process of message production. This might eventually trigger the introduction of extraneous comments and derailments while generating a story.

Conclusions

The linguistic production of older adults is characterized by a gradual linguistic weakness which is, at least in part, influenced by their cognitive decline. It is important to take into account the typology of tasks used to elicit language production in the elderly as different approaches can provide very different results. For example, Schmitter-Edgecombe et al. [12] compared word-finding skills in three groups of adults with different ages by administering the Boston Naming Test and a spontaneous discourse production task. The group of older participants (in their 70, 80s, and 90s) produced more errors than younger participants only in the latter task as in the naming test they were surprisingly even more accurate than younger participants. This suggests that ecological tasks such as the discourse production task used in this experiment may be highly informative about the actual linguistic difficulties experienced by a given individual.

Key Points

- The linguistic production of older adults is characterized by a gradual linguistic weakness.
- Such weaknesses are influenced also by the cognitive decline.
- Discourse production tasks are highly informative about the actual linguistic difficulties experienced by speakers.

References

1. Marini A, Andreetta S, Del Tin S, Carlomagno S (2011) A multi-level approach to the analysis of narrative language in aphasia. Aphasiology 25(11):1372–1392. doi:10.1080/02687038.2011.584690
2. Thornton R, Light LL (2006) Language comprehension and production in normal aging. In: Birren JE, Schaie KW (eds) Handbook of the psychology of aging. Academic, San Diego, CA, pp 261–287. doi:10.1016/B978-012101264-9/50015-X
3. Marini A, Andreetta S (2016) Age-related effects on language production: a combined psycholinguistic and neurolinguistic perspective. In: Wright HH (ed) Cognition, language and aging. John Benjamins Publishing Company, Amsterdam, Netherlands, pp 55–79
4. Schroeder DH, Salthouse TA (2004) Age-related effects on cognition between 20 and 50 years of age. Personal Individ Differ 36:393–404. doi:10.1016/S0191-8869(03)00104-1
5. Lindenberger U, Baltes PB (1997) Intellectual functioning in old and very old age: cross-sectional results from the Berlin aging study. Psychol Aging 12:410–432. doi:10.1037/0882-7974.12.3.410
6. Connor LT, Spiro A, Obler LK, Albert ML (2004) Change in object naming ability during adulthood. J Gerontol Ser B 59(5):203–209. doi:10.1093/geronb/59.5.P203
7. Feyereisen P (1997) A meta-analytic procedure shows an age-related decline in picture naming: comments on Goulet, Ska, and Kahn (1994). J Speech Lang Hear Res 40(6):1328–1333. doi:10.1044/jslhr.4006.1328
8. Shadden B (1997) Discourse behaviours in older adults. Semin Speech Lang 18(2):156–147. doi:10.1055/s-2008-1064069

9. Heller RB, Dobbs AR (1993) Age differences in word finding in discourse and nondiscourse situations. Psychol Aging 8:443–450. doi:10.1037/0882-7974.8.3.443
10. Marini A, Boewe A, Caltagirone C, Carlomagno S (2005) Age-related differences in the production of textual descriptions. J Psycholinguist Res 34(5):439–463. doi:10.1007/s10936-005-6203-z
11. Kemper S, Sumner A (2001) The structure of verbal abilities in young and older adults. Psychol Aging 16:312–322. doi:10.1037/0882-7974.16.2.312
12. Schmitter-Edgecombe M, Vesneski M, Jones DW (2000) Aging and word-finding: a comparison of spontaneous and constrained naming tests. Arch Clin Neuropsychol 15(6):479–493
13. Pushkar Gold D, Arbuckle TY (1995) A longitudinal study of off-target verbosity. J Gerontol Psychol Sci 50B:307–315
14. Wills CL, Capilouto GJ, Wright HH (2012) Attention and off-topic speech in the recounts of middle-age and elderly adults: a pilot investigation. Contemp Issues Commun Sci Disord 39:105–112
15. Hasher L, Zacks RT (1988) Working memory, comprehension, and aging: a review and a new view. Psychol Learn Motiv 22:193–225. doi:10.1016/S0079-7421(08)60041-9

Rehabilitation of Older People with Swallowing Disorders

38

Emelyne Grech, Erwan de Mones, and Isabelle Bourdel-Marchasson

38.1 Introduction

In European countries, life expectancy in the elderly is increasing, particularly in men. However, in Sweden the estimated number of years of life with either severe or mobility disability has remained relatively constant over the last 20 years [1]. The prevalence of swallowing disorders differs across populations and settings but is probably the highest in those with severe disability or who are living in nursing homes. Estimations of prevalence of dysphagia in older people vary according to health status. We previously estimated that one in five inpatients in geriatric acute care wards has swallowing disorders [2], and the prevalence can reach 60% in nursing homes [3]. The consequences of these difficulties are severe, including aspiration pneumonia, malnutrition, dehydration, poor quality of life [4], and increased mortality.

E. Grech
Speech Language Therapy Department, University of Bordeaux, Bordeaux, France
e-mail: emelyne.grech@hotmail.fr

E. de Mones
Otorhinolaryngology Department, CHU of Bordeaux, Bordeaux, France
e-mail: erwan.de-mones-del-pujol@chu-bordeaux.fr

I. Bourdel-Marchasson (✉)
Department of Clinical Gerontology, CHU Bordeaux, Bordeaux, France

CNRS, RMSB, UMR 5536, Bordeaux, France

University Bordeaux, RMSB, UMR 5536, Bordeaux, France
e-mail: isabelle.bourdel-marchasson@chu-bordeaux.fr

© Springer International Publishing AG 2018

S. Masiero, U. Carraro (eds.), *Rehabilitation Medicine for Elderly Patients*, Practical Issues in Geriatrics, DOI 10.1007/978-3-319-57406-6_38

38.2 Specific Features of Dysphagia in Older Patients

This chapter focuses on oropharyngeal dysphagia. Although frequent in older people, esophageal dysphagia is not concerned by rehabilitation. The main causes of dysphagia in older people are peripheral or central neurological difficulties. Otorhinolaryngological causes include anatomical and functional diseases such as cancers, pharyngoesophageal diverticula, local compression, and cervical osteophytes. Iatrogenic causes are also frequent. Moreover, several drugs can amplify and decompensate baseline subclinical difficulties owing to their negative effect on motility (neuroleptic, benzodiazepine), xerostomia (anticholinergic drugs), or excessive sedation. Wearing a nasogastric tube can also disturb the ability to swallow. In fact, dysphagia is frequent in the elderly owing to their increasing frailty. Other factors include behavioral problems, episodes of delirium, poor oral health including loss of teeth and mycosis, oropharyngeal pain, or gastroesophageal reflux.

Physiological aging can lead to swallowing difficulties, aka presbyphagia. Presbyphagia can alter each of the swallowing phases, oral, pharyngeal, and esophageal phase, but usually the difficulties are combined [5]. During the oral phase, chewing can be altered by a decrease in biting force, poor oral health, or impaired anteroposterior tongue motility. As a result, preparation of the food bolus is slowed down and less efficient. Additionally, decreased salivary production leads to further poor food bolus quality. Salivary or food leakage may result from a defect in lip closure and weak labial tone. Failure to close the velolingual sphincter may result in premature leakage of food bolus to the pharynx. Finally, the oropharyngeal sensory loss that decreases feeding pleasure and interest may also disturb laryngopharyngeal movement. An increase in the sensory detection threshold may result in the subsequent triggering of swallowing reflex. Ossification of the laryngeal cartilage may reduce the magnitude of laryngeal elevation and thus alter the protective capacity of the airways. Pharyngeal peristalsis is slowed down, thereby increasing transit time and the risk of food stasis in the vallecula or piriform sinus. Esophageal movement may also be disturbed with increased transit time or functional impairment of the lower esophageal sphincter.

The global mobility or breathing that is involved in swallowing is also modified with aging. Cough reflex can be diminished or less efficient. Presbyphagia can thus be considered as an aggravating but not a causative factor. Indeed, complications are not observed in healthy older people who are able to compensate these difficulties [6].

38.3 The Multidisciplinary Team

In view of the multifactorial causes of swallowing disorders in older people, management of dysphagia should be **multidisciplinary** with a central role for the **medical practitioner** (MP), both for the coordination of those involved and for diagnosis and treatment. He collects symptoms and signs of dysphagia from the patients and caregivers and conducts the diagnostic procedure including prescription of radiographic exams or clinical dysphagia workup performed by a speech therapist or physiotherapist. He may also refer to a dentist, otorhinolaryngologist, and gastroenterologist for comprehensive management. His first concern is the respiratory or nutritional complications of swallowing disorders. The MP will propose etiological treatment that is either medical, such as dopamine in Parkinsonian dysphagia, or surgical such as extraction of diverticula and if needed rehabilitation. He also performs a global health assessment and functional and nutritional assessment and will likely work with the pharmacist in order to modify the treatment plan. **Professional caregivers**, nurses, or assistants should be trained to screen for dysphagia. They will implement the recommendations resulting from the dysphagia assessment. They are in a position to observe changes in dysphagia symptoms and the efficiency of the recommended changes. They also are in charge of oral health in subjects who are unable to look after themselves. In general, rehabilitation is conducted by **speech therapists** and **physiotherapists**. The speech therapist is trained in dysphagia workup, rehabilitation of swallowing, and the implementation of an individualized palliative care plan. To this end, he collaborates with the patient, his relatives, and caregivers. The physiotherapist helps patients with breathing, either in the event of pulmonary complications or if impaired breathing is an aggravating factor. Furthermore, he is in charge of tonus and motility rehabilitation which can help the patient to adopt adequate head and trunk positions during meals to improve independence. **Occupational therapists** can propose adaptive techniques during meals to facilitate self-feeding along with rehabilitation of hand grip. The role of the **dietician** is to modify the texture of food to facilitate feeding with regard to the patient's needs as demonstrated by the dysphagia workup. He has to ensure the best diet for the patient that takes into account his tastes and habits. Swallowing disorders often affect the strength required to eat, resulting in fastidious and tiring meals that go unfinished. Consequently, food fortification is often necessary to meet the nutritional needs of the patient [7].

38.4 General Objectives

Care for the dysphagic patient can be summarized in three points: prevention of respiratory complications, improvement of nutritional status, and establishing the best quality of life as possible [8]. There are essentially two ways to achieve these goals. First, **rehabilitation** requires personal investment and active participation of the older patient. The programs include exercises to promote automatisms in motor processes using intensive long-lasting training. Second, **adaptive care** aims to ensure safety during meals. The implementation of compensatory strategies is to be considered as palliative care.

38.5 Analytical Rehabilitation

These exercises are designed to improve the motor, sensitive, and sensorial functions of organs concerned. To benefit from such a program, the patient has to be personally committed; he should have good general health and good somatic and psychological status and have sufficient cognitive resources to understand the aim and issues involved. In this chapter we give some examples of exercises.

On the other hand, the relevance of the rehabilitation program relies on the accuracy of the previous assessment of the patient's impairments. The action of eating and swallowing is itself a rehabilitation exercise, soliciting the whole sensorimotor loop in a real situation. Some reflexes have to be stimulated, such as the swallowing reflex which could be delayed or the cough reflex which is an efficient airway unblocking mechanism. Conversely, other reflexes must be inhibited, such as primary reflexes, i.e., biting and sucking. The gag reflex, which is the opposite of the swallowing reflex, should be controlled when exacerbated.

Among the rehabilitation techniques, facial massage is important in the event of palsy and thermo-active stimulation, or cryotherapy can be used to reinforce the nervous system arousal. Thermal and tactile stimulation of the pillars of the soft palate using the technique of Logemann [9] is done before meals. Cryotherapy is also done before meals and consists in oral cavity massaging with iced tips to favor the swallowing reflex by stimulation of the structures sensitive to cold. Voluntary processes can also be used to improve swallowing. Swallowing maneuvers that at the first glance appear as compensatory may in the long term modify the physiology of swallowing. They can be performed during meals with food or in between with saliva or water. According to Logemann and colleagues [10], the supraglottal swallowing exercise aims to protect the airways. It involves a number of successive steps: inspiring while holding one's breath, taking the food bolus, swallowing, expiring, and then coughing. The Mendelsohn maneuver consists in voluntary prolongation of laryngeal elevation to protect the airways and to assist the opening of the cricopharyngeal sphincter during swallowing. Effortful swallowing is proposed in the event of lingual dysfunction with vallecular stasis. It consists in voluntary use of all mouth and throat muscles with maximal intensity around the bolus to improve the propulsive force and pharyngeal contraction, resulting in pharyngeal clearance [11].

Analytical exercises complete the rehabilitation program according to the difficulties identified. They focus on several anatomical structures: the lips and cheek muscles, the tongue, the soft palate, and the larynx. Work on apraxia allows the sensorimotor sequence to be mobilized, leading to automatization of some movements. It also aims at reinforcing the laryngeal muscular structures that are frail and difficult to access. The Shaker technique is used to improve the opening of the upper esophageal sphincter while exercising the suprahyoid muscles [12]. The subject is supine and is instructed to perform a series of three sustained head lifts for 1 min each as an isometric exercise and successive head lifts as an isokinetic exercise. Furthermore, it is sometimes useful to work against the resistance to optimize muscle strength of the previously hypotonic structures.

Whenever possible, biofeedback tools help the patient to perceive the efficiency of exercising. The subject can exercise in front of a mirror or using signals from an accelerometer [13] or surface electromyography from the various structures involved in dysphagia [14].

Sequencing the swallow can be useful in some older patients with apractophagia, i.e., apraxia of swallowing [15]. Taking into account the cognitive and motor capacities of the patient, the swallowing sequence is shown to the patient during meals so that they become automatic. Finally, telling the subject to swallow may be efficient in subjects with the "rolling" phenomenon associated with Parkinsonian palsy.

38.6 Adaptive Care

This model of care involves personalized adaptation corresponding to the results of the dysphagia workup of the older patient. Taste and uses in daily living are as far as possible taken into account as well as the motor and cognitive capacities of the patient to apply the adaptive measures. Furthermore, adaptation should rely on the resources of the patients, financial resources and social support, including caregiver availability.

In the event of degenerative disease or failure to recover after analytical rehabilitation, compensatory strategies will be the keystone of care for swallowing difficulties. Unfortunately the majority of older dysphagic people are concerned: exhaustion, poor general health, cognitive difficulties, and depression prevent actual rehabilitation. These compensatory strategies have a palliative goal to allow feeding while ensuring adequate nutrition or pleasure as safely as possible.

Textural adaptations aim to change the consistency of food according to the ability of the older subject [16]. When chewing is difficult, a texture easily swallowed is proposed (Fig. 38.1).To facilitate swallowing, it is preferable to propose well-homogenized food with a smooth mouth feel. According to the changes in each patient, some

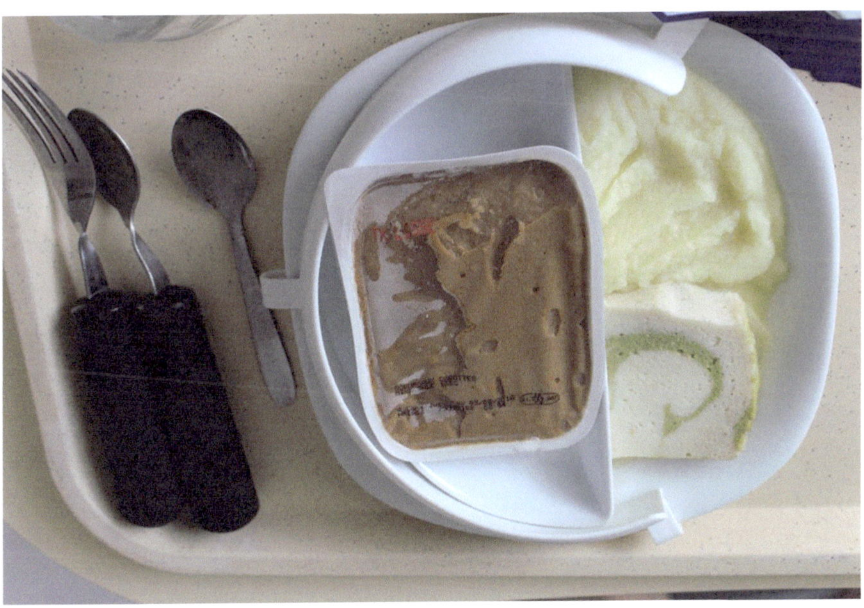

Fig. 38.1 Technical aids and modified meal texture. Note that vegetables, meat, and starch are separated for better tasting

textures will be preferred and others excluded. Solid food may need to be definitively avoided. Indeed, the risk of suffocation due to aspiration of a piece of food is great and life-threatening. Furthermore, a change in texture may necessitate long food bolus preparation (chewing, salivating) and propulsion strength. It is possible either to cut the food into small pieces or to grind it. To improve its cohesion in the mouth and to facilitate its propulsion, the bolus may be coated with sauce or fat. However, shredded or mixed textures are often used because they facilitate swallowing. It should be remembered that production of saliva will decline with permanent use of mixed textures. Some textures are dangerous, e.g., crumbled food that is dispersible in the mouth and may be aspired during the inspiratory whoop. Fibrous textures (leeks, lettuce) also have the same disadvantage. In addition, food that is both liquid and solid like fruit salad is also to be avoided because it requires oral strength and rapid swallowing. Liquid foods can be thickened if the patient has a delayed swallow reflex. The thickness may range from that of fruit nectar to the consistency of stewed fruit. Indeed, liquid has minimal adhesiveness so the speed of the liquid flowing is high, resulting in aspiration before swallowing. Temperature and taste may also be modified. For example, hot or iced liquid or food and sparkling or sweet liquids amplify the reflex response to the oral presence of food compared to tasteless or lukewarm products. Special attention must be paid to adapting the pharmaceutical form of drugs with the help of the pharmacist to be sure of their efficiency and safety.

Postural adaptations first concern global posture (Figs. 38.2 and 38.3). The subject should not be lying down to eat. In a sitting or semi-sitting position, the

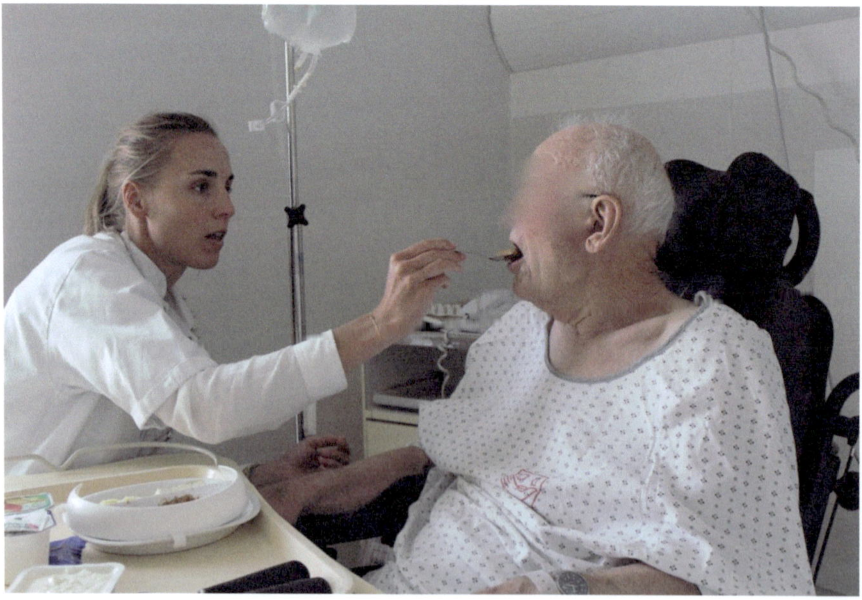

Fig. 38.2 A patient with right-side hemiplegia and right-side laryngeal paralysis in the adequate position for assisted feeding

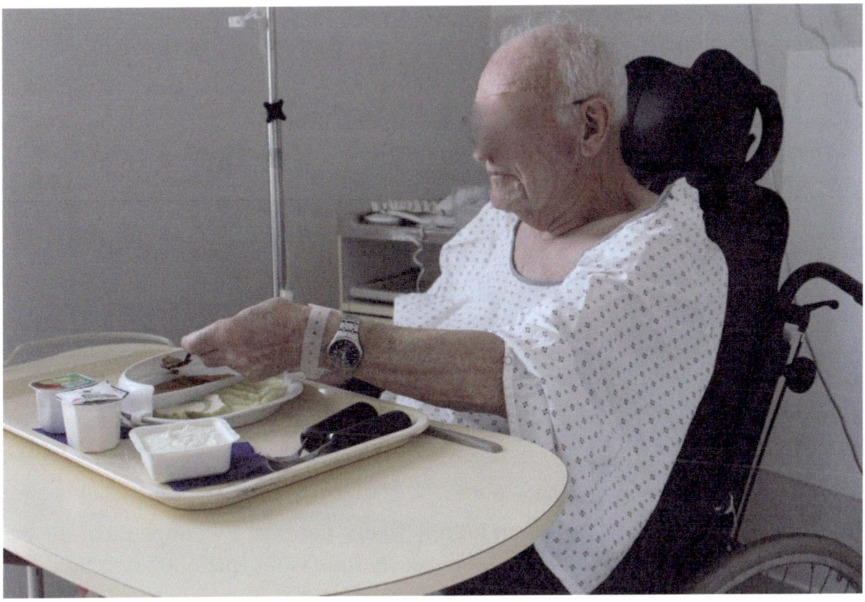

Fig. 38.3 Use of technical aids for easier and safe self-feeding

trunk is properly supported. After the meal it is recommended to stay in this position and not to immediately lie down in order to reduce the risk of acid regurgitation. Neck posture directly impacts swallowing. Lateral bending or hyperextension of the neck which leads mechanically to opening of the larynx should be avoided because they decrease the efficiency of pharyngeal propulsion. The patient should be encouraged to flex the neck as this avoids aspiration on its own in 55% of dysphagic subjects [17]. Furthermore, this position allows the epiglottis to move posteriorly, thus enlarging the vallecular space. In the event of hemilarynx, palsy rotation on the side of the palsy allows better glottal closing and airway protection. Additionally this posture leads to better relaxation of the upper esophageal sphincter and reduces the possibility of stasis in the pharynx and piriform recess.

Environmental adaptations can also be made during the meals of dysphagic subjects. The direct environment should be quiet with few distractors such as TV and radio. The subject is also instructed to focus all his attention on swallowing and to avoid speaking during the meal. The risk of aspiration during the inspiratory whoop is real. Instructions given to the subject should be short and clear or even illustrated. Technical aids may be necessary to facilitate swallowing or to optimize autonomy during the meal (Fig. 38.1). A slip-resistant pad maintains the plate in place; plastic cutlery diminishes the risk of oral injuries in the event of tremor; a foam sleeve facilitates grip; a bended spoon facilitates access to the oral cavity; a plate with edges makes it easier to guide the food to the spoon. For liquids cups with a spout lid are to be avoided because they induce hyperextension of the neck, which could be harmful for the airways. Nosey cups or check straws

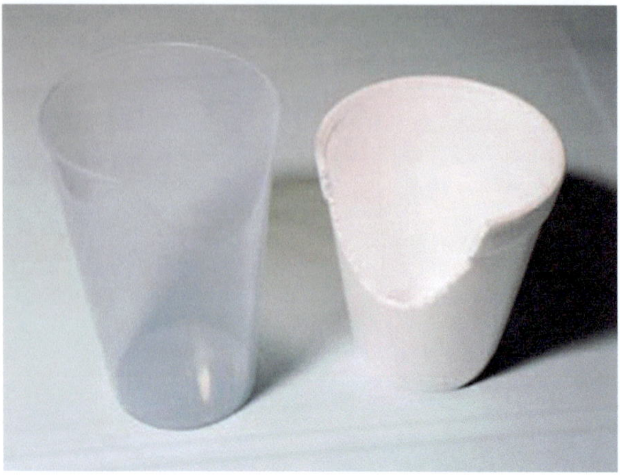

Fig. 38.4 Nosey cups: these cups have a special cutout for the nose in order to drink liquids without bending the neck. They are also used for monitoring fluid intake during meal

are preferable (Fig. 38.4). Human help is likely necessary to implement all the abovementioned recommendations. For all these reasons, patients, families, and caregivers need to be aware of these measures. Caregivers should be trained for a range of uses and technical procedures such as sitting in front of the patient and below him during feeding and bringing the spoon downward to avoid hyperextension. Since older people get tired rapidly, food intake should be split up into at least five snacks per day.

38.7 Training, Information, and Education for Health

Training and education for health are essential in the management of swallowing disorders in older people. Dysphagia and the adaptive process lead to numerous changes in daily life with psychological and social consequences [18]. Implementing changes in this intimate symbolic field can be difficult. At first glance textural adaptations may be seen as infantilizing, for example, and globally the quality of life is impaired. Dysphagic subjects and caregivers find it difficult to make the connection between swallowing and other health issues, and they often minimize the consequences on their health. They may consider that the changes they need to make are just not worthwhile in view of the benefit they may derive for them. For adaptations to be efficient, they require personal energy, money, and time, with the result that both subjects and relatives are often exhausted. All these factors reinforce the lack of compliance and increase the risk of complications and multiple hospitalizations.

We propose that education for health should be taken into account whenever a person undergoes rehabilitation. This program complies with the recommendations of the French High Authority of Health (HAS, Haute Autorité de Santé, http://www.has-sante.fr/portail/upload/docs/application/pdf/etp_-_definition_finalites_-_recommandations_juin_2007.pdf).

The first phase is devoted to informing the patient about his pathology and recognizing the signs of dysphagia. The aim is to lead the subject step by step to making the connection between his swallowing disorders and the actual complications he has had or may have. Support during mealtime is a way to transfer this knowledge to the patient. Caregivers should also be familiarized with these principles, be they professional or familial. The key for success is to meet the subject's needs as much as possible and to identify his abilities. The family is met before the end of the rehabilitation process not only to give them personalized recommendations but to negotiate with them what they can do in their own personal circumstances. The medical team also needs to be trained in this regard because the initial training of professional caregivers in the field of dysphagia is often incomplete. Nursing staff may express their compassion as family members do and may be frustrated by feeding limitations. To deal with these difficulties, formal education is not sufficient, while bedside teaching is efficient but time-consuming.

These multidisciplinary principles and the idea of placing the patient in the center of a personalized and flexible project are the core of educational therapy (Fig. 38.5). This is not limited to technical training or psychological support. Education for health aims to build a therapeutic alliance and promote the patient's insight, which are fundamental for compliance, notably in older people [19].

Education for health in swallowing disorders can be organized in three sessions during a rehabilitation stay or in a day hospital, as in our institution group sessions are preferable after completion of individual analytical work because they save time

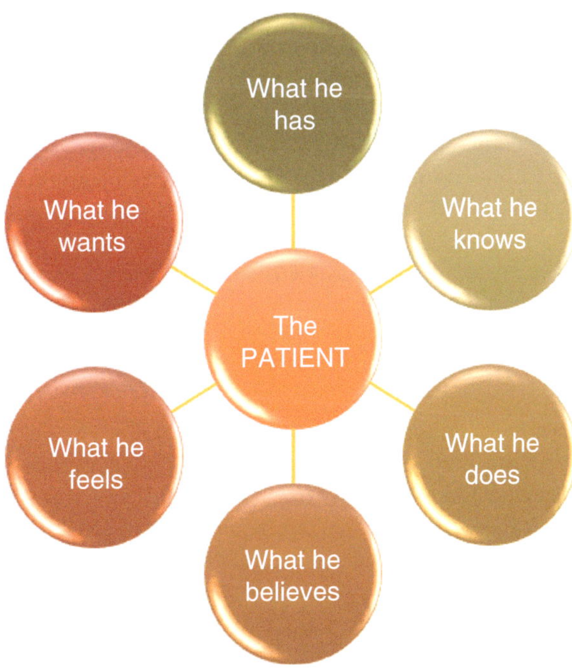

Fig. 38.5 The educational diagnosis

and are likely to increase compliance. The first theme is the link between swallowing and breathing; the second focuses on postures, textures, and adapted environment; and the third concerns warning signs and emergency measures. Patients first have an educational interview to establish with their active participation an educational diagnosis and to allow them to establish personalized goals that take into account their own difficulties and way of life.

During the first session entitled "signs of the wrong way of swallowing and breathing," patients receive information about functional swallowing and chat informally with staff and other patients. This is the opportunity to express their own beliefs. In this way, they can find out how other people cope with the problem and how they feel about it. They have to understand the importance of safe swallowing and how breathing and swallowing work together. At the end they should be able to identify the warning signs in breathing. They receive information about safety techniques (clear throat, cough) and emergency measures (Heimlich maneuver, call to emergency medical service). Patients and family have to establish an action plan in the event of problems, and they have to learn who the key contacts are.

During the second session called "texture workshop," the acquisition of knowledge and actual skills is emphasized. Patients and relatives are trained to use the right technical procedures to adapt their food to their needs. The choice of the food best suited to their difficulties, preferences, and nutritional needs, recognizing those they should not eat, is also a subject of training.

The third session named "posture and environment" aims to lead patients and relatives to a better understanding of the effects of posture and environment on the quality of swallowing. Patients alone or with caregivers can perform technical gestures able to modify their posture in a real situation. For example, caregivers are invited to sit in the right position to feed their relatives. This forms the basis of general group discussion about what constitutes a favorable environment for swallowing.

At the end of this program, each participant is interviewed about what he/she thought of the program and whether the initial goals were achieved. A second program can be recommended thereafter, if necessary.

A positive effect on quality of life (QOL) is expected after adaptive rehabilitation, particularly with education for health given on an individual or collective basis. We use the French version [20] of a QOL questionnaire for patients with oropharyngeal dysphagia (SWAL-QOL) [21, 22] to explore the efficiency of rehabilitation to improve quality of life. The SWAL-QOL is a self-report questionnaire of QOL specific to dysphagic patients. It contains 44 items and explores the burden of difficulties, food selection, eating duration, eating desire, fear, sleep, fatigue, communication, mental health, and social impact of swallowing disorders. We use the total SWAL-QOL score, the "burden" score, and the "symptoms of dysphagia" QOL score. We interviewed eight older patients who were matched for age, cognitive level, and social support. Four patients received the dysphagia education for health program in group, and four were seen individually. They were assessed at admission and 3 months after following the program or at discharge. The scores were low in all

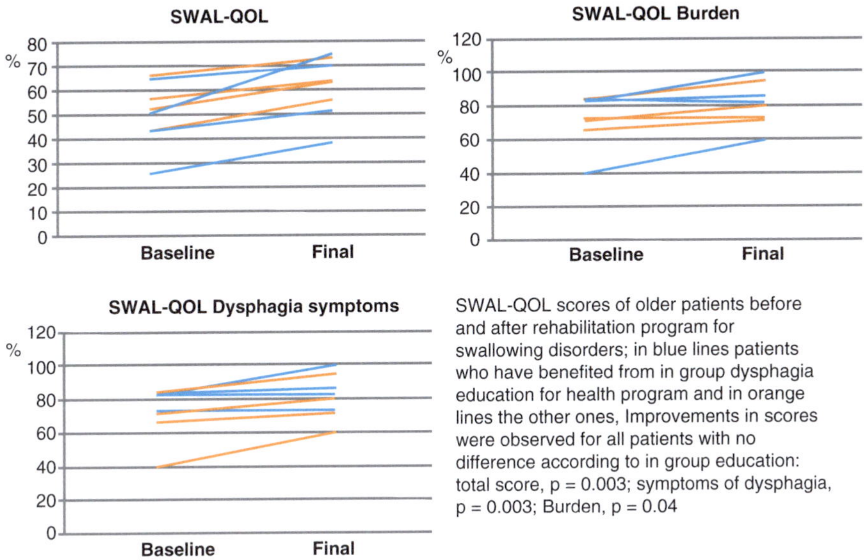

Fig. 38.6 SWAL-QOL changes after rehabilitation

subjects. After rehabilitation scores of all patients improved (Fig. 38.6). Indeed, we may expect better improvement in patient compliance owing to the dynamic of the group although this was not observed; during group sessions subjects have the possibility to face other patients with similar symptoms they have; they recognized themselves in other patients for a better involvement in the learning. Real-life feedback is also a means to link the swallowing disorders and complications that some of them may have experienced. In addition, the exchange of information and impressions between participants helps them to work out new recipes that combine pleasure on the palate and safe eating.

38.8 Sharing of Information

The way information is written down and passed on from one person to another is a critical issue in the management of older dysphagic patients, so that quality of care and safe eating are ensured. Material can be in the form of written instructions but also photos or drawings of adequate postures or food textures. These instructions must be updated as the patient's situation changes. These documents should be easy to find and to use and close to where meals are prepared and eaten.

In conclusion, care for elderly dysphagic subjects is not limited to specific rehabilitation which is sometimes difficult to administer owing to their exhaustion, cognitive and mood disorders, as well as to the frequently multifactorial causes of their difficulties. Beyond curative medical or surgical treatment, adaptive strategies should seek to limit the occurrence of complications and to offer satisfying taste and nutrition. It may be difficult for patients and families to accept and implement these recommendations because the topic is highly personal and has symbolic overtones. Thus, each member of the multidisciplinary team has his own role to play to ensure the long-term efficiency of rehabilitation. Education for health that is centered on the patient and involves the family may promote active participation and have a greater effect on quality of life and safety.

References

1. Sundberg L, Agahi N, Fritzell J, Fors S (2016) Trends in health expectancies among the oldest old in Sweden, 1992–2011. Eur J Pub Health 26(6):1069–1074. doi:10.1093/eurpub/ckw066. PubMed PMID: 27175003
2. Poisson P, Laffond T, Campos S, Dupuis V, Bourdel-Marchasson I (2014) Relationships between oral health, dysphagia and undernutrition in hospitalised elderly patients. Gerodontology 33(2):161–168. doi:10.1111/ger.12123. PubMed PMID: 24612262
3. Rofes L, Arreola V, Almirall J, Cabre M, Campins L, Garcia-Peris P et al (2011) Diagnosis and management of oropharyngeal Dysphagia and its nutritional and respiratory complications in the elderly. Gastroenterol Res Pract 2011. doi:10.1155/2011/818979. PubMed PMID: 20811545; PubMed Central PMCID: PMCPMC2929516
4. Timmerman AA, Speyer R, Heijnen BJ, Klijn-Zwijnenberg IR (2014) Psychometric characteristics of health-related quality-of-life questionnaires in oropharyngeal dysphagia. Dysphagia 29(2):183–198. doi:10.1007/s00455-013-9511-8. PubMed PMID: 24590284
5. Humbert IA, Robbins J (2008) Dysphagia in the elderly. Phys Med Rehabil Clin N Am 19(4):853–66, ix–x. doi:10.1016/j.pmr.2008.06.002. PubMed PMID: 18940645; PubMed Central PMCID: PMCPMC3182519
6. Woisard-Bassols V, Puech M (2011) La réhabilitation de la déglutition chez l'adulte: le point sur la prise en charge fonctionnelle. Solal, Marseille
7. Wright L, Cotter D, Hickson M, Frost G (2005) Comparison of energy and protein intakes of older people consuming a texture modified diet with a normal hospital diet. J Hum Nutr Diet 18(3):213–219. doi:10.1111/j.1365-277X.2005.00605.x. PubMed PMID: 15882384
8. Singh S, Hamdy S (2006) Dysphagia in stroke patients. Postgrad Med J 82(968):383–391. doi:10.1136/pgmj.2005.043281. PubMed PMID: 16754707; PubMed Central PMCID: PMCPMC2563739
9. Lazzara G, Lazarus C, Logemann J (1986) Impact of thermal stimulation on the triggering of the swallowing reflex. Dysphagia 1:73–77
10. Logemann JA, Gibbons P, Rademaker AW, Pauloski BR, Kahrilas PJ, Bacon M et al (1994) Mechanisms of recovery of swallow after supraglottic laryngectomy. J Speech Hear Res 37(5):965–974. PubMed PMID: 7823564
11. BJW M (1994) Treatment of dysphagia in adults. In: Cherney LR (ed) Clinical management of dysphagia in adults and children. Aspen Publishers, Inc., Gaithersburg, pp 153–183
12. Shaker R, Easterling C, Kern M, Nitschke T, Massey B, Daniels S et al (2002) Rehabilitation of swallowing by exercise in tube-fed patients with pharyngeal dysphagia secondary to abnormal UES opening. Gastroenterology 122(5):1314–1321. PubMed PMID: 11984518
13. Reddy NP, Simcox DL, Gupta V, Motta GE, Coppenger J, Das A et al (2000) Biofeedback therapy using accelerometry for treating dysphagic patients with poor laryngeal elevation: case studies. J Rehabil Res Dev 37(3):361–372. PubMed PMID: 10917268
14. Bogaardt HC, Grolman W, Fokkens WJ (2009) The use of biofeedback in the treatment of chronic dysphagia in stroke patients. Folia Phoniatr Logop 61(4):200–205. doi:10.1159/000227997. PubMed PMID: 19590219
15. Larsen GL (1973) Conservative management for incomplete dysphagia paralytica. Arch Phys Med Rehabil 54(4):180–185. PubMed PMID: 4697225

16. Steele CM, Alsanei WA, Ayanikalath S, Barbon CE, Chen J, Cichero JA et al (2015) The influence of food texture and liquid consistency modification on swallowing physiology and function: a systematic review. Dysphagia 30(1):2–26. doi:10.1007/s00455-014-9578-x. PubMed PMID: 25343878; PubMed Central PMCID: PMCPMC4342510
17. Terre R, Mearin F (2012) Effectiveness of chin-down posture to prevent tracheal aspiration in dysphagia secondary to acquired brain injury. A videofluoroscopy study. Neurogastroenterol Motil 24(5):414–9, e206. doi:10.1111/j.1365-2982.2011.01869.x. PubMed PMID: 22309385
18. Plowman-Prine EK, Sapienza CM, Okun MS, Pollock SL, Jacobson C, Wu SS et al (2009) The relationship between quality of life and swallowing in Parkinson's disease. Mov Disord 24(9):1352–1358. doi:10.1002/mds.22617. PubMed PMID: 19425089; PubMed Central PMCID: PMCPMC3614344
19. Barofsky I (1978) Compliance, adherence and the therapeutic alliance: steps in the development of self-care. Soc Sci Med 12(5A):369–376. PubMed PMID: 705382
20. Khaldoun E, Woisard V, Verin E (2009) Validation in French of the SWAL-QOL scale in patients with oropharyngeal dysphagia. Gastroenterol Clin Biol 33(3):167–171. doi:10.1016/j.gcb.2008.12.012. PubMed PMID: 19250781
21. McHorney CA, Bricker DE, Kramer AE, Rosenbek JC, Robbins J, Chignell KA et al (2000) The SWAL-QOL outcomes tool for oropharyngeal dysphagia in adults: I. Conceptual foundation and item development. Dysphagia 15(3):115–121. doi:10.1007/s004550010012. PubMed PMID: 10839823
22. McHorney CA, Bricker DE, Robbins J, Kramer AE, Rosenbek JC, Chignell KA (2000) The SWAL-QOL outcomes tool for oropharyngeal dysphagia in adults: II. Item reduction and preliminary scaling. Dysphagia 15(3):122–133. doi:10.1007/s004550010013. PubMed PMID: 10839824

The Aging Effects in Spinal Cord Injury Rehabilitation

39

H.A. Cerrel Bazo, E. Demertzis, and A. Musumeci

39.1 Introduction

Over the past decades, the prevalence of spinal injuries among older adults has been increasing. In fact, the occurrence of spinal cord injuries among individuals aged 70 and older has increased almost fivefold, passing from 4 to 15% in the past 30 years [1].

The increasing survival trend of the elderly population in Westernized countries due to "*traumatic*" *spinal cord injury* (TSCI) which is secondary to falls and car accidents is not only due to increased life expectancy but also to a better and prompt intervention of the emergency medical system (EMS) [2]. As for the general population, the elder SCI patient requires not only specialized medical care and rehabilitation but also easy access to environments suitable for wheelchairs, appropriate homecare, adequate equipment, transportation, and financial support. SCI specialists will need to be aware that older individuals may have an increased incidence of other cumulative illnesses (e.g., ischemic heart disease, hypertension, cardiac failure, diabetes mellitus, anemia, cerebrovascular, etc.) and the identification of the SCI may be delayed, the symptoms manifested being difficult to understand and examine. Indeed delays in presentation of illness can be related to communication disturbances (deafness, confusion, aphasia, dysarthria), impaired memory (many times difficulties in obtaining a clear history), and lack of understanding of own symptoms: "It's only my age."

Assessment in elder subjects may be hampered by restlessness or fatigue, and diseases may present in atypical ways because of altered physiology (e.g., impaired homeostatic control of blood pressure or temperature) or others.

H.A. Cerrel Bazo (✉)
Spinal Cord Injury and Severe Acquired Brain Injury Center, Rehabilitation Hospital at High Level of Specialization of Motta di Livenza, Treviso, Italy
e-mail: hcb57@yahoo.com

E. Demertzis • A. Musumeci
Rehabilitation Unit, Department of Neurosciences, University of Padua, Padua, Italy
e-mail: sunny.elena@libero.it; alfredomusumeci@yahoo.com

© Springer International Publishing AG 2018

S. Masiero, U. Carraro (eds.), *Rehabilitation Medicine for Elderly Patients*, Practical Issues in Geriatrics, DOI 10.1007/978-3-319-57406-6_39

According to Menter and Hudson, normal aging involves three processes [3]: (1) the physiologic changes of the body itself, (2) the individual's change in social roles, and (3) self-realization, all overlapped but distinctly different. As individuals age, they experience a variety of new and unanticipated issues; these may include medical, functional, socioeconomic, and support problems. Individuals experience changes and functional declines in all body systems as they age. The rates of decline vary from individual to individual, depending on genetics, body habitus, lifestyle, and general state of health. Williams and Hadler have demonstrated the variation in the rate of decline for the different organ systems in the body [4]. Katzman has also illustrated the differing rates of decline between the pulmonary system and the peripheral nervous system; the study demonstrated a 60% decline in pulmonary function for individuals by age 80 and 15% decline of nerve conduction velocity. All this considerations may also apply for the people as they get older and become ill having a trauma and/or a spinal cord injury; in this regard, elders with spinal cord injury seem to show worst outcomes in personal and social life as well as of life satisfaction, showing greater vulnerability after SCI [5].

39.2 What Is a Spinal Cord Injury?

While there is debate about what is contemplated as "spinal cord injury" (SCI) and/or "spinal cord disorder" (SCI/D), all lesions to the *spinal cord*, *conus medullaris*, and *cauda equina* (inside the vertebral canal) are considered within the context of this definition.

The spinal cord injury (SCI) affects conduction of sensory, motor, autonomic nervous system (ANS) signals across the site(s) of lesion(s), generating a clinical picture of paraplegia [sensory and/or motor loss (paralysis) in the trunk and legs] or quadriplegia [sensory and motor loss in the arms, body, and legs] both accompanied by dysfunctional bowel and bladder activity and/or cardiorespiratory and circulatory malfunction, temperature/sweating disturbances as well as sexual/erectile dysfunction.

SCI is a medically complex and life-disrupting condition, one of the most invalidating pathologies in the field of rehabilitation.

Damage to the spinal cord may be traumatic or non-traumatic. Traumatic SCI (TSCI) can result from many different causes—including falls, motor vehicle injuries, occupational and sports injuries, and violence. Non-traumatic SCI (NTSCI) or spinal cord disorder, on the other hand, usually involves an underlying pathology—such as infectious disease, oncology disorders, musculoskeletal disease such as osteoarthritis, and congenital problems such as spina bifida. Generally speaking, the higher up the spinal cord injury, the more extensive the range of impairments will be.

The extent and severity of the SCI depends not only on the level of injury but also on whether the lesion is *complete* or *incomplete*. According to the International Standards for Neurological Classification of SCI [6], a spinal cord injury is considered complete if there is absence of the *sacral sparing*, meaning loss of voluntary motor and/or sensory control of the anal sphincter and deep anal region (S4/5). On the contrary, the presence of the *sacral sparing* is true for the incomplete lesions.

Table 39.1 The following is the International Standards for Neurological Classification of SCI and the American Spinal Injuries Association Impairment Scale (AIS)

A—No motor or sensory function below the level of the lesion
B—No motor function below the level of the lesion but sensory function that continues into the sacral segments
C—Most motor function below the level of the lesion preserved, and more than half of key muscles have a motor grade of 3 or less
D—Most motor function below the level of the lesion preserved, and more than half of key muscles have a motor grade of greater than 3
E—Normal motor and sensory function

The neurologic examination (motor and sensory index) within the first 20–40 days (after the spinal shock) following a spinal cord injury is able to predict neurologic recovery with great accuracy. According to the International Standards for Neurological Classification of SCI [6] and the American Spinal Injuries Association Impairment Scale (AIS), the SCI can be classified as complete or incomplete. Complete lesions are defined as AIS A, and incomplete lesions are defined as AIS B, AIS C, AIS D, or AIS E (see Table 39.1).

The neurological recovery below the level of SCI is possible, but patients in Asia A generally show no significant recovery (5% or less) in this area a year after SCI. Individuals who are classified ASIA B have approximately a 35% chance of improving to grade C or D and almost none (statistically significant) to grade E 1 year after the SCI. Instead, those classified initially with grades C can improve to grade D with a likelihood of 60–70% [7].

In addition to physical examination, MRI examination of the spinal cord can provide information regarding future recovery. Hemorrhage within the cord is suggestive of an unfavorable prognosis, with a better prognosis for improvement suggested by (in order) contusion, edema, and a normal appearance of the cord.

39.3 An Onset View of the SCI in the Elderly and Its Medical Complications Resulting Therefrom

Early onset SCI differs from late onset SCI in elderly patients can occur in (A) those injured when young but with a long history of SCI who then have reached old age, known as *early onset*, and (B) those whose SCI onset have arrived when senior, known as *late onset* (see Table 39.2). While both types can be the result of TSCI or NTSCI causes, TSCI happens less frequently in older patients in whom SCI is a consequence of falls or motor vehicle accident (MVA).

Early Onset SCI elderly by early onset differ from SCI seniors from late onset. In this sense, SCI can exacerbate the physical and physiologic declines—including in the musculoskeletal system, cardiovascular, gastrointestinal (GI), pulmonary, and integumentary accompanied by the aging process. A number of long-term follow-up studies and many authors have documented the tendency for individuals with SCI to

Table 39.2 Elderly with spinal cord injury and clinical onset

	Early onset	Late onset
1. SCI?	Injured young, long history of SCI, have reached old age	Those whose SCI onset have arrived when senior
2. Physical and physiologic declines	SCI onset ≤15 years old, the **maintenance phase** last ≥20 years SCI onset ≥20 years old, the **functional decline phase** is "quick" and aging speed at a much younger age	The **acute phase** can last longer, the **maintenance phase** is short, **and** the **functional decline phase** is "quick"
3. SCI perpetuating degenerative effects	Present	Present
4. Physical capacity reduction	Reduced	Incredibly reduced
5. Pneumonia, kidney stone, decubitus ulcer	Often in tetraplegia	Often in paraplegia/tetraplegia
6. Premorbid medical conditions	Is rare, minor	Frequent and complicated

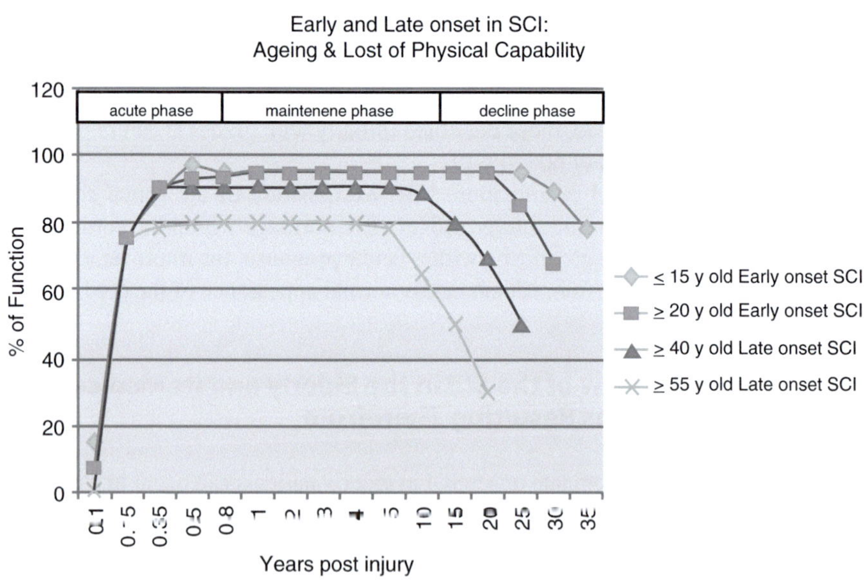

Fig. 39.1 Aging and loss of physical capability (capacity) in SCI individuals

age more rapidly than the population of able-bodied. That means, individuals with SCI develop characteristics and medical problems commonly associated with the aging process at a much younger age. Kempt talking about Long-Term Outcomes with Disability, during the Rancho Los Amigos Seminar in 1998, said that younger individuals whose SCI onset was during or prior to adolescence may enjoy a maintenance phase of 20 years prior to experiencing functional decline (see Fig. 39.1).

Cushman and Hassett found that, in people with SCI of 15 years or more, 93% of them had experienced a decline in functional status [8]. A study by Smith et al. found that in adults with long-term disability—specifically, SCI, multiple sclerosis, muscular dystrophy, or post-polio syndrome—the development of chronic comorbid medical conditions is associated with factors such as body mass index, waist circumference, and the existence of another chronic comorbidity [9].

Late Onset According to Kempt (Rancho Los Amigos Seminar 1998), individuals who are aged 55 years at the onset of their SCI may only have 5–7 years of relatively stable functioning status prior to experiencing a decline. In fact older people may have premorbid medical conditions associated that can determine poorer end results of the rehabilitation process. In one US study conducted during the 1970s and 1980s, 24.3% of persons with SCI who were above 60 years old at injury had arthritis, 8.6% had significant heart disease, 4.3% had diabetes, and 4.3% were obese [10, 11]. Above age 61, there is a greater risk of diabetes, heart disease, obesity and arthritis, poorer outcomes with respect to walking, and more difficulties with bladder and bowel independence. Long-term medical complication rates increase with both older age and greater injury severity [12–16]. During the 5th post-injury year, among persons who are >60 years of age, 7.1% develop pneumonia, and 29.5% have abnormal renal function. The corresponding figures for persons >40 years of age are 2.2% for pneumonia and 10.2% for abnormal renal function. The long-term odds of developing a kidney stone are 50% higher for persons who are at least 55 years of age compared with those who are aged 25–34 and 90% higher for persons with complete tetraplegia compared with persons with AIS D injuries [13]. There is also an increased risk of pressure ulcers among the elderly, and they play an important role in rehabilitation outcomes [17–19]. The odds of developing a pressure ulcer are 30% higher among persons who are at least 50 years of age compared with those who are aged 15–29 [20]. However, advanced age appears to be related not only to the frequency of pressure ulcers but also to their severity. In fact an aging-related decrease in muscle mass and vascularity may reduce the tolerance of aged skin to pressure and shearing forces, consequently leading to the development of pressure ulcers [21]. In any case, the vast majority of young and/or seniors with SCI after discharge from an intensive rehabilitation center can become sedentary on a wheelchair, not participating much in physical activities [22, 23], exposed to *severe degenerative effects* that perpetuate (see Table 39.3).

Table 39.3 Degenerative effects in spinal cord injury individuals

Perpetuating degenerative effects in SCI
Severe muscle atrophy [24–28], edema [29], deep vein thrombosis [30]
Restrictive lung disorders [31], reduction of the cardiopulmonary fitness [32, 33]
Depression, chronic pain syndrome [27]
Recurrent urinary tract infection (UTI), sexual dysfunction [34]
Obesity and HDL reduction [35–39]
Osteoporosis [40], fractures [40, 41]
Spasticity [42, 43]
Decubitus ulcer [11, 44]

Table 39.4 Secondary medical complications in SCI

Thromboembolic disease: **DVT** Decubitus ulcer
Autonomic dysfunction: • **Orthostatic hypotension** • **Bradycardia** • **Autonomic dysreflexia**
Neurogenic bladder and sex dysfunction
Neurogenic bowel dysfunction
Heterotopic ossification Spasticity Depression

Despite the age of SCI onset, a consequent physical capacity (capability) reduction, like in the sedentary lifestyle from SCI, is a condition that definitively can offer health deterioration, increasing the risk of medical complications secondary to a chronic disability status [34]. It's known that the physical capability in individuals with spinal cord injury is directly related to independence in ADLs (activities of daily living), and it's extremely necessary to keep the physical capacity of these individuals after discharge. In contrary, self-independence in a wheelchair is not enough to keep the patient healthy. Studies on wheelchair users with SCI indicated that those who maintain a more active lifestyle by regularly participating in exercise and sports programs can increase their muscle strength, aerobic fitness, and physical performance to levels well above those of their sedentary cohorts [45–48]. As in the able-bodied population, physical capability for SCI appears to decline with age [10]. Among SCI in general and in particular in persons >60 years of age at injury, 47% had at least one pressure sore during initial hospitalization, 30% developed pneumonia, 11.4% had deep vein thrombosis, 10% had a gastrointestinal hemorrhage, and 5.7% had a renal stone [10, 11] (see Table 39.4).

39.4 Effects of Aging in Spinal Cord Injury

The aging process for some groups of people with disabilities begins earlier than usual. Some people with developmental disabilities show signs of premature aging in their 40s and 50s [21], and they may experience age-related health conditions more frequently. The aging process and associated changes (presbycusis, deconditioning, loss of strength and balance, osteoporosis) may have a greater impact on people with disabilities. Those with existing mobility impairments (like in SCI individuals) may increasingly experience functional loss as they age [49] (see Fig. 39.1). Generally speaking, normal aging is associated with a reduction in functional reserve capacity in tissues and organs. The following are some of the physiological changes that may be expected with aging in the SCI population:

Cardiovascular Changes The incidence of cardiovascular disease among individuals with SCI is over 200% higher than the expected incidence in an age- and gender-matched control population (Kocina et al.) [50]. In individuals surviving 30 years or longer following SCI, nearly 50% of all deaths occur due to premature cardiovascular disease (CVD) [51].

Besides the autonomic dysfunction in SCI, hypertension, HDL decrease, reduced exercise tolerance, platelet aggregation, obesity, and reduced venous return (due to decrease in sympathetic tone and a reduction in the muscular pumping action of the lower extremities) are some of the causes that lead to myocardial infarcts and diabetes in elderly SCI individuals. Up to 75% of the SCI population are overweight or obese [52] and have adipose tissue deposited particularly around the abdomen, increasing the risk for developing CVD. Disruption of the autonomic nervous system and from the normal cardiovascular control mechanisms also contributes to heightened cardiovascular risk, with changes to peripheral vasculature, blood pressure abnormalities, heart rate variability, occurrence of cardiac arrhythmias, and a blunted cardiovascular response to exercise, limiting the capacity to perform physical activity [53].

Pulmonary Changes Following SCI, respiratory complications are the most common cause of death [54–57]. The spectrum of pulmonary complications following SCI includes respiratory failure, pneumonia, atelectasis, pulmonary thromboembolism, sleep apnea disorders, dyspnea, and dysphonia. But, what are the pathophysiological issues that are at the basis of respiratory problems in spinal cord injury? In these patients, the reduction in lung compliance was attributed to reduced lung volume and changes in the mechanical properties of the lung due to alterations in the surfactant, which can occur quickly with low lung volume ventilation [56]. The inefficiency of the respiratory system contributes to the risk of respiratory muscle fatigue, particularly during pneumonia and/or airway obstruction. During inspiratory resistive-loaded inhalation in tetraplegia, the causes of inefficiency during the inspiratory acts are due to the decrease of the lower transverse dimension of the rib cage; the diaphragm does not work close to its optimal length for the tension production. In complete C2 SCI and below, there is a reduction of predicted vital capacity (VC) of 20–50%, inefficiency in ventilation, and markedly impaired cough, due to changes in lung compliance, chest-wall distortion, and impairment in both muscles of inhalation and exhalation.

Diminished pulmonary function can result from restrictive disease, obstructive disease, or a combination of these. In spinal cord injury (SCI), restrictive lung disease occurs as a result of respiratory muscle paralysis. The higher the level of SCI, the greater the restrictive impairment. Weakened muscles of inhalation prevent deep breaths, and some patients with quadriplegia may not sigh, leading to atelectasis and related gas-exchange and lung-compliance abnormalities. Dysfunctional muscles of exhalation cause impaired cough and secretion clearance (with associated atelectasis), increase in airways resistance, and persistence of infection when it occurs [56] (see Fig. 39.2).

The development of kyphosis, scoliosis, or increasing spasticity can cause further restrictive disease as the individual with SCI ages.

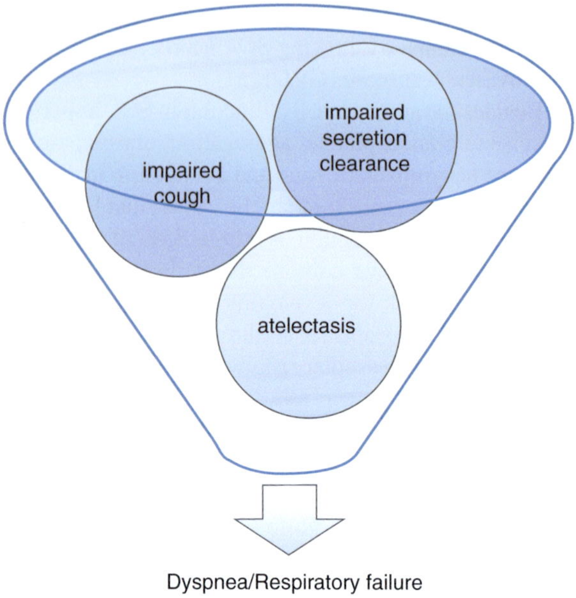

Fig. 39.2 Dysfunctional muscles of exhalation in SCI can cause respiratory failure

Sleep apnea reportedly occurs in 40% of individuals with SCI. The frequency of obstructive sleep apnea increases with age. Of those individuals with SCI who experience sleep apnea, only 25% have been found to be obese. The long-term use of baclofen may be associated with the development of obstructive sleep apnea.

Neurological Changes The peripheral nervous system (PNS) acts as the trait d'union for communication between the central nervous system (CNS)/brain and the limbs, organs, and tissues of the rest of the body, transmitting signals to coordinate actions. The reaction time which these signals coordinate the aforementioned actions seems to deteriorate during the aging process. In SCI individuals, there is little evidence to show that neither the PNS nor CNS prematurely declines in these people [58].

Neuropathic pain (NP) is common following SCI and can substantially reduce the person's ability to function and their quality of life. Neuropathic pain typically occurs at the SCI level or below of the lesion being characterized by physical characteristics such as temperature (e.g., hot, burning, sunburned, frostbitten) and electricity (e.g., an electric shock, tingling, stabbing, shooting pain). Pain can be apart from any external stimulus (rest pain) or can result from a stimulus that, under normal conditions, wouldn't cause pain (allodynia), or pain can be excessive in response to a painful stimulus (hyperalgesia). The NP may be intermittent or constant and may fluctuate in intensity. These symptoms may result from a reactive synaptogenesis changes in central neuronal function, altering thresholds of the pain response. The evaluation of neuropathic pain following SCI requires knowledge about spine biomechanics, spine neurophysiology, and differentiation between mechanical versus neuropathic origin of the pain. The underlying condition many times is not identified but sometimes may be due to syringomyelia, scar tissue, tethering cord, unstable spine, posttraumatic cyst formation, and others. NP may be exacerbated by the weather change and at times by an unrelated disease or medical complications (e.g., renal stone, urinary tract infection, fecaloma). Patients are relieved to be informed that their pain need not reflect any active problem and need not cause them to curtail their activities. Indeed, an increased level of activity may decrease suffering [59]. Neuropathic pain can be exacerbated by many conditions, but there is no evidence to suggest that neuropathic pain increases with age [60]. Early onset of pain in people with SCI is a strong predictor of future pain. Approximately two-thirds of people with SCI experienced some form of pain, with one-third of these reporting severe pain [61]. People with pain related to their SCI are often unable to gain significant relief from pharmacological medications or have to discontinue their use due to side effects [61]. Psychosocial and environmental factors have been shown to play a key part in the experience of chronic pain in people with SCI [62].

Posttraumatic syringomyelia is a progressive enlargement of a cystic cavity (or syrinx), which originates at the site of injury in the spinal cord, and may also occur in people with SCI, causing neurologic deterioration [63]. Onset may take months to years after injury, being heralded by changes in neuropathic pain, or spasticity, deterioration in function with an ascending sensory loss with or without motor weakness, or, sometimes, autonomic symptoms such as increased sweating.

According to Young, spasticity (SPS) is a "velocity dependent increase in muscle tone with exaggerated tendon jerks resulting in hyper-excitability of the stretch reflex" in combination with other features of the upper motor neuron syndrome [43]. Furthermore, Young had divided the characteristic signs of upper motor neuron damage in positive and negative. The positive ones include increase of muscle tone and tendon jerks, clonus, extensor stretch reflexes, and released flexor reflexes such as Babinski reflex. The negative ones are paresis, loss of fine motor control and loss of dexterity, increased fatigability of muscles, and hypotonia in early phase of upper motor neuron damage.

Clinically, spasticity causes resistance to passive motion of the limbs, exaggerated deep tendon reflexes, clonus, and involuntary co-contraction of muscle groups. SPS can follow complete and incomplete SCI. Usually SCI is immediately followed by a period of flaccidity, with spasticity developing over weeks. SPS has favorable effects as well as unfavorable. It can be used to assist with mobility, can improve circulation, and may be useful for decreasing the risk of deep venous thrombosis and osteoporosis. On the other hand, spasticity can interfere with positioning, mobility, and hygiene, and spasms can be painful. When making a decision to intervene, one must take into consideration both the positive and the negative aspects of a patient's spasticity and the degree and type of the patient's spasticity.

According to our knowledge, there is no evidence to show the change of the symptoms of spasticity in SCI individuals during the years or a long-term effect of the treatment of spasticity.

Immediately after SCI, the presence of pain appears to be the best predictor of future pain, and this likely does not change significantly over time [64, 65].

In general, there is a continued dearth of knowledge regarding the aging SCI nervous system.

Depression and Cognitive Functioning In people with SCI, depression affects the subject in different ways. It affects mood, ambition, outlook, problem solving, and energy levels. It works against wellness and health and against having a good quality of life. Individuals with SCI who are depressed often have more difficulty looking after themselves and managing their medical condition; they may have difficulty managing a correct diet, drinking sufficient water, taking care of their skin, taking medications, and posturing correctly on a wheelchair. Although depression is common among people with SCI, many people with SCI never experience an episode of depression. Aging with an SCI/D is more difficult for women. McColl [66] found that age, gender, and disability result in an excess of depression among older women with SCI. Krause [67] and co-workers suggested that minorities in SCI are at greater risk for depression, particularly minority women, but that education and income largely account for the elevated risk. This study also reported that individuals who were older at SCI onset, beginning with the ages of 30–39, were at greater risk for both presence of clinically significant symptoms of depression and major depression. They conclude saying that "symptoms of depression are highly prevalent after SCI and are related to aging, gender or ethnicity, and socioeconomic status indicators (education and income)." The older the individual at SCI, the more dramatic the adaptation required.

In response to aging with SCI, it is difficult to say that those who have lived the longest with SCI have experienced the higher levels of depression or if the onset of depression is consequent to the secondary conditions resulting from aging [8]. In our experience, working with SCI for a long time, like for the general population, behavior and emotion in response to an injury are a complex interaction of own personality, social/family support, level of education, and economic possibilities. In essence, every SCI, and every person with SCI, is different, and the coping mechanism to the SCI seems to depend more to the social support of the individual, level of education, and economic support rather than his or her unique personality or his level of injury; currently, no one can accurately predict who or when one of these individuals will become depressed. Healthcare providers need to look out for the signs and symptoms of psychological stress and provide quality information and support to people in a time-appropriate manner. Recommendations for maintaining psychological health include maintaining social connections and being proactive within the community, doing physical activity, encouraging the uptake of a hobby/activity, and making sure the person with SCI knows when to ask for help, should he need it.

Cognitive impairment following SCI is high and seems to reach 40–50% of SCI [68]. However, such deficits are frequently attributed to concomitant brain injury [69–73] or to premorbid conditions such as poor intellectual or occupational functioning [74], previous brain injuries, alcoholism or drug abuse [69], low blood pressure [75], and psychiatric disorders. Some studies exploring cognitive functioning following SCI in the absence of the abovementioned conditions report deficits in processing speed, learning, memory, and attention [71, 76]. When concomitant head injury is ruled out, one prominent explanation for such deficits involves secondary changes to brain organization or activity resulting from SCI [77]. Reactive depression has also been highlighted as a possible source of cognitive decline [78–80] and negative influence on cognitive performance [81]. Finally, recent research showing changes in spinal excitability [82] and plasticity [83] during learning supports the possibility that decline in certain cognitive functions is linked to spinal cord damage directly. Kowalczyk et al. [84] demonstrated that the alterations found in motor function in cervical myelopathy secondary to degenerative disease and spinal cord compression are due not only to local effects of spinal compression but also to distal effects related to cortical reorganization and decreased N-acetylaspartate/creatine in the motor cortex. This study may shed light about some important changes that can happen with aging with SCI. Myelopathy secondary to degenerative disease in older individuals may well represent a model of aging with SCI. In this sense, changes in brain function that may occur may not only be a fruit of natural aging, but instead SCI and spinal cord compression can influence not only the spinal cord and its functions but also the brain function, determining a change in the reorganization of the cortical motor cortex.

Gastrointestinal Changes Bowel disturbances such as constipation, distension, abdominal pain, rectal bleeding, hemorrhoids, bowel accidents, and autonomic hyperreflexia occur in 27–62% of SCI patients. With the aging process, the SCI aggravates the dysfunctions of neurological intestine [85].

(a) *Dysphagia*: This is present in 22.5–30% of patients with SCI and is related to age, to the presence of a tracheostomy, to the effects of mechanical ventilation [86], and to cervical spinal surgery (anterior approach). As a result, dysphagia can be the consequence of three pathological causes: (a) direct compression of the aerodigestive tract and associated nerves, as well as local inflammation that leads to mucosal edema, formation of adhesions, fibrosis, and cricopharyngeal spasms; (b) swelling of prevertebral soft tissue, due to repetitive mechanical trauma (i.e., dynamic constant movement of the pharyngo-laryngo-esophageal complex over a rigid structure/bony protuberance), causing a small movement of the pharyngeal wall, altered upper esophageal sphincter opening, incomplete epiglottic deflection, and a vallecular, piriform sinus and posterior pharyngeal wall food residue; and (c) presence of several anatomical structures at risk of damage during the anterior cervical spine surgery. Surgical procedures involving the cervical spine C3 or higher can lead to damages of cranial nerves glossopharyngeal (IX) and hypoglossal (XII), while those made in the C3–4 region endanger the superior laryngeal nerve (SLN).

    A deficit in the oral phase of swallowing points out a possible damage of cranial nerves hypoglossal and glossopharyngeal, compromising the propulsive action of the tongue. Weakened pharyngeal swallowing suggests disruption of pharyngeal plexus and the pharyngeal muscles, which can occur with injury to the SLN [87]. The vagus nerve, although normally protected by the carotid sheath during anterior cervical exposures, is vulnerable to retraction injury at any subaxial cervical levels.

(b) *Pýrōsis or heartburn*: This symptom is the result of incomplete upper esophageal sphincter relaxation, while resting upper and lower esophageal sphincter pressures may be normal. Delay with gastric emptying (GE), recumbency position, immobilization, and the use of certain drugs (such as anticholinergics and meperidine) predispose to pýrōsis. Heartburn may predispose some SCI patients to lung aspiration or "ab ingestis" pneumonia. Gastric emptying (GE) times increase directly with the higher level of the SCI and the increased duration of injury. Intravenous metoclopramide, a potent dopamine receptor antagonist with prokinetic properties, corrects impaired GE [88, 89].

(c) *Fecal impaction*: This is a common GI complication in SCI [90, 92]. It is related to reduction of colonic mass movements and inability to use abdominal muscles to assist in defecation. Inadequate dietary fiber and water intake is the primary cause, but lack of mobility and the inability to use abdominal muscles in the aging population of SCI patients can predispose to this disorder more often. Constipation in complete SCI may also be related to previous urinary outlet surgery and the use of anticholinergic agents to manage the neurogenic bladder [88].

Patients may present with loss of appetite and nausea and are mistakenly given antinausea preparations, most of which have anticholinergic and constipating properties. Liquid stool may pass around the blockage. Plain films of the abdomen show the feces and abnormal air patterns. Treatment involves digital disimpaction and proximal or distal washout and anal fragmentation of the hardened stool palpable in the rectum. At times manual disimpaction may be aided by the use of an anal retractor.

Oral solution of polyethylene glycol (PEG) solutions is used to soften or wash out proximal stool. Oral regimens vary from 1 to 2 L of PEG with electrolytes or 17 g of PEG 3350 in 120 to 240 mL of water every 15 min until the patient begins passing stool or eight glasses have been consumed [91]. This technique is contraindicated when a bowel obstruction exists.

Enemas and suppositories are used as distal softening agents. Most enema solutions contain water and an osmotic agent (one of such combinations contains water, docusate sodium syrup, and sorbitol). When the impaction has been adequately treated, possible etiologies are explored. A total colonic evaluation (colonoscopy or barium enema) should be performed to reveal anatomic abnormalities (stricture or malignancy). Endocrine and metabolic screening, including thyroid function tests, is also indicated [92].

When the abovementioned methods of fecal evacuation have failed, cisapride, a 5-HT4 serotoninergic agonist drug facilitating the release of acetylcholine at the myenteric plexus, can be used. Cisapride is able to increase gastrointestinal motility especially in the small intestine and colon, but one of its most feared adverse effects is the appearance of a long QT syndrome that can predispose the individual to torsades de pointes and often fatal arrhythmia (for that reason it has been taken off the market in the USA).

Neostigmine is a drug, which increases cholinergic tone by blocking the metabolism of acetylcholine by acetylcholinesterase and can be effective in the treatment of constipation. It was tested in combination with glycopyrrolate (an anticholinergic agent that reduces bradycardia and bronchoconstriction caused by neostigmine) [93].

(d) *Megacolon*: Although SCI age over 50 years presented an almost threefold increase in risk for the presence of megacolon, the origin of megacolon is not well understood. Two hypotheses seem to support the origin; the first is the acquired origin, and the second is the level of spinal cord injury.

In supporting the acquired origin hypothesis of megacolon, Harari and Minaker reported that, in the first 5 years of SCI, it is rare for the phenomenon of constipation to occur and a post-injury period of 10 years or more placed patients at an almost fourfold greater risk of having megacolon. This finding supports the abovementioned hypothesis, stating that the problem is acquired, possibly through degeneration or decompensation of smooth muscle in the intestine [94]. Following the paralysis of the peristaltic movements of the intestine, the colon loses its shape acquiring an abnormal dilated form. Distressing symptoms such as prolonged and difficult evacuation, recurrent abdominal distension, and abdominal pain tend to develop, and standard treatments for constipation become less effective. As the use of laxatives and suppositories increases, so does the incidence of bowel bloating, nausea, and fecal impaction, and as a consequence, the megacolon develops.

The second hypothesis finds its support studying the chronic SCI; some researchers believe that most likely the pathophysiological events responsible for the abnormal dilatation of the colon depend from the level of SCI [90, 94, 95].

Potential complications of megacolon in SCI are colonic volvulus, sigmoid volvulus following sigmoid colectomy, fecal impaction, autonomic dysreflexia, dyspnea, weight loss, malnutrition, feelings of anxiety, and loss of self-confidence. The management from megacolon can end with surgical treatment, and the colostomy is the suggested treatment.

The Malone antegrade continence enema [96] is an operation whereby the appendix is brought out to the skin forming an appendicostomy. Through the small stoma, patients can introduce a catheter and administer an enema that washes out the colon and rectum. The overall success rate in patients with SCI who were dissatisfied with conservative treatment was very high (between 74 and 87.5%). Complications occur in 12.5 and 67% of patients, including wound infection, small bowel obstruction, and stomal stenosis [96].

(e) *Hemorrhoids and colorectal carcinoma* [96–98]: Hemorrhoids are prevalent in those SCI individuals who strain and use suppositories, enemas, or chemical stimulation for bowel management; hemorrhoidal bleeding occurs in up to 76% of patients, in particular in those who use digital stimulation. Conservative therapy, banding, and sclerotherapy of hemorrhoids reduce bleeding and/or symptoms [97].

Colorectal carcinoma when discovered is more advanced in SCI than in non-paralyzed subjects, and morbidity after surgery may be higher [98]. A delay in diagnosis may occur since the distension, constipation, and pain may be attributed to GI complications of SCI; in addition, the difficulty of bowel preparation in these patients may result in an avoidance of screening colonoscopies.

(f) *Gallstones*: Gallstones or complications from previous cholecystectomy occur in 17–31% of SCI patients [99, 100], some of whom have risk factors such as diabetes, obesity, and/or family history of gallbladder disease [99]. The reason for the increase in gallstones in SCI is unknown, but different reasons are suspected. Some researchers have reported an impaired gallbladder filling due to impaired gallbladder relaxation in SCI lesions above T5. Others implicate the gastroduodenal and colonic motility disorders seen in these patients [101], with altered bile acid and impaired biliary lipidic secretion [102].

Acute acalculous cholecystitis presents with a right upper quadrant mass, steady fever, tachycardia, and cholestasis. Predisposing factors include narcotics use, mechanical ventilation with positive end-expiratory pressure, and hyperalimentation. Complications include a gangrenous gallbladder and the presence of an inflammatory mass [103].

In any case, it is not easy to make diagnosis of gallbladder disease in SCI individuals, due to sensory and motor impaired functions. Symptoms and signs of gallbladder disease may be atypical or even absent so that pathologic processes are often advanced at diagnosis.

Endocrine and Metabolic Changes The rate of diabetes has been reported to be higher in SCI patients than in the general population. In SCI individuals, the predisposition to carbohydrate (diabetes mellitus type 2) and lipid abnormalities is thought to be largely a consequence of extreme inactivity (paralysis and immobilization), and the constellation of metabolic findings (i.e., growth hormone deficiency, testosterone deficiency) appears to occur prematurely in persons with SCI.

Some studies suggested that serum insulin-like growth factor 1 levels are impaired in persons with SCI compared to the population, and this may be a sign of premature aging (Level 5 evidence) [107]. Glucose tolerance is lower after SCI, and diabetes mellitus occurs prematurely in men with SCI (Level 5 evidence) [104]. Bauman reported that after oral glucose tolerance testing (OGTT) in SCI patients, 38% of those with quadriplegia and 50% of those with paraplegia had normal OGTT. Twenty-two percent of SCI patients were diabetic according to the criteria established by the World Health Organization (WHO). Bauman also found abnormally decreased levels of human growth hormone and testosterone in individuals with SCI. Low levels of these hormones can result in a reduced capacity for cellular repair and a reduced capacity for maintaining lean muscle mass and strength. In addition, low levels of these hormones can prolong healing and soft tissue repair following injuries [105]. Low levels of testosterone are due to a dysfunction in the hypothalamic-pituitary-testicular axis, which in the general male population can lead to decreased libido, impotence, insomnia, fatigue, hot flushes, poor memory, anxiety, depression, and irritability [106].

Some experts reported that persons with SCI have higher levels of fat mass and experience significantly faster rates of age-related declines of lean tissue (Level 5 evidence) [110].

Lipid abnormalities, especially a depressed serum HDL-cholesterol concentration with or without elevated serum triglyceride values, may be present in association with impaired glucose tolerance and/or diabetes mellitus [107].

Musculoskeletal Changes (see Table 39.5) (a) *Muscles*: Regardless of the level of SCI, during the aging process, the muscles lose strength, the motor gesture and posture fail, the body loses coordination and balance control, and joint capsules may tighten and lose flexibility consequently and can develop contractures. As a result of immobilization, muscle fibers and connective tissues are maintained in a shortened position; they adapt to the shortened length (by the contraction of collagen fibers and a decrease in muscle fiber sarcomeres); moreover, loose connective tissue in muscles and around the joints gradually changes into dense. Kern et al., Carraro et al., Camagnini et al., Protasi et al., and Cerrel Bazo et al. [25–28] have shed light on the main factors inhibiting muscle recovery after an SCI in paralyzed limbs. Lean muscle mass is lost and is replaced with adipose tissue in SCI patients [25–28].

(b) *Pain*: Chronic musculoskeletal pain, a type of nociceptive pain, may occur with abnormal posture, gait, and overuse of structures such as the arm and shoulder. For example, using a manually operated wheelchair increases the risk of developing shoulder pain; carpal tunnel syndrome and ulnar nerve entrapment at the cubital tunnel and Guyon canal are also seen. Muscle spasm pain is often seen in patients with incomplete SCI [108–111].

Table 39.5 Musculoskeletal changes in spinal cord injury individuals

Musculoskeletal changes	
Muscles	Lose strength, lean muscle mass, decreased muscle fiber size, reduced number of myofibrils, reduced concentration of mitochondrial enzymes, and reduced number of the excitatory-contractile structures
Pain	Musculoskeletal pain, nociceptive pain, overuse of shoulder-arm-wrist joints and shoulder-arm-wrist pain. Carpal tunnel syndrome and ulnar nerve entrapment. Upper extremities degenerative joint diseases, rotator cuff tears, rotator cuff tendinitis, subacromial bursitis, and capsulitis
Osteoporosis	Decreased osteoblastic activity associated with a dramatic increase in bone degradation. Disuse bone loss (distal to the neurological level of injury). Neural lesions and hormonal changes also seem to be involved in this process
Bone fractures	Loss of bone biomechanical strength Biosynthesis of a structurally modified matrix unable to sustain normal mechanical stress
Skin and soft tissue	Thinning of the subcutaneous tissues over weight-bearing surface, thinning of the skin, and a loss of elasticity. The aging-related decrease in muscle mass and vascularity may reduce the tolerance of aged skin to breakdown. Difficulty healing once a pressure sore has developed

Visceral pain is a less distinct category of SCI-related pain. It arises from damage, irritation, or distension of internal organs. This type of pain is reported in 15% of patients with chronic SCI [108, 109]. Older people with dementia, other forms of cognitive impairment, or severe mental illness may not be able to communicate effectively about pain. In such cases, it is important to attend to nonverbal communication and behaviors including altered interpersonal interactions, changes in activity patterns or routines, mental status changes, and physiological changes.

Subbarao and colleagues reported that more than 70% of individuals with chronic SCI suffered pain in their upper extremities [112]. Pain has been reported to increase with time after the onset of the injury and is more common and severe in older individuals. The most common overuse syndromes causing pain in the upper extremities are degenerative joint diseases, rotator cuff tears, rotator cuff tendinitis, subacromial bursitis, and capsulitis [113]. Most of SCI patients require some sort of pain treatment or modification of their activities at some point of life. Activities that commonly contribute to overuse are transfers, wheelchair pushing, pressure releases, movements that require sustained arm positions above-shoulder level, and crutch walking in individuals with incomplete SCI.

It is critical, therefore, to consider joint and limb preservation strategies even in the initial phases of rehabilitation training because, by the time shoulder pain is severe enough to cause dysfunction, it may be too late to reverse it and the functional losses associated may become permanent [114].

(c) *Osteoporosis and bone fractures*: In patients who have a complete SCI, bone loss develops distal to the neurological level of injury.

The pathogenesis of osteoporosis after SCI is generally considered due to disuse; however, neural lesion and hormonal changes also seem to be involved in this process. Uebelhart [115] believes that osteoporosis in the spinal cord injury subjects is a matter of decreased osteoblastic activity associated with a dramatic increase in bone degradation. The development of a rapid and severe osteoporosis is only observed in the paralyzed part of the body, and the peak of this severe process of bone loss reaches the plateau 6–9 months after the onset of the SCI. Garland et al. corroborate in some ways the results from Uebelhart in a study performed in women with SCI. They found the bone mineral density in the spine either was maintained or was increased in relation to the time since the injury. The bone mineral density in the hips of the injured patients initially decreased approximately 25%; thereafter, the rate of loss was similar to that in the control group. The bone mineral density in the knees of the injured patients rapidly decreased 40–45% and then further decreased only minimally [116]. This finding is unlike that seen in healthy women, in whom bone mineral density decreases with age. Osteoporosis in aging with SCI is still controversial, and still further investigations are necessary to elucidate the problem.

The loss of bone biomechanical strength and the biosynthesis of a structurally modified matrix, which is unable to sustain normal mechanical stress, increase dramatically the risk of fractures. Clinically, the majority of pathological fractures in patients with SCI occur in the knee [41, 117–119]. Supracondylar fracture of the femur was so prevalent in the series reported by Comarr et al. that they termed it "the paraplegic fracture" [117]. Pharmacological treatment with diphosphonates has been proposed, and some timid results in preventing bone loss have been obtained. Further studies will need to elucidate long-term treatment results in early onset and in elderly SCI. The benefit of non-pharmacological treatment methods such as standing up, orthotically aided walking, weight-bearing physical exercises, functional electrical stimulation, and pulsed electromagnetic field is controversial. Risk factor modification such as reducing caffeine intake and tobacco or alcohol use and increasing calcium intake and vitamin D levels can be helpful.

(d) *Soft tissue changes*: Body composition changes can be summarized as a loss of lean muscle mass and an increase percentage of body adipose tissue that occurs as a function of time. Most SCI subjects experience weight gain that increases with time and that eventually results in a level of obesity that puts significant limitations on the patients' functional capabilities. Furthermore, as a result of aging, SCI subjects experience a loss or thinning of the subcutaneous tissues [120] over weight-bearing surfaces (the buttocks), and this results in loss of elasticity. Soft tissue changes associated to the aging-related decrease in muscle mass and vascularity may reduce the skin tolerance of aged skin to pressure and shearing forces leading to the development of pressure ulcers: skin is more subject to breakdown and difficulty in healing once a pressure sore or decubitus ulcer has developed [14, 105, 121, 122].

Functional Decline The literature suggests that persons with SCI may be more susceptible to earlier age-related functional declines when compared to the able-bodied (AB) population [123]. Adkins reported that SCI results in physiological and functional changes and potentially accelerates bodily declines at approximately the time of injury, after which the effect of aging is said to proceed at a normal rate [124].

Menter and Hudson [3] have developed a model of aging that predicts the functional decline of individuals and allows us to determine when these changes may occur. Immediately following the SCI onset, the individual incurs on a phase of maximum invigoration and acquires capable function for ADL allowed by the level of SCI and neurological recovery, maximizing the functional potential through rehabilitation. This phase is call acute restoration and lasts approximately 1 ½ year; this stage is followed by the maintenance phase or plateau. SCI may reach a symbiosis between capacities and functional activities and the vestiges from disability; this period may last for many years. A functional decline phase may follow in which overuse, physiological, and degenerative changes of age may present.

After having evaluated individuals with SCI of at least 15 years, Cushman and Hassett [8] found that 93% had experienced a decline in functional status by the time of the first evaluation. According to Kempt (Long-Term Outcome with Disability, Rancho Los Amigos Seminar, 1998), individuals of age 55 years at the onset of their SCI may only have 5–7 years of relatively stable functioning status prior to experiencing a decline.

It has been reported by Liem et al. [125] that constipation, pressure ulcers, female gender, and years post-injury were associated with the need of more aid with the activities of daily living (ADLs). There was a 42% increased odds of needing more help with ADLs per decade after SCI. In females SCI, the higher rates of divorce, separation, and single (remaining) mean that they are more likely than men to receive personal care from an attendant [67].

Regarding the functional outcome of a person with SCI, many factors will come together to determine which patients will bloom or will be prostrate by the challenges of SCI/D. Certainly, proper medical care, physical therapy, occupational therapy, recreational therapy, vocational rehabilitation, nursing care, sufficient family, friends and community resources facilitated by social work, and direct and indirect interventions by psychologists will make a major impact on outcomes.

Another aspect to be reckoned with is the interaction between the patient's own developmental strengths and his/her vulnerabilities, the significance that the SCI holds for the individual, influencing readiness to accept our interventions and the ability to realize their own potential following injury or disease.

In conclusion, the aging process and the influences of SCI over it should be taken under account when planning SCI rehabilitation in the elderly. Besides the above-mentioned difficulties, personal adversities in coping with the injury and dissatisfaction with life will decrease the possibilities of good living. This limits the "sick" old SCI patient (in addition to the young) to return home and reintegrate into society, increasing, at the same time, medical and social costs of our society.

Key Points

- Traumatic SCI is less frequent in older patients, and non-traumatic SCI usually involves an underlying organic disease.
- Clinical course of spinal cord injury (SCI) patients depends on age at onset of the spinal injury, CIR (cumulative illness rating), and incompleteness of the SCI: the more the age of onset is earlier, the lower the CIR, and the better the motor index return due to the incompleteness of the injury, the better will be the functional result after rehabilitation.
- Several organs are affected by degenerative and pathological changes after SCI, and respiratory complications are the most common cause of death.
- Physical capability and functioning after SCI may follow three phases: (1) the acute functional restoration, (2) the maintenance phase, and (3) the functional decline.
- Older adults may have premorbid medical conditions associated and frequently show worst outcomes if not appropriately and timely treated.
- The vast majority of young and/or seniors with SCI can become sedentary on a wheelchair, not participating much in physical and social activities. Proper medical multidisciplinary treatment associated to patient's cognitive and socioeconomic status, environmental support, and willingness to overcome his condition largely impact on SCI outcomes.

References

1. Thomas Jefferson University (2007) Elderly spinal cord injuries increase five-fold in 30 years, neurosurgeons find. Science Daily 2007. Available at www.sciencedaily.com/releases/2007/03/070319111256.htm
2. Kannus P, Palvanen N, Niemi S, Parkkari J (2007) J Gerontol A Biol 62:180–183
3. Menter RR, Hudson LM (1995) In: Stover S (ed) Spinal cord injury clinical outcomes from the model systems. Aspen, New York, p 272
4. Williams ME, Hadler NM (1983) Sounding board. The illness as the focus of geriatric medicine. N Engl J Med 308(22):1357–1360
5. Franceschini M, Cerrel Bazo H, Lauretani F et al (2011) Age influences rehabilitative outcomes in patients with spinal cord injury (SCI). Aging Clin Exp Res 23(3):202–208
6. Waring WP III, Biering-Sorensen F, Burns S, Donovan W, Graves D, Jha A et al (2010) Review and revisions of the international standards for the neurological classification of spinal cord injury. J Spinal Cord Med 33:346–352
7. Fawcett JW, Curt A, Steeves JD, Coleman WP, Tuszynski MH, Lammertse D, Bartlett PF, Blight AR, Dietz V, Ditunno J, Dobkin BH, Havton LA, Ellaway PH, Fehlings MG, Privat A, Grossman R, Guest JD, Kleitman N, Nakamura M, Gaviria M, Short D (2007) Guidelines for the conduct of clinical trials for spinal cord injury as developed by the ICCP panel: spontaneous recovery after spinal cord injury and statistical power needed for therapeutic clinical trials. Spinal Cord 45:190–205
8. Cushman LA, Hassett J (1992) Spinal cord injury: 10 and 15 years after. Paraplegia 30(10):690–696
9. Smith AE, Molton IR, Jensen MP (2016) Self-reported incidence and age of onset of chronic comorbid medical conditions in adults aging with long-term physical disability. Disabil Health J 9:533
10. Sawka MN, Glaser RM, Laubach LL, Al-Samkari O, Suryaprasad AG (1981) Wheelchair exercise performance of the young, middle-aged, and elderly. J Appl Physiol 50(4):824–828
11. Byrne DW, Salzberg CA (1996) Major risk factors for pressure ulcers in the spinal cord disabled: a literature review. Spinal Cord 34:255–263
12. Vidal J, Sarrias M (1991) An analysis of the diverse factors concerned with the development of pressure sores in spinal cord injured patients. Paraplegia 29:261–267
13. Elliott TR, Kurylo M, Chen Y, Hicken B (2002) Alcohol abuse history and adjustment following spinal cord injury. Rehabil Psychol 47:278–290
14. Bennett L, Kavner D, Lee BK, Trainor FA (1979) Shear vs pressure as causative factors in skin blood flow occlusion. Arch Phys Med Rehabil 60:309–314
15. DeVivo MJ, Kartus PL, Rutt RD, Stover SL, Fine PR (1990) The influence of age at time of spinal cord injury on rehabilitation outcome. Arch Neurol 47:681–691
16. Chen Y, DeVivo MJ, Jackson AB (2005) Pressure ulcer prevalence in people with spinal cord injury: age-period-duration effects. Arch Phys Med Rehabil 86:1208–1213
17. McKinley WO, Jackson AB, Cardenas DD, DeVivo MJ (1999) Long-term medical complications after traumatic spinal cord injury: a regional model systems analysis. Arch Phys Med Rehabil 80:1402–1410
18. Sekar P, Wallace DD, Waites KB, DeVivo MJ, Lloyd LK, Stover SL et al (1997) Comparison of long-term renal function after spinal cord injury using different urinary management methods. Arch Phys Med Rehabil 78:992–997
19. Chen Y, DeVivo MJ, Roseman JM (2000) Current trend and risk factors for kidney stones in persons with spinal cord injury: a longitudinal study. Spinal Cord 38:346–353
20. DeVivo MJ, Fine PR (1986) Predicting renal calculus occurrence in spinal cord injury patients. Arch Phys Med Rehabil 67:722–725
21. Australian Institute of Health and Welfare (2000) Disability and ageing: Australian population patterns and implications. Australian Institute of Health and Welfare, Canberra
22. Ragnarsson KT, Lammertse DP (1991) Rehabilitation in spinal cord disorders. 2. Anatomy, pathogenesis, and research for neurologic recovery. Arch Phys Med Rehabil 72:S295–S297
23. Brown M, Gordon WA, Ragnarsson KT (1987) Unhandicapping the disabled: what is possible? Arch Phys Med Rehabil 68:206

24. Burke RE (1980) Motor units: anatomy, physiology and functional organization. In: Brooks U (ed) Handbook of physiology I: the nervous system, vol 1. American Physiology Society, Bethesda
25. Kern H, Hofer C, Mödlin M, Mayr W, Vindigni V et al (2008) Stable muscle atrophy in long-term paraplegics with complete upper motor neuron lesion from 3- to 20-year SCI. Spinal Cord 46:293–304
26. Kern H et al (2004) Long-term denervation in humans causes degeneration of both contractile and excitation-contraction coupling apparatus, which is reversible by functional electrical stimulation (FES): a role for myofiber regeneration? J Neuropathol Exp Neurol 63:919–931
27. Boncompagni S, Kern H, Rossigni K, Hofer C, Mayr W, Carraro U, Protasi F (2007) Structural differentiation of skeletal muscle fibers in the absence of innervation in humans. Proc Natl Acad Sci U S A 104(49):19339–19344
28. Cerrel Bazo HA, Carraro U, Helmut K (2007) The role of regenerative miogenesis in motor recovery of plegic muscles through FES. Research thesis for the Physical Medicine and Rehabilitation Residency program & specialty. University of Verona School of Medicine, Verona, Italy
29. Trieschmann RB (1987) Aging with a disability. Demos, New York
30. Katz RT et al (1987) Functional electrical stimulation to enhance fibrinolytic activity in spinal cord injury patients. Arch Phys Med Rehabil 68:423
31. Fugl-Meyer AR (1971) Effects of respiratory muscle paralysis in tetraplegic and paraplegic patients. Scand J Rehabil Med 3:141
32. Dearwater S et al (1979) Assessment of physical activity in inactive populations. Med Sci Sports Exerc 17:67
33. Figoni SF (1984) Spinal cord injury and maximal aerobic power. Am Correct Ther J 38:44
34. Green D (ed) (1996) Medical management of long-term disability. Rehabilitation Institute of Chicago, Don Olson, 2nd edn. Butterworth-Heinemann, Newton
35. Heldenberg D et al (1981) Lipid concentrations in young quadriplegic patients. Atherosclerosis 39:163
36. LaPorte RE et al (1983) HDL cholesterol across a spectrum of physical activity from quadriplegia to marathon running. Lancet 1:1212
37. Brenes G et al (1986) HDL serum concentrations in physically active and sedentary spinal cord injured patients. Arch Phys Med Rehabil 67:445
38. George C, Dugan N, Porter J (1987) Body composition and exercise tolerance in spinal cord injury. Presented at the ASIA meeting, Boston, 20–22 March 1987
39. Bauman WA, Adkins RH, Spungen AM, Herbert R et al (1999) Is immobilization associated with an abnormal lipoprotein profile? Observations from a diverse cohort. Spinal Cord 37:485–493
40. Garland DE, Steward CA, Adkins RH et al (1992) Osteoporosis after spinal cord injury. J Orthop Res 10:371
41. Ragnarsson KT, Sell GH (1981) Lower extremity fractures after spinal cord injury: a retrospective study. Arch Phys Med Rehabil 62:413–423
42. Adams MM, Hicks AL (2005) Spasticity after SCI. Spinal Cord 43:577–586. doi:10.1038/sj.sc.3101757
43. Young RR (1994) Spasticity: a review. Neurology 44:512–520
44. Daniel RK, Wheatley D, Priest D (1985) Pressure sores and paraplegia: an experimental model. Ann Plast Surg 15:41
45. Eriksson P, Lofstrom L, Ekblom B (1988) Aerobic power during maximal exercise in untrained and well-trained persons with quadriplegia and paraplegia. Scand J Rehabil Med 20(4):141–147
46. Kofsky PR, Shephard RJ, Davis GM, Jackson RW (1985) Muscle strength and aerobic power: a study of lower-limb disabled males. Int Rehabil Med 7(4):151–155
47. Davis GM, Shephard RJ (1988) Cardiorespiratory fitness in highly active versus inactive paraplegics. Med Sci Sports Exerc 20(5):463–468

48. Glaser RM, Davis GM (1989) Wheelchair-dependent individuals. In: Franklin BA, Gordon S, Timmis GC (eds) Exercise in modern medicine. Williams & Wilkins Co., Baltimore, pp 237–267
49. Field MJ, Jette AM (eds) (2007) The future of disability in America. The National Academies Press, Washington
50. Kocina P (1997) Body composition of spinal cord injured adults. Sports Med 23(1):48–60
51. Szlachcic Y, Carrothers L, Adkins R, Waters R (2007) Clinical significance of abnormal electrocardiographic findings in individuals aging with spinal injury and abnormal lipid profiles. J Spinal Cord Med 30(5):473–476
52. Groah SL, Nash MS, Ward EA, Libin A, Mendez AJ, Burns P et al (2011) Cardiometabolic risk in community-dwelling persons with chronic spinal cord injury. J Cardpulm Rehabil 31(2):73–80
53. Myers J, Lee M, Kiratli J (2007) Cardiovascular disease in spinal cord injury: an overview of prevalence, risk, evaluation, and management. Am J Phys Med Rehabil 86(2):142–152
54. DeVivo MJ, Chen Y (2011) Trends in new injuries, prevalent cases, and aging with spinal cord injury. Arch Phys Med Rehabil 92(3):332–338
55. Lidal IB, Snekkevik H, Aamodt G, Hjeltnes N, Biering-Sørensen F, Stanghelle JK (2007) Mortality after spinal cord injury in Norway. J Rehabil Med 39(2):145
56. Brown R, DiMarco AF, Hoit JD, Garshick E (2006) Respiratory dysfunction and management in spinal cord injury. Respir Care 51(8):853–870
57. Arora S, Flower O, Murray NP, Lee BB (2012) Respiratory care of patients with cervical spinal cord injury: a review. Crit Care Resusc 14(1):64–73
58. Hitzig SL, Sakakibara BM, Miller WC, Eng JJ (2012) Aging following spinal cord injury. In: Eng JJ, Teasell RW, Miller WC, Wolfe DL, Townson AF, Hsieh, JTC et al (eds) Spinal cord injury rehabilitation evidence version 40. Vancouver, pp 1–82
59. Richards JS, Siddall P, Bryce T, Dijkers M, Cardenas DD (2007) Spinal cord injury pain classification: history, current trends, and commentary. Top Spinal Cord Inj Rehabil 13(2):1–19
60. Widerström-Noga EG, Finnerup NB, Siddall PJ (2009) Biopsychosocial perspective on a mechanisms-based approach to assessment and treatment of pain following spinal cord injury. J Rehabil Res Dev 46(1):1–12
61. Siddall PJ (2009) Management of neuropathic pain following spinal cord injury: now and in the future. Spinal Cord 47(5):352–359
62. Goossens D, Dousse M, Ventura M, Fattal C (2009) Chronic neuropathic pain in spinal cord injury patients: what is the impact of social and environmental factors on care management? Ann Phys Rehabil Med 52(2):173–179. Epub 2009/11/17
63. Edgar R, Quail P (1994) Progressive post-traumatic cystic and non-cystic myelopathy. Br J Neurosurg 8(1):7–22. Epub 1994/01/01
64. Jensen MP, Hoffman AJ, Cardenas DD (2005) Chronic pain in individuals with spinal cord injury: a survey and longitudinal study. Spinal Cord 43:704–712
65. Rintala DH, Hart KA, Priebe MM (2004) Predicting consistency of pain over a 10-year period in persons with spinal cord injury. J Rehabil Res Dev 41:75–88
66. McColl MA (2002) A house of cards: women, aging and spinal cord injury. Spinal Cord 40:371–373
67. Krause JS, Kemp B, Coker J (2000) Depression after spinal cord injury: relation to gender, ethnicity, aging, and socioeconomic indicators. Arch Phys Med Rehabil 81:1099–1109
68. Bloch A, Tamir D, Vakil E, Zeilig G (2016) Specific deficit in implicit motor sequence learning following spinal cord injury. PLoS One 11(6):e0158396. doi:10.1371/journal.pone.0158396
69. Davidoff GN, Morris J, Roth E, Bleiberg J (1985) Cognitive dysfunction and mild closed head injury in traumatic spinal cord injury. Arch Phys Med Rehabil 66:489–491
70. Dowler RN, Harrington DL, Haaland KY, Swanda RM, Fee F, Fiedler K (1997) Profiles of cognitive functioning in chronic spinal cord injury and the role of moderating variables. J Int Neuropsychol Soc 3:464–472
71. Schueneman AL, Morris J (1982) Neuropsychological deficits associated with spinal cord injury. Sci Dig 4:64–69

72. Wilmot CB, Cope DN, Hall KM, Acker M (1985) Occult head injury: it's incidence in spinal cord injury. Arch Phys Med Rehabil 66:227–231
73. Trieschmann RB (1988) Spinal cord injuries: psychological, social, and vocational rehabilitation, 2nd edn. Demos, New York
74. Warren AN, Pullins J, Elliott TR (2008) Concomitant cognitive impairment in persons with spinal cord injuries in rehabilitation settings. In: Gontovsky ST, Golden CJ (eds) Neuropsychology within the inpatient rehabilitation environment. Nova Science Publishers, Inc, Hauppauge, pp 79–98
75. Jegede AB, Rosado-Rivera D, Bauman WA, Cardozo CP, Sano M, Moyer JM et al (2010) Cognitive performance in hypotensive persons with spinal cord injury. Clin Auton Res 20:3–9. doi:10.1007/s10286-009-0036-z
76. Craig A, Nicholson Perry K, Guest R, Tran Y, Middleton J (2015) Adjustment following chronic spinal cord injury: determining factors that contribute to social participation. Br J Health Psychol 20:807–823. doi:10.1111/bjhp.12143
77. Sabbah P, de Schonen S, Leveque C, Gay S, Pfefer F, Nioche C et al (2002) Sensorimotor cortical activity in patients with complete spinal cord injury: a functional magnetic resonance imaging study. J Neurotrauma 19:53–60. doi:10.1089/089771502753460231
78. Bonanno GA, Kennedy P, Galatzer-Levy IR, Lude P, Elfström ML (2012) Trajectories of resilience, depression, and anxiety following spinal cord injury. Rehabil Psychol 57:236. doi:10.1037/a0029256
79. Craig AR, Hancock KM, Dickson H (1994) A longitudinal investigation into anxiety and depression over the first two years of spinal cord injury. Paraplegia 33:221–230
80. Kennedy P, Rogers BA (2000) Anxiety and depression after spinal cord injury: a longitudinal analysis. Arch Phys Med Rehabil 81:932–937. doi:10.1053/apmr.2000.5580
81. Castaneda AE, Tuulio-Henriksson A, Marttunen M et al (2008) A review on cognitive impairments in depressive and anxiety disorders with a focus on young adults. J Affect Disord 106:1–27. doi:10.1016/j.jad.2007.06.006
82. Lungu O, Frigon A, Piché M et al (2010) Changes in spinal reflex excitability associated with motor sequence learning. J Neurophysiol 103:2675–2683. doi:10.1152/jn.00006.2010
83. Vahdat S, Lungu O, Cohen-Aded J, Marchand-Pauvert V, Benali H, Doyon J (2015) Simultaneous brain-cervical cord fMRI reveals intrinsic spinal cord plasticity during motor sequence learning. PLoS Biol 13:e1002186. doi:10.1371/journal.pbio.1002186
84. Kowalczyk I, Duggal N, Bartha R (2012) Proton magnetic resonance spectroscopy of the motor cortex in cervical myelopathy. Brain 135:461–468
85. Lynch AC, Wong C, Anthony A et al (2000) Bowel dysfunction following spinal cord injury: a description of bowel function in a spinal cord-injured population and comparison with age and gender matched controls. Spinal Cord 38:717–723
86. Kirshblum S, Johnston MV, Brown J, O'Connor KC, Jarosz P (1999) Predictors of dysphagia after spinal cord injury. Arch Phys Med Rehabil 80:1101–1105
87. Martin RE, Neary MA, Diamant NE (1997) Dysphagia following anterior cervical spine surgery. Dysphagia 12(1):2–8
88. Segal JL, Milne N, Brunnemann SR, Lyons KP (1987) Metoclopramide-induced normalization of impaired gastric emptying in spinal cord injury. Am J Gastroenterol 82:1143–1148
89. Zhang RL, Chayes Z, Korsten MA, Bauman WA (1994) Gastric emptying rates to liquid or solid meals appear to be unaffected by spinal cord injury. Am J Gastroenterol 89:1856–1858
90. Gore RM, Mintzer RA, Calenoff L (1981) Gastrointestinal complications of spinal cord injury. Spine 6:538–544
91. DiPalma JA, Smith JR, Cleveland M (2002) Overnight efficacy of polyethylene glycol laxative. Am J Gastroenterol 97:1776–1779
92. Wrenn K (1989) Fecal impaction. N Engl J Med 321:658–662
93. Rosman AS, Chaparala G, Monga A, Spungen AM, Bauman WA, Korsten MA (2008) Intramuscular neostigmine and glycopyrrolate safely accelerated bowel evacuation in patients with spinal cord injury and defecatory disorders. Dig Dis Sci 53:2710–2713

94. Harari D, Minaker KL (2000) Megacolon in patients with chronic spinal cord injury. Spinal Cord 38:331–339
95. Banwell JG, Creasy GH, Aggarwal AM, Mortimer JT (1993) Management of the neurogenic bowel in patients with spinal cord injury. Urologic Clin North Am 20:517–526
96. Ebert E (2012) Gastrointestinal involvement in spinal cord injury: a clinical perspective. J Gastrointestin Liver Dis 21(1):75–82
97. Scott D, Papa MZ, Sareli M, Velano A, Ben-Ari GY, Koller M (2002) Management of hemorrhoidal disease in patients with chronic spinal cord injury. Tech Coloproctol 6:19–22
98. Stratton MD, McKirgan LW, Wade TP et al (1996) Colorectal cancer in patients with previous spinal cord injury. Dis Colon Rectum 39:965–968
99. Moonka R, Stiens SA, Resnick WJ et al (1999) The prevalence and natural history of gallstones in spinal cord injured patients. J Am Coll Surg 189:274–281
100. Ketover SR, Ansel HJ, Goldish G, Roche B, Gebhard RL (1996) Gallstones in chronic spinal cord injury: is impaired gallbladder emptying a risk factor? Arch Phys Med Rehabil 77:1136–1138
101. Fealey RD, Szurszewski JH, Merritt JL, DiMagno EP (1984) Effect of traumatic spinal cord transaction on human upper gastrointestinal motility and gastric emptying. Gastroenterology 87:69–75
102. Apstein MD, Dalecki-Chipperfield K (1987) Spinal cord injury is a risk factor for gallstone disease. Gastroenterology 92:966–968
103. Romero Ganuza FJ, La Banda G, Montalvo R, Mazaira J (1997) Acute acalculous cholecystitis in patients with acute traumatic spinal cord injury. Spinal Cord 35:124–128
104. Lavela SL, Weaver FM, Goldstein B, Chen K, Miskevics S, Rajan S, Gater DR Jr (2006) Diabetes mellitus in individuals with spinal cord injury or disorder. J Spinal Cord Med 29:387–395
105. Bauman WA, Spungen AM (1994) Disorders of carbohydrate and lipid metabolism in veterans with paraplegia or quadriplegia: a model of premature aging. Metabolism 43(6):749–756
106. Tenover JL (1997) Testosterone and the aging male. J Androl 18(2):103–106
107. Hitzig SL, Eng JJ, Miller WC, Sakakibara M, SCIRE Research Team (2011) An evidence-based review of aging of the body systems following spinal cord injury. Spinal Cord 49(6):684–701. doi:10.1038/sc.2010.178
108. Chiodo AE, Scelza WM, Kirshblum SC, Wuermser LA, Ho CH, Priebe MM (2007) Spinal cord injury medicine. 5. Long-term medical issues and health maintenance. Arch Phys Med Rehabil 88:S76–S83. doi:10.1016/j.apmr.2006.12.015
109. McKinley WO, Gittler MS, Kirshblum SC, Stiens SA, Groah SL (2002) Spinal cord injury medicine. 2. Medical complications after spinal cord injury: identification and management. Arch Phys Med Rehabil 83:S58–S64, S90–S98
110. Rekand T, Hagen EM, Grønning M (2012) Chronic pain following spinal cord injury. Tidsskr Nor Laegeforen 132:974–979. doi:10.4045/tidsskr.11.0794
111. Siddall PJ, Middleton JW (2006) A proposed algorithm for the management of pain following spinal cord injury. Spinal Cord 44:67–77
112. Subbarao JV, Klopfstein J, Turpin R (1995) Prevalence and impact of wrist and shoulder pain in patients with spinal cord injury. J Spinal Cord Med 18(1):9–13
113. Kirshblum S, Druin E, Planten K (1997) Musculoskeletal conditions in chronic spinal cord injury. Top Spinal Cord Inj Rehabil 2:23–35
114. Dalyan M, Cardenas DD, Gerard B (1999) Upper extremity pain after spinal cord injury. Spinal Cord 37:191–195
115. Uebelhart D, Demiaux-Domenech B et al (1995) Bone metabolism in spinal cord injured individuals and in others who have prolonged immobilisation. A review. Paraplegia 33(11):669–673
116. Garland DE, Adkins RH, Stewart CA, Ashford R, Vigil D (2001) Regional osteoporosis in women who have a complete spinal cord injury. J Bone Joint Surg Am 83-A(8):1195–1200
117. Comarr AE, Hutchinson RH, Bors EB (1962) Extremity fractures of patients with spinal cord injuries. Am J Surg 103:732–739

118. Eichenholtz SN (1963) Management of long-bone fractures in paraplegic patients. J Bone Joint Surg Am 45:299–310
119. Freehafer AA (1995) Limb fractures in patients with spinal cord injury. Arch Phys Med Rehabil 76:823–827
120. Rossier AB, Favre H, Valloton MB (1991) Body composition of spinal cord injured adults. In: The spinal cord injured patient: comprehensive management. WB Saunders, Philadelphia, pp 163–170
121. Bauman WA, Garland DE, Schwartz E (1997) Calcium metabolism and osteoporosis in individuals with spinal cord injury. Top Spinal Cord Inj Rehabil 2:84–96
122. Bauman WA, Waters RL (2004) Aging with a spinal cord injury. In: Kemp BJ, Mosqueda L (eds) Aging with a disability: what the clinician needs to know. Johns Hopkins University Press, Baltimore, pp 153–174
123. Thompson L, Yakura J (2006) Aging related functional changes in persons with spinal cord injury. Top Spinal Cord Inj Rehabil 6:69–82
124. Adkins RH (2004) Research and interpretation perspectives on aging related physical morbidity with spinal cord injury and brief review of systems. NeuroRehabil 19:3–13
125. Liem N, McColl M, King W, Smith K (2004) Aging with a spinal cord injury: factors associated with the need for more help with activities of daily living. Arch Phys Med Rehabil 85(10):1567–1577

Peripheral Neuropathies and Rehabilitation of Older Patients

40

Chiara Briani and Luca Padua

40.1 Introduction

Aging is associated with an increased incidence of peripheral neuropathy, with consequent gait impairment and increased incidence of falls. A recent prospective population-based study showed that the prevalence of polyneuropathy in the general middle-aged and elderly population is at least 4% and increases with age [1]. The most common causes of neuropathy in elderly are idiopathic, diabetic, iatrogenic (mainly secondary to chemotherapy), or due to nutritional deficiencies.

A systematic review by Ward et al. including eight epidemiologic studies (six cross-sectional and two longitudinal) in older adults showed that abnormal sensory and motor peripheral nerve function not only is associated with reduced lower limb motility and general mobility but is also predictive of poor physical function and disability [2].

It has been calculated that almost one-third of people >65 years complain of sensory symptoms due to neuropathy [3] and this is associated with greater morbidity and mortality [4].

Physical rehabilitation is frequently recommended in patients affected with peripheral neuropathy, although evidence-based efficacy is lacking. In the only Cochrane review on exercise in patients with peripheral neuropathy, which included any randomized or quasi-randomized controlled trial comparing the effect of exercise with no exercise therapy or drugs or nondrug treatment on functional ability, it resulted that there is inadequate evidence to evaluate the effect of exercise on

C. Briani (✉)
Department of Neuroscience, University of Padua, Padua, Italy
e-mail: chiara.briani@unipd.it

L. Padua
Department of Geriatrics, Neurosciences and Orthopaedics, Università Cattolica del Sacro Cuore, Rome, Italy

Don Carlo Gnocchi Onlus Foundation, Milan, Italy

© Springer International Publishing AG 2018

S. Masiero, U. Carraro (eds.), *Rehabilitation Medicine for Elderly Patients*, Practical Issues in Geriatrics, DOI 10.1007/978-3-319-57406-6_40

functional ability in people with peripheral neuropathy [5]. Also a review on physical rehabilitation for critical illness myopathy and neuropathy has found no proper studies to be considered [6].

The main reasons accounting for the scarce evidence-based data are likely the absence of standardized rehabilitation protocols and the lack of proper, reliable, and sensitive outcome measures. Moreover, the heterogeneity of the neuropathies, the common presence of comorbidities in older patients, the natural course of the neuropathy, and the physiological aging are all concurrent factors that make it difficult to identify specific rehabilitative programs and outcome measures sensitive to changes.

Keeping in mind these limitations, we will address the role of rehabilitation in the most common neuropathy with known cause, that is, diabetic polyneuropathy, and other peripheral nervous system disorders for which sound studies are available in the literature.

40.2 Diabetic Neuropathy

Despite diabetes mellitus is the most common cause of peripheral neuropathy worldwide, no evidence-based data are available for rehabilitative programs in diabetic peripheral neuropathy.

A recent systematic review [7], which included patients with different causes of neuropathy besides diabetes, identified 11 studies (seven randomized controlled trials, four controlled clinical trials), most of them performed in older diabetic patients with peripheral neuropathy. Oxford levels of evidence and corresponding grade of recommendation were provided for each considered study. The authors concluded that balance training appears to be the most effective exercise intervention and also endurance training is important especially in diabetic neuropathy, helping also glycemic control and body weight. A further small uncontrolled study (12 weeks of moderate or intense aerobic exercise) in diabetic patients with and without neuropathy showed improvement in gait, reaction time, and postural stability in older adults with type 2 diabetes [8]. However, the small size of the study and the lack of an age-matched control group limit the power of the data.

Moreover Davies et al. performed a systematic review on the role of physical activity and psychological coping strategies in the management of painful diabetic neuropathy [9].

Of 1306 studies identified, only 4 (2 investigating physical activity and 2 investigating psychological coping) were considered. However, the studies enrolled small sample size and applied different outcome measures. The lack of blinding was a further limitation.

Concerning pain and generally symptoms due to diabetic neuropathy, physical therapy and especially transcutaneous electrical nerve stimulation (TENS) appear useful in two meta-analyses showing reduction of pain. Both studies concluded that large multicenter RCTs are needed to evaluate the long-term effect of TENS [10, 11].

40.3 Chemotherapy-Induced Peripheral Neuropathy (CIPN)

Chemotherapy-induced peripheral neuropathy (CIPN) is a major and potentially dose-limiting adverse event of several chemotherapeutic agents. CIPN is characterized by distal symmetrical numbness, tingling, paresthesias, dysesthesias, pain, and/or weakness which significantly impact functionality and quality of life (QoL).

Streckmann et al. performed the first RCT focused on balance control and polyneuropathy in cancer patients. The study was a prospective, single-center, two-armed, open randomized, controlled trial on 61 lymphoma patients with CIPN who underwent a 36-week exercise (sensorimotor, endurance, and strength training) rehabilitation protocol [12]. The patients had a wide range of age (20–67 years), and old patients were also included. The primary end point of the study was the improvement of QoL. Secondary end points included balance control on static and dynamic surface, movement coordination, endurance, strength, and therapy side effects. The results of the study showed that exercise, especially sensorimotor training, improved patients' QoL, balance control, and general physical performance and reduced limitations secondary to side effects of chemotherapy.

Conclusions

Despite the lack of evidence-based data to support specific rehabilitative programs in old patients with peripheral neuropathy, still physical exercise has a general positive role in patients' well-being and motility. The primary aim of the rehabilitation scientific world should be an adequate planning of prospective controlled trials in order to identify not only specific rehabilitative programs but also reliable outcome measures.

Finally, technological rehabilitation is a new and stimulating field with promising tools, as virtual reality and robotics [13–15]. Besides the demonstration of the efficiency of this approach, it is necessary to check the safety of these tools considering the clinical features and fragilities of old patients.

Key Points

- Peripheral neuropathy is common in elderly and may contribute to increased incidence of falls.
- Physical rehabilitation is frequently recommended in patients with peripheral neuropathy, although evidence-based efficacy is lacking and proper outcome measures are missing.
- Balance and endurance trainings seem to be effective exercises in diabetic neuropathy.
- Virtual reality and robotics are new tools that might help rehabilitative programs, provided that efficiency and safety are proved in old, and often fragile, patients.

References

1. Hanewinckel R, Drenthen J, van Oijen M et al (2016) Prevalence of polyneuropathy in the general middle-aged and elderly population. Neurology 87(18):1892–1898. [Epub ahead of print]
2. Ward RE, Caserotti P, Cauley JA et al (2015) Mobility-related consequences of reduced lower-extremity peripheral nerve function with age: a systematic review. Aging Dis 7(4):466–478
3. Mold JW, Vesely SK, Keyl BA et al (2004) The prevalence, predictors, and consequences of peripheral sensory neuropathy in older patients. J Am Board Fam Pract 17(5):309–318
4. Mold JW, Lawler F, Roberts M et al (2008) The health consequences of peripheral neurological deficits in an elderly cohort: an Oklahoma Physicians Resource/Research Network Study. J Am Geriatr Soc 56(7):1259–1264
5. White CM, Pritchard J, Turner-Stokes L (2004) Exercise for people with peripheral neuropathy. Cochrane Database Syst Rev 4:CD003904
6. Mehrholz J, Pohl M, Kugler J, Burridge J et al (2015) Physical rehabilitation for critical illness myopathy and neuropathy: an abridged version of Cochrane Systematic Review. Eur J Phys Rehabil Med 51(5):655–661
7. Streckmann F, Zopf EM, Lehmann HC et al (2014) Exercise intervention studies in patients with peripheral neuropathy: a systematic review. Sports Med 44(9):1289–1304
8. Morrison S, Colberg SR, Parson HK et al (2014) Exercise improves gait, reaction time and postural stability in older adults with type 2 diabetes and neuropathy. J Diabetes Complicat 28(5):715–722
9. Davies B, Cramp F, Gauntlett-Gilbert J et al (2015) The role of physical activity and psychological coping strategies in the management of painful diabetic neuropathy – a systematic review of the literature. Physiotherapy 101(4):319–326
10. Jin DM, Xu Y, Geng DF et al (2010) Effect of TENS on symptomatic diabetic peripheral neuropathy: a meta-analysis of randomized controlled trials. Diabetes Res Clin Pract 89(1):10–15
11. Pieber K, Herceg M, Paternostro-Sluga T (2010) Electrotherapy for the treatment of painful diabetic peripheral neuropathy: a review. J Rehabil Med 42(4):289–295
12. Streckmann F, Kneis S, Leifert JA et al (2014) Exercise program improves therapy-related side-effects and quality of life in lymphoma patients undergoing therapy. Ann Oncol 25(2):493–499
13. Schwenk M, Grewal GS, Honarvar B et al (2014) Interactive balance training integrating sensor-based visual feedback of movement performance: a pilot study in older adults. J Neuroeng Rehabil 11:164
14. Grewal GS, Schwenk M, Lee-Eng J et al (2015) Sensor-based interactive balance training with visual joint movement feedback for improving postural stability in diabetics with peripheral neuropathy: a randomized controlled trial. Gerontology 61(6):567–574
15. Schwenk M, Grewal GS, Holloway D et al (2016) Interactive sensor-based balance training in older cancer patients with chemotherapy-induced peripheral neuropathy: a randomized controlled trial. Gerontology 62(5):553–563

Rehabilitation of Older Patients with Mental Disorders

41

Raffaele Gimigliano, Antimo Moretti, Francesca Gimigliano, Anna Mazzola, and Giovanni Iolascon

41.1 Brain and Ageing

The effects of ageing on the brain and cognitive functions can cause significant impairment affecting autonomy and quality of life (QoL) of older people [1].

41.1.1 Pathology

It has been widely shown that brain volume and weight decrease with age at a rate of about 5% per decade after the age of 40 [2], with a decline rate that increases with ageing, particularly after 70 years old [3]. Neurons' death is often the main cause of reduced grey matter [4]. However, also a deterioration of white matter can occur in people over 40 years, particularly involving the frontal lobe [5].

These anatomical and histological findings are associated with impaired brain functions, such as memory (the ability to encode, store and retrieve information), learning, specific motor, coordination and balance functions.

Many factors may influence the ageing brain, such as genetics, neuroendocrinology, lifestyle and nutrition, as well as social and cultural milieu [1].

R. Gimigliano • A. Moretti • A. Mazzola • G. Iolascon (✉)
Department of Medical and Surgical Specialties and Dentistry, University of Campania "Luigi Vanvitelli", Naples, Italy
e-mail: giovanni.iolascon@unicampania.it

F. Gimigliano
Department of Mental and Physical Health and Preventive Medicine, University of Campania "Luigi Vanvitelli", Naples, Italy

© Springer International Publishing AG 2018

S. Masiero, U. Carraro (eds.), *Rehabilitation Medicine for Elderly Patients*, Practical Issues in Geriatrics, DOI 10.1007/978-3-319-57406-6_41

41.2 General Definitions and Epidemiology of Mental Disorders in the Elderly

Mental disorders are defined as psychiatric illness or diseases manifested by breakdowns in the adaptational process expressed primarily as abnormalities of thought, feeling and behaviour producing either distress or impairment of function. Dementia, delirium and major depression are the most commonly diagnosed psychiatric conditions in elderly.

According to DSM-5, delirium and dementia are neurocognitive disorders (NCDs). NCDs include conditions characterized by acquired primary cognitive impairments, such as Alzheimer's disease, vascular dementia, Lewy body dementia, Parkinson's disease dementia, frontotemporal dementia, post-traumatic dementia and other less common types of dementia.

However, cognitive impairment could be present as a complication of many, if not all, mental disorders [6].

Diagnostic criteria of NCDs include the decline in one or more cognitive domains (attention, execution, learning and memory, speech, perception). To be defined as major, cognitive impairments have to be documented through specific neuropsychological assessment tools and have to interfere with the activities of daily living (ADLs) [6].

The term dementia is used to define the major NCD with a degenerative aetiology that mainly affects older people; when the same symptoms are present in young individuals as a complication of a traumatic brain injury or HIV infection, we prefer to use the general term NCD [6].

41.3 Dementia: Definition and Epidemiology

Dementia is one of the most relevant global health problems, considering its high prevalence and huge burden in terms of disability and mortality. It was estimated that over 44 million of individuals worldwide are affected by this condition and it is expected that this number will grow to more than 135 million in 2050, as a result of the ageing population [7].

In senile dementia (>60 years of age), the major causes are in the 60% cases of Alzheimer's disease and in the 15–20% cases of vascular dementia or Lewy body disease (LBD). Other less common type of dementia are Parkinson's dementia, secondary to multiple sclerosis and AIDS Huntington's disease, Korsakoff's syndrome and Creutzfeldt-Jakob disease (CJD) are even less frequent [8].

41.4 Diagnosis and Assessment

Accurate clinical diagnosis of dementia and its underlying causes is crucial for the prognosis and the pharmacological and rehabilitative management. The cognitive manifestations of dementia can be detected by neuropsychological assessment, with specific batteries that are based on a combination of instruments assessing cognitive and behavioural functions. The process should examine the three functional systems determining behaviour: cognition, emotion and executive functions.

In addition to patient history and functional and cognitive evaluation, biohumoural and neuroimaging assessments might give interesting information.

41.5 Delirium: Definition and Epidemiology

Delirium is a transient reversible cerebral dysfunction clinically characterized by clouding of consciousness with fluctuating attention and a wide range of neuropsychiatric abnormalities [6]. This condition is very common in frail institutionalized older persons with a prevalence of 10–30%, growing up to 70–80% in patients in an intensive care unit (ICU) [9].

The presence of delirium causes a significant increase of risk of complications, prolonged hospitalization and mortality, with a consequent impact on health-care costs [10].

41.6 Diagnosis and Assessment

The DSM-5 suggests that diagnosis of delirium requires the presence of the following criteria [6]:

- Disturbances of attention: impairment in the ability to direct, focus, sustain and shift attention
- Disorder of awareness: reduced orientation to the environment or at times even to oneself that develops over a short period and tends to fluctuate during the course of the day
- Cognitive impairments, such as memory deficit and language alterations
- Perceptual disturbance, including misinterpretations, illusions or hallucinations

All abovementioned impairments should be attributed to general medical condition, intoxication, drug use or more than one cause.

The gold standard for the screening of delirium is the Confusion Assessment Method (CAM) that is a structured interview investigating the main clinical issues of delirium, such as acute change in mental status with fluctuating course (1), attention deficit (2), disorganization of thought (3) and consciousness impairment (4). The presence of both impairments 1 and 2 and at least one of the other two suggests the diagnosis of delirium.

Lipowski proposed three subtypes of delirium depending on the psychomotor state: hypoactive, hyperactive and mixed, the first one showing the worst prognosis [11].

It has been suggested that the physiopathology of delirium depends on several factors, such as disruptions of neurotransmission, inflammation or acute stress responses.

According to current data, the management of delirium requires the use of antipsychotics and non-pharmacological approaches.

Early diagnosis and treatment of modifiable factors, such as malnutrition, dehydration, insomnia and immobilization, would prevent the development of delirium [12].

41.7 Depression: Definition and Epidemiology

Depression is an affective disorder characterized by either a dysphoric mood or loss of interest or pleasure in usual activities. The presence of a sad, empty or irritable mood or somatic and cognitive impairments affecting the functional performance is a common finding of a depressive disorder [13].

Major depression is characterized by episodes lasting 2 weeks or more with significant mood, cognitive and neurovegetative changes. This condition has a prevalence of 10–20% [14] and is one of the main causes of disability, considering that 40.5% of the total disability-adjusted life years (DALYs) due to mental disorder and drug abuse is attributable to major depressive disorder (MDD) [15].

41.8 Diagnosis and Assessment

The DSM-5 recently proposed new criteria to make diagnosis of MDD. At least five of the following symptoms during a 2-week period must be present: depressed mood, anhedonia, significant weight change or appetite disturbance, sleep disorders, psychomotor agitation or retardation, fatigue, feelings of worthlessness, loss of concentration, indecisiveness and recurrent thoughts of death or of suicidal ideation with or without a specific plan [13]. One of the symptoms must be either the depressed mood or the loss of interest or pleasure in almost all activities (anhedonia).

In older people, the gold standard for the assessment of depression is the original version of the Geriatric Depression Scale (GDS) that consists of 30 items, but several short versions of this screening tool are also available The treatment of the acute phase may include pharmacotherapy, psychotherapy, the combination of medication and psychotherapy or other treatments such as electroconvulsive therapy (ECT) or transcranial magnetic stimulation (TMS) and light therapy.

41.9 Physiatric Approach to Mental Disorders in the Elderly

The physiatric approach is by definition holistic and patient-centred. This approach is ideal for an elderly patient with mental disorders. The first step in the formulation of the rehabilitation plan is the rehabilitative diagnosis aimed to identify and quantify the patient's functional alterations. In view of the chronic progressive and irreversible deterioration of the demented, the rehabilitative approach depends on the clinical phase of the dementia.

41.10 Dementia

Onset and progression of dementia are highly variable and depend on the aetiology. NCDs are also characterized by the presence of functional limitation in ADLs and neuropsychiatric symptoms, such as euphoria, disinhibition, hallucination or agitation. In the analysis of the different components of functional status of the patients, we should perform first the analysis of cognitive and non-cognitive impairments, then the assessment of functional limitation in ADLs and in the end the evaluation of the level of social participation and QoL.

41.11 Cognitive Impairments in Dementia

Dementia is characterized by multiple cognitive impairments due to the involvement of many areas of the brain, but memory and executive function deficits represent a dominant part and their progressive worsening defines the progressive stages of the disease (Table 41.1).

Executive functions are controlled by the frontal cortex; thus, the decrease of volume and function of this region explains the reduction of these functions. Language comprehension, especially of complex texts, is based on working memory, and this decreases in the elderly due to the brain atrophy of hippocampus, a structure of the medial temporal lobe involved in memory formation [17].

In dementia usually there is an alteration of memory or orientation functions associated with at least one of the following impairments: language, perception, attention, apraxia, problem-solving and abstract thinking.

41.12 Neuropsychological Assessment and Rehabilitation

The neuropsychological rehabilitation is the branch of the rehabilitation medicine that aims to rehabilitate cognitive impairments and the resulting limitations in daily living activities and social participation in patients suffering from disorders of the central nervous system.

Table 41.1 Clinical features of dementia according to disease stages

Dementia	MCI	Moderate	Severe	End stage
Memory loss	Short term	Most short term and some long term	Most short and long term	Almost all short and long term
Functional loss	IADLs	Most IADLs and some basic ADLs	Basic ADLs	Bed bound

Adapted from [16]

Abbreviations: *MCI* mild cognitive impairment, *IADLs* instrumental activities of daily living, *ADLs* activities of daily living

The neuropsychological rehabilitation is based on a preliminary assessment consisting in a battery approach, which involves tests of a variety of cognitive ability area, such as memory, attention, processing speed, reasoning, judgement, problem-solving and spatial and language functions.

The main steps of the neuropsychological evaluation are the collection of medical history, the clinical interview with the patient and family members, administration of cognitive and functional assessment instruments, analysis and interpretation of the results from the tests and preparation of the report aimed at the construction of an individual rehabilitation plan.

The Mini-Mental State Examination (MMSE) is a very useful tool for analysing the general framework of cognitive impairment in a patient suffering from mental illness, particularly in dementia [18]. A viable alternative to the MMSE in the primary care setting can be the administration of the clock-drawing test (CDT) and the Mini-Cog test. The CDT is performed by giving the patient a sheet of paper with a large (relative to the size of handwritten numbers) pre-drawn circle on it and instructing the patient to draw numbers in the circle to make it look like the face of a clock and then draw the hands of the clock to read "10 after 11". The score ranges from 1 to 6 with higher scores reflecting a greater number of errors and degree of impairment. A score of ≥3 represents a cognitive deficit, while a score of 1 or 2 is considered normal [19]. The Mini-Cog test is a 3-min instrument to screen for cognitive impairments in older adults in a primary care setting. The Mini-Cog uses a three-item recall test for memory and a simply scored clock-drawing test (CDT). It is as effective as or better than established screening tests and faster than the Mini-Mental State Examination. It detects many people with mild cognitive impairment (MCI).

41.13 Functional Assessment

In a hospital setting, the functional assessment of patients with dementia is generally performed by administering the Barthel Index (BI), which is one of the most widely used rating scales for the measurement of activity limitations in patients with neuromuscular and musculoskeletal conditions.

For outpatient, functional status assessment begins with a review of the two key divisions of functional ability: ADLs and instrumental activities of daily living (IADLs). The two instruments for assessing ADLs and IADLs, respectively, are the Katz ADL scale and the Lawton IADL scale.

41.14 Pharmacological Therapy in NCDs

An appropriate drug therapy of NCDs requires the knowledge of the disease aetiology.

Medications can revert the underlying cause of dementia in only a small percentage of cases (potentially reversible dementia). Generally, drugs can only slow the course of an irreversible dementia, such as the tacrine in Alzheimer's disease, or prevent worsening of the disease, such as aspirin for vascular dementia. Psychotropic drugs could revert depression or behavioural symptoms associated with dementia.

In irreversible forms of dementia, the treatment focuses on maximizing the residual functions of the patient, to restore some of the lost functions and to educate and support the family and caregivers [20].

41.15 Rehabilitation of Dementia

The global outcome of the individual rehabilitation plan (IRP) for the patients affected by NCDs is to keep him/her autonomous and safe in the execution of ADLs and IADLs for as long as possible. In the early stages of the disease, it was observed that learning is possible by giving appropriate support, leading to the hypothesis that cognition-based interventions, including reality orientation therapy (ROT) and non-specific cognitive training, could exert beneficial effects [21].

Four rehabilitative approaches for the people with dementia were described [22]:

- Reality orientation and skills training approaches
- Emotion-oriented approaches
- Behaviour-oriented approaches
- Stimulation-oriented approaches

The first approach aims to address cognitive deficits, whereas the other three aim to maximize patients' mood and to reduce the impact of behavioural problems, such as aggression or incontinence.

The ROT aims to improve orientation and behavioural skills through cognitive activities and interpersonal and social interactions, combined with the use of aids and facilities to assist in encoding, storing and retrieving information. With repeated multimodal stimulation (music, visual, verbal), the ROT could reinforce the patient's information about his/her personal history and space/time orientation. The ROT was designed from Folsom in 1958 and later developed by Taulbee and Folsom in the 1960s as a rehabilitation approach targeted to patients confused or with cognitive impairments [23]. In particular, the interventions aimed to reorientation in time consists of stimulating memory skills through the use of writing supports to encode/retrieve data about the day, month and year, or holidays, or other meaningful events in patients' life; spatial reorientation is preferentially obtained by stimulating the encode/retrieve of meaningful meeting place for patients, using verbal cues to reinforce memory. Moreover, several aids, such as digital watches with 24-h dial, specific signs placed in various rooms (e.g. bathroom, kitchen, bedroom, etc.) for orientation around house, should be useful in order to enhance encoding/retrieving activities.

During a session of ROT, the therapist repeatedly presents basic personal and current information to each patient beginning with the patient's name, where he or she is and the date. When the patient has relearned these basic facts, others are presented such as age, home town and former occupation [22]. Generally ROT is applied as a group therapy (4–6 patients with similar cognitive impairment), where caregivers are trained to give treatment at home. The number and duration of sessions are variable, ranging from 45 to 60 min for two to four times a week [24].

In addition to this formal modality, an informal ROT approach is required, consisting of the introduction of temporal and spatial facilities in the patient's environment with the involvement of caregivers and/or family members. The best candidates to ROT are patients with mild to moderate cognitive impairment, without sensory and/or behavioural disorders that may affect compliance to rehabilitation programmes.

Skills training aims to help patients to improve cognitive functioning, albeit only temporarily, in an attempt to stop or slow cognitive decline. The memory training is done by an operator in the presence of a caregiver, and it consists of performing daily activities, such as self-care, clothing, cooking, communicative strategies and so on. The duration of a single session of skills training ranges from 8 to 45 min.

Cognitive training is useful for the treatment of specific cognitive impairments based on individual and group sessions, including computer training. The latter is reserved to patients affected by MCI aiming to stimulate and enhance sustained and selective attention and visuospatial associative memory. Cognitive training is performed using board games that increase brain function, such as Advanced Progressive Matrix (or Raven's Progressive Matrix, RPM), puzzles and computer games. Each session has to be conducted in a neuropsychological laboratory, for a duration of 60 min. Speech rehabilitation is common to treat language impairments in patients affected by NCDs. It consists essentially of stimulation of the spare capacity and the use of the compensatory strategies of communication and provision of appropriate education and counselling of the patient and family members.

Another option to treat language impairments in patients with moderate to severe NCDs is music therapy. This approach is based on musical activities, both vocal and instrumental, designed to acquire cognitive abilities that facilitate the retrieving process and enhance verbal and non-verbal communication skills. The duration of each one-to-one session is 1 h. However, it is possible to perform a group session of music therapy in case of mild to moderate NCDs.

Global reactivation therapy (GRT) is another cognitive stimulation intervention based on 12 group sessions, of 1 h each performed three times per week. It consists in training memory, attention, language, reasoning and learning strategies in order to preserve temporal orientation as well as personal autonomy.

Considering that current evidences suggest that, for people with NCDs, ADL skill training can promote independence in personal care tasks and social participation [25], occupational therapy (OT) should be considered a gold standard for the management of these patients. The OT aims to stimulate functional capacity (e.g. hand dexterity), cognitive abilities (e.g. attention, learning) and creativity using a variety of materials and turning them into finished products through manipulative and decorative techniques. The rehabilitative intervention is carried out in an outpatient setting and lasts 1 h per day for 4 weeks.

The methods used in rehabilitation practice are commonly based on empirical approaches.

41.16 Rehabilitation of Delirium

Delirium management includes pharmacological and supportive therapy and rehabilitative approach [26]. Environmental monitoring of intensive care and pain management are milestones of the conservative treatment. Fluid, electrolyte balance and nutrition should be evaluated and eventually given carefully.

The most commonly used medications are haloperidol, α2-adrenergic receptor agonist (dexmedetomidine, clonidine) and sedatives.

The environment should be quiet (i.e. using earplugs for sleeping) and well lighted. Caregivers and family members should be encouraged to reinforce the patient orientation.

During daylight situations of sensory deprivation must be avoided, correcting sensory deficits, if necessary, with eyeglasses and hearing aids.

Hyperactive type of delirium is characterized by agitation, fear and perceptual impairments. Physical restraints, if possible, should be avoided. These patients should always be supervised and, if possible, assisted by a family member.

Reorientation therapy and/or skills training approaches may be helpful. Early exercise and mobilization were recently found to be safe and well tolerated by critically ill patients [27]. The Society of Critical Care Medicine (SCCM) published the guidelines for pain, agitation and delirium (PAD) which suggest that it is essential to treat delirium in the broader management of patients in intensive care units.

41.17 Rehabilitation of Major Depression

MDD is the most prevalent and disabling form of depression, but only 20% of patients receive adequate treatment, which includes drug therapy and/or psychotherapy [28]. However, the role of physical exercise in addition to conventional therapy is gaining attention, as many recent studies have shown that it can be as effective in reducing depressive symptoms as medical therapy or psychological interventions.

A programme lasting 10–14 weeks, with 45–59-min sessions, performed five times a week, demonstrated the greatest efficacy in a population with depressive syndrome. Both aerobic and strength exercises, regardless of the intensity, provided similar benefits. In the recent guidelines for management of depression in adults, the UK National Institute for Health and Clinical Excellence (NICE) recommends a group physical activity programme based on three sessions a week (lasting 45 min to 1 h) over 10–14 weeks for patients affected by mild to moderate depression [29].

Robertson et al. in a meta-analysis of trials exploring the effects of walking as a treatment for depression reported that this intervention could be beneficial in reducing symptoms by nearly 50% [30].

According to the results of the literature and clinical experience, we recommend a tailored exercise programme (aerobic exercise in group sessions of 150 min per week) for patients affected by mild to moderate depression.

41.18 Caregiver Stress

Caregiver stress could be intended as the physical and emotional strain of a person who provides direct care, particularly assistance for basic ADLs and IADLs and medical (i.e. managing medication, planning and accompanying to medical appointments) and emotional support. Caregiver or family members usually provide almost the 90% of long-term care needs in chronic diseases, including NCDs and MDD [31]. In the USA, in 2009, 65.7 million of people received assistance (two thirds were elderly patients) by a caregiver [32].

The rapid increase of caregiver burden is a consequence of the growing number of elderly people, particularly those affected by chronic conditions, and the lack of professional support that should help family members and/or caregivers. Most caregivers are women who take care of a family member (86%) or a friend (14%), with an average time of about 20.5 h per week spent in this activity [31]. A recent cohort study estimated that the cost of informal caregiving for a patient with dementia was $56,290 per year [33], which is higher than the expenditure for home health care and medical care in a nursing home.

Caregivers are subjected to significant discomfort, as suggested by a survey in which one third of the caregivers interviewed reported high level of stress [31]. It was found that the caregiver stress is a pathological condition with clinical manifestations and biohumoural milieu modifications similarly to those suffering from post-traumatic stress disorders. Furthermore, aged caregivers have a higher risk of mortality compared with non-caregivers in the same age group [34].

Caring for a person with an NCD represents a challenging issue considering that caregivers see a progressive deterioration of patient's mental and physical health over time. On the other hand, the chronic mental and physical burden on caregivers might lead to reduced quality of care for patients with NCDs, with worsening of patient's health status, particularly of psycho-behavioural symptoms of dementia. The patient factors that most commonly affect the caregiver burden are sleep disturbances, urinary disturbance/incontinence, older age and male gender and diarrhoea/constipation.

It was demonstrated a correlation between behavioural and psychological symptoms of dementia (BPSD) and caregiver stress, and at the same time, it is well known that BPSD is also strictly related to comorbidity and medications in patients with dementia; therefore, the number and type of comorbidities and administered drugs affect the risk of developing a caregiver stress condition.

41.18.1 Prevention and Treatment of Caregiver Stress

The management of caregiver stress is based on interventions directed to caregivers and family members and to patients affected by NCDs. Several studies demonstrated that tailored educational and support programmes for caregivers are effective to reduce the burden of caregiver stress. Educational programmes should be based on information about signs and symptoms, prognosis and natural history of the pathology and also considering the effect of both pharmacological and non-pharmacological approaches.

Physical therapy for NCD patients can significantly reduce the caregivers' burden because it is effective not only for the prevention of gait/motor impairment but also for the improvement of mood, apathy and day/night reversal typical features of patients with NCDs.

The treatment of comorbidities and the modification of pharmacological treatment could result in improvement of BPSD, thus reducing the caregiver stress.

Recently, Adelman et al. [35] proposed a practical approach to manage the caregiver burden, including the following interventions:

- Encourage the caregiver to consider himself/herself as a member of the care team.
- Encourage caregivers to maintain an adequate level of self-care and health status, particularly if they are elderly and/or affected by a chronic condition. Caregivers have to engage in health-promoting behaviours such as regular exercise and other activities that improve QoL.
- Educate caregivers by providing them information about patient's disease and therapy. Moreover caregivers should receive a training for proper lifting and transferring patients to avoid back injuries. Furthermore, counselling about coping strategies for caregiver stress might be useful. Educational interventions should be provided by physical and occupational therapists, nurses and social workers.
- Technological support could be used to facilitate patient's autonomy. Emergency alert systems could be useful for the management of patients with MCI, thus reducing the presence of caregiver at patient's home. Also home intercom systems or a webcam may be used for monitoring patients with dementia. New technologies may offer additional supportive measures, such as drug dispenser alarms or voice reminders. Moreover, educational programmes can be provided using integrated phone or mobile system technologies.
- Implementation of assistance services that provide volunteer programmes (e.g. Alzheimer Association), non-medical home care services (e.g. housekeeping) and home safety modification. Access to respite care services may provide relief for caregivers of patients affected by dementia.
- Coordination of health-care services, including physical and neuropsychological rehabilitation.

Key Points

- Ageing can significantly impair the cognitive functions affecting older people's autonomy and quality of life.
- Dementia, delirium and major depression are the most common psychiatric conditions of elderly people.
- The rehabilitative approach to patients with mental disorders should be multidisciplinary, holistic and patient centred and includes the formulation of the individual rehabilitation plan.
- Caregivers or family members should be considered as members of the care team. Health-care professionals who deal with older patients with chronic mental disorders should be taking into account also the caregiver stress.

References

1. Peters R (2006) Ageing and the brain. Postgrad Med J 82:84–88
2. Svennerholm L, Boström K, Jungbjer B (1997) Changes in weight and compositions of major membrane components of human brain during the span of adult human life of Swedes. Acta Neuropathol 94:345–352
3. Scahill R, Frost C, Jenkins R et al (2003) A longitudinal study of brain volume changes in normal ageing using serial registered magnetic resonance imaging. Arch Neurol 60:989–994
4. Raz N (2004) The ageing brain: structural changes and their implications for cognitive ageing. In: Dixon R, Bäckman L, Nilsson L (eds) New frontiers in cognitive ageing. Oxford University Press, Oxford, pp 115–134
5. Tullberg M, Fletcher E, DeCarli C et al (2004) White matter lesions impair frontal lobe function regardless of their location. Neurology 63:246–253
6. Diagnostic and statistical manual of mental disorders: DSM-5.—5th ed. p.; cm. 2013 American Psychiatric Association. Available from: http://psy-gradaran.narod.ru/lib/clinical/DSM5.pdf. Accessed 27 June 2016
7. Alzheimer's Disease International. Dementia Statistics; 2014. Available from: http://www.alz.co.uk/research/statistics. Accessed 27 Mar 2014
8. Plassman BL, Langa KM, Fisher GG et al (2007) Prevalence of dementia in the United States: the aging, demographics, and memory study. Neuroepidemiology 29(1–2):125–132
9. Marcantonio ER (2011) In the clinic delirium. Ann Intern Med 154:ITC 6–ITC16
10. Rizzo JA, Bogardus ST Jr, Leo-Summers L (2001) Multicom-ponent targeted intervention to prevent delirium in ho-spitalized older patients: what is the economic value? Med Care 39:740–752
11. Lipowski ZJ (1989) Delirium in the elderly patient. N Engl J Med 320(9):578–582
12. Saxena S, Lawley D (2009) Delirium in the elderly: a clinical review. Postgrad Med J 85:405–413
13. American Psychiatric Association (2013) Diagnostic and statistical manual of mental disorders, 5th edn. American Psychiatric Association, Washington
14. Andrade L, Caraveo-Anduaga JJ, Berglund P, Bijl RV, De Graaf R, Vollebergh W et al (2003) The epidemiology of major depressive episodes: results from the International Consortium of Psychiatric Epidemiology (ICPE) surveys. Int J Methods Psychiatr Res 12:3e21
15. Whiteford HA, Degenhardt L, Rehm J, Baxter AJ, Ferrari AJ, Erskine HE et al (2013) Global burden of disease attributable to mental and substance use disorders: findings from the Global Burden of Disease Study 2010. Lancet 382:1575–1586
16. Delirium and dementia. Available at: http://me.aapmr.org/kn/article.html?id=74. Accessed 25 July 2016
17. Glisky EL (2007) Changes in cognitive function in human aging. In: Riddle DR (ed) Brain aging: models, methods, and mechanisms. CRC Press, Boca Raton, pp 3–20
18. Folstein MF, Folstein SE, McHugh PR (1975) "Mini-mental state". A practical method for grading the cognitive state of patients for the clinician. J Psychiatr Res 12(3):189–198
19. Shulman KI, Gold DP, Cohen CA, Zucchero CA (1993) Clock drawing and dementia in the community: a longitudinal study. Int J Geriatr Psychiatry 8:487–496
20. Mace NL, Rabins PV (1981) The 36 hour day-a family guide to caring for persons with Alzheimer's disease, related dementing diseases and memory loss in later life. Johns Hopkins University Press, Baltimore
21. Bäckman L (1992) Memory training and memory improvement in Alzheimer's disease: rules and exceptions. Acta Neurol Scand Suppl 139:84–89
22. Carrion C, Aymerich M, Baillés E, López-Bermejo A (2013) Cognitive psychosocial intervention in dementia: a systematic review. Dement Geriatr Cogn Disord 36(5–6):363–375
23. Taulbee LR, Folsom JC (1966) Reality orientation for geriatric patients. Hosp Community Psychiatry 17(5):133–135

24. Spector A, Thorgrimsen L, Woods B, Royan L, Davies S, Butterworth M et al (2003) Efficacy of an evidence-based cognitive stimulation therapy programme for people with dementia: randomised controlled trial. Br J Psychiatry 183:248–254
25. National Institute for Health and Clinical Excellence: Guidance (2007) Dementia: A NICE-SCIE guideline on supporting people with dementia and their carers in health and social care. Editors National Collaborating Centre for Mental Health (UK). Source Leicester (UK): British Psychological Society
26. Jackson P, Khan A (2015) Delirium in critically ill patients. Crit Care Clin 31:589–603
27. Schweickert WD, Pohlman MC, Pohlman AS et al (2009) Early physical and occupational therapy in mechanically ventilated, critically ill patients: a randomised controlled trial. Lancet 373(9678):1874–1882
28. Gelenberg AJ (2010) The prevalence and impact of depression. J Clin Psychiatry 71(3):e06
29. NICE Depression: the treatment and management of depression in adults (update) NICE clinical guideline 90, 2009. Available from: www.nice.org.uk/CG90. Accessed 2 Nov 2012
30. Robertson R, Robertson A, Jepson R et al (2012) Walking for depression or depressive symptoms: a systematic review and meta-analysis. Ment Health Phys Act 5(1):66–75
31. National Alliance for Caregiving and AARP. Caregiving in the United States 2009. http://www.caregiving.org/data/04finalreport.pdf. Accessed 19 Feb 2014
32. Arno PS, Levine C, Memmott MM (1999) The economic value of informal caregiving. Health Aff (Millwood) 18(2):182–188
33. Hurd MD, Martorell P, Delavande A, Mullen KJ, Langa KM (2013) Monetary costs of dementia in the United States. N Engl J Med 368(14):1326–1334
34. Schulz R, Beach SR (1999) Caregiving as a risk factor for mortality: the Caregiver Health Effects Study. JAMA 282(23):2215–2219
35. Adelman RD, Tmanova LL, Delgado D, Dion S, Lachs MS (2014) Caregiver burden: a clinical review. JAMA 311(10):1052–1060

Cardiac Rehabilitation in the Elderly Patients

42

Francesco Cacciatore and Pasquale Abete

42.1 Introduction

Cardiac rehabilitation (CR) is a complex intervention offered to patients with heart disease, which includes components of health education, advices on cardiovascular risk reduction, physical activity, and stress management. Cardiac rehabilitation reduces mortality (27% reduction in all-cause mortality and 31% reduction in CHD mortality), morbidity, and unplanned hospital admissions in addition to improvements in exercise capacity, quality of life, and psychological well-being. [1]. Current indications for CR are the following: post-myocardial infarction (MI), post-coronary artery bypass grafting (CABG), angina, percutaneous transluminal coronary angioplasty (PTCA), valve replacement or repair, heart transplant, heart failure (HF) II-III New York Heart Association (NYHA) class and recently also HF end stage, and left ventricular assisting device (LVAD) implant [1]. In the recent years, patients admitted to cardiac rehabilitation are characterized by a growing clinical instability, with a complex comorbidity scenario due to the aging process and the unsolved acute phase of the disease that require the need of rehabilitation [2, 3]. In a short period of years, in all western countries, there has been a radical change in the rehabilitation world, with a relevant change in elderly proportion. In the USA the mean age increased from 60.6 to 63.4 years, and the proportion of patients 75 years or older increased by 59% [4]. These changes

F. Cacciatore, MD, PhD
Department of Translational Medical Sciences, University of Naples Federico II, Naples, Italy

Heart Transplant Unit, Azienda Ospedaliera Specialistica dei Colli, Naples, Italy
e-mail: Francesco.cacciatore@fsm.it

P. Abete, MD, PhD (✉)
Department of Translational Medical Sciences, University of Naples Federico II, Naples, Italy
e-mail: pasquale.abete@unina.it

© Springer International Publishing AG 2018

S. Masiero, U. Carraro (eds.), *Rehabilitation Medicine for Elderly Patients*, Practical Issues in Geriatrics, DOI 10.1007/978-3-319-57406-6_42

prompted the physician to acquire a more specialized approach for the management of elderly complex patient to be rehabilitated. The Cardiac Rehabilitation 1996 AHCPR Guidelines identified smoking cessation, lipid management, weight control, blood pressure control, improved exercise tolerance, symptom control, return to work, and psychological well-being/stress management as outcomes to be reached by rehabilitation program [5]. These outcomes are still to be the goal to achieve in an adult patient but are far from the real needs of the elderly, especially the oldest-old where disability is the main problem to manage [6]. Care of elderly patients in rehabilitation starts from the assessment of active problems at admission, continues through the phase of clinical stabilization and prevention of adverse clinical events, and then continues in the recovery of frailty and disability through rehabilitation recovery paths, guided by careful clinical and functional assessment based on comprehensive geriatric assessment (CGA) [7]. Multidimensional assessment is a tool capable of identifying the multiple dimensions of the older person and to assess the diseases (comorbidity) and the function (cardiovascular, physical, and cognitive) and any deficit (nutritional, disability, and frailty), considering also the social support [8]. It identifies, then, a new concept relating to the elderly patient, or that of the polyfactorial deficiency, the relative recovery, and therefore the complexity. The concept of clinical complexity in the past was identified with the severity or difficulty of the clinical case, then taking on a totally subjective value. Thus, the clinical judgment refers to the diagram "certainty-consent," introduced by Stacey for the analysis of complex systems [9] and applied to and Zimmerman et al. [10] and by Goldberger [11] in clinical models. The Stacey diagram and Zimmerman define "simple" the system toward which there is the maximum of knowledge together with the maximum of consent by the operators; opposite the "chaos" characterizes the system in which the minimum of knowledge is accompanied by the minimum consensus; the "complex systems" are distributed in the area between simplicity and chaos. By transferring these concepts to clinical medicine, we can agree that the knowledge that we derive from the "evidence-based medicine" (EBM) serve to broaden the scope of "the simple medicine" and the "complexity" is identified with clinical medicine and chronic disability, characterized by the simultaneous presence of several clinical problems, for which the scientific knowledge is not yet complete and the solution of which is not the clinical cure but the patient's functional recovery. We have to agree that the demographic revolution seen at the end of the last century in industrialized countries and in particular in Italy [12] resulted in a revolution in the field of clinical medicine and rehabilitation, with a need of a more complex diagnostic evaluation approach [13] and a therapeutic individual rehabilitation, able to maintain continuing care facilities at different levels of health and social health organization. In advancing age, in fact, there is high prevalence of multiple diseases, often in terminal stage, with atypical clinical presentation [14, 15], and therefore the diagnostic-evaluative and therapeutic approach to these patients should be driven by a comprehensive geriatric assessment. Several studies have shown that the CGA limits the incidence and severity of outcomes such as disability and mortality in elderly patients [16].

It should also be emphasized that the comorbidity can take very complex issues: in the elderly cardiac patient, the simultaneous detection of extra-cardiac comorbidities and multiple cardiovascular diseases in the same patient (cardiovascular comorbidity) is frequent [17]. The clinicians have to assess the role of "active comorbidity" as clinically relevant and capable of compromising the functional state. The association of comorbidity with disability is explained by the progressive loss of the anatomical and functional reserve of various organs and systems (vulnerability), characterizing the physiology of the different stages of geriatric age. Faced with these various biological conditions, it is clear that the result on the functional state is different when the same disease affects adults or elderly subjects and expresses different frames of disability as it increases the degree of vulnerability, which reduces the anatomical and functional reserve [18]. Furthermore, a complex situation can become simple when it is managed in an organized system, capable of absorbing the different aspects that make the situation complex. Hence, it becomes essential to avoid the "chaos" of the system improving the facilities which in recent years have grown their "complexity" of care, such as intensive rehabilitation; they can adapt their systems to more complex standards and suited to the frail elderly population. Therefore, the medicine of complexity is identified with the geriatric medicine: from a clinical point of view, in fact, the patient of geriatric interest is a very old patient characterized by age-related reduced functional reserve (vulnerability), by comorbidity, disability, polipharmacy with the relative increase in the risk of adverse drug reactions and by critical socioeconomic and environmental conditions; these findings define the "frail status" of the geriatric patient [7]. This concept, only recently identified, outlines a particular risk condition, i.e., by a reduction in capacity to perform basic activities of daily living, from a high comorbidity and loss of functional reserve of organs and systems. Frailty is also considered as a result of changes in the neuromuscular, endocrine, and immune systems. The criteria for identifying vulnerable people are not universally accepted. Numerous authors define frailty as the sum of a number of biological and clinical markers, which also can be seen in a dynamic position between a healthy condition and a condition of extreme fragility. Frailty further destabilizes clinic status and is necessary to be prevented and treated not only in an "acute" setting but also in the field of post-acute rehabilitation and ongoing care.

42.2 Rehabilitation Project and the Functional Recovery Program

The possibility of functional recovery is established through a preliminary evaluation by the rehabilitation team establishing the possible benefits of rehabilitation and the time required for this to happen. Rehabilitation should take place in the hospital soon after a heart attack, heart surgery, or other major heart problems (phase 1). After the disease stabilization, at a stage where the clinical instability of the acute phase makes possible the patient's participation to rehabilitation program, it will start the phase 2. The cardiac rehabilitation program could continue at an outpatient facility. Phase 2 of cardiac rehabilitation usually lasts from 3 to 6 weeks and involves continued monitoring of cardiac responses to exercise and activity. This opportunity is in this epidemiological scenario even less frequent due to the severe stage of the disease in the elderly patient, and rehabilitation is preferred in specialized setting as inpatients. The assessment will also serve to identify the most suitable rehabilitation setting for the elderly (hospital, ambulatory, or at home); having important studies demonstrated efficacy in postinfarction of home rehabilitation for low-risk patients [19] and in 75 years older patients with a moderate frailty level [20, 21] (intensive outpatient therapy, phase 3; independent ongoing conditioning, phase 4).

The clinical and functional examination allows quantifying the deficit tied to the active issue on admission and active and passive comorbidity and directs the team on the rehabilitation needs and diagnostic, therapeutic, and patient management. Therefore, screening assessment at the entrance is the first step for the elaboration of a Rehabilitation Project and the functional recovery program. Initial evaluation also allows evaluating the social and environmental factors, family conditions and therefore social support, housing conditions for the structural home changes for protected discharge at home, and the availability of medical support.

42.3 Comprehensive Geriatric Assessment (CGA)

The comprehensive geriatric assessment (CGA) is a key tool in the approach to the elderly patient. The CGA allows analyzing the various components of the patient (physical, cognitive, and social) at admission, during rehabilitation, and at discharge. The CGA identifies and prioritizes clinical problems, identifies the functional recovery objectives and planning care interventions, transfers the assistance program to the rehabilitation team, and verifies the implementation of the interventions during the rehabilitation process (Fig. 42.1). In the functional evaluation, the elderly will be oriented mainly on its degree of residual acute event skills. Some authors have suggested rehabilitation programs vary according to the meters walked

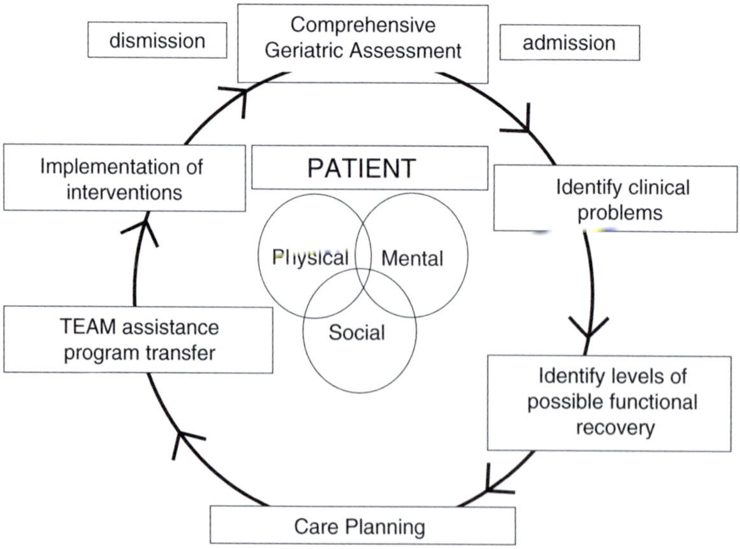

Fig. 42.1 Comprehensive geriatric assessment—from the assessment to interventions

in 6-minute walking test, which took into account, in addition to demographic variables, clinical variables such as ejection fraction and the presence of comorbidities. The proposed algorithm identifies specific functional recovery routes to functional residual capacity [22, 23]. Other models are based on levels of frailty, built on the frailty staging system which identifies three classes and therefore different needs of functional rehabilitation [8].

The CGA uses tools of different grading: the most commonly used in rehabilitative environment are the Activity of Daily Living (ADL), [24] Barthel Index [25], Cumulative Illness Rating Scale (CIRS) [26], Geriatric Depression Scale (GDS) [27], Mini-Mental State Examination (MMSE) [28], and functional assessment (6-minute walking test) [29], more oriented to the evaluation of cardiac patients, while the Tinetti [30] and the Short Physical Performance Battery (SPPB) [31] are tests used to evaluate balance and gait and physical functioning (Fig. 42.2).

The evaluation of these functions is of great importance especially in the very elderly. In this regard, Lavie et al. showed that the cardiovascular rehabilitative intervention leads to an improvement of the health status in general and the quality of life and a decrease in perceived pain. Furthermore, hostility, depression, and anxiety are reduced to a greater extent in the oldest-old than in adults after cardiovascular rehabilitation [20, 21].

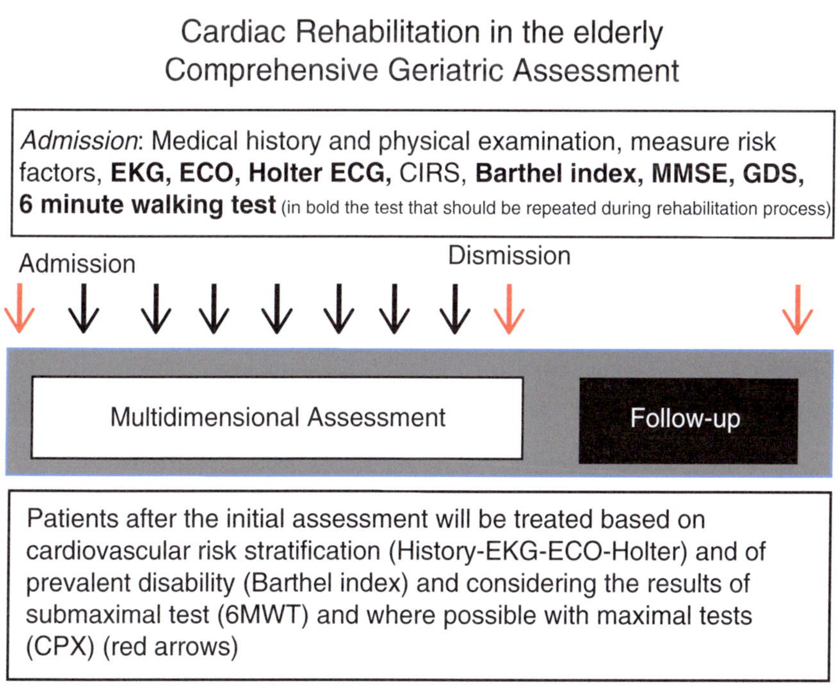

Fig. 42.2 Comprehensive Geriatric Assessment in elderly patient underwent cardiac rehabilitation.

42.4 Specific Protocols for Elderly Patients

To set the subdivision criteria of elderly subjects, in order to identify the best targets to be pursued with rehabilitation, we can refer, in a schematic way, to the cognitive and motor functions that are respectively expressed in the ability to perform, despite the presence of cognitive impairment, a functional recovery path, and preserved autonomy in performing IADL and ADL. At the moment, however, no known studies using the multidimensional assessment oriented to rehabilitation have demonstrated the effectiveness of particular rehabilitation protocols. The questions that need answering are oriented to understanding if this population with conditions such as cognitive impairment, disability, and frailty get a clinical and functional improvement with protocols designed to these special populations.

Physical rehabilitation, implemented in accordance with the risk assessment criteria related to the exercise and adapted to the different disease patterns, is an integral part of management of patient with cardiovascular disease. For rehabilitation purposes we have to make a distinction in the context of this population considering the burden of disability. As already mentioned, the patient with disability tends to coincide with the complex patient, embracing a wide spectrum of cardiovascular conditions and possibly extra-cardiac comorbidity associated with the underlying cardiac disease, characterized by varying degrees of impairment of functional capacity. This impairment arises from a disability, which, through a limitation of usual and, therefore, a restriction of the individual's participation in his social life, determines different degrees of disability.

The rehabilitative intervention may be configured in patients less compromised in a physical training program, while the more functionally limited patients may be subjected to physical activity that, as controlled and programmed, cannot constitute a classical exercise program of effective workout. In any case, the patient's physical cardiovascular rehabilitation configures an operational framework "TEAM" involving in various reasons many actors (doctor, nurse, physiotherapist, etc.), with loads and different goals depending on the degree of disability. The rehabilitation process of these patients will be strictly individualized in relation to their functional impairment/disability at admission and the usual functional capacity. The following proposed protocols do not follow the traditional approach of rehabilitation nosology in cardiology (i.e., different protocols for different events or acute or chronic diseases), but rather suggest a transversal criterion for various conditions, based on different levels of disability of patients.

42.5 The Patient with Severe Chronic Disability

The patient with severe chronic disability is defined as a patient with at least 3 ADL lost [32] even present before the acute event. Patients in this category have to be defined as chronic disable. This category includes complex patients chronically bedridden for cardiac causes (refractory heart failure) or noncardiac causes (neurological complications with severely disabling outcomes, severe cognitive impairment, severe orthopedic limitations, etc.). The approach to severe chronic disability patient starts from the assessment and management of clinical stability and prevention of adverse events. In fact, soon after the acute phase of various clinical pictures (i.e., myocardial infarction, unstable angina, pulmonary edema, stroke, etc.), a passive mobilization of the patient is at least advisable for the prevention of thromboembolic event due to bedridden, passing then, if possible, a physical activity program based on the procedures showed in Table 42.1.

The physiotherapy load in these patients is high.

The objectives and outcomes of the rehabilitation for the patient with severe chronic disability are showed in Tables 42.2 and 42.3.

Table 42.1 Individualized protocols of training based on disability status

Severe chronic disability	Temporary severe disability	Mild/moderate disability	Without disability
Mobilization sessions: active/passive	Mobilization sessions: active/passive	Training sessions of variable load exercise with assistive movement training apparatus	Sessions of variable load exercise using bike and treadmill as effective workout stimulus increasing intensity and sessions
Diaphragmatic respiratory gymnastics	Diaphragmatic respiratory gymnastics	Diaphragmatic respiratory gymnastics	Diaphragmatic respiratory gymnastics
Posture changes	Posture changes	Sessions of breathing exercises and calisthenics at a reduced energy expenditure, low, medium, or high	Sessions of breathing exercises and calisthenics at a reduced energy expenditure, low, medium, or high
Reeducation sessions in motor impairment	Reeducation sessions in motor impairment	Sessions of strengthening of individual muscle groups	Sessions of strengthening of individual muscle groups
Sessions of bronchial unblocking	Sessions of bronchial unblocking		
Sessions of calisthenics exercises	Sessions of calisthenics exercises		
Sessions with a muscle stimulation	Sessions with a muscle stimulation		
Muscle strengthening sessions	Muscle strengthening sessions		
	Training sessions gait and walk		

Table 42.2 Objectives of the rehabilitation based on disability status

Severe chronic disability	Temporary severe disability	Mild/moderate disability	Without disability
Improve the patient's ability to perform ADL	Improve the patient's ability to perform ADL	Improve the patient's ability to carry out the usual ADL	Increase the patient's functional capacity through training of the resistance and/or strength
Reduce the level of supervision in ADL	Increase, if possible, the patient's functional capacity	Increase the patient's functional capacity through training of the resistance and/or strength	Determine a training load applied at home once the patient has been discharged
Minimize the deconditioning due to loss of muscle tone	Reduce the level of supervision	If possible, determine a training load applied at home once the patient has been discharged	
Reduce adverse events	Minimize the deconditioning due to loss of muscle tone		
	Resolution of the bedridden and for the continued rehabilitation intervention as physical training		

Table 42.3 Outcome of the rehabilitation based on disability status

Severe chronic disability	Temporary severe disability	Mild/moderate disability	Without disability
Increase in the score of disability scales administered at the beginning of the rehabilitation process	Increase in the score of disability scales administered at the beginning of the rehabilitation process	Increase in the score of disability scales administered at the beginning of the rehabilitation process	The increase of 6-minute walking test distance
	If possible, the formal documentation of the termination of the setting bed using 6-minute walking test	If possible, increasing the distance of 6MWT	The increase of work capacity assessed by TE or CPX
		If possible, increase the cardiovascular capacity assessed by TE or CPX	

42.6 Temporary Severe Disability

This category includes complex patients with 3 or more ADL lost due to the acute event, but free of disability before the acute event, temporarily bedridden for cardiac causes (heart failure instability, complex ventricular arrhythmias, acute ischemia, etc.) or noncardiac causes (neurological complications, severe bedsores, poor evolution of surgical wounds, significant pulmonary complications with possible need for ventilatory support, febrile systemic infections, need of nutritional support, acute renal failure, delirium, severe pleural and/or pericardial effusion, severe anemia, etc.) for which it is estimated an improvement and/or resolution of symptoms. The level of disability of these patients will initially be quantified in a formal way through Barthel Index (BI). In addition, it will be appropriate to quantify the level of former habitual physical activity and comorbidities. The approach to the temporary severe disabled patient is based on the assessment and management of clinical stability. In this kind of patient a passive mobilization should be at least considered for the prevention of thromboembolic events, passing then (or immediately if the cause of the bedridden was not clinical instability) to a physical activity program based on the procedures showed in Table 42.1.

The physiotherapy load in these patients is moderate/high.

The objectives and outcomes of the rehabilitation of the patient with temporary severe disability complex are showed in Tables 42.2 and 42.3.

42.7 The Mild/Moderate Disabled Patient

Patient with ADL lost less than 3 is defined as mild/moderate disabled. This means that these patients may be functionally limited and sometimes even to a significant extent, but still lower than that of patient's severe disabilities. In this category are included patients in waiting list for heart transplantation during hemodynamic compensation, and possibly those recently transplanted patients with large pleural effusion and/or pericardial effusion and with significant anemia and patients with LVAD implantation where the limitation in ADL are also due to the ability to use the mechanical support.

Depending on the clinical condition, the functional evaluation of complex mild/moderate disabilities of patients can take advantage of the following tools:

1. Barthel Index (ADL)
2. 6-minute walking test (WT)
3. Conventional exercise testing (TE) or cardiopulmonary (CPX)

The exercise program will be based on the procedures showed in Table 42.1, variously associated with each other.

The physiotherapy load in these patients is low/moderate.

The objectives and outcomes of the rehabilitation of the patient with mild/moderate disabilities are showed in Tables 42.2 and 42.3.

42.8 The Patient Not Disabled

It defines a patient without disability in ADL. This means that these patients are not limited in the basic activities of their daily lives. They will still be functionally limited to higher-intensity activities depending on the severity of their underlying disease and/or comorbidities and their level of muscle conditioning (sedentary/active life). Depending on the clinical condition, the functional evaluation of non-disabled patients can take advantage of the following tools:

1. 6-minute walking test
2. Conventional CPX

The exercise program will be based on the procedures showed in Table 42.1, variously associated with each other. The physiotherapy load during management of these patients is low/moderate. The objectives and outcomes of the patient's rehabilitation without a disability are showed in Tables 42.2 and 42.3.

Conclusion

The rehabilitation process in the elderly should be implemented in accordance with the risk assessment criteria related to the exercise and adapted to the different disease patterns and disabilities. The patient's disability tends to coincide with a state of complexity, embracing a wide spectrum of cardiovascular and non-cardiovascular conditions associated with the underlying cardiac disease, characterized by varying degrees of impairment in functional capacity. This impairment arises from a disability, which, through a limitation of usual and, therefore, a restriction of the individual's participation in his social life, determines different degrees of frailty. Therefore, the rehabilitative intervention may be driven by multidimensional assessment, configured in patients less compromised in a classical physical training program, while the more functionally limited patients may be subjected to physical activity that even if they do not constitute an effective workout stimulus is still effective in the disability prevention. In any case, the cardiac rehabilitation configures an operational team framework involving various reasons of many professions depending on the degree of disability and the different needs of the patient. The rehabilitation process of these patients will be strictly individualized in relation to their functional impairment/disability at admission and the usual functional capacity. The proposed protocols do not follow the traditional approach of rehabilitation in cardiology (i.e., different protocols for different events or acute or chronic diseases), but rather suggest a transversal criterion for various clinical scenarios, based on different levels of patients' disability.

The combination of these procedures in terms of duration, frequency, and intensity will be individualized based on the patient's clinical condition. In any case, at least two daily sessions of the same procedure or two procedures seem applicable in the majority of patients. The progression of the load of physical activity criteria privileges first an increase of duration of individual sessions and then the frequency and finally intensity. For patients with mild/moderate disability and for those who are not disabled, the assessment of the current functional capacity will be appropriate for an assessment of habitual physical activity and comorbidities.

Key Points

- Cardiac rehabilitation is an intervention for the patients with heart disease, which includes health education and physical activity and aims to reduce mortality, morbidity, and hospital admission of the patients.
- Cardiac rehabilitation programs in the elderly should be based on comprehensive geriatric assessment and should be also driven by the specific disability of the patient and not only by the disease.
- Elderly patients, especially if frail, require a tailored rehabilitative intervention.

References

1. Dalal HM, Doherty P, Taylor RS (2015) Cardiac rehabilitation. BMJ 351:h5000
2. Annual report on the activity of a hospital admission. Admissions for rehabilitation and long-term care. www.Ministerosalute.it
3. Ottenbacher KJ, Smith PM, Illig SB et al (2004) Trends in length of stay, living setting, functional outcome, and mortality following medical rehabilitation. JAMA 292:1687–1695
4. Audelin MC, Savage PD, Ades PA (2008) Changing clinical profile of patients entering cardiac rehabilitation/secondary prevention programs: 1996 to 2006. J Cardiopulm Rehabil Prev 28:299–306
5. Balady GJ, Ades PA, Comoss P, Limacher M, Pina IL, Southard D, Williams MA, Bazzarre T (2000) Core components of cardiac rehabilitation/secondary prevention programs. A statement for healthcare professionals from the American Heart Association and the American Association of Cardiovascular and Pulmonary Rehabilitation Writing Group. Circulation 102:1069–1073
6. Manton KJ, Corder L, Stallard S (1997) Chronic disability trends in elderly United States populations: 1982–1994. Proc Natl Acad Sci 94:2593–2598
7. Fried LP, Ferrucci L, Darer J et al (2004) Untangling the concepts of disability, frailty, and comorbidity: implications for improved targeting and care. J Gerontol A Biol Sci Med Sci 59:255–263
8. Cacciatore F, Abete P, Mazzella F, Viati L, Della Morte D, D'Ambrosio D, Gargiulo G, Testa G, De Santis D, Galizia G, Ferrara N, Rengo F (2005) Frailty predicts long-term mortality in elderly subjects with chronic heart failure. Eur J Clin Invest 35:723–730
9. Stacey RD (1999) Strategic management and organizational dynamics: the challenge of complexity. Financial Times, London
10. Zimmerman B, Lindberg B, Pisek P (1988) Insight from complexity science for health care leaders. VHA Press, Irving
11. Goldberger AL (1996) Nonlinear dynamics for clinicians; chaos theory, fractals, and complexity at bedside. Lancet 347:1312–1314
12. The World health report 2006: working together for health. World Health Organization, Geneva, 2006. http://www.who.int/whr/2006/annex/en
13. Giannuzzi P, Mezzani A, Saner H et al (2003) Physical activity for primary and secondary prevention. Position paper of the Working Group on cardiac rehabilitation and exercise physiology of the European Society of Cardiology. Eur J Cardiovasc Prev Rehabil 10:319–332
14. Galizia G, Cacciatore F, Testa G et al (2011) Role of clinical frailty on long-term mortality of elderly subjects with and without chronic obstructive pulmonary disease. Aging Clin Exp Res 23:118–125

15. Cacciatore F, Testa G, Galizia G et al (2013) Clinical frailty and long-term mortality in elderly subjects with diabetes. Acta Diabetol 50:251–260
16. Stuck AE, Egger M, Hammer A et al (2002) Home visits to prevent nursing home admission and functional decline in elderly people: systematic review. JAMA 287:1022–1028
17. Cacciatore F, Gallo C, Ferrara N, Abete P, Paolisso G, Canonico S, Signoriello G, Terracciano C, Napoli C, Varricchio M, Rengo F (1998) Morbidity patterns in aged population in southern Italy. A survey sampling. Arch Gerontol Geriatr 26:201–213
18. Min LC, Elliott MN, Wenger NS et al (2006) Higher vulnerable elders survey scores predict death and functional decline in vulnerable older people. J Am Geriatr Soc 54:507–511
19. Marchionni N, Fattirolli F, Fumagalli S et al (2003) Improved exercise tolerance and quality of life with cardiac rehabilitation of older patients after myocardial infarction: results of a randomized, controlled trial. Circulation 107:2201–2206
20. Lavie CJ, Milani RV (1995) Effects of cardiac rehabilitation programs on exercise capacity, coronary risk factors, behavioral characteristics, and quality of life in a large elderly cohort. Am J Cardiol 76:177–179
21. Lavie CJ, Milani R (2004) Benefits of cardiac rehabilitation in the elderly. Chest 126:1010–1012
22. Opasich C, De Feo S, Pinna GD et al (2004) Distance walked in the 6-minute test soon after cardiac surgery: toward an efficient use in the individual patient. Chest 126:1796–1801
23. Cacciatore F, Abete P, Mazzella F, Furgi G, Nicolino A, Longobardi G, Testa G, Langellotto A, Infante T, Napoli C, Ferrara N, Rengo F (2012) Six-minute walking test but not ejection fraction predicts mortality in elderly patients undergoing cardiac rehabilitation following coronary artery bypass grafting. Eur J Prev Cardiol 19:1401–1409
24. Katz S, Ford AB, Moskowitz RW et al (1963) Studies of illness in the aged. The index of ADL; a standardized measure of biological and psychological functions. JAMA 185:94–99
25. Mahoney FI, Barthel DW (1965) Functional evaluation: the Barthel Index. Md State Med J 14:61–65
26. Parmelee PA, Thuras PD, Katz IR et al (1995) Validation of the Cumulative Illness Rating Scale in a residential geriatric population. J Am Geriatr Soc 43:130–137
27. Yesavage JA, Brink TL, Rose TL et al (1983) Development and validation of a geriatric depression screening scale: a preliminary report. J Psychiatr Res 17:37–49
28. Folstein MF, Folstein SE, McHugh PR (1975) "Mini-mental state": a practical method for grading the cognitive state of patients for the clinician. J Psychiatr Res 12:189–196
29. Bittner V (1997) Six-minute walk test in patients with cardiac dysfunction. Cardiology 42:897–902
30. Tinetti ME (1986) Performance-oriented mobility assessment of problems in elderly patients. J Am Geriatr Soc 34:119–126
31. Guralnik JM, Simonsick EM, Ferrucci L, Glynn RJ, Berkman LF, Blazer DG, Scherr PA, Wallace RB (1994) A short physical performance battery assessing lower extremity function: association with self-reported disability and prediction of mortality and nursing home admission. J Gerontol 49:M85–M94
32. Ferrucci L, Guralnick JM, Simonsick E et al (1996) Progressive versus catastrophic disability: a longitudinal view of the disablement process. J Gerontol A Biol Sci Med Sci 51:M123–M130

Rehabilitation in Older Patients with Peripheral Arterial Disease

43

Adriana Visonà

43.1 Introduction

Cardiovascular diseases (CVDs) are the leading cause of death and disability in Europe, posing a great social and economic burden. The sedentary lifestyle strongly promotes and accelerates age-related conditions, such as frailty and disability, representing an independent risk factor for cardiovascular disease and all causes related to morbidity and mortality. Moreover, the time devoted to physical activity linearly decreased with age. Peripheral arterial disease (PAD) itself, both asymptomatic and symptomatic, represents an important risk factor for cardiovascular morbidity and mortality. The striking increase in both the incidence and prevalence of PAD with increasing age is apparent from epidemiological data, and it has been estimated that the biennial incidence rate of intermittent claudication (IC) is 26.6 per 1000 men and 13.3 per 1000 women. Physical activity is one of the cornerstones for prevention of cardiovascular disease and for the treatment of PAD. However, most studies demonstrated that the relationship between physical fitness and vascular disease was mainly performed with middle-aged adults, and relatively few studies have been conducted among elderly subjects [1].

43.2 Mechanisms of Rehabilitation

The benefit and possible mechanisms of rehabilitation, also in old patients, include improvements in endothelial function, skeletal muscle metabolism, and blood viscosity. In addition to hemodynamic and metabolic mechanisms, improved biomechanisms

A. Visonà
Angiology Unit, San Giacomo Hospital, Castelfranco Veneto, TV, Italy

President, Italian Society for Angiology and Vascular Medicine (SIAPAV), Italy

Past President, European Society for Vascular Medicine (ESVM), Italy
e-mail: adrianavisona@gmail.com

© Springer International Publishing AG 2018

S. Masiero, U. Carraro (eds.), *Rehabilitation Medicine for Elderly Patients*, Practical Issues in Geriatrics, DOI 10.1007/978-3-319-57406-6_43

of walking also contribute to increase walking ability by decreasing the oxygen requirements to sustain a given level of constant load exercise. Many studies have also documented an improvement of general physical capability with a reduction in heart rate, respiration, and oxygen consumption with the same workload. Patients acquire the capability to walk for longer distance and duration at higher speed [2]. Indeed, PAD patients with IC had improved endothelial-dependent vasodilation measured in the upper extremity after engaging in a treadmill walking rehabilitation program [3].

The beneficial effects of low to moderate aerobic exercise training programs on improving functional capacity in old patients with PAD have been documented. Such patients could improve claudication symptoms after only a couple of months of rehabilitation and are likely to experience continual improvement thereafter. In addition to improving endothelial function and exercise tolerance, 6 months of exercise rehabilitation improves calf blood flow after an ischemic response. The severity of PAD may adversely impact the beneficial effects of an exercise rehabilitation program on flow-mediated endothelial function, and there was a trend for less improvement in patients with the lowest ankle to brachial index. Moreover, patients with the lowest baseline calf blood flow (maximal blood flow and postocclusive hyperemic response) had the smallest improvement in endothelial function. This suggests that in patients with severe PAD, adverse effects of atherosclerosis on endothelial function may be, in part, irreversible, or a different treatment design may be needed to see significant improvements [3].

43.3 Modification of Risk Factors

Cardiovascular risk factor modification is a pivotal element of the treatment of PAD. Although extensive evidence showed that exercise improves hypertension, glucose intolerance, and hyperlipidemia in patients without PAD, it remains unclear whether exercise rehabilitation has an impact on cardiovascular risk factors in patients with PAD. Even if large functional gains occur in patients with IC after exercise rehabilitation, it is possible that the absolute amount of exercise in debilitated population (old age and PAD) is insufficient to induce favorable alterations in cardiovascular risk factors [1]. Anyhow, it has been demonstrated that exercise rehabilitation program, in older patients with PAD, lowers LDL-C levels by 8%, total cholesterol levels by 5%, and systolic BP by 6%. These beneficial changes in the cardiac risk factor profiles may potentially reduce the rate of progression of atherosclerosis, as well as the associated complications. Therefore, exercise rehabilitation should be considered an integral part of the management of older patients with PAD [1]. Physical training should represent the primary therapeutic approach also in the subjects with a cluster of risk factors as metabolic syndrome (MS) [1, 4]. Smoking adversely affects exercise capacity in PAD patients, who are the prime candidates for exercise rehabilitation. Anyhow their relatively low baseline physical function does not impair their ability to regain lost functional independence to levels similar to those of nonsmoking patients with PAD.

43.4 Exercise Rehabilitation and Overall Strategy

Patients with IC experience reversible muscle ischemia during walking that is characterized by cramping and aching in the affected muscle. These symptoms result in a severe limitation in exercise performance and walking ability in elderly as well. The exercise limitation is associated with marked impairments in walking distance, walking speed, and overall function. Therefore, the treatment goals are to relieve symptoms and improve exercise performance and daily functional abilities. The initial approach to the treatment of limb symptoms should focus on structured exercise. According to the Trans-Atlantic Inter-Society Consensus (TASC) recommendations, supervised exercise should be part of the treatment of patients with PAD and IC. The most effective programs employ treadmill or track walking that is of sufficient intensity to bring on claudication and near-maximal pain, followed by rest, over the course of 30–60 min session. Exercise sessions are typically conducted three times a week for 3 months. How intensive should training be to prevent harmful effects? The crucial point is when and at what workload should exercise be stopped during a single training session. The guidelines suggest to encourage exercise to near-maximal pain, and TASC document indicates that pain during the exercise is predictive of the best results [2, 5]. The best workload in training of patients with PAD and IC should be aerobic and submaximal. The use of protocols providing a workload with a single well-defined fraction of training (60–70% of maximum walking capacity measured during the test), which is near-maximal pain, but without reaching claudication pain, is advisable [5, 6]. Different mechanisms appear to explain the exercise-mediated increase in ambulatory function. Improvements in walking economy and calf perfusion are two mechanisms that act synergistically to relieve claudication by decreasing the metabolic demand of walking and increasing oxygen delivery, respectively. However, exercise-mediated improvements in peripheral circulation in PAD patients with IC are not a consistent finding, as some studies report an increase, although others report no change in perfusion. The better energy utilization in the calf may be the factor which contributes to a delay in the development of claudication, therefore, manifested by increased distances walked. Furthermore, exercise training improved the self-reported quality of life (QOL) as assessed by the medical outcomes short form (MOS SF)-36 and the disease-specific walking impairment questionnaire (WIQ) instrument. Exercise training improves ambulatory function, perceived walking ability, and health-related QOL in older PAD patients with IC and supports current recommendations for exercise training in this patient population. The efficacy of whole-body progressive resistance training as a treatment for the symptoms of PAD in older adults was also evaluated. High-intensity progressive resistance training (H-PRT) significantly improved 6 min walk ability in older patients with PAD and IC, whereas low-intensity nonprogressive resistance training and unsupervised walking did not [7]. Improvement in walking ability is based on TASC evidence, which suggests that a change in distance of more than 50 m is clinically significant in most disease states. The finding of a greater than 60 m improvement in 6 min walking distance (6MWD) in the H-PRT group would be associated with a reduction in cardiovascular mortality and would thus be considered clinically significant. Furthermore, a 6MWD of less than 350 m is predictive of high risk of cardiovascular mortality across cardiopulmonary disorders [5, 7]. Also in older adults, a 6-month spinning training combined with proper diet has proved useful in ameliorating metabolic syndrome.

Although some experts believe that spinning could be too much intense for elderly, some others support spinning also in elderly, considered safe and useful if performed cautiously, with a careful monitoring of heart rate, blood pressure, pulse oximeter, and glycemia [4]. Spinning exerts several systemic beneficial effects, improving the muscle strengthening and the body coordination, the ventilator and maximal aerobic capacities, and vascular compliance.

Physical activity reduces the risk of fall, and fractures, optimize the cardiorespiratory performances, and ameliorate the coronary perfusion. Both standard physical training and spinning added to diet significantly improved lipid and glycemic profile. The patients receiving only diet probably require more time to achieve the same results. Moreover, standard physical training plus diet significantly lower plasma total cholesterol and triglycerides. In patients who performed spinning, a significant reduction of waist circumference, body mass index, and blood pressure was found, as well as improvement of glucose homeostasis.

The most frequent *contraindications* to physical activities in elderly patients with PAD are: (1) rest pain, (2) history of exertional angina, (3) exercise tolerance limited by leg pain of nonvascular origin (e.g., arthritis, orthopedic pain) and by factors other than intermittent claudication (e.g., dyspnea, fatigue, dizziness), (4) surgery related to PAD during the preceding 3 months, (5) myocardial infarction within the preceding 3 months, and (6) unstable claudication symptoms during the preceding 3 months. The major limitation of exercise rehabilitation is the lack of availability of a supervised setting to refer patients. Though exercise therapy is of proven effectiveness, some patients are simply not willing to persist with an exercise program in order to maintain the benefit. In addition, a claudication exercise program in a patient with diabetes who has severe distal neuropathy may precipitate foot lesions in the absence of proper footwear [5]. In conclusion, vascular rehabilitation, in particular supervised aerobic exercise, improves the risk factor profile and represents a cornerstone for the treatment also in older patients with PAD, considered subjects at higher risk for cardiovascular morbidity and mortality. Exercise therapy should be pursued and promoted in clinical and research field in older patients.

Key Points

- PAD frequent in elderly, beneficial effects of aerobic supervised exercise, amelioration of risk profile and quality of life, improvement of disease-specific walking impairment in elderly patients with PAD.

References

1. Izquierdo-Porrera AM, Gardner AW, Powell CC, Katzel LI (2000) Effects of exercise rehabilitation on cardiovascular risk factors in older patients with peripheral arterial occlusive disease. J Vasc Surg 31(4):670–677
2. Andreozzi GM, Kalodiki E, L Gašpar L, Martini R, Minar E, Angelides N, Nicolaides AN, Novo S, Visonà A, Prior M, Arosio E, Hussein EA, Poredos P, Antignani PL, Avram R, Roztocil K, Stvrtinova V, Kozak M, Vacula I; Central European Vascular Forum; Mediterranean League of Angiology and Vascular Surgery; North Africa and Middle East Chapter of International Union of Angiology (2014) Consensus Document on Intermittent Claudication from the Central European Vascular Forum (C.E.V.F.)-3rd revision (2013) with the sharing of the Mediterranean League of Angiology and Vascular Surgery, and the North Africa and Middle East Chapter of International Union of Angiology. Int Angiol 33(4):329–347
3. Brendle DC, Joseph LJ, Corretti MC, Gardner AW, Katzel LI (2001) Effects of exercise rehabilitation on endothelial reactivity in older patients with peripheral arterial disease. Am J Cardiol 87(3):324–329
4. Verrusio W, Andreozzi P, Renzi A, Martinez A, Longo G, Musumeci M, Cacciafesta M (2016) Efficacy and safety of spinning exercise in middle-aged and older adults with metabolic syndrome: randomized control trial. Ann Ist Super Sanita 52(2):295–300
5. Norgren L, Hiatt WR, Dormandy JA, Nehler MR, Harris KA, Fowkes FG; TASC II Working Group (2007) Inter-Society Consensus for the Management of Peripheral Arterial Disease (TASC II). J Vasc Surg 45(Suppl S):S5–S67
6. Tsai JC, Chan P, Wang CH, Jeng C, Hsieh MH, Kao PF, Chen YJ, Liu JC (2002) The effects of exercise training on walking function and perception of health status in elderly patients with peripheral arterial occlusive disease. J Intern Med 252(5):448–455
7. Parmenter BJ, Raymond J, Dinnen P, Lusby RJ, Fiatarone Singh MA (2013) High-intensity progressive resistance training improves flat-ground walking in older adults with symptomatic peripheral arterial disease. J Am Geriatr Soc 61(11):1964–1970

Exercise Training Modalities in Lower Limb Peripheral Artery Disease

44

Stefano Lanzi, Lucia Mazzolai, and Luca Calanca

Lower limb peripheral artery disease (LLPAD) is a chronic atherosclerotic disease which leads to narrowing and/or occlusion of arteries supplying the legs. The most characteristic symptom of LLPAD is intermittent claudication (IC), a cramping lower limb (buttocks, thighs, calf, or foot) pain occurring during exercise and resolving with rest. IC is characterized by inadequate oxygen supply (from impaired blood flow) to meet metabolic demand [1]. Based on a large population study, IC prevalence increases from about 2% in a population aged 40–44 years to 7% in a population aged 70–74 years [2]. It has previously been shown that LLPAD patients have a significant reduction in muscle strength [3], walking performance [4], and physical functioning [5] compared to subjects without LLPAD. Moreover, LLPAD patients are also generally less implicated in regular exercise [6] and in daily life activities [5, 7]. These significant reductions may cause decreased quality of life [8] and contribute to increase in mortality risk [9].

Regular exercise training is recommended as one of the primary baseline measures in LLPAD with the aim to improve walking capabilities and contribute to reduce cardiovascular risk [1, 10]. There is a large body of evidence supporting the pivotal role of regular exercise training in improving walking performance [i.e., pain-free walking distance (PFWD), maximal walking distance (MWD), and six-minute walking distance (6MWD)], physical functioning, and quality of life in LLPAD patients [1, 10, 11]. Moreover, it has recently been shown that exercise training also leads to significant improvement in aerobic fitness [peak oxygen uptake ($V'O_{2peak}$)] [12]. This is relevant, as poor aerobic fitness has been suggested to be a strong mortality predictor in patients with LLPAD [13]. In general, exercise training sessions have a duration which varies between 30 and 60 min (depending

S. Lanzi (✉) • L. Mazzolai • L. Calanca
Division of Angiology, Heart and Vessel Department, University Hospital Lausanne, Lausanne, Switzerland
e-mail: Stefano.Lanzi@chuv.ch; Lucia.Mazzolai@chuv.ch; Luca.Calanca@chuv.ch

© Springer International Publishing AG 2018

S. Masiero, U. Carraro (eds.), *Rehabilitation Medicine for Elderly Patients*, Practical Issues in Geriatrics, DOI 10.1007/978-3-319-57406-6_44

on individual exercise tolerance) and are performed two to three times per week for a total of 3 or 6 months [1]. To achieve maximal benefits, exercise training should be supervised by physiotherapists or sport trainers [14]. As blood flow and pressure (ankle-brachial index) are unaffected by exercise training [12], other potential mechanisms, such as changes in microcirculation, endothelial function, muscle metabolism, inflammation, and walking economy, seem to be implicated in the improvement of walking performance [10].

Walking and lower extremity aerobic training (strengthening and aerobic training focused on lower limbs) are the most common modes of training [1, 15]. However, by reason of more severe claudication pain, lower pain tolerance, increased risk of fall linked with an impaired balance, and/or other comorbidities (diabetes, orthopedic, and rheumatic diseases), elderly LLPAD patients cannot always complete a walking training session and/or have a limited enthusiasm with regard to regular exercise. Therefore, in order to allow elderly LLPAD patients to benefit from rehabilitation programs, alternative modes of training (e.g., arm crank ergometer, resistance training, Nordic pole walking, cycling) have also been evaluated, and promising results were described [12, 15, 16].

As the impaired blood flow induces lower limb skeletal muscle ischemia and leg pain during walking, upper limb exercise performed with an arm crank ergometer (Fig. 44.1) may be an interesting pain-free and well-supported training modality [17]. Indeed, it has been demonstrated that 12-week arm crank exercise training performed at 60–70% of the peak work rate (2 min of exercise followed by 2 min of rest for 40 min) may increase walking performance and $V'O_{2peak}$ [17]. This was explained, at least in part, by an increased lower limb oxygen delivery during walking and suggests that circulatory adaptations may also occur in untrained limbs [17]. Indeed, it has been shown that upper limb exercise training may have a systemic anti-inflammatory effect in LLPAD patients [18], which could positively impact endothelial function and reduce cardiovascular risk. Therefore, upper limb training may be especially useful in elderly LLPAD patients with concomitant lower limb diseases affecting walking capacity (orthopedic, rheumatic). Although to our knowledge this type of training has not been evaluated in more severe stage of LLPAD [Fontaine stages III (rest pain) and IV (ischemic ulcers or gangrene)], this might be an interesting opportunity to improve aerobic fitness and reduce the cardiovascular risk.

Resistance exercise training has also been suggested as an effective training modality [19–23]. Indeed, LLPAD patients have a significant reduction in calf muscle area [24] and also have lower leg strength which is associated with walking capabilities [22]. It has been demonstrated that 12-week whole-body (e.g., calf raise on leg press machine, leg press, leg curl, leg extension, crunches, seated row, bench press) resistance training [3 sets of 10 repetitions performed at the intensity between 11 and 13 (light and somewhat hard, respectively) on Borg's scale (rating of perceived exertion to monitor level of intensity during exercise)] improves walking performance to a similar extent as treadmill exercise training [21]. Interestingly, compared to walking, this mode of exercise elicits lower pain during the training sessions [23]. Furthermore, longer resistance training programs have also been

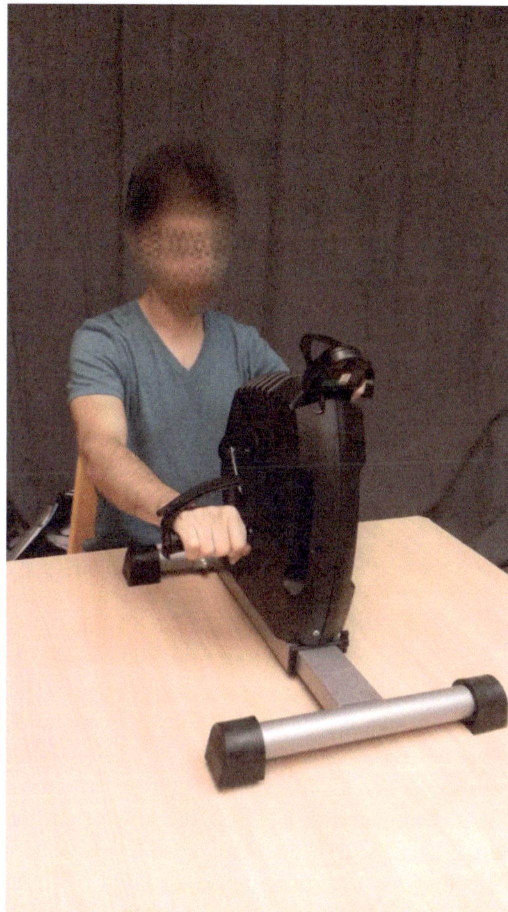

Fig. 44.1 Arm crank ergometer

evaluated. It has been shown that 24-week whole-body resistance training [2 sets of 8–15 repetitions performed at approximately 70% of one repetition maximum (1RM)] significantly improves walking performance and strength compared to control group [20]. Another study [19] showed that 24-week lower limb progressive resistance training (3 sets of 8 repetitions performed at 50–80% 1RM) improves walking performance on treadmill and quality of life (assessed by questionnaire) compared to control group. However, there were no significant changes in the 6MWD compared to control group [19]. Finally, it has recently been demonstrated that intensity of resistance training may also have an impact on the improvement of walking performance. Indeed, 24-week whole-body high-intensity progressive resistance training (3 sets of 8 repetitions performed at 50–80% 1RM) significantly improved the 6MWD and whole-body strength compared to whole-body low-intensity resistance training (3 sets of 8 repetitions performed at 20–30% 1RM) and control group. The adaptations in the high-intensity progressive resistance training group were related to significant changes in bilateral calf and hip extensor skeletal muscle endurance [22].

Nordic pole walking has been shown to increase the PFWD and the MWD compared to walking without poles, suggesting that this type of exercise may improve walking performance despite a higher cardiovascular stimulation [25]. The use of poles may increase the walking speed and reduce the lower extremity load, which seems to be relevant in LLPAD patients [26]. In addition, as elderly LLPAD patients may have an impaired balance [27], the use of poles might also be useful. It has been demonstrated that 24-week Nordic pole walking exercise training, performed at maximal or near to maximal claudication pain, increases walking performance, $V'O_{2peak}$, and physical functioning (assessed by questionnaire) in LLPAD patients [28]. Nordic pole walking training was found to be as effective as treadmill training for the improvement in walking performance [29].

Cycling exercise might also be a safe and feasible training modality [30]. Although 6-week cycling exercise training performed at vigorous intensity showed a significant increase in cycling time, no significant improvement was observed in walking performance in response to cycling exercise compared to treadmill exercise training (performed at the same relative exercise intensity) in LLPAD patients [30]. However, in a subgroup of patients who experienced similar (anatomic location) exercise-limiting symptoms during walking and cycling, walking performance was improved after cycling training. This suggests a cross-transfer effect of training modalities and highlights the potential role of cycling in some LLPAD patients [30].

In conclusion, data suggest that different training modalities (other than walking) are safe, feasible, and effective in LLPAD patients. These allow elderly LLPAD patients to benefit from rehabilitation programs taking into account their specific needs. Compared to walking, the lower pain induced by other training modalities during exercise may encourage patients to better adhere to regular exercise training. To better optimize training prescription in all LLPAD patients, further research is needed using combined or varied training modalities.

Key Points

- Regular exercise training is recommended as one of the primary baseline measures in LLPAD patients.
- Other than walking, different training modalities (e.g., arm crank ergometer, resistance training, Nordic pole walking, and cycling) are safe, feasible, and effective in LLPAD patients.

References

1. Lane R, Ellis B, Watson L, Leng GC (2014) Exercise for intermittent claudication. Cochrane Database Syst Rev 7:CD000990

2. Norgren L, Hiatt WR, Dormandy JA, Nehler MR, Harris KA, Fowkes FG et al (2007) Inter-Society Consensus for the Management of Peripheral Arterial Disease (TASC II). J Vasc Surg 45(Suppl S):S5–S67
3. Camara LC, Ritti-Dias RM, Meneses AL, D'Andrea Greve JM, Filho WJ, Santarem JM et al (2012) Isokinetic strength and endurance in proximal and distal muscles in patients with peripheral artery disease. Ann Vasc Surg 26:1114–1119
4. Regensteiner JG, Wolfel EE, Brass EP, Carry MR, Ringel SP, Hargarten ME et al (1993) Chronic changes in skeletal muscle histology and function in peripheral arterial disease. Circulation 87:413–421
5. McDermott MM, Liu K, Greenland P, Guralnik JM, Criqui MH, Chan C et al (2004) Functional decline in peripheral arterial disease: associations with the ankle brachial index and leg symptoms. JAMA 292:453–461
6. Bartelink ML, Stoffers HE, Biesheuvel CJ, Hoes AW (2004) Walking exercise in patients with intermittent claudication. Experience in routine clinical practice. Br J Gen Pract 54:196–200
7. McDermott MM, Liu K, O'Brien E, Guralnik JM, Criqui MH, Martin GJ et al (2000) Measuring physical activity in peripheral arterial disease: a comparison of two physical activity questionnaires with an accelerometer. Angiology 51:91–100
8. Regensteiner JG, Hiatt WR, Coll JR, Criqui MH, Treat-Jacobson D, McDermott MM et al (2008) The impact of peripheral arterial disease on health-related quality of life in the Peripheral Arterial Disease Awareness, Risk, and Treatment: New Resources for Survival (PARTNERS) Program. Vasc Med 13:15–24
9. Criqui MH, Langer RD, Fronek A, Feigelson HS, Klauber MR, McCann TJ et al (1992) Mortality over a period of 10 years in patients with peripheral arterial disease. N Engl J Med 326:381–386
10. Stewart KJ, Hiatt WR, Regensteiner JG, Hirsch AT (2002) Exercise training for claudication. N Engl J Med 347:1941–1951
11. Parmenter BJ, Dieberg G, Phipps G, Smart NA (2015) Exercise training for health-related quality of life in peripheral artery disease: a systematic review and meta-analysis. Vasc Med 20:30–40
12. Parmenter BJ, Dieberg G, Smart NA (2015) Exercise training for management of peripheral arterial disease: a systematic review and meta-analysis. Sports Med 45:231–244
13. Leeper NJ, Myers J, Zhou M, Nead KT, Syed A, Kojima Y et al (2013) Exercise capacity is the strongest predictor of mortality in patients with peripheral arterial disease. J Vasc Surg 57:728–733
14. Fokkenrood HJ, Bendermacher BL, Lauret GJ, Willigendael EM, Prins MH, Teijink JA (2013) Supervised exercise therapy versus non-supervised exercise therapy for intermittent claudication. Cochrane Database Syst Rev CD005263
15. Parmenter BJ, Raymond J, Dinnen P, Singh MA (2011) A systematic review of randomized controlled trials: walking versus alternative exercise prescription as treatment for intermittent claudication. Atherosclerosis 218:1–12
16. Lauret GJ, Fakhry F, Fokkenrood HJ, Hunink MG, Teijink JA, Spronk S (2014) Modes of exercise training for intermittent claudication. Cochrane Database Syst Rev CD009638
17. Tew G, Nawaz S, Zwierska I, Saxton JM (2009) Limb-specific and cross-transfer effects of arm-crank exercise training in patients with symptomatic peripheral arterial disease. Clin Sci 117:405–413
18. Saxton JM, Zwierska I, Hopkinson K, Espigares E, Choksy S, Nawaz S et al (2008) Effect of upper- and lower-limb exercise training on circulating soluble adhesion molecules, hs-CRP and stress proteins in patients with intermittent claudication. Eur J Vasc Endovasc Surg 35:607–613
19. McDermott MM, Ades P, Guralnik JM, Dyer A, Ferrucci L, Liu K et al (2009) Treadmill exercise and resistance training in patients with peripheral arterial disease with and without intermittent claudication: a randomized controlled trial. JAMA 301:165–174
20. McGuigan MR, Bronks R, Newton RU, Sharman MJ, Graham JC, Cody DV et al (2001) Resistance training in patients with peripheral arterial disease: effects on myosin isoforms, fiber type distribution, and capillary supply to skeletal muscle. J Gerontol A Biol Sci Med Sci 56:B302–B310

21. Meneses AL, de Lima GH, Forjaz CL, Lima AH, Silva GQ, Cucato GG et al (2011) Impact of a supervised strength training or walking training over a subsequent unsupervised therapy period on walking capacity in patients with claudication. J Vasc Nurs 29:81–86
22. Parmenter BJ, Raymond J, Dinnen P, Lusby RJ, Fiatarone Singh MA (2013) High-intensity progressive resistance training improves flat-ground walking in older adults with symptomatic peripheral arterial disease. J Am Geriatr Soc 61:1964–1970
23. Ritti-Dias RM, Wolosker N, de Moraes Forjaz CL, Carvalho CR, Cucato GG, Leao PP et al (2010) Strength training increases walking tolerance in intermittent claudication patients: randomized trial. J Vasc Surg 51:89–95
24. McDermott MM, Hoff F, Ferrucci L, Pearce WH, Guralnik JM, Tian L et al (2007) Lower extremity ischemia, calf skeletal muscle characteristics, and functional impairment in peripheral arterial disease. J Am Geriatr Soc 55:400–406
25. Oakley C, Zwierska I, Tew G, Beard JD, Saxton JM (2008) Nordic poles immediately improve walking distance in patients with intermittent claudication. Eur J Vasc Endovasc Surg 36:689–694; discussion 95-6
26. Willson J, Torry MR, Decker MJ, Kernozek T, Steadman JR (2001) Effects of walking poles on lower extremity gait mechanics. Med Sci Sports Exerc 33:142–147
27. Gardner AW, Montgomery PS (2001) Impaired balance and higher prevalence of falls in subjects with intermittent claudication. J Gerontol A Biol Sci Med Sci 56:M454–M458
28. Collins EG, Langbein WE, Orebaugh C, Bammert C, Hanson K, Reda D et al (2005) Cardiovascular training effect associated with polestriding exercise in patients with peripheral arterial disease. J Cardiovasc Nurs 20:177–185
29. Bulinska K, Kropielnicka K, Jasinski T, Wojcieszczyk-Latos J, Pilch U, Dabrowska G et al (2015) Nordic pole walking improves walking capacity in patients with intermittent claudication: a randomized controlled trial. Disabil Rehabil:1–8
30. Sanderson B, Askew C, Stewart I, Walker P, Gibbs H, Green S (2006) Short-term effects of cycle and treadmill training on exercise tolerance in peripheral arterial disease. J Vasc Surg 44:119–127

Lymphedema Rehabilitation of the Elderly

45

Gert Apich

45.1 Introduction

Lymphedema is a chronic disease, due to an insufficient lymph transport capacity caused by an insufficient number or function of lymph vessels or their malformation. Therefore, the waste products, which are normally removed with lymph, cannot be transported, and this provokes lymph congestion and lymphostasis, in which fluid and protein levels in the interstitial space increase. The clinical sign is swelling, which left untreated can progress and provoke tissue hardening and/or adiposity; this process can lead to several complications and disability.

Lymphedema classification is shown in Table 45.1.

45.2 Classification

Table 45.1 Lymphedema classification

Classification according to etiology [1]	
Primary (congenital) lymphedema	Are based on a genetic developmental disorder of lymphatic vessels and/or lymph nodes (aplasia, atresia, hypoplasia, hyperplasia, lymphangioma). They can occur in combination with other dysplasia/syndromes (e.g., Turner syndrome, Noonan syndrome, Klippel-Trenaunay-Weber syndrome) or isolated
Secondary (acquired) lymphedema	Are due to an acquired injury to the lymph vessel system (e.g., post-traumatic, post-inflammatory, artificial, post-reconstructive, or caused by malignant tumors or metastases)

(continued)

G. Apich
Physical Medicine and General Rehabilitation,
KABEG LKH and Lymphklinik Wolfsberg, Wolfsberg, Austria
e-mail: gert.apich@kabeg.at

© Springer International Publishing AG 2018

S. Masiero, U. Carraro (eds.), *Rehabilitation Medicine for Elderly Patients*, Practical Issues in Geriatrics, DOI 10.1007/978-3-319-57406-6_45

Table 45.1 (continued)

Classification according to clinical stages [2]	
Stage 0 (interval stage)	There is no edema, but a pathological scintigraphical finding indicating reduced transport capacity
Stage 1	Is spontaneously reversible, and the swelling may resolve overnight
Stage 2 (spontaneous irreversible stage)	The swelling persists without resolving
Stage 3 (elephantiasis)	There is a monstrous swelling
Classification according to localization [2]	
Localized lymphedema	Head, arm, leg, or genital lymphedema or lymphostatic enteropathy
Generalized lymphedema	The whole body can be affected

45.3 Diagnosis

A diagnosis of lymphedema can be based on both basic and advanced diagnostic measures [3].

Basic measures comprise medical history, examination, palpation, and measurement.

Taking a **medical history** involves asking about malignant disease, surgery, erysipelas infections, soft tissue lesions, venous and arterial disease, medication intake, hereditary factors, and pain—although classic lymphedema is pain-free. If a patient is experiencing pain, this may point to malignant lymphedema.

Examination: Which parts of the body are affected by the swelling? Asymmetry is one of the salient clinical signs of lymphedema. Bilateral swelling normally indicates a systemic cause, e.g., cardiogenic, nephrogenic, hepatogenic, or from medicine intake. Localization of primary lymphedema is mainly peripheral. In secondary lymphedema, proximal localizations are more typical. The presence of skin signs of lymphedema such as deep skin creases, box-shaped teeth, hyperkeratosis, papillomatosis cutis lymphostatica (Fig. 45.1), lymph cysts, or lymph fistulae confirms the diagnosis.

Palpation: Fibrosis can be detected using the skinfolding test. The skinfold between the thumb and index finger is compared with the thickness of the skinfold with the opposite side. If there is a lymphedema, the skinfold is always thicker (Fig. 45.2). A thickened skinfold detected in the region of the second or third toe is referred to as a positive Stemmer sign (Fig. 45.3).

The measurement can be done with a measuring tape (Kuhnke method) or with an optoelectronic device (Perometer) [4].

45.3.1 Advanced Diagnostic Measures

If medical history, physical examination, and palpation yield no clinical findings and if it's still unsure as to whether or not the patient has lymphedema, then diagnostic measures [5] using high-resolution ultrasound, indirect lymphography,

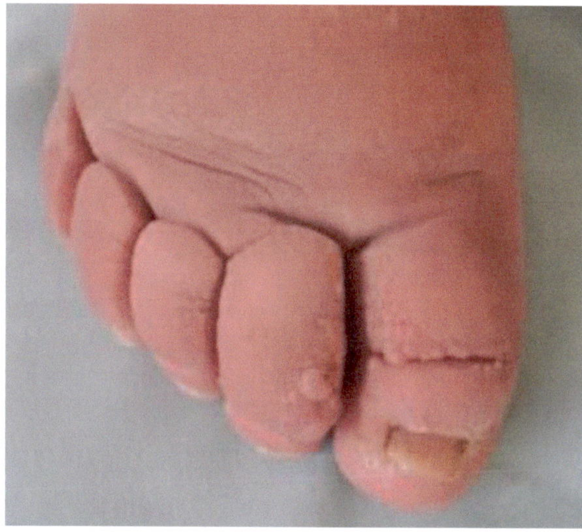

Fig. 45.1 Deep skin creases, box-shaped teeth, and papillomatosis cutis lymphostatica at the first and second toe (picture: ©Apich)

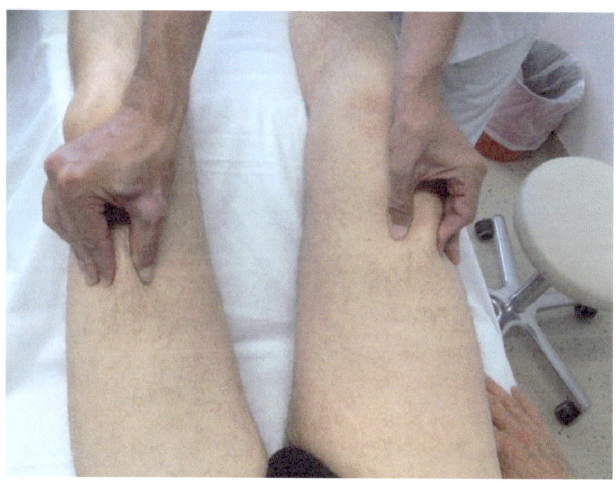

Fig. 45.2 Positive skinfolding test of the right thigh (picture: ©Apich)

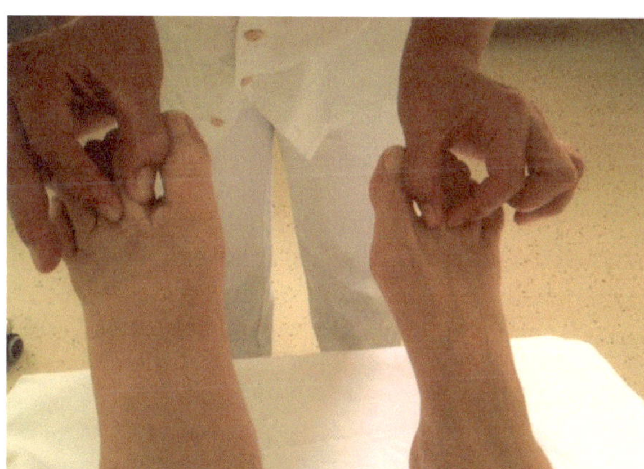

Fig. 45.3 Positive Stemmer sign on the right second toe (picture: ©Apich)

scintigraphic quantification of lymphatic function (gold standard), computed tomography (CT), magnetic resonance imaging (MRI), near-infrared fluorescence (NIRF) imaging methods, or bioelectrical impedance analysis should be used.

45.4 Differential Diagnosis

45.4.1 Asymmetrical Edema

These may occur in venous thromboses, post-thrombosis syndrome, post-reconstructive edema, status following supination trauma of the ankle, inflammatory edema attributable to polyarthritis, in Sudeck's atrophy, a ruptured Baker's cyst can lead to asymmetric swelling—to name but a few.

45.4.2 Symmetrical Edema

It can be cardiac, nephrogenic, or hepatogenic or can be found in cases of lipoedema or obesity or by taking medication.

Especially elderly patients might have the so-called mixed edema, a combination of lymphedema (asymmetric) and symmetrical edema in generalized systemic diseases.

45.5 Therapy Options for Lymphedema

45.5.1 Conservative Therapy

Complete decongestive therapy (CDT) has the following purposes:

- Reducing the current stage of lymphedema to a lower stage
- Edema and volume reduction (Fig. 45.4)
- Consistency normalization
- Improving muscle and joint pump function
- Instructing patients in self-treatment techniques such as performing manual lymph drainage on their own, the lymphological compression bandage technique, and decongesting exercises

This treatment aims to reintegrate the patients into their social and work environment, to obtain a psychological stabilization [6, 7] and an improved quality of life [8]. Furthermore, it avoids the onset of complications such as erysipelas infections, mycosis, papillomatosis cutis lymphostatica, and lymphangiosarcoma and reduces the need for nursing care.

CDT can be performed on an outpatient and inpatient basis and consists of two phases.

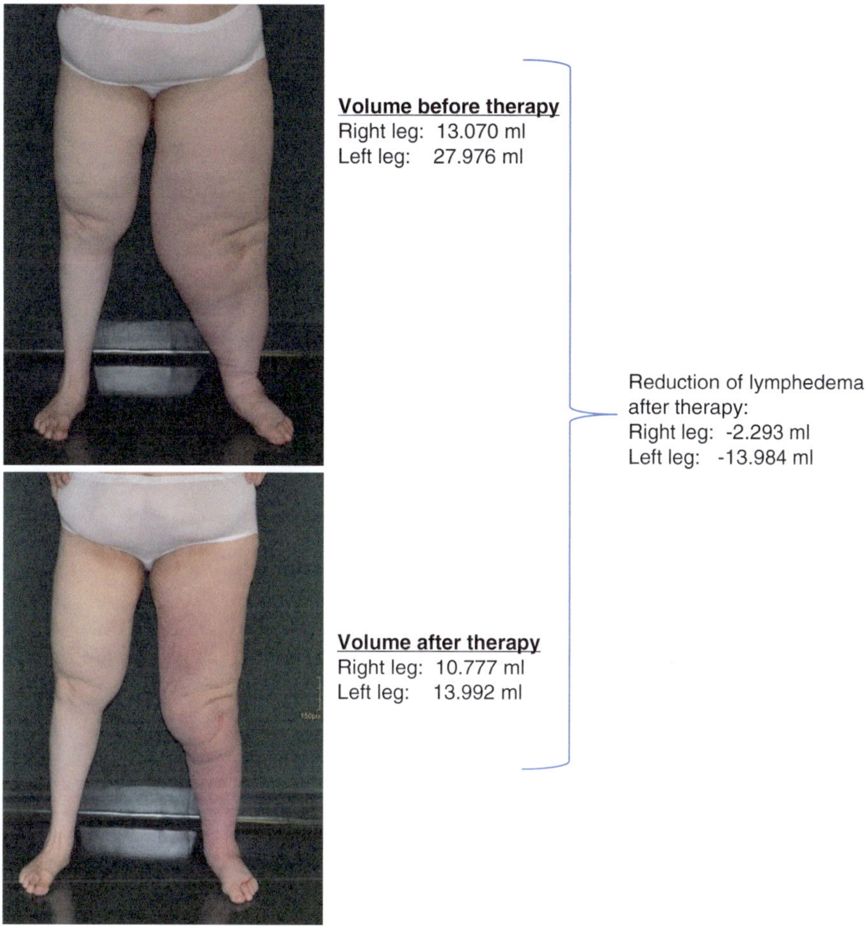

Fig. 45.4 Edema and volume reduction after successful conservative lymphedema therapy with the complex decongestive physical therapy (CDT) using the example of a secondary lymphedema of the left leg (picture: ©Apich)

45.5.2 Phase 1 of Manual Decongestion Therapy

It allows the mobilization and drainage of accumulation of protein-rich fluid in the interstitium. This phase includes skin rehabilitation, antisepsis, and care, **manual lymph drainage (MLD)**, **compression therapy**, and **decongestion movement therapy.**

Regular skin care is essential, in fact, aging skin tends to dry out due to drugs, lack of hydration, and various comorbidities. This can be further enhanced by the mechanical effect and the suction of the compression treatment.

Manual lymph drainage (MLD) promotes anastomosis formation, an increase in the motor unit of lymph drainage, and increased transport capacity. General contraindications for MLD [9] are acute diseases such as cardiac failure, infections, and thrombophlebitis and venous thrombosis.

Compression therapy is done with compression bandages and aims to increase the interstitial pressure, to reduce ultrafiltration, to augment reabsorption, to enhance transport capacity, and to loosen fibrosclerotic tissue.

First of all, skin care, using a well-tolerated skin care product, is crucial, because otherwise the compression bandage will provoke skin degreasing and dryness. The second purpose is to protect the skin, by using a knitted tube over the affected part; this tube absorbs perspiration and protects the skin. Then, a fleece padding is applied to avoid unevenness, to distribute compression pressure evenly, and to compensate for wrapping glitches. A short-stretch bandage finishes the compression bandage.

Absolute contraindications for compression bandages are very poorly compensated cardiac insufficiency in the presence of acute cardiac failure, peripheral arterial occlusive disease (PAOD) stages III and IV, scleroderma, Sudeck's atrophy, abscesses, boils, and the loss of skin sensitivity [10].

The decongestion movement therapy, wearing compression bandages or compression stockings, stimulates the muscle and joint pumps and thus promotes venous and lymphatic drainage.

At the end of phase 1, the patient wears medical compression stockings, which were previously measured by an experienced technician (a flat knitwear for the stockings should be used).

Contraindications to the use and the compliance to wear the stockings are to be considered, especially in elderly patients. It should be noted that bedridden patients require a lower pressure bandage than ambulatory active patients.

45.5.3 Phase 2 of Manual Decongestion Therapy

The main purpose of phase 2 is the preservation of the therapeutic success achieved thus far. This phase is identical to phase 1, except that compression therapy is carried out using custom-made medical compression stockings that the patient should wear during the day. During the night, if necessary, the extremities can be bandaged. Patients should do decongestion exercises while wearing the compression stockings (e.g., Nordic walking, swimming, or training with a cross-trainer in the presence of an arm lymphedema; walking, Nordic walking, biking, hiking, and using a cross-trainer, in case of leg lymphedema).

The implementation of the CDT should be stage-adjusted but depends also on the location (arm, leg, genital, head, or combined) and on coexisting comorbidities (e.g., congestive heart failure, muscular-skeletal disorders, mental illness, frailty). The therapy should be modified especially for the elderly persons and for patients with malignant lymphedema.

45.5.4 Medications

Currently, no medication cures lymphedema. In the event of complications such as erysipelas infections, penicillin is prescribed, usually for 14 days or more [11]. For patients who are allergic or resistant to penicillin, clindamycin or a macrolide antibiotic such as erythromycin is prescribed. Diuretics are unsuitable for lymphedema management, because they decrease fluid content in the interstitial space without reducing protein levels; thus, they have the reverse of the desired effect—because the proteins determine a stronger fibrotic reaction.

45.5.5 Instructions

Patients can be trained on how to apply their own bandages, to do lymph drainage; they also acquire some information on skin antisepsis, skin care, nutritional counseling, lifestyle changes (e.g., reduce weight, stop smoking), and psychological self-help techniques. If necessary, relatives can also receive a training in some skills, such as compression bandaging.

45.5.6 Additive Physical Therapy [12]

45.5.6.1 Specific Therapies for Lymphedema

The intermittent pneumatic compression [13] promotes the displacement of interstitial fluid. It is no substitute for manual lymph drainage. Mechanical negative pressure therapy, known as LymphaTouch, loosens tissue that deteriorated due to fibrosclerosis, and it stimulates the motor unit of lymph drainage. The low-level laser therapy works on the same principle and also acts as an anti-inflammatory [14]. Lymph taping also enhances the motor unit of lymph drainage. All these therapies lead to a lymphedema volume reduction.

45.5.6.2 Non-specific Therapies for Lymphedema

Conditions such as obesity, muscular impairment, and movement restrictions can undermine or even cancel the therapeutic effects of CDT and need to be managed. In this regard, highly hyperemizing measures should be avoided in the edematous regions, as they can provoke an increase in the lymph-dependent load and thus exacerbate existing lymphedema. However, these measures can be applied outside the affected regions and include strength and endurance training (Nordic walking), movement therapy involving decongestion exercises, and physical modalities such as electrotherapy, ultrasound, heat therapy, laser therapy, magnetic field therapy [15], respiration therapy, sensory-motor training, ergotherapy, speech therapy (particularly in head, neck, and facial lymphedema), and exercises for swallowing disorders, breathing, and voice. Physical modalities are also helpful and necessary for pain therapy, if present.

45.5.6.3 Operative Management

Surgery is used as alternative measure only after all conservative therapeutic options have been exhausted and only if therapeutic success has been too low or if therapy has failed completely. The surgical treatments are resection and drainage procedures, as well as reconstructive procedures.

45.5.6.4 Follow-Up Visits

Lymphological follow-up visits should be performed once a year and, in the event of complications, earlier, to ensure the preservation of the therapeutic success over the long term. Medical visits include medical examinations, checking volume changes, the patient's skin, and his medical compression stockings.

Conclusion

Lymphatic rehabilitation of the elderly is a multimodal and interdisciplinary therapy. Especially in the older patient, it is important to modify the therapy according to the individual characteristics, in order to obtain a long-term improvement and to ameliorate the quality of life.

Key Points

- Lymphedema is a chronic disease, due to an insufficient lymph transport capacity, that can lead to several complications and disability.
- Lymphatic rehabilitation of the elderly is a multimodal and interdisciplinary therapy.
- Conservative lymphedema therapy is the most important treatment in the lymphedema rehabilitation.
- Physical modalities can be used as additive measures to treat lymphedema and pain, if present.
- Surgery is indicated only when all conservative therapeutic options have been exhausted.

References

1. Földi E, Földi M (2010) Lymphostatische Krankheitsbilder. In: Földi E, Földi M (Hrsg.) Lehrbuch Lymphologie für Ärzte, Physiotherapeuten und Masseure/med. Bademeister. 7. Auflage. Urban & Fischer Verlag, Stuttgart, pp 175–263 (Földi M, Földi E, Strößenreuther C, Kubik S (2012) Földi's textbook of lymphology: for physicians and lymphedema therapists (English))
2. Pritschow H, Schuchhardt C (2014) Das Lymphödem und die Komplexe Physikalische Entstauungstherapie. Ein Handbuch für die Praxis in Wort und Bild; 4. Auflage_2014_Köln_ Viavital Verlag GmbH, pp 44–67 (Pritschow H, Schuchhardt C (2008) Lymphedema – management and complete physical decongestive therapy: a manual for treatment (English))
3. AWMF-Leitlinien: Diagnostik und Therapie der Lymphödem - S2k Leitlinie, Reg.Nr.058.001. Online: http://www.awmf.org/leitlinien/aktuelle-leitlinien.html (2009) [May 2017]

4. Herpertz U (2014) Ödeme und Lymphdrainage. Diagnose und Therapie; Lehrbuch der Ödematologie; 5. Auflage. Schattauer Verlag, pp 70–75
5. Weissleder H, Schuchardt C (2011) Erkrankungen des Lymphgefäßsystems. 5. Auflage. Viavital Verlag GmbH, Köln, pp 79–160 (Weissleder H, Schuchardt C (2007) Lymphedema – diagnosis and therapy (English))
6. Flaggl F, Döller W, Jäger G, Apich G (2006) Prävalenz komorbider psychischer Störungen bei Lymphödempatienten in der medizinischen Rehabilitation. Praxis Klinische Verhaltensmedizin und Rehabilitation 71:75–82
7. Jäger G, Döller W, Roth R (2006) Quality of life and body image impairments in patients with lymphedema. Lymphology 39:193–200
8. Quendler S (2008) Lebensqualität von Lymphödempatienten und ihre emotionalen und kognitiven Komponenten. Diplomarbeit Universität Wien
9. Herpertz U (2014) Ödeme und Lymphdrainage. Diagnose und Therapie; Lehrbuch der Ödematologie; 5. Auflage. Schattauer Verlag, pp 303–306
10. Asmussen PD, Söllner B (2004) Kompressionstherapie. Prinzipien und Praxis. Urban & Fischer Verlag, München, p 104
11. Weissleder H, Schuchardt C (2011) Erkrankungen des Lymphgefäßsystems. 5. Auflage. Viavital Verlag GmbH, Köln, p 173 (Weissleder H, Schuchardt C (2007) Lymphedema – diagnosis and therapy (English))
12. Fialka-Moser V (Hrsg.) (2013) Kompendium physikalische Medizin und Rehabilitation. Diagnostische und therapeutische Konzepte. 3 Auflage. Springer Verlag, Wien
13. Weissleder H, Schuchardt C (2011) Erkrankungen des Lymphgefäßsystems. 5. Auflage. Viavital Verlag GmbH, Köln, pp 187–206 (Weissleder H, Schuchardt C (2007) Lymphedema – diagnosis and therapy (English))
14. Weissleder H, Schuchardt C (2011) Erkrankungen des Lymphgefäßsystems. 5. Auflage. Viavital Verlag GmbH, Köln, pp 605–608 (Weissleder H, Schuchardt C (2007) Lymphedema – diagnosis and therapy (English))
15. Strößenreuther RHK (2010) Entstauende Bewegungs- und Atmungstherapie, Krankengymnastik sowie weitere Maßnahmen der physikalischen Therapie. In: Földi E, Földi M (Hrsg.) Lehrbuch Lymphologie für Ärzte, Physiotherapeuten und Masseure/med. Bademeister. 7. Aufl. Urban & Fischer, Stuttgart, pp 497–508

Pulmonary Rehabilitation in the Elderly

46

Beatrice Nordio, Marco Poletti, Silvia Iovino, and Andrea Vianello

46.1 Introduction

Dyspnea, fatigue, lower exercise tolerance, peripheral muscle dysfunction, and mood disorders are commonly noted in elderly patients with chronic obstructive pulmonary disease (COPD) and other chronic respiratory disorders who may benefit from a pulmonary rehabilitation program (PRP) aiming to achieve personalized goals as far as symptoms, physical functioning, quality of life (QoL), hospitalization, and morbidity are concerned.

According to the most recent recommendations and guidelines, pulmonary rehabilitation (PR) can be defined as a comprehensive patient-tailored intervention including exercise training, education, and behavioral change that is prescribed on the basis of an exhaustive personalized assessment and that aims to improve the physical and psychological conditions of persons with chronic respiratory diseases and to promote their long-term adherence to health-enhancing behavior and activities [1].

Commonly managed by a specialized, interdisciplinary team, PR can be initiated at any stage of a respiratory disorder, even during an acute exacerbation phase, and is being prescribed to an increasing number of elderly patients with COPD and/or other respiratory disorders (e.g., bronchiectasis, interstitial lung diseases, neuromuscular diseases, etc.). Although rare, contraindications to PR include severe cognitive dysfunction or psychiatric illness, unstable comorbidity (e.g., unstable angina, uncompensated congestive heart failure, etc.), severe exercise-induced hypoxemia, inability to exercise, lack of motivation, nonadherence, inadequate financial resources, and persistence of smoking [1–3].

B. Nordio • M. Poletti • S. Iovino • A. Vianello (✉)
Division of Respiratory Pathophysiology, University-City Hospital of Padua, Padua, Italy
e-mail: marcopoletti88@gmail.com; andrea.vianello@sanita.padova.it

© Springer International Publishing AG 2018

S. Masiero, U. Carraro (eds.), *Rehabilitation Medicine for Elderly Patients*, Practical Issues in Geriatrics, DOI 10.1007/978-3-319-57406-6_46

As candidates for PRP show significant differences in underlying pathophysiology, symptoms, and disease course, an individualized approach is preferred to a standard rehabilitation plan. PR can produce many benefits in both inpatients and outpatients, as well as in housebound patients; the ideal location depends on the patient's preference, its cost, and availability. The minimum duration for an effective PRP is 8 weeks, but longer programs almost certainly produce greater benefits. Withdrawal from these kinds of rehabilitation plans seems to range from 10% to 32%, and the causes seem to be linked to exacerbation of the underlying disease, depressive symptoms, lack of family support, and/or transportation problems.

46.2 Technical Aspects

The main components of a PRP are listed in Table 46.1. PR is implemented by a specialized, interdisciplinary team, including physicians and other healthcare professionals such as physiotherapists, respiratory therapists, nurses, psychologists, behavioral specialists, exercise physiologists, nutritionists, occupational therapists, and social workers, depending on the characteristics of the individualized program (Table 46.2). In most cases, a pulmonologist heads the PR team. While a physical therapist provides a specific exercise regimen personalized to the patient's individual goals and needs, an occupational therapist is usually responsible for teaching conservation measures and assesses the need for prosthetic devices or

Table 46.1 Components of a pulmonary rehabilitation program

Assessment
Symptom evaluation
Quality-of-life measurements
Pulmonary function tests
Comorbidities and therapy
Exercise training
Endurance training
Interval training
Resistance/strength training
Flexibility training
Upper limb training
Inspiratory muscle training
Neuromuscular electrical stimulation
Maximizing the effects of exercise training
Pharmacotherapy
Oxygen and helium–oxygen hyperoxic gas mixtures
Noninvasive positive pressure ventilation
Education
Behavior change
Collaborative self-management
Addressing motivational issues
Breathing strategies
Pursed-lip breathing
Computer-aided breathing feedback

Table 46.2 Multidisciplinary team participants in a pulmonary rehabilitation team

Pulmonologist
Respiratory therapist
Physical therapist
Educational therapist
Nurse/exercise physiologists
Nutritionist
Social worker
Psychologist/behavioral specialist
Occupational therapist
Social worker

wheelchairs. A respiratory therapist supervises the exercise program and teaches the patient how to do breathing exercises, as well as the proper use of aerosol medication and oxygen therapy. Every candidate needs to undergo a thorough assessment before beginning a PRP so that the most beneficial exercises can be identified and prescribed, to rule out comorbidities, to make appropriate adjustments to the program, and to optimize medical therapy. Once underway, all the professionals involved in the PRP should meet on a regular basis to examine each patient's individual progress and to discuss variations that could help him/her to reach the goals established [1–3].

46.2.1 Assessment

As mentioned above, a complete, comprehensive evaluation of the patient's physical, psychological, and lung function status should be performed to establish the candidate's suitability for PRP. The most frequently reported symptoms are fatigue, cough, weakness, and dyspnea at rest and/or during exertion. St. George's Respiratory Questionnaire (SGRQ), the Chronic Respiratory Disease Questionnaire (CRQ), and the COPD Assessment Test (CAT) are the most common questionnaires that are used for symptom assessment. The presence of depression and anxiety should also be evaluated, as both conditions can adversely affect a patient's ability to participate in a PRP. The patient's capacity to complete activities of daily living (ADL) can be rated using performance scales, including the Manchester Respiratory Activities of Daily Living Scale, the Pulmonary Functional Status and Dyspnea Questionnaire, and the London Chest Activity of Daily Living Scale. Physicians should also evaluate if the patient is following an optimal medical regimen usually consisting in inhaled bronchodilators and corticosteroids, and if need be, long-term oxygen therapy.

Pulmonary function tests (PFT) should be routinely included in a candidate's comprehensive pre-PR evaluation since they are essential to confirm the diagnosis of the underlying disease, to assess the level of ventilatory impairment, and to evaluate the effect of pharmacologic therapy. Static and dynamic lung volumes including total lung capacity (TLC), forced vital capacity (FVC), forced expiratory volume in first second (FEV_1), and FEV_1/FVC ratio can be utilized to identify an obstructive and/or restrictive ventilatory defect (Figs. 46.1 and 46.2). While a reduction in the FEV_1/FVC ratio below the predicted value is consistent with an obstructive ventilatory impairment, the lack of response to inhaled bronchodilator therapy may contribute to establishing a diagnosis of COPD (Fig. 46.3). A specific evaluation of respiratory muscle strength is mandatory for patients with neuromuscular disorders (e.g., amyotrophic lateral sclerosis, myasthenia gravis, muscular dystrophies, etc.), which is based on the measurement of maximal inspiratory and expiratory pressure

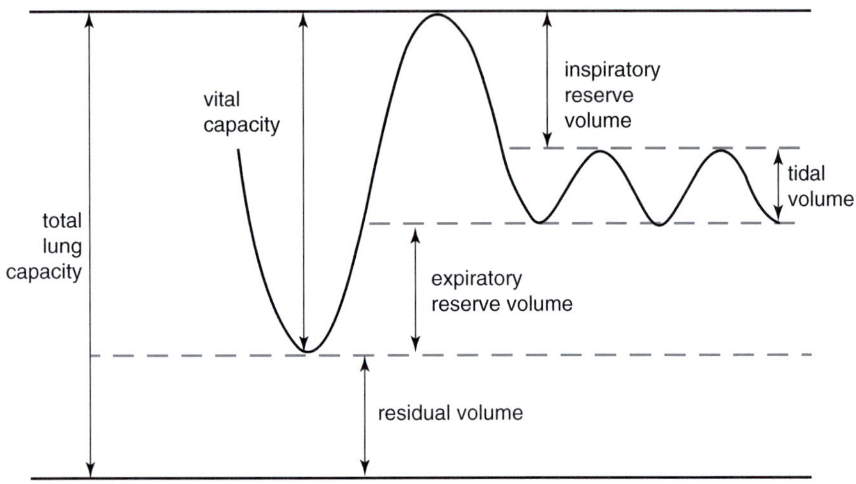

Fig. 46.1 Lung volumes and capacities according to spirometry

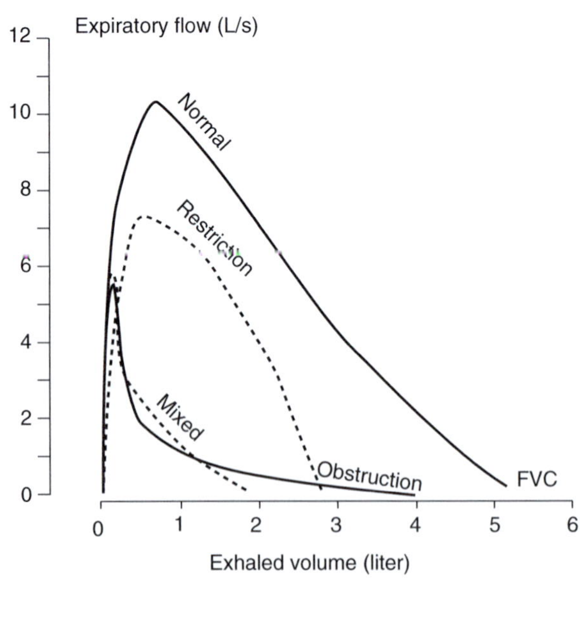

Fig. 46.2 Flow/volume curve recorded by a spirometric challenge test during a forced expiration, showing a normal FVC/VC ratio and obstructive, restrictive, and mixed alterations

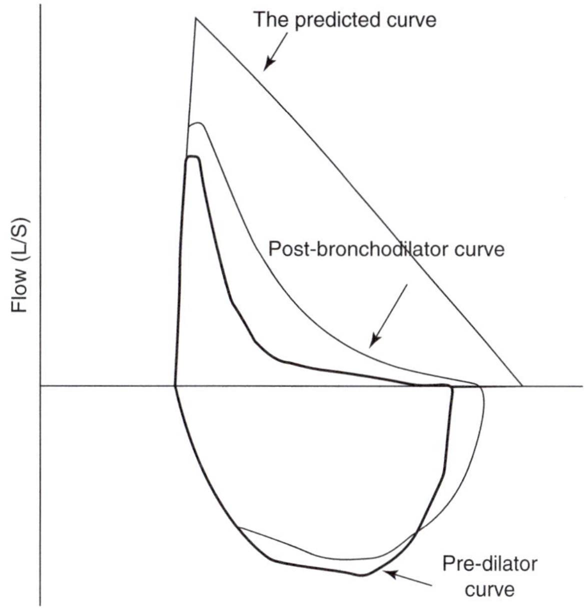

Fig. 46.3 Flow/volume curve recorded during a forced expiratory spirometric challenge before and after bronchodilator administration

(MIP, MEP); a high negative MIP value (<−80 cm H_2O) or a high positive MEP value (>+90 cm H_2O) can, respectively, exclude clinically relevant inspiratory or expiratory muscle weakness. Functional tests should also include a maximal cardiopulmonary exercise testing (CPET) that may provide essential data to identify factors contributing to exercise limitation, assess the safety of exercise, and establish the patient's maximal work rate.

46.2.2 Exercise Training

Patients with chronic respiratory disorder commonly show shortness of breath leading to inactivity which, in turn, leads to a loss of muscle strength, mobility problems, sarcopenia, and cardiac dysfunction. Age-related pulmonary function decline and the presence of comorbidities may limit exercise even further. Considered the cornerstone of PR, exercise training is the best method to improve muscle function. An improvement in skeletal muscle function after exercise training leads to greater exercise capacity despite the absence of changes in lung function. The improved oxidative capacity and efficiency of the skeletal muscles lead, moreover, to a lower ventilatory requirement for a given submaximal work rate, which, in turn, may reduce dynamic hyperinflation and exertional dyspnea. Although the total amount of work should be individualized depending on the patient's specific need to ameliorate aerobic capacity and muscle strength, training on a regular basis with activity loads exceeding those of everyday life is essential to improve exercise performance.

A variety of exercise regimens are available for exercise training [1–3]:

1. **Endurance training**. Endurance training can improve aerobic capacity and reduce breathlessness and fatigue by ameliorating cardiorespiratory function. High-intensity endurance training performed by cycling or walking is usually prescribed five times per week, at an intensity of continuous exercise (>60% of maximal work rate) for 20–60 min sessions. Work intensity can be established on the basis of the results of the Borg Dyspnea Scale (target 4–6) or the Rating of Perceived Exertion (RPE) (target 12–14). The benefits expected include improvement in exercise tolerance, muscle function, and bioenergetics.
2. **Interval training**. Interval training combines high-intensity exercise with periods of rest or low-intensity work to help the patient achieve a high training load while avoiding the onset of dyspnea and fatigue. The strategy is particularly indicated for patients with severe exercise-induced dyspnea and/or severe comorbidities.
3. **Resistance/strength training**. As patients with chronic respiratory diseases can also show reduced muscle mass and strength that may, in turn, limit exercise tolerance, they may benefit from strength training of specific muscle groups, in particular repetitive lifting of heavy weights. Interestingly, a combination of resistive and endurance training has been found to be extremely effective in increasing exercise capacity, with the additional advantage of counteracting an abnormal loss of bone mineral density that is common among COPD patients.
4. **Flexibility training**. Postural abnormalities such as thoracic kyphosis, increased chest anterior-posterior diameter, shoulder elevation, and protraction or trunk flexure may accelerate pulmonary function decline, increase the work of breathing, and worsen QoL in COPD patients. Upper and lower body flexibility programs, including stretching of the major muscle groups, at least 2–3 days per week, can improve thoracic posture and mobility.
5. **Upper limb training**. Aerobic upper limb resistance training should help the patient with self-care activities including dressing, bathing, and simple household tasks.
6. **Inspiratory muscle training**. Elderly patients with respiratory impairment may show diminished pressure-generating capacity by the inspiratory muscles that may reduce exercise tolerance and contribute to dyspnea. Inspiratory muscle training in this case could be particularly advantageous.
7. **Transcutaneous neuromuscular electrical stimulation (NSE)**. NSE, which can improve skeletal muscle strength and exercise capacity and decrease dyspnea and fatigue, can be utilized in deconditioned individuals with severe ventilatory or cardiac limitations. This technique may be beneficial to individuals with cognitive and psychological difficulties and/or severe dyspnea who are not eligible for standard PRPs.

Frequency, intensity, and specificity of exercise sessions are the most important variables determining the impact of training:

1. **Frequency**. For pragmatic reasons, most PRPs organize sessions two or three times weekly. Although some evidence indicates that two sessions per week may be inadequate to produce effects, it is also true that most therapists instruct patients to exercise at home in between sessions.
2. **Intensity**. Most studies indicate that there is a threshold for the training effect. An improvement in endurance seems to be a virtual certainty if a level of intensity corresponding to 60–75% of the maximum oxygen uptake can be sustained for at least 20–30 min a few days per week.
3. **Specificity**. Training regimens are prescribed that are specific to the patient's needs. For example, walking endurance activities increase walking endurance and thus the lower extremities but not the upper ones. Furthermore, endurance exercises improve endurance capabilities more than strength, whereas strength training (i.e., weightlifting) increases strength but not necessarily endurance or other outcomes such as exercise capacity or health status. Most programs, thus, incorporate a variety of training regimens.

46.2.2.1 Maximizing the Effects of Exercise Training

The effect of exercise training can be enhanced by a number of measures aiming to improve ventilatory capacity and blood gas exchanges, including the utilization of bronchodilators, oxygen and helium–oxygen hyperoxic gas mixtures, and noninvasive mechanical ventilation.

1. **Pharmacological agents**. Pharmacologic therapy is one of the key components of a treatment management plan for subjects with chronic airflow limitation aiming to prevent and control symptoms, reduce exacerbations, and improve exercise tolerance and general health status. Inhaled bronchodilators can increase expiratory flow and reduce dynamic hyperinflation by acting on the airway smooth muscles. Since it increases exercise tolerance, bronchodilators are an essential component of PRP in elderly patients with COPD [4]. Although studies on anabolic hormonal supplementation, and in particular testosterone analogs, have demonstrated that they produce a positive effect on muscle mass, they do not seem to induce a significant increase in muscle strength and endurance in individuals with COPD [1].
2. **Supplemental oxygen therapy**. Oxygen therapy is usually considered a routine supplementary measure in patients with respiratory diseases enrolled in a PRP as it tends to improve exercise tolerance and reduce breathlessness. Studies evaluating the efficacy of oxygen supplementation during exercise training have, nevertheless, produced conflicting results. In fact, while oxygen therapy with respect to compressed air results in higher training intensity in normoxic individuals with moderate to severe COPD, supplemental oxygen does not improve exercise tolerance and/or health status in individuals with severe COPD and exercise-induced hypoxemia. Given these considerations, it is not entirely clear if supplemental oxygen therapy is beneficial during exercise training. Of interest, patients administered with long-term oxygen therapy commonly require augmented oxygen flow rate during exercise to maintain adequate oxygenation [5]. With respect to

room air, heliox, which is helium–oxygen mixture, may reduce gas density and lower airway resistance and air trapping in patients with obstructive disease, thereby enhancing exercise tolerance. Although heliox theoretically appears to be an effective tool to augment maximal work rate during training, evidence suggesting that it can have a beneficial impact on exercise training is still inconsistent [6].

3. **Noninvasive positive pressure ventilation**. Recent studies have shown that long-term use of noninvasive positive pressure ventilation (NPPV) can improve functional status, prevent deterioration of gas exchanges, and reduce hospitalization in patients with severe COPD. NPPV can, moreover, reduce the work of breathing and improve exertional dyspnea during exercise, making it possible to prolong a training session. Due to expiratory flow limitation and a higher respiratory rate, COPD patients may, in fact, experience air trapping during exercise, leading to elevated end-expiratory lung volume (EELV). This phenomenon, also known as "dynamic hyperinflation," which may significantly increase the elastic work of breathing, worsen exertional dyspnea, and reduce exercise tolerance, can be effectively counteracted by NPPV [7]. Used as an integral part of PRP, NPPV also allows respiratory muscles to rest at the end of a training session. Despite results demonstrating its efficacy, provided that its application is labor-intensive, the use of NPPV as an adjunctive component of a PRP is still uncommon and requires the supervision of experienced personnel. Interestingly, NPPV can be also used to improve exercise tolerance during recovery from an acute exacerbation of COPD [8].

46.2.3 Education

One of the aims of PR is to cover the educational needs of participants, in particular COPD patients. Specific educational and self-management information is furnished to patients in the attempt to promote positive changes in health habits and behaviors, such as reducing exposure to risks, maximizing compliance to medications, and adhering to a more active lifestyle. The effectiveness of educational programs for COPD patients has not been specifically studied, although a Cochrane review concluded that it is associated with improvement in QoL and lower hospitalization rate. Actual scientific evidence has not, however, confirmed the value of self-management education in COPD patients [9, 10].

46.2.4 Other Interventions

1. Breathing Strategies

   As stated earlier, individuals with obstructive lung disease, and particularly COPD, may have dynamic hyperinflation, which limits exercise capacity. Because breathing retraining focuses on slowing the respiratory rate, primarily through prolonged expiration, it may be beneficial in reducing dyspnea via diminishing exercise-induced dynamic hyperinflation. Adaptive breathing strategies using yoga breathing techniques, pursed-lip breathing, and computer-aided breathing feedback have been employed.

2. Nutritional Support
   Nutritional support is an important aspect of PR. Indeed, patients with chronic respiratory conditions are frequently either over- or underweight, and a low body mass index correlates with a worse prognosis. Survival analysis studies have shown that body weight has an independent effect on survival in COPD, and the negative effect of low body weight can be reversed by appropriate therapy in some patients. A number of studies have reported that nutritional interventions improve outcomes. In particular, creatine supplementation has been associated with improvements in fat-free muscle mass, strength, and QoL score.

46.3 Clinical Applications

46.3.1 COPD

According to the American Thoracic Society (ATS)/European Respiratory Society (ERS) definition, COPD is a preventable, treatable disease state characterized by airflow limitation that is not fully reversible. The airflow limitation is usually progressive and is associated with an abnormal inflammatory response of the lungs to noxious particles or gases, primarily caused by cigarette smoking. Although COPD affects the lungs, it also produces significant systemic consequences. Symptoms such as fatigue, shortness of breath, and weight loss are commonly present and contribute to the patient's overall health status burden. In addition, acute disease exacerbations and hospitalizations may significantly contribute to progressive disability. Nearly all symptomatic COPD patients could benefit from PR to help maintain functional capacities and to substantially reduce symptoms. The presence of depressive symptoms should not prevent the patient from participating in PR, and the therapist should be aware that it may even have a positive physical and psychological effect.

Elderly COPD patients often have difficulty in carrying out tasks used to measure physical capacity (e.g., treadmill maximal exercise test) due to their muscle strength limitation which does not permit them to achieve maximal exercise performance. Surrogate and/or submaximal tests such as the six-minute walking test (6MWT) could be utilized in this population. Indeed, since patients are free to walk at their preferred intensity during this test and most daily activities are performed at submaximal levels of strength and intensity, the 6MWT may perfectly reflect the individual's functional adaptation to exercise during these activities. A cutoff value below 350 walked meters is generally considered the threshold limit predicting poor prognosis in these patients [11]. A standard PRP for these patients should include exercise training, smoking cessation, nutrition counseling, and education. Aerobic exercise is, in particular, the best comprehensive intervention, as it involves the upper and lower extremities and aims to enhance muscle strength and endurance. The combination of resistance and endurance training seems to be able to increase muscle strength and mass, to restore the highest possible level of independent function, and to substantially reduce symptoms. A standard PRP can be feasible and operational in a variety of settings, including the patients' home, even if patients present severe chronic respiratory insufficiency or following acute decompensation and/or hospitalization. Although there have been reports that PR improves patients' general health status and physical performance, its effect on the rate of exacerbations is controversial. A significant increase in muscle strength, gait speed, and stair climbing has been reported in most frail COPD patients older than 80 who have participated in a PRP including at least 4 weeks of exercise training. Supervised programs have led to greater benefit with respect to unsupervised ones. A short comprehensive program including education, exercise, physiotherapy, and occupational therapy in elderly COPD inpatients recovering from acute exacerbation has been found to be associated with lower readmission rates over the following year with respect to untreated ones.

46.3.2 Non-COPD Disorders

Benefits linked to PRP can also be found in elderly patients with non-COPD respiratory disorders (Table 46.3), but precisely because these patients may have particular requirements, the PRP needs to be individually tailored for them.

1. **Interstitial lung diseases**. Interstitial lung diseases (ILDs), functionally characterized by a restrictive ventilatory pattern, are a heterogeneous group of diseases affecting the pulmonary interstitium. Exercise intolerance, which is a key feature of ILDs, is often associated with marked dyspnea on exertion. Poor exercise tolerance is associated with reduced QoL and poor survival. Exercise limitation in ILD is due to altered respiratory mechanics, impaired gas exchange, and circulatory limitation. Exercised-induced hypoxia and pulmonary hypertension are common in ILDs. Physical deconditioning probably plays a role in ILD, just as it does in other chronic respiratory diseases. Avoidance of activities and breathlessness may likewise, in turn, provoke dyspnea and fatigue and further curtailment of physical activity. Emerging evidence suggests that PR may result in relevant short-term benefits in patients with ILD. Although the pathophysiologic mechanisms in respiratory limitation in COPD and ILD differ, the similarities in clinical problems (exercise intolerance, muscle dysfunction, dyspnea, impaired QoL) suggest that PR could produce substantial improvements in these patients as well. Sporadic studies on the effect of PR in ILD patients have indicated that they need close supervision and that appropriate adjustments must be made to standard program outlines. They have also demonstrated that in many cases improvements are not

Table 46.3 Non-COPD chronic lung disorders and respiratory conditions that may benefit from a pulmonary rehabilitation program in the elderly patients

• Chest wall disease
• Interstitial lung disease; post-ARDS pulmonary fibrosis
• Lung cancer
• Non-cystic fibrosis bronchiectasis
• Neuromuscular diseases such as post-polio syndrome
• Pulmonary vascular disease

maintained at the 6-month follow-up assessment. Supplemental oxygen should be made available to ILD patients during exercise training given the high risk of severe hypoxemia and pulmonary hypertension [12, 13].

Although recent studies have not shown that PR produces significant effects in patients with idiopathic pulmonary fibrosis (IPF), current guidelines for its management recommend that it should be prescribed to most patients. Given dramatic disease progression, timely referral to a PRP is particularly important in patients in whom it is essential to maintain muscle strength and endurance [14]. Besides exercise training, advance care planning to optimize activities of daily living and management of mood disorders should also be taken into consideration [1, 13].

2. **Non-cystic fibrosis-related bronchiectasis**. Bronchiectasis refers to the abnormal, irreversible dilatation of the bronchi caused by chronic inflammatory changes in the bronchial walls, leading to parenchymal structural alterations, progressive airflow obstruction, and dynamic hyperinflation. Their predominant symptoms include chronic cough with purulent sputum, recurrent pulmonary infections, dyspnea, exercise limitation, and reduction of QoL. Many patients experience recurrent exacerbations, and a higher frequency predicts a poorer prognosis. Additionally, reduction in exercise capacity has been associated with progressive airflow obstruction, dyspnea secondary to dynamic hyperinflation, and psychological impairment. International guidelines recommend that these patients be provided PR aiming to improve physical capacity and QoL. A PRP is commonly based on endurance exercise training combined with inspiratory muscle training (IMT) and airway clearance techniques. A large retrospective study concluded that the magnitude and duration of benefits in exercise capacity and QoL are similar to those observed in COPD. A PRP may also provide an ideal opportunity to initiate or optimize airway clearance, with regular monitoring and technique review. Although airway clearance techniques have positive effects on sputum expectoration, their impact on lung function and QoL warrants further studies [1, 2, 15].
3. **Neuromuscular disorders (NMDs)**. NMDs include a heterogeneous group of approximately 600 different diseases, showing various symptoms, functional limitations, and prognoses. Pulmonary complications caused by respiratory muscle dysfunction are commonly a source of morbidity and mortality in patients with NMD: indeed, due to the progressive weakening of inspiratory muscles, a large proportion of patients are known to develop a severe restrictive ventilatory impairment requiring periodic monitoring of lung volumes and maximal respiratory pressures. Muscle weakness can lead to the progressive onset of alveolar hypoventilation and a severe inability to cough. Patients with NMDs are frequently referred to a PR team for adaptation to NPPV: respiratory support provided by long-term mechanical ventilator, in fact, can be effective in relieving respiratory distress symptoms, reversing or stabilizing hypoventilation, improving sleep quality, enhancing QoL, prolonging survival, and providing long-term care benefits. Chronic, progressive hypercapnia and associated symptoms may

be resolved in patients with adequate bulbar muscle strength and cognitive function who use NPPV, via a mouthpiece or a nasal mask. Additional insufflation and exsufflation support should be made available by means of manually and/or mechanically assisted coughing which can eliminate bronchial secretions. A number of patients with NMD may benefit from a comprehensive PRP including exercise training, and in particular inspiratory muscle training (IMT). Related improvements in inspiratory muscle performance associated with a subjective amelioration in the capacity to perform ADL and higher levels of well-being have been reported in patients with post-poliomyelitis syndrome [16]. The impact of training protocols on force and endurance in patients with NMDs remains, however, controversial, and no improvement associated with IMT has been reported in those patients who are already retaining CO_2. In conclusion, exercise training should be prescribed with caution in NMD individuals, as the potential for further muscle damage cannot be excluded.

4. **Lung cancer**. Mostly caused by tobacco smoking, lung cancer is one of the most common cancers worldwide. It is generally classified into non-small cell lung cancer (NSCLC) and small cell lung cancer, with the former representing 85–90% of all cases. Treatment of lung cancer (i.e., surgery, radiotherapy, and/or chemotherapy) depends on disease stage but also on the presence of comorbidities, functional performance, QoL, and peak aerobic capacity. Cancer-related symptoms include deconditioning, muscle weakness, fatigue, cachexia, and anxiety, frequently resulting in disability. Dyspnea and depressed mood also contribute to impaired QoL. Preoperative peak exercise treadmill tests often need to be curtailed because of leg discomfort in 70% of patients with NSCLC, suggesting that extra-pulmonary features, just as lower limb muscle dysfunction, may contribute to poor exercise performance. Physical activity levels generally do not spontaneously return to pre-surgery levels and often remain impaired for 6 months or longer due to leg discomfort in a majority of patients. It would be important thus to consider referring lung cancer patients to pre- and postoperative PRPs [1–3]. Preoperative PR can optimize patients' exercise tolerance and overall medical stability before undergoing cancer resection surgery. Improvement in exercise performance could also help an inoperable patient become a fit candidate for potentially curative surgery. Moreover, a lower incidence of postoperative respiratory morbidity and a shorter postoperative stay have been associated with preoperative PR. Data on the optimal length of preoperative PR are, however, scarce. Implementing PR in the period between diagnosis and treatment may be challenging, as patients and healthcare professionals are reluctant to delay lung resection. As a result, the duration of preoperative rehabilitation must be dictated by medical necessity. Even a short (2–4 week) preoperative PR (including self-efficacy-based exercise prescription, IMT, and the practice of slow breathing) can have positive effects on preoperative functional exercise capacity and shorten hospital stay with respect to usual care [1, 17]. Evidence on the efficacy of postoperative PR in lung cancer patients is

limited. While aerobic and strength training programs in the immediate postoperative period have been found to improve strength in some studies, they do not seem to have any effect on the 6MWT or on QoL. Most postoperative exercise training programs are based on existing COPD training programs. Supervised programs usually consist in cycle ergometry, treadmill walking, weight training, gymnastics, or a combination of these. For those who are unable to follow these exercise training modalities due to dyspnea or fatigue, NSE could be a reasonable alternative. In addition to exercise training, nutritional and psychosocial counseling, behavioral change, occupational therapy, and progressive relaxation techniques should be considered [1, 18]. The influence of chemotherapy on the success of postoperative PR also needs to be clarified. Preliminary data suggest that improvements in QoL, exercise performance, and fatigue are limited in patients not receiving chemotherapy. Alternative forms of exercise training may be effective in enhancing participation in people undergoing chemotherapy. Depending on their clinical complexity, postoperative lung cancer patients should begin PR after a comprehensive assessment during which comorbidities are evaluated by a specialized rehabilitation team using validated objective measurements to establish a tailored PRP.

Conclusions

PR may reduce the sensation of dyspnea, increase functional exercise capacity, and improve the QoL in elderly patients with COPD; patients with chronic respiratory diseases other than COPD may also benefit from a comprehensive, interdisciplinary PRP.

Despite the availability of robust evidence supporting the efficacy of PRPs, further studies are needed to fill the gaps in our knowledge. The mechanisms and components of PRP that are essential for success, the specific exercise prescriptions that produce the greatest benefits, how to sustain and maintain long-term benefits, and what non-COPD causes of respiratory impairment respond more favorably to PR are important questions that require urgent answers.

Key Points

- Pulmonary rehabilitation (PR) including exercise, education, and nutritional support is the first choice treatment option for elderly patients with chronic respiratory disorders.
- Exercise training is the cornerstone of PR.
- PR programs should be individualized according to the specific needs of every patient.
- PR can improve the symptoms, general health status, physical performance, and quality of life in individuals with COPD as well as in many patients with non-COPD respiratory disorders.

References

1. Spruit MA, Singh SJ, Garvey C et al (2013) An official American Thoracic Society/European Respiratory Society statement: key concepts and advances in pulmonary rehabilitation. Am J Respir Crit Care Med 108:13–64
2. Bolton CE, Bevan-Smith EF, Blakey JD et al (2013) British Thoracic Society pulmonary rehabilitation guideline group/BTS guideline on pulmonary rehabilitation in adults. Thorax 68:ii1–i30
3. American Association of Cardiovascular and Pulmonary Rehabilitation (2004) Guidelines for pulmonary rehabilitation programs. Human Kinetics, Champaign
4. Rabe KF, Hurd S, Anzueto A et al (2007) Global initiative for chronic obstructive lung disease. Global strategy for the diagnosis, management, and prevention of chronic obstructive pulmonary disease: GOLD executive summary. Am J Respir Crit Care Med 176:532–555
5. Emtner M, Porszasz J, Burns M et al (2003) Benefits of supplemental oxygen in exercise training in non-hypoxemic chronic obstructive pulmonary disease patients. Am J Respir Crit Care Med 168:1034–1042
6. Scorsone D, Bartolini S, Saporiti R et al (2010) Does a low-density gas mixture or oxygen supplementation improve exercise training in COPD? Chest 138:1133–1139
7. O'Donnell DE, Webb KA (2008) The major limitation to exercise performance in COPD is dynamic hyperinflation. J Appl Physiol 105:753–755
8. Köhnlein T, Schönheit-Kenn U, Winterkamp S et al (2009) Noninvasive ventilation in pulmonary rehabilitation of COPD patients. Respir Med 103:1329–1336
9. Nici L, ZuWallack R (2012) American Thoracic Society Subcommittee on Integrated Care of the COPD Patient. An Official American Thoracic Society Workshop Report: the integrated care of the COPD patient. Proc Am Thorac Soc 9:9–18
10. Effing T, Monninkhof EM, van der Valk PD et al (2007) Self-management education for patients with chronic obstructive pulmonary disease. Cochrane Database Syst Rev 4:CD002990
11. Crisafulli E, Morandi A, Olivini A, Malerba M, Clini EM (2014) Rehabilitation and supportive therapy in elderly patients with chronic obstructive pulmonary disease. Eur J Intern Med 25:329–335
12. Holland AE (2010) Exercise limitation in interstitial lung disease – mechanisms, significance and therapeutic options. Chron Respir Dis 7:101–111
13. Holland AE, Hill CJ, Conron M et al (2008) Short term improvement in exercise capacity and symptoms following exercise training in interstitial lung disease. Thorax 63:549–554
14. Nishiyama O, Kondoh Y, Kimura T et al (2008) Effects of pulmonary rehabilitation in patients with idiopathic pulmonary fibrosis. Respirology 13:394–399
15. Ong HK, Lee AL, Hill CJ et al (2011) Effects of pulmonary rehabilitation in bronchiectasis: a retrospective study. Chron Respir Dis 8:21–30
16. Cup EH, Pieterse AJ, Ten Broek-Pastoor JM et al (2007) Exercise therapy and other types of physical therapy for patients with neuromuscular diseases: a systematic review. Arch Phys Med Rehabil 88:1452–1464
17. Benzo R, Wigle D, Novotny P et al (2011) Preoperative pulmonary rehabilitation before lung cancer resection: results from two randomized studies. Lung Cancer 74:441–445
18. Cesario A, Ferri L, Galetta D et al (2007) Post-operative respiratory rehabilitation after lung resection for non-small cell lung cancer. Lung Cancer 57:175–180

Postoperative Rehabilitation of Elderly Patients

47

Jannis V. Papathanasiou

47.1 Introduction

According the World Health Organization, the aim of physical and rehabilitation medicine (PRM) is to maximize function and minimize limitation of activity and restriction of participation, resulting from an underlying impairment or disease [1]. Rehabilitation was defined as inpatient multidisciplinary programs with active physiotherapy or occupational therapy, or both, according to the WHO ICF framework. Rehabilitation has been also described as the "secret weapon" of geriatric medicine and, in tandem with comprehensive clinical assessment, is among the most effective interventions. Usually, geriatric PRM is multidisciplinary care, because there are a myriad of health-related and contextual factors in complex interaction that must be addressed in a coordinated fashion [2]. The PRM team is usually led by a PRM specialist who has expertise to treat a wide range of pathologies and functional deficits. PRM specialists also have to provide pain and spasticity managing and to prescribe appropriate prosthetics and orthotics [3]. The PRM interventions are well accepted in younger adults with neurological, orthopedic, musculoskeletal, cardiovascular, and surgical diseases. Compared to PRM interventions in younger adults, the nature of PRM in elderly individuals differs in many aspects related with special needs of aging such as multiple comorbidities, causes of disability, frailty, polypharmacy, and cognitive nutritional and depression problems. Because of multidisciplinary care of elderly patients, the PRM team includes therapists (physical, occupational, speech), nurses, prosthetists, psychologist/psychiatrists, orthotists, dieticians, and social workers [4].

J.V. Papathanasiou, MD, PhD
Department of Kinesitherapy, Faculty of Public Health, Medical University of Sofia, Sofia, Bulgaria

Department of Medical Imaging, Allergology and Physiotherapy, Faculty of Dental Medicine, Medical University of Plovdiv, Plovdiv, Bulgaria
e-mail: giannipap@yahoo.co.uk

© Springer International Publishing AG 2018
S. Masiero, U. Carraro (eds.), *Rehabilitation Medicine for Elderly Patients*, Practical Issues in Geriatrics, DOI 10.1007/978-3-319-57406-6_47

One of the greatest challenges of geriatric rehabilitation is to improve functional status and quality of life (QoL) of elderly patients prior to surgery, as well to reduce the postoperative complications (PC) and the mortality rate [5]. Apart from decreased physical activity and sedentary lifestyle in the elderly and the so-called surgical stress syndrome, there is an increasing recognition of the multiple deleterious effects of hospitalization on elderly individuals as contributors to functional decline and iatrogenic complications. The adaptive capacity of elderly patients decreases, especially before and after major life events like hospital admissions and surgical interventions, making them vulnerable to loss of functioning and reduced societal participation [6, 7]. Loss of functioning is observed in up to 50% of hospitalized elderly individuals before admission, as a result of decreased functional capacity [8]. The majority of elderly inpatients spend 80% of the hospital stay lying in bed. Bed rest without medical reason leads to a rapid loss of aerobic capacity and lower extremity strength [9, 10].

The effectiveness of geriatric PRM interventions was demonstrated through numerous studies [11]. The PRM approach of elderly patients has many variations and will be different in different phases of the diseases, as the service is based on what the PRM physician assessed as needed for the patient.

The PRM management of elderly patients can be divided into preoperative PRM interventions, defined as "the process of enhancing the functional capacity of the individual to enable him or her to withstand a stressful event," and postoperative PRM interventions, defined as "a treatment designed to facilitate the process of recovery from injury, illness and disease" [12]. Currently, clinical studies indicated that interdisciplinary preoperative and postoperative PRM interventions during hospitalization may improve functional capacity, physical performance, and QoL of elderly patients [13].

The involvement of interdisciplinary PRM team in the whole rehabilitation process has the goal of accurately diagnosing medical conditions and optimizing functional capabilities of frail elderly patients, including early discharge plan implementation during inpatient hospital stay [14].

Surgical and medical interventions target the health issues, whereas PRM interventions (preoperative and postoperative) are designed to augment the functional capacity and well-being of the elderly patients. However, we lack evidence of whether such PRM interventions also may affect the risks of death and readmissions [15, 16].

47.2 Preoperative PRM Management of Elderly Patients

The preoperative PRM management of elderly patients is fundamental in identifying risk factors for the development of PC and prescript preoperative PRM program. The PRM process ideally begins with a comprehensive preoperative assessment of the older patient, which is the multidisciplinary assessment of medical, functional, and psychosocial issues including cardiopulmonary exercise testing (CPET), six-minute walk test (6MWT), activities of daily living (ADLs), fall risk, polypharmacy,

Table 47.1 Preoperative assessment of elderly surgical patient

In addition to conducting a complete history and physical examination of the elderly patient, the following assessments are recommended:
• Assess the elderly patient's cognitive ability
• Screen the elderly patient's depression
• Identify the elderly patient's risk factors for developing postoperative delirium
• Screen for alcohol or drug abuse/dependence
• Perform a preoperative cardiac evaluation according to the American College of Cardiology/ American Heart Association algorithm for patients undergoing noncardiac surgery
• Prevent the elderly patients from postoperative pulmonary complications
• Document the patient's functional status
• Document the patient's history of falls
• Determine baseline frailty score
• Assess the elderly patient's nutritional status
• Take an accurate and detailed medication history and monitor for polypharmacy
• Determine the elderly patient's treatment goals and family's expectations

Adapted from "Chow WB, Rosenthal RA, Merkow RP" et al. Optimal preoperative assessment of the geriatric surgical patient: a best practices guideline from the American College of Surgeons National Surgical Quality Improvement Program and the American Geriatrics Society. J Am Coll Surg 2012; 215:453–66

cognition, mood, social support, etc. In preoperative PRM assessment, additional components as nutritional status, continence, vision, hearing, dentition, living situation, and spirituality can be also assessed [17]. The range and depth of the preoperative PRM assessment depend on the expertise of the PRM team members. The American College of Surgeons and American Geriatric Society promulgated recommendations for preoperative assessment of geriatric surgical patients, which encompass a wide breadth of health issues (Table 47.1) [18]. 6MWT is a well-validated preoperative measure applied in elderly patients that does not require sophisticated equipment or extensive training. It is proven that 6MWT has excellent test-retest reliability and predicts risk for mortality and mobility loss, as well the development of PC in elderly patients [19]. Jones et al. found that falls are significantly and strongly associated with PC and readmissions [20].

The PRM team must take into account that elderly patients often underreport disability because of lack of self-awareness and cognitive impairment or simply minimize their functional limitations [3, 8]. Usually, the elderly patients and their families have their own expectations, and these should be reconciled with the PRM team's assessment. Once the preoperative PRM assessment is completed, it is important to educate patients and families regarding options for PRM and to set expectations in accordance with enhanced recovery programs (ERP), and preoperative PRM interventions produce less anxiety, pain improvement, and patient's satisfaction in educated elderly [5, 21]. In general, preoperative PRM interventions aim to improve physical function of elderly patients prior to surgery, as well to reduce PC, length of hospital stay, and negative effects of the surgical stress syndrome. Preoperative PRM programs for elderly surgery patients have been shown to be beneficial and safe, and they may include aerobic exercise training, e.g., thoracic expansion exercises, taught shoulder exercises, as well as marching on the spot for varying amounts of time, once a day. Aerobic exercise training is associated with improved physical fitness of elderly patients before and improved functional recovery after abdominal and thoracic surgery [22]. Evidence demonstrates that respiratory muscle training decreases the incidence of PC after abdominal and thoracic surgery [23]. The use of different forms of exercise training including endurance and interval has been shown to improve musculoskeletal and cardiovascular function in the elderly patients [24].

Instructions for deep breathing, splinted coughing exercises, and shoulder exercises, as well as exercises for prevention of deep vein thrombosis, are included in the information booklet and DVD shared among elderly patients preoperatively. It's proven that patients who are educated prior to surgery have less anxiety, improved pain, and patient satisfaction [11, 21, 25].

Elderly patients are encouraged to record data concerning their physical function, ADL, and QoL in the diary section of the information booklet, which sets out what they achieved each day of their hospital stay [5, 6].

47.3 Postoperative PRM Management of Elderly Patients

Postoperative PRM interventions have been shown to be beneficial among elderly individuals following surgery procedures. In many studies, it was demonstrated that exercise training significantly increases strength and functional and motor performance among elderly patients and may also improve the balance and psychological factors [26]. In this phase it is beneficial for the PRM team to counsel patients and their families on the expected outcomes and various postoperative alternatives. The prescription of an appropriate postoperative PRM program tailored to the elderly's specific needs is a part of a multidisciplinary postoperative PRM approach [6]. Several high-quality studies have highlighted the early mobilization as the fundamental cornerstone of the postoperative PRM management in elderly patients. Schweickert et al. found that patients receiving early physical training and occupational therapy enjoyed better functional outcomes and had a shorter duration of delirium and more ventilator-free days, when they were discharged [27]. In general, it was prooven in many studies that included eledrly patients, early physical training after surgery is feasible and tolerable, resulting in improvement of QoL, physical fitness and well-being. Elderly patients should receive the PRM specialist's advice on the first postoperative day and, then, at minimum once a day, until they are able to exercise independently [28]. In order to improve the mobility of elderly patients who underwent surgery, wall or portable suction drains are used. For elderly patients who are unable to leave the bed space, portable exercise bikes or step-ups are used. Patients must be encouraged to perform the individual tailored mobilization program, which requires a minimum of 60 m walking four times on the first day, 80 m on the second day, 100 m on the third day, and then increasing this according to the individual [29].

During postoperative mobilization program, elderly patients are encouraged to perform posture and arm exercises four times daily. The training intensities are predominately based on heart rate reserve and rated perceived exertion using commonly the modified Borg scale. It seems that posture and arm exercises may significantly reduce the shoulder dysfunction and regain functional ADL [30, 31]. Various training modalities (i.e., endurance, resistive, and interval training) may be included in postoperative rehabilitation of elderly patients. It has been shown that these training modalities are able to improve musculoskeletal and cardiovascular function of the elderly individuals [24].

Additional components like pain management and dietary guidance are incorporated in current postoperative PRM programs for elderly patients. Pain management is crucial for the PRM team which deals with pain using various modalities, such as analgesic medications, transcutaneous electrical nerve stimulation (TENS), and heat and cold applications.

One of the most important issues of postoperative PRM is the discharge of elderly patients. Before discharge, elderly surgical patients are checked for functional capacity, functional independence, pain, balance, walking, grip strength, and general well-being. Elderly patients are encouraged to record data concerning their physical function, ADL, and QoL in the diary section of the information booklet, which sets out what they achieved each day of their hospital stay [5, 6]. An individual postoperative PRM program is suggested to be followed after discharge in order to achieve a fully functional QoL of the elderly patients.

Conclusion

The effectiveness of geriatric PRM interventions in elderly surgical patients was demonstrated through numerous studies. The PRM approach of elderly patients has many variations. Currently, clinical studies indicated that interdisciplinary preoperative and postoperative PRM interventions during hospitalization may improve functional capacity, physical performance, and QoL of elderly patients. There is high-quality evidence that preoperative and postoperative PRM programs, provided to elderly patients undergoing thoracic, abdominal, and major joint replacement surgery, are well tolerated, safe, and effective.

Key Points

- The adaptive capacity of elderly patients decreases, especially before and after major life events like hospital admissions and surgical interventions.
- The physical and rehabilitation medicine (PRM) in elderly individuals differs in many aspects compared to PRM in younger adults.
- One of the greatest challenges of geriatric rehabilitation is to improve functional status and quality of life (QoL) of elderly patients prior to surgery.
- The early mobilization has been highlighted as the fundamental cornerstone of the postoperative PRM management in elderly patients.
- It's proven that preoperative and postoperative PRM programs, provided to elderly patients undergoing surgery, are well tolerated, safe, and effective.

References

1. WHO Expert Committee on Disability Prevention and Rehabilitation (1981) Disability prevention and rehabilitation. World Health Organ Tech Rep Ser 668:1–39
2. Biffl WL, Biffl SE (2015) Rehabilitation of the geriatric surgical patient: predicting needs and optimizing outcomes. Surg Clin North Am 95:173–190
3. Gutenbrunner C, Lemoine F, Yelnik A, Joseph PA, de Korvin G, Neumann V, Delarque A (2011) The field of competence of the specialist in physical and rehabilitation medicine (PRM). Ann Phys Rehabil Med 54:298–318
4. Federspiel C, Keipes M (2014) Geriatrics from the 19th to the 21st century. 150 years of geriatric medicine: from increasing life expectancy to improving quality of life for the very old. Bull Soc Sci Med Grand Duche Luxemb:69–78
5. Simpson JC, Moonesinghe SR, Grocott MP, Kuper M, McMeeking A, Oliver CM et al (2015) Enhanced recovery from surgery in the UK: an audit of the enhanced recovery partnership programme 2009–2012. Br J Anaesth 115:560–568
6. Wells JL, Seabrook JA, Stolee P, Borrie MJ, Knoefel F (2003) State of the art in geriatric rehabilitation. Part II: clinical challenges. Arch Phys Med Rehab 84:898–903
7. Brown CJ, Flood KL (2013) Mobility limitation in the older patient: a clinical review. JAMA 310:1168–1177
8. Palleschi L, Fimognari FL, Pierantozzi A, Salani B, Marsilii A, Zuccaro SM, Di Cioccio L, De Alfieri W (2014) Acute functional decline before hospitalization in older patients. Geriatr Gerontol Int 14:769–777
9. Brown CJ, Redden DT, Flood KL, Allman RM (2009) The underrecognized epidemic of low mobility during hospitalization of older adults. J Am Geriatr Soc 57:1660–1665
10. Welvaart WN, Paul MA, Stienen GJ, van Hees HW, Loer SA, Bouwman R, Niessen H, de Man FS, Witt CC, Granzier H, Vonk-Noordegraaf A, Ottenheijm CA (2011) Selective diaphragm muscle weakness after contractile inactivity during thoracic surgery. Ann Surg 254:1044–1049
11. Vidan M, Serra JA, Moreno C et al (2005) Efficacy of a comprehensive geriatric intervention in older patients hospitalized for hip fracture: a randomized, controlled trial. J Am Geriatr Soc 53:1476–1482
12. Ditmyer M, Topp R, Pifer M (2002) Prehabilitation in preparation for orthopaedic surgery. Orthop Nurs 21:43–51
13. Cruise CM, Sasson N, Lee MH (2006) Rehabilitation outcomes in the older adult. Clin Geriatr Med 22:257–67; viii
14. Prestmo A, Hagen G, Sletvold O et al (2015) Comprehensive geriatric care for patients with hip fractures: a prospective, randomised, controlled trial. Lancet 385:1623–1633
15. Patel BK, Hall JB (2013) Perioperative physiotherapy. Curr Opin Anaesthesiol 26:152–156
16. Hoogeboom TJ, Dronkers JJ, Hulzebos EH, van Meeteren NL (2014) Merits of exercise therapy before and after major surgery. Curr Opin Anaesthesiol 27:161–166
17. Levett DZ, Grocott MP (2015) Cardiopulmonary exercise testing for risk prediction in major abdominal surgery. Anesthesiol Clin 33:1–16
18. Chow WB, Rosenthal RA, Merkow RP et al (2012) Optimal preoperative assessment of the geriatric surgical patient: a best practices guideline from the American College of Surgeons National Surgical Quality Improvement Program and the American Geriatrics Society. J Am Coll Surg 215:453–466
19. Santos BF, Souza HC, Miranda AP, Cipriano FG, Gastaldi AC (2016) Performance in the 6-minute walk test and postoperative pulmonary complications in pulmonary surgery: an observational study. Braz J Phys Ther 20:66–72
20. Jones TS, Dunn CL, Wu DS et al (2013) Relationship between asking an older adult about falls and surgical outcomes. JAMA Surg 148:1132–1138
21. Kiyohara LY, Kayano LK, Oliveira LM, Yamamoto MU, Inagaki MM, Ogawa NY, Gonzales PE, Mandelbaum R, Okubo ST, Watanuki T, Vieira JE (2004) Surgery information reduces anxiety in the pre-operative period. Rev Hosp Clin Fac Med Sao Paulo 59:51–56

22. Nagarajan K, Bennett A, Agostini P, Naidu B (2011) Is preoperative physiotherapy/pulmonary rehabilitation beneficial in lung resection patients? Interact Cardiovasc Thorac Surg 13:300–302
23. Dronkers JJ, Chorus AM, van Meeteren NL, Hopman-Rock M (2013) The association of preoperative physical fitness and physical activity with outcome after scheduled major abdominal surgery. Anaesthesia 68:67–73
24. Valkenet K, van de Port IG, Dronkers JJ, de Vries WR, Lindeman E, Backx FJ (2011) The effects of preoperative exercise therapy on postoperative outcome: a systematic review. Clin Rehabil 25:99–111
25. Dronkers J, Veldman A, Hoberg E et al (2008) Prevention of pulmonary complications after upper abdominal surgery by preoperative intensive inspiratory muscle training. A randomised controlled pilot study. Clin Rehab 22:134–142
26. Jack S, West M, Grocott MP (2011) Perioperative exercise training in elderly subjects. Best Pract Res Clin Anaesthesiol 25:461–472
27. Schweickert WD, Pohlman MC, Pohlman AS et al (2009) Early physical and occupational therapy in mechanically ventilated, critically ill patients: a randomized controlled trial. Lancet 373:1874–1882
28. Kosse NM, Dutmer AL, Dasenbrock L, Bauer JM, Lamoth CJ (2013) Effectiveness and feasibility of early physical rehabilitation programs for geriatric hospitalized patients: a systematic review. BMC Geriatr 13:107
29. Kaneda H, Saito Y, Okamoto M, Maniwa T, Minami K, Imamura H (2007) Early postoperative mobilization with walking at 4 hours after lobectomy in lung cancer patients. Gen Thorac Cardiovasc Surg 55:493–498
30. Kendrick KR, Baxi SC, Smith RM (2000) Usefulness of the modified 0-10 Borg scale in assessing the degree of dyspnea in patients with COPD and asthma. J Emerg Nurs 26:216–222
31. Li WW, Lee TW, Yim AP (2004) Shoulder function after thoracic surgery. Thorac Surg Clin 14:331–343

Rehabilitation of Older Patients with Chronic Kidney Diseases

48

Domenico Intiso

48.1 Introduction

Population is dramatically changing as the elderly represent the fastest-growing demographic segment, and by 2050, Italian National Institute of Statistics (ISTAT) forecasts each of the three persons will be older than 65 years. The incidence of chronic kidney diseases (CKD) has been shown to increase with age, and nearly half of old people suffer from this condition [1]. CKD has been defined as the presence of kidney damage or reduced glomerular filtration rate (GFR) less than 60 mL/min/1.73 m^2 that is present for 3 months or more [2]. According to GFR, CKD is graded in five stages from 1 to 5 with 1 indicating a GFR > 90 mL/min/1.73 m^2 that represent kidney damage with normal or increased kidney function and 5 indicating a GFR < 15 mL/min/1.73 m^2. This renal functionality is the expression of kidney failure and end-stage renal disease requiring hemodialysis. The prevalence of CKD varies from 23.4% to 35.8% in people aged 64 years or older [3]. However, as mentioned above because the elder population is dramatically growing, it is predictable that a larger number of old subjects suffering from CKD will need care and assistance. With respect, it is essential to plan and organize reforms of National Health System, making it more resilient to the impact of aging population with CKD in order to prevent frailty and to reduce disability. In elders, CKD may be associated with the development of disability regardless of body composition, physical performance, and comorbidity because well-functioning old people with CKD can develop functional limitation. The mechanism may be related to a heightened inflammatory state in CKD [4]. Furthermore, in comparison with those with normal renal function, the elderly patients with CKD are more likely to have increased comorbidities, walking impairments, and decrement in quality of life. Therefore, structured and

D. Intiso
Unit of Physical Medicine and Rehabilitation, Unit of Neuro-rehabilitation, IRCCS "Casa Sollievo della Sofferenza", San Giovanni Rotondo, FG, Italy
e-mail: d.intiso@operapadrepio.it

© Springer International Publishing AG 2018

S. Masiero, U. Carraro (eds.), *Rehabilitation Medicine for Elderly Patients*, Practical Issues in Geriatrics, DOI 10.1007/978-3-319-57406-6_48

well-resourced primary prevention programs based on reducing the risk factors for CKD and rehabilitative strategies adjunct to proper interventions during the renal disease could make a big difference in reducing the impact that CKD will predictably have on disability occurrence and related social cost.

48.2 Rehabilitation Role

Rehabilitation has been defined by the World Health Organization (WHO) as "the use of all means aimed at reducing the impact of disabling and handicapping conditions and at enabling people with disabilities to achieve optimal social integration." This definition incorporates clinical rehabilitation but also endorses the concept of social participation as requiring a matching of the social environment to the needs of people with disabilities. The overall aim of rehabilitation is to enable people with disabilities to lead the life that they would wish, given any restriction imposed on their activities by impairments resulting from illness or injury as well as from their personal context [5]. Rehabilitation has been demonstrated effective and efficient in reducing the burden of disability and enhancing the opportunities for disabled people. Since body impairments and functional limitations can be multiform and variable, an individualized and tailored rehabilitative project has to be planned to reduce disability. The rehabilitation project should be tailored on the individual effective needs of CKD people considering stage of disease, complications, and comorbidities. Individualized rehabilitative project should list the procedures that will be applied to obtain functional recovery including type of exercises, rehabilitative techniques, and timing and duration of application. Furthermore functional goals that can be reached and the role of involved personnel staff should also be reported. The rehabilitative process is unique in treating people according to a holistic approach or a biopsychosocial model with the aim of supporting a person's independent living and autonomy. As a patient-centered process, it has to be appropriate to optimize both activity and participation to ameliorate person's quality of life.

48.3 Rehabilitation in Elder Subjects with CKD

Exercise capacity and quality of life are markedly impaired in chronic kidney disease. In the early stages of elder people suffering from CKD, musculoskeletal impairment and multi-organ disturbances can cause higher risk of mobility reduction. This condition could lead to a greater decline in gait speed with functional limitation [6]. Walking ability reduction and capacity to move to outside one's home and neighborhood may cause lesser participation in family, religious services, and social activities. CKD old people can develop earlier these functional limitations compared to elders without CKD. Therefore, they could more prone to isolation and to conditions that promote reduced stimulation and motivation as well as mood and cognitive disorders. Furthermore, old patients with CKD are more likely to have decrement in quality of life compared to elders with normal renal function. Elders with GFR less than 45 mL/min/1.73 m^2 have a decline in basic activities of daily living (BADL) greater than those without CKD [7]. Several rehabilitative strategies and approaches can be engaged in these people to delay the functional limitation and to ameliorate the residual abilities, in particular physical activity including aerobic and resistance exercises that produce positive effects on cardiorespiratory fitness, physical function, and self-reported health.

Elders with early stage of CKD and not severe limitations have to perform regular aerobic exercises. Among these, also resistance training exercises should be performed. This type of exercises has been demonstrated to reduce the malnutrition-inflammation complex syndrome of CKD improving physical performance, muscle mass, and quality of life in subjects with CKD [8] as well as in older hemodialysis patients. Of course, not all CKD subjects have to perform regular exercises, in particular subjects with severe comorbidities. In addition to that reported by American College of Cardiology Foundation/American Heart Association [9], several contraindications to exercise are specific to CKD patients such as symptomatic hearth arrhythmias, pulmonary congestion, and peripheral edema. On the other hand, specific rehabilitative interventions have to be tailored whenever multiple comorbidities such as multi-joint arthritis, sarcopenia, heart failure, and neurological disturbances contribute to the disability. Occupational therapy can be an essential rehabilitative strategy in those suffering from CKD and multiple comorbidities that affect functional abilities and ADLs. The use of assistive devices is a common intervention used to meet the goal of maintaining independence, and assistive tools are commonly recommended for ADLs. They include dressing sticks, long-handled shoe horns, long-handled sponges, button hooks, shower seats, and three-in-one commodes. These items have been shown to be effective in minimizing energy output and improving function with self-care and ADLs in patients with functional deficits from orthopedic and neuromuscular diseases. Correct techniques can save energy, increase time efficiency, and decrease frustration. Rehabilitative intervention can help to find the best technique or equipment for particular situation and recommend when a caregiver will have to provide more assistance. A further essential role of occupational therapy is environmental and home living adaptation for CKD elders with functional limitation and comorbidities who are at risk of falls that are the leading cause of injury and associated morbidity in elderly. In these subjects, proper programs include home hazard assessments by trained individuals, removal or modification of identified hazards, installation of safety devices such as handrails on stairs and grab bars on bathrooms, and improvements in lighting. Falls may lead to decreased mobility, hospitalization, depressive symptoms, functional decline, decreased social activity, and poor quality of life [10]. All older adults with and without CKD at risk of falling should be offered an exercise program incorporating balance, gait, and strength training. Since fall risk can depend on several factors, a single approach can be insufficient. To date, several trials have demonstrated that multicomponent and multifactorial interventions resulted in an approximately 30% relative risk reduction in fall rate [11]. Recently a different model has been proposed in caring elder CKD people that should change from traditional disease-based model to individualized patient-centered approach [12].

People with CKD could complain of complex functional impairments and multisystem clinical disorders needing of specialized care and specific rehabilitative interventions. An individualized approach prioritizes patient preferences and embraces the notion that observed signs and symptoms often do not reflect a single unifying disease process and instead reflect the complex interplay between many different factors. This care method could result particularly positive in frail old people with CKD. These subjects are mostly inclined toward hospitalization, disability, and death. Generally, frailty refers to a condition characterized by a gradual physiologic decline in multiple body systems, by loss of function, loss of physiologic reserve, and increased vulnerability to disease and death. The loss of skeletal muscle mass (sarcopenia) is probably a key component of these conditions. Thus, it is crucial to develop interventions in decreasing adverse health outcomes. A large number of papers have reported that also frail elder people can benefit from regular physical activity including aerobic or endurance exercise training [13].

Among frailty factors, one of the most important is loss of muscle mass. Although data remain controversial, studies have revealed that aerobic exercises can increase muscular mass of extremities in elderly [14]. The right rehabilitative interventions should be planned on the functional ability of elders and tailored by more structured and interdisciplinary approaches as functional decline advances [15]. Interdisciplinary care team including physiatrist, geriatrician, nephrologist, and other medical practitioner knowledgeable in the care of older adults such as nurses, social worker, and occupational or physical therapist could be more effective than the usual single- or disease-centered approach in treating multisystem disorders of frail old people with CKD in order to obtain the best benefit by the one's own expert and the professional's competent contribution.

Key Points

- The elder population is dramatically growing; therefore it is predictable that a larger number of old subjects suffering from chronic kidney disease (CKD) will need care and assistance.
- Exercise capacity and quality of life are markedly impaired in old people with CKD, but the rehabilitation can improve the functional limitation reducing the impact of disabling and handicapping conditions.
- The rehabilitative approach should be tailored on the individual effective needs of CKD people considering stage of disease, complications, and comorbidities. Interdisciplinary care team could be more effective than the usual single- or disease-centered strategy in treating frail old people with CKD.

References

1. Stengel B, Metzger M, Froissart M, Rainfray M, Berr C, Tzourio C, Helmer C (2011) Epidemiology and prognostic significance of chronic kidney disease in the elderly—the Three-City prospective cohort study. Nephrol Dial Transplant 26:3286–3295
2. Levey AS, de Jong PE, Coresh J, El Nahas M, Astor BC, Matsushita K, Gansevoort RT, Kasiske BL, Eckardt KU (2011) The definition, classification, and prognosis of chronic kidney disease: a KDIGO controversies conference report. Kidney Int 80:17–28
3. Zhang QL, Rothenbacher D (2008) Prevalence of chronic kidney disease in population-based studies: systematic review. BMC Public Health 8:117
4. Fried LF, Lee JS, Shlipak M, Chertow GM, Green C, Ding J, Harris T, Newman AB (2006) Chronic kidney disease and functional limitation in older people: health, aging and body composition study. J Am Geriatr Soc 54:750–756
5. Negrini S, Ceravolo MG (2008) The white book on physical and rehabilitation medicine in Europe: a contribution to the growth of our specialty with no boundaries. Am J Phys Med Rehabil 87:601–606
6. Liu CK, Lyass A, Massaro JM, D'Agostino RB Sr, Fox CS, Murabito JM (2014) Chronic kidney disease defined by cystatin C predicts mobility disability and changes in gait speed: the Framingham Offspring Study. J Gerontol A Biol Sci Med Sci 69(3):301–307
7. Bowling CB, Sawyer P, Campbell RC, Ahmed A, Allman RM (2011) Impact of chronic kidney disease on activities of daily living in community-dwelling older adults. J Gerontol A Biol Sci Med Sci 66(6):689–694
8. Castaneda C, Gordon PL, Parker RC, Uhlin KL, Roubenoff R, Levey AS (2004) Resistance training to reduce the malnutrition-inflammation complex syndrome of chronic kidney disease. Am J Kidney Dis 43:607–616
9. Nelson ME, Rejeski WJ, Blair SN, Duncan PW, Judge JO, King AC, Macera CA, Castaneda-Sceppa C, American College of Sports Medicine, American Heart Association (2007) Physical activity and public health in older adults: recommendation from the American College of Sports Medicine and the American Heart Association. Circulation 116(9):1094–1105
10. Brenneman SK, Barrett-Connor E, Sajjan S, Markson LE, Siris ES (2006) Impact of recent fracture on health-related quality of life in postmenopausal women. J Bone Miner Res 21:809–816
11. Panel on Prevention of Falls in Older Persons, American Geriatrics Society and British Geriatrics Society (2011) Summary of the Updated American Geriatrics Society/British Geriatrics Society clinical practice guideline for prevention of falls in older persons. J Am Geriatr Soc 59(1):148–157
12. Bowling CB, Muntner P, Sawyer P, Sanders PW, Kutner N, Kennedy R, Allman RM (2014) Community mobility among older adults with reduced kidney function: a study of life-space. Am J Kidney Dis 63(3):429–436
13. Chin A, Paw MJ, van Uffelen JG, Riphagen I, van Mechelen W (2008) The functional effects of physical exercise training in frail older people: a systematic review. Sports Med 38(9):781–793
14. Sugawara J, Miyachi M, Moreau KL, Dinenno FA, DeSouza CA, Tanaka H (2002) Age-related reductions in appendicular skeletal muscle mass: association with habitual aerobic exercise status. Clin Physiol Funct Imaging 22(3):169–172
15. Intiso D, Di Rienzo F, Russo M, Pazienza L, Tolfa M, Iarossi A, Maruzzi G (2012) Rehabilitation strategy in the elderly. J Nephrol 25(Suppl 19):S90–S95

49 Pelvic Floor Rehabilitation of the Elderly

Paolo Di Benedetto

49.1 Introduction

Pelvic floor rehabilitation (PFR) is nowadays an important strategy for the treatment of many pelvic floor disorders in adults and in older people. The recognized pioneer of PFR is the American gynecologist Arnold H. Kegel who in the years 1948–1951 proposed pelvic floor muscle (PFM) exercises to prevent and/or treat female urinary incontinence and genital prolapse. Kegel's techniques were also used successfully by other authors, but as the years passed, they sank into unjustified oblivion, until the 1980s of the last century when many European authors rekindled in Europe the interest of PFR techniques [1, 2].

In 1992 the International Continence Society (ICS) published its seventh report on the standardization of terminology devoted to rehabilitation techniques of the lower urinary tract: PFR thus acquired its scientific dignity, and PFM exercises or PFM training (PFMT) became considered a fundamental part of therapeutic programs in the field of urinary incontinence (UI) [3]. In 1996 American guidelines on the management of UI in adults emphasized the role of rehabilitation treatment, and, finally, in 1998 the ICS during the first International Consultation on Incontinence (ICI) proposed the algorithms of UI suggesting PFMT as the initial most important therapeutic strategy [4, 5]. In the following years, many researchers showed the efficacy of behavioral interventions, especially designed for frail older people with cognitive and physical impairments and now considered the mainstay of UI treatment in these cases. Contemporaneously PFR has been more and more indicated in many other functional disorders of pelvic floor, both in women and males (prevention and treatment of fecal incontinence, pelvic organ prolapse, chronic pelvic pain and sexual dysfunction, UI after radical prostatectomy) [6].

P. Di Benedetto
University Tor Vergata, Rome, Italy
e-mail: mrsart@libero.it

© Springer International Publishing AG 2018

S. Masiero, U. Carraro (eds.), *Rehabilitation Medicine for Elderly Patients*,
Practical Issues in Geriatrics, DOI 10.1007/978-3-319-57406-6_49

Rehabilitation techniques, appropriately chosen according to the specific problem, all have the primary objective of improving pelvic floor performance in order to allow the perineum to best carry out its functions of pelvic visceral support, bladder inhibition, strengthening of the urethral and anal sphincters, and counteracting intra-abdominal pressure rises. Whatever the indications or the therapeutic program used, the general and specific aims of PFR are the following:

(a) General aims:

- To support pelvic organs
- To improve pelvic floor and bladder proprioception
- To improve the continence-micturition cycle (in cases of complex bladder sphincter and pelvic floor dysfunction)
- To increase or relax the tone of the levator ani consensually activating the periurethral striated muscles and external urethral and anal sphincters
- To improve the perineal closure reflex to abdominal stress
- To lay the bases for good vaginal sensitivity and optimal orgasmic sensation

(b) Specific aims:

- Gynecological aim: prevention and/or treatment of pelvic organ prolapse
- Urogynecological aim: prevention and/or treatment of urinary incontinence
- Coloproctological aim: prevention and/or treatment of fecal incontinence
- Psychosexual aim: positive effect on the quality of sexual life

PFR consists of biofeedback (BFB), functional electrical stimulation (FES), pelvic floor muscle training (PFMT), vaginal cones (VC) in female patients, and behavioral interventions [2, 7, 8].

BFB allows the subject to modify the unconscious physiological events, while FES and PFMT are aimed to inhibit overactive bladder, improve pelvic *awareness*, and strengthen the pelvic floor muscles (PFM).

PFMT plays an extremely important role in the conservative treatment of overactive bladder (OAB), UI, mild degree of pelvic organ prolapse (POP), and chronic pelvic pain (CPP), but in the near future, it should also be proposed as an actual secondary and primary prevention of pelvic floor dysfunction. VC are used to improve the strength of PFM in women, mainly in cases of self-treatment.

The core of PFMT is a correct PFM contraction that results in a ventral and cranial movement of the perineum and an upward movement of the pelvic organs together with an anterior movement caused primarily by the vaginal and rectal parts of the levator ani muscle. When the PFM contract, the urethra closes as do the anus and the vagina; this contraction is important in preventing involuntary loss of urine or rectal contents.

PFMT is indicated particularly in stress urinary incontinence (SUI) where we recommend a "sequential" protocol of PFMT: increasing awareness of the pelvic floor, PFM strengthening after correction of agonist and antagonist synergies, and, eventually, increasing the reflex contraction of PFM during the raises of abdominal pressure [8]. A normal function of PFM is also important in the inhibition of detrusor activity.

Age is no barrier to the benefits of PFMT: there is evidence to suggest that older people are just as likely to benefit from pelvic floor muscle exercises for incontinence as younger people.

Behavioral interventions, also called urinary voiding programs, are used for inhibiting bladder overactivity (bladder retraining) and, predominantly, in frail elderly: they require active caregiver participation and include prompted and timed voiding. Prompted voiding involves prompts to toilet when the patients have micturition urgency. Timed or scheduled voiding involves toileting an individual at fixed intervals, such as every 2–3 h.

49.2 Pelvic Floor Dysfunction in the Elderly

Pelvic floor dysfunction (PFD) is abnormal functioning of the pelvic floor. The following conditions may occur as a result of PFD in the elderly:

1. Overactive bladder (urgency, high frequency of micturitions, nocturia)
2. Urinary incontinence (stress, urge or urgency, and mixed incontinence)
3. Urinary retention (complete or incomplete)
4. Fecal incontinence
5. Chronic constipation
6. Pelvic organ prolapse
7. Sexual dysfunction
8. Chronic pelvic pain syndromes.

Among these conditions, *overactive bladder (OAB) and UI* are very common disorders in older adults. According to the Agency for Healthcare Research and Quality (AHRQ), 13 million Americans are incontinent. UI is two to three times more common in women than men. High-risk groups for developing UI include prior hysterectomy, obesity, history of stroke, chronic obstructive pulmonary disease, women with POP, men treated for prostate cancer, frail elderly, and nursing home residents. In Italy the overall prevalence rate of UI in an institutionalized population is 55%, higher in women than in men.

OAB is a syndrome characterized by frequency of urination (more than eight times during the day or the night) and almost one episode of urgency, with or without urgency urinary incontinence [5].

UI can have significant negative impact on self-esteem and has been associated with increased rates of depression; it also affects quality of life and activities of daily living and may result in increased dependence on caregivers. Cognitive impairment and gait abnormalities have been linked to increased rates of both isolated UI and combined urinary and fecal incontinence. Tinetti et al. demonstrated a strong association between urinary incontinence and an increased risk of falls.

UI is defined as an involuntary loss of urine: it may be either acute (reversible or transient) or chronic (persistent or established). Transient UI is typically caused by non-urologic factors such as delirium, infection, atrophic urethritis, pharmaceuticals, psychological factors, excess urine output, reduced mobility, and stool impaction (diapers). Correction of the underlying problem often leads to resolution of the UI. There are a variety of forms of chronic UI, including stress incontinence, urge incontinence, mixed incontinence, overflow incontinence, and functional incontinence.

Stress urinary incontinence is (SUI) caused by a decrease in outlet resistance at the level of the bladder neck: leakage occurs when the pressure in the bladder exceeds the outlet closure pressure. Patients describe episodes of incontinence with activities that increase intra-abdominal pressure, such as coughing, sneezing, or laughing. This may be caused by either urethral hypermobility or intrinsic sphincter deficiency, very common in women, mainly in the elderly.

Urgency urinary incontinence (UUI) is typically caused by overactivity of the detrusor muscles in the bladder wall. Abnormal contractions during bladder filling lead to a sensation of urgency, and if strong enough, these contractions may cause urinary leakage. Urgency incontinence is often (but not necessarily) associated with neurologic disorders, such as prior stroke.

Mixed urinary incontinence (MUI) is involuntary urine leakage associated with both urgency and effort.

The incidence of UI after radical prostatectomy (RP) ranges from 6 to 87%. The cause of post-prostatectomy UI might be due to intrinsic sphincter deficiency, OAB, and/or decreased bladder compliance.

Overflow incontinence is caused by an inability to completely empty the bladder with each voiding attempt. This is often caused by poor detrusor contractility and may be associated with chronic conditions such as diabetes mellitus and some neurologic disorders. Patients typically describe constant dribbling incontinence caused by leakage from the full bladder. Sensation is often diminished, and patients may not sense a high post-void residual (PVR) volume.

A unique form of UI in the elderly population is detrusor hyperactivity with impaired contractility (DHIC): described by Resnick and Yalla, this syndrome is particularly common in frail elderly people and is essentially a combination of UUI and bladder voiding failure [9]. In these cases, the bladder demonstrates abnormal detrusor contractions with filling but diminished contractile function during the voiding effort. Functional UI is defined as the urinary leakage associated with inability to use the toilet because of impairment of cognitive and/or physical functioning, psychological unwillingness, or environmental barriers. With regard to this type of UI, Fonda proposed the classification of patients' toileting capacity, defining:

- *Independent continence* is that of persons not being wet and being able to void independently during the day and night.
- *Dependent continence* is that of persons with cognitive or physical disabilities who can be dry because of assistance given.

- *Social continence* is that of persons who are incontinent, but the problem is well contained with appropriate aids, maintaining personal dignity and caregiver morale [5].

Moreover, in the geriatric population, the underlying causes of UI are often multiple and interact with each other. Common causes of mobility limitations include arthritis and gait disturbances. UI seen in people with dementia is often functional in origin. Nocturia is another very common complaint in older adults and is generally associated with functional incontinence. Nocturia can have significant physical and psychosocial impacts, including a higher risk of falls and sleep deprivation. The pathophysiology in older adults is still not completely understood.

Urinary retention (complete or incomplete *UR*) can be defined as the inability to void the bladder; it is the result of dysfunctional voiding that is related to bladder underactivity or bladder outlet obstruction (bladder neck/urethral sphincter/PFM overactivity). UR is not infrequent in older people.

Fecal incontinence (FI) rates are more difficult to estimate: prevalence rates vary between 2 and 10% in community-dwelling elderly aged without gender difference. The most common types of FI in frail older people are related to urgency and passive leakage. Passive leakage can refer to seepage and staining followed by bowel movements that are not associated with fecal urgency and may also occur with fecal impaction. *Chronic constipation*, instead, is more frequent in the elderly (40%), but it remains poorly defined: it is not easy to identify functional constipation (slow transit time through the colon) and obstructed defecation syndrome (ODS) that often are associated. In patients with ODS, the anal sphincter and PFM often fail to relax, or even contract, at the defecation.

The incidence of *pelvic organ prolapse (POP)* increases with age. Approximately 50% of all women over the age of 50 years complain of symptomatic POP. Some studies found that in women evaluated for genital prolapse, 73% reported UI, 34–62% voiding dysfunction, and 31% fecal incontinence. Surgery for POP is common also in elderly (11.1 at 80 years) and is not successful for all women.

There are no data regarding the incidence of *chronic pelvic pain (CPP)*; the prevalence of multisystem etiology has been estimated at 3.8% of all women. CPP may be associated with the concomitant increase in depressive symptoms in the elderly: the acronym UPOINT identifies the possible causes of pelvic pain (urinary, psychosocial, organ specific, infections, neurologic/systemic, and tenderness of PFM), and in this context PFMs and urethral and anal sphincters have to be assessed. In the last years, the pivotal role of the short, painful, and/or hypertonic pelvic floor in the development of several life-altering and chronic genitourinary conditions has been recognized. It is prudent finally to consider pudendal nerve entrapment in all patients with CPP.

Sexual dysfunction (SD) occurs in both men and women, and the overall prevalence of these disorders increases with age. Panser et al. conducted a population-based cross-sectional study of 2115 men and found that, in comparison with men aged 40–49 years, older men (70–79 years) are more worried about their overall sexual function (24.9 versus 46.6%), reporting higher levels of dissatisfaction, decreased libido, and impaired erectile function. They also found that risk factors for erectile dysfunction include comorbid disease (such as diabetes mellitus, heart disease, and hypertension) and their pharmacological treatment. Very little is known about the psychosocial and physiologic aspects of female sexual dysfunction. Several studies have documented that female sexual dysfunction increases with age, but the causes of these changes are still poorly understood, even if hyperactivity of the PFM is often causally associated with this dysfunction, namely, dyspareunia and vaginismus.

49.3 Diagnostic Evaluation of UI and FI

Unless terminally or severely medically ill with short remaining life expectancy (RLE), all elderly patients with UI and FI (the most bothersome conditions) should undergo a basic evaluation that includes history (including bladder and bowel diary), physical examination, measurement of post-void residual (PVR) volume in selected cases, and urinalysis. The usual baseline assessment for UI and FI in frail older patients should also include assessment of cognition, neurological and physical state, activities of daily living (ADL), and social environmental factors. The role of urodynamic tests in the evaluation of geriatric UI is controversial: they are sometimes uncomfortable and relatively invasive and expensive. Simplified diagnostic tests (e.g., bedside *eyeball* cystometry) can provide important diagnostic information about bladder capacity, PVR, and detrusor overactivity and allow a stress test at a known volume: in other words they are useful to diagnose and appropriately treat many elderly patients with UI. In the majority of geriatric females, the basic evaluation with stress maneuvers will exclude other conditions and allow a presumptive diagnosis of urge incontinence due to detrusor instability and/or stress incontinence upon which an appropriate treatment can be performed. Diagnosis without specialized tests is often more difficult in geriatric males, in whom detrusor instability can be associated with outlet obstruction, even in the absence of an elevated PVR. Generally basic evaluation provides the most valuable information not only for diagnosis but also for therapeutic planning.

If older people have other significant conditions (pain, hematuria, recurrent symptomatic UTI, pelvic mass, pelvic irradiation, POP beyond introitus, suspected fistula, weight loss, chronic diarrhea, fecal impaction, inflammatory bowel disease), specialist referral should be considered, and it is not correct to plan a rehabilitation program [6].

49.4 The Role of PFR and Behavioral Techniques in Wealthy and Frail Elderly

People in the elderly may be considered as wealthy or frail. In contrast to wealthy, the term "frail older persons" defines the people over the age of 65 years with a clinical presentation of impaired physical activity, mobility, balance, muscle strength, motor processing, cognition, and feelings of fatigue. Frailty is not, however, synonymous with disability and comorbidity, even if frail people usually have multiple chronic medical conditions, take multiple drugs, and have difficulties in the personal activities of daily life (ADLs) and a high risk of intercurrent diseases, hospitalization, and death. This clarification is very important in order to plan therapeutic programs for pelvic floor dysfunction in the elderly. No differences exist among the rehabilitation treatments for adult and wealthy older people.

Initial management should be individualized and influenced by goals of care, treatment preferences, and estimated RLE, as the most likely clinical diagnosis. PFMT is considered as fist-line therapy in many pelvic floor dysfunctions, notably in UI. In association with other conservative measures, it has a relevant role in the improvement of quality of life (QoL). Age is no barrier to the benefits of PFR. There is evidence to suggest that older people are just as likely to benefit from PFMT for incontinence as younger people.

49.4.1 Urinary Incontinence

A variety of behavioral therapies have been developed to address UI, including bladder retraining, PFMT, VC in women, prompted or assisted voiding routines, BFB, FES, and complementary therapies (hypnosis and acupuncture). These conservative therapies are usually recommended as first-line treatment options, particularly for geriatric patients. PFMT is better than no treatment, a placebo drug, or an inactive control treatment for women with OAB, SUI, UUI, or MUI (level of evidence = 1; Moore et al.) [6]. Women treated with PFMT were more likely to report a cure or improvement and a better QoL; they also indicated fewer daily leakage episodes and had less urine leakage on the pad test than those in the control group in immediately after treatment and in the long term. The effect of PFMT in women with SUI does not seem to decrease with increased age: in trials with older women with SUI, it appeared both primary and secondary outcome measures were comparable to those in trials focused on younger women.

The International Consultation on Incontinence (ICI) recommends that supervised PFMT should be offered as a first-line conservative therapy for women of all ages with SUI, UUI, or MUI (grade of recommendation, A), therefore also in wealthy old people.

In frail elderly, instead, prompted voiding techniques have been developed and used successfully, in particular with nursing home residents. Ouslander et al. demonstrated an overall response rate of 41% in a cohort of 191 elderly incontinent nursing home residents (mean age 84.5 years) who underwent a prompted toilet training program [10]. These researchers found that the overall wet percentage went from 26.7 to 6.4% and was sustained at 9.6% after 9 weeks. Obviously multidisciplinary teamwork is usually needed to reach the best results [11]. Prompted voiding should be continued in eligible persons after a 3-day trial only in those that achieve more than a 20% reduction in wet checks or reach at least two thirds of appropriate toileting rates (the number of times the person void into the toilet divided by the total number of voids). All other people should be managed by "check and change" (Waggs et al.) [6]. In patients with dementia, UI occurs in 30–100%, and the degree of UI is strongly associated with patient's general status and ambulation. In case of ambulatory patients, prompted voiding, PFMT, and oral antimuscarinics seem to be the treatment of choice. In this regard, several studies have examined the differences between drugs and behavioral therapies. In a randomized controlled trial comparing PFMT with BFB to anticholinergic medication (oxybutynin) for treatment of UUI, Burgio et al. demonstrated superior results for the PFMT [12, 13]. The overall efficacy of the combination of oxybutynin and PFR was found to be superior to that of placebo or of either medical or behavioral therapy alone. On this point, pharmacotherapy has been widely used to treat UI, particularly for the treatment of OAB and UUI (Table 49.1). Antimuscarinics have shown efficacy in older adults, but their use can be associated sometimes with significant side effects, including dry mouth, constipation, blurred vision, and confusion. Newer drugs (as mirabegron, β3-agonist) may have fewer systemic side effects in older adults and the same efficacy of antimuscarinics.

Few pharmacologic agents are available for the treatment of SUI. Phenylpropanolamine (often used in the past) has been removed from the market because of an associated increased risk of stroke. At this time, the only medications that show some efficacy in the treatment of SUI are topical vaginal estrogen (but the studies are controversial) and duloxetine hydrochloride. This latter drug is a

Table 49.1 Pharmacological treatment

Indication/action	Drug name	Dosage	Side effects & precautions	Level of evidence[a]	Grade of recommendation[a]
OAB/UUI/MUI To modulate/reduce and/or suppress bladder overactivity and prevent UI	Oxybutynin IR	2.5–5 mg tds	Dry mouth, blurred vision, nausea constipation, tachycardia	1	A
	Oxybutynin ER	5–30 mg od		1	A
	Oxybutynin TDS	3.9 mg od		1	A
	Oxybutynin IV	5 mg od/tds		1	A
	Propantheline	15–30 mg tds/qds		2	B
	Tolterodine	2 mg bd		1	A
	Tolterodine ER	4 mg		1	A
	Trospium	20 mg bd/tds		1	A
	Solifenacin	5–10 mg od		1	A
	Darifenacin	7.5–15 mg od		1	A
	Imipramine	10–25 mg bd/tds	Tachycardia Hypotension	3	C
	Mirabegron	25–50 mg od		1	A
OAB (nocturia)	Desmopressin	0.1–0.2 mg od		1	A
	Desmopressin IN	20 µg od		1	A
Bladder outflow overactivity To decrease bladder outflow resistance	Phenoxybenzamine	10–20 mg od	Orthostatic hypotension, dizziness, fatigue, nasal congestion, retrograde ejaculation	2a	B
	Prazosin	1 mg od/bd		2a	B
	Doxazosin	1–2 mg od/bd		2a	B
	Alfuzosin ER	10 mg od			
	Terazosin	5–10 mg od			
	Tamsulosin	0.4 mg od			

od once daily, *bd* twice daily, *tds* three times daily, *qds* four times daily, *IR* immediate release, *ER* extended release, *TDS* transdermal, *IV* intravesically, *IN* intranasally

[a]Assessments according to the Oxford system (modified)

combined norepinephrine and serotonin reuptake inhibitor, which has been shown to significantly increase sphincter muscle activity during the filling/storage phase of micturition of women [6]. The pharmacologic therapy in the elderly should follow these rules: carefully evaluate the cognitive and cardiovascular state of the patient; start with low dosage and build up the dose slowly; and review regularly the outcome and the side effects.

49.4.2 Voiding Dysfunction (Urinary Retention)

Sometimes, mainly in females, dysfunctional bladder voiding is associated with CPP: relaxing PFM and BFB therapy may be beneficial. In males drugs like the α-adrenoceptor antagonists are used to improve the flow rate and reduce the post-void residual (PVR) of urine (Table 49.1). In case of significant PVR, intermittent catheterization is the treatment of choice. Sometimes incomplete bladder voiding is associated with OAB or UUI or MUI: in this case the treatment is not easy, mainly in men, and treatment options are based on accurate functional diagnosis including drugs (antimuscarinics, α-adrenoceptor antagonists, myorelaxants), behavioral interventions, PFR, and intermittent catheterization.

49.4.3 Urinary Incontinence After Radical Prostatectomy

PFMT, in association or no with BFB and FES (with a rectal or transcutaneous electrode), is the most commonly recommended conservative treatment for UI after radical prostatectomy (RP). Some reviews demonstrated that PFMT is better than no treatment, because it can reduce the frequency of incontinence episodes. Another study showed that an early PFMT after RP significantly reduces continence recovery time [14]. The rationale of this treatment is that PFM contraction may improve the strength of the external urethral sphincter during the raises of intra-abdominal pressure and inhibits the OAB. The value of PFMT for the treatment of UI after RP remains unclear; the efficacy of additional BFB or FES has not been proven.

49.4.4 Fecal Incontinence

For the cognitively intact older persons, PFMT can be considered (in isolation or in association with BFB and FES therapy), but few studies exist among frail older patients. Improving stool consistency can be done with dietary and supplementary fibers; loperamide at low doses may be considered to improve stool consistency.

49.4.5 Obstructed Defecation Syndrome (ODS)

The treatment of ODS is problematic and controversial. However, the patients should be given conservative treatment before considering invasive procedures.

BFB training seems indicated to teach these patients in managing their anorectal musculature during defecation. Other advices are essential: adequate hydration, high fiber intake, use of probiotics, regular physical activity, enemas, and laxatives.

49.4.6 Pelvic Organ Prolapse

PFMT may have a role in treating women with symptomatic POP, but there are no objective evidence-based studies to support this. In general any factor that leads to chronic increases in abdominal pressure should be avoided: constipation, chronic chest pathologies, and smoking. PFMT in our opinion is necessary also after surgery, considering that recurrence of POP after surgery is correlated with a reduced PFM contraction strength and an increased genital hiatus [13].

49.4.7 Chronic Pelvic Pain and Sexual Dysfunction

Rehabilitation of the pelvic floor can involve more than strengthening of atrophic PFMs of normal length. Different techniques are required to restore the short and/or painful PFMs to full function (active and passive stretching, neuromuscular reeducation, and progressive strengthening, transvaginal manual therapy in women, connective tissue manipulation, BFB training) [15]. Analgesic electrical stimulation (transcutaneous electrical neurostimulation or TENS and interferential currents) and drug and lifestyle interventions (patients' education, improved sleep patterns, and breathing relaxation exercises) can be done to reduce pelvic pain allowing a comprehensive PFMT, including pelvic floor muscle exercises (PFM contraction/relaxation and proprioceptive neuromuscular facilitation) and myofascial therapy.

Conclusions

After Kegel, PFR has acquired an undoubted scientific consensus in all the world in the field of female UI. Moreover in the last 30 years, many other pelvic disorders have been treated by appropriately utilized conservative techniques, such as PFMT, BFB training, and FES. The ICI in 1998 suggested PFMT as first-line option in the treatment of UI in women, men, and wealthy older people. In frail disabled patients, conservative management can often be directed to achieving *dependent* continence by use of behavioral approach (prompted and timed voiding). Pharmacotherapy often helps PFMT to improve urinary continence. Surgery, if necessary, should be indicated, mainly when PFR failed, as age per se is not a contraindication to surgery.

Key Points

- Urinary incontinence has a high prevalence, is often underestimated, and is not inevitable in older adults.
- The initial management of urinary incontinence includes bladder retraining and pelvic floor rehabilitation (biofeedback, electrical stimulation, and pelvic floor exercises).
- Pelvic floor muscle training is the initial most important therapeutic strategy.
- The pharmacologic therapy is used in addition to pelvic floor rehabilitation, mainly in the treatment of urge urinary incontinence.

References

1. Kegel AH (1948) Progressive resistance exercises in the functional restoration of perineal muscles. Am J Obstet Gynecol 56:238
2. Bourcier A (1989) Le plancher pelvien. Vigot Ed, Paris
3. Fantl JA, Newman DK, Colling J et al (1996) Urinary incontinence in adults: acute and chronic management. Clinical practice guideline, No 2, 1996 Update. Rockville, MD: U.S. Department of Health and Human Services. Public Health Service, Agency for Health Care Policy and Research. AHCPR Publication No. 96-0682
4. Abrams P, Cardozo L, Fall M et al (2002) The standardization of terminology of lower urinary tract function: report from the Standardization Sub-Committee of the International Continence Society. Neurourol Urodyn 21(2):167–178
5. Fonda D, Benvenuti F, Castleden M et al (1998) Conservative management of incontinence in older people. 1st International Consultation on Incontinence, 28 June–1 July 1998
6. Abrams P, Cardozo L, Khoury S, Wein A (2013) Incontinence. 5th International Consultation on Incontinence. EAU-ICUD
7. Bø K, Hagen RH, Kvarstein B et al (1990) Pelvic floor muscle exercise for the treatment of female stress urinary incontinence. III. Effects of two different degrees of pelvic floor muscle exercise. Neurourol Urodyn:489–502
8. Di Benedetto P (1999) Treatment of urinary stress incontinence with pelvic floor exercises. In: Appell RA, Bourcier AP, La Torre F (eds) Pelvic floor dysfunction – investigation and conservative treatment. CESI, Roma, pp 211–218
9. Resnick NM, Yalla SV (1987) Detrusor hyperactivity with impaired contractile function: unrecognized but common cause of incontinence in elderly patients. JAMA 257:3076
10. Ouslander JG, Zarit SH, Orr NK, Muira SA (1990) Incontinence among elderly community-dwelling dementia patients. Characteristics, management, and impact on caregivers. J Am Geriatr Soc 38:440–445
11. Der-Sheng H, Yen-Ho W (2008) Urinary incontinence in dementia. Incont Pelvic Floor Dysfunct 2:63–66

12. Burgio KL, Locker JL, Goode PS et al (1998) Behavioral vs drug treatment for urge incontinence in older women: a randomized controlled trial. JAMA 280:1995–2000
13. Sherburn M (2007) Evidence for pelvic floor physical therapy in the elderly. In: Bø K, Berghmans B, Mørkved S, Van Kampen M (eds) Evidence based physical therapy for the pelvic floor. Bridging science and clinical practice. Elsevier, Churchill, Livingstone, Chap. 12, pp 345–367
14. Filocamo MT, Li Marzi V, Del Popolo G, Cecconi F, Marzocco M, Tosto A, Nicita G (2005) Effectiveness of early pelvic floor rehabilitation treatment for post-prostatectomy incontinence. Eur Urol 48:734–738
15. FitzGerald MP, Kotarinos R (2003) Rehabilitation of the short pelvic floor. II. Treatment of the patient with the short pelvic floor. Int Urogynecol J 14:269–275

Physical Activity and Sexual Function in Older People

50

Paolo Di Benedetto

50.1 Introduction

The number of people 65 years of age and older continues to rise in the Unites States of America (USA) and in the Western countries. In the USA in particular from approximately 35 million in 2000, the persons aged over 65 by 2030 will be 71 million, 20 million of whom will exceed the age of 80.

Almost 75% of elderly persons have at least one chronic illness, and about 50% have at least two chronic illnesses. The well-being and quality of life (QoL) of older people are often seriously compromised even in subjects not complaining of degenerative or vascular neurological diseases, psychiatric disorders, or oncological problems. A healthy lifestyle lowers risks of many diseases and promotes a feeling of well-being: a balanced diet and regular physical activity can help prevent some of the health problems associated with aging and reduced mobility.

In this context, multiple studies found that sexuality continues to be an important aspect of life for many adults throughout midlife and into old age [1–3]. The American Association of Retired Persons reported in 2005 that 62% of men and 51% of women between ages 60 and 69 believed sexual activity is an important component of a good relationship and an acceptable QoL: these figures declined slightly after age 70. With regard to that, the National Council of Aging (NCOA) reported that 71% of men in their sixties, over 57% in their seventies, and 27% in their eighties engaged in sexual activity at least once a month; these percentages were lower for women (51%, 30%, and 18%, respectively). The study of Bretschneider and McCoy concluded that the majority of women and men over eighties continued to fantasize about intimate contact with a partner, even if there

P. Di Benedetto
University Tor Vergata, Rome, Italy
e-mail: mrsart@libero.it

© Springer International Publishing AG 2018

S. Masiero, U. Carraro (eds.), *Rehabilitation Medicine for Elderly Patients*, Practical Issues in Geriatrics, DOI 10.1007/978-3-319-57406-6_50

are gender differences (41.2% of males aged 75–85 showed an interest in sex compared with 11.4% of females the same age [4, 5]). Then, it has been stated that many elderly persons enjoy an active sex life in contrast with the general perception of an "asexual" old age and the prevailing myth that aging and sexual dysfunction (SD) are inexorably linked.

The purpose of this chapter is to provide an overview of aging on the sexual life of "healthy" men and women and to describe the role of physical activity and exercise training as an important aspect of prevention and treatment of SD in the elderly.

50.2 Sexuality in Older Men and Women

Although erectile functioning tends to decline progressively beginning in midlife, it should not be inferred that erectile failure is an inevitable consequence of aging. Certainly older men suffer from multiple typical changes in erectile dysfunction (ED) and ejaculatory and orgasmic disorders: lengthier delay in reaching a full erection, less rigidity of the erect penis, fewer or no erections during sleep, increase latency to ejaculation, less forceful ejaculation, reduced volume of sperm expelled at each ejaculation, and lengthened refractory period following ejaculation (spanning sometimes as long as a few days). ED is prevalent among men and its presence is often an indicator of systemic disease. Risk factors for ED include cardiovascular disease, hypertension, diabetes mellitus (DM), tobacco use, hyperlipidemia, hypogonadism, lower urinary tract symptoms, metabolic syndrome, and depression. Addressing the modifiable risk factors frequently improves a patient's overall health and increases life span. The literature suggests that smoking cessation, treatment of hyperlipidemia, and increasing physical activity will improve erectile function in many patients. How the treatment of DM, depression, and hypogonadism impacts erectile function is less clear. Clinicians need to be aware that certain antihypertensive agents can adversely impact erectile function. Androgen serum levels gradually decrease in men beginning around age 50 and are often implicated in the decline of sexual responsiveness; some studies suggest that the benefits of testosterone treatment for improving sexual function are limited to those whose testosterone levels fall below a relatively low "threshold" value that seems to be necessary to maintain an adequate sexual function.

Unlike men, whose sexual performances generally decrease after early adulthood, women's sexual responsiveness does not show such a consistent pattern over the life span: the incidence of sexual problems in women may actually decrease after early adulthood, and sexual satisfaction among older women may remain somewhat higher that in men. Menopause is characterized by a dramatic reduction in estrogen, progesterone, and androgen levels. Sexual changes are well known: low desire (43%), reduction of vaginal lubrication (39%), lining of the vaginal wall thins, shortening of the vagina, atrophy of the genital tissues, orgasmic dysfunction, or inability to climax (34%) [6]. All these factors may lead to painful sexual intercourse (dyspareunia, vaginismus, and vulvar vestibulitis). Age-related changes in women somewhat mirror those that occur in men: these changes are related to vaginal lubrication, clitoral responses, and orgasm that tends to be briefer and associated with fewer muscular contractions. These declines in sexual responsiveness may be reduced sometimes by a regular sexual activity, although the mechanism of benefit is not understood. The role of estrogen and androgen supplementation in women is not clear: there are insufficient data for a clear risk-benefit of hormone treatment [7]. For reducing the risk of systemic estrogen therapy, localized estrogen preparations can be effective alternatives in order to improve vaginal dryness and irritation. There is not enough evidence that any of the complementary therapies available are any better than placebo for menopausal vasomotor symptoms and few safety data exist [8].

We have also to consider that women often avoid sexual intercourse because of pelvic floor dysfunction: not only overactive bladder and urinary incontinence (urgency, stress, or mixed urinary incontinence) but also, and more frequently, chronic pelvic or low back pain conditions may interfere with a good sexuality. Irrespective of the site of pain, women complaining of chronic pain generally are depressed, with higher pain scores associated with greater depression.

50.3 Sexuality as an Aspect of Healthy Aging

Clinical studies suggest that many elderly couples discontinue sexual activity due to illnesses, particularly in the male partner. Some chronic medical conditions among aged patients (including cardiovascular diseases, hypertension, and DM) are associated with various sexual problems in men and women. Sexual dysfunction heightens anger, frustration, and depression with the involvement of the partners that often present with similar symptoms. Patients with chronic heart failure (CHF) have sexual dysfunction that impairs QoL: recent trials have demonstrated that exercise training (ET) improves QoL of CHF patients, but it is not established whether this benefit may be associated with an improvement in SD.

Moreover, several drugs are commonly associated with sexual dysfunction. Besides benzodiazepines, tricyclic antidepressants and selective serotonin reuptake inhibitors (SSRIs), used for the treatment of depression, may have well-documented side effects: decreased sexual interest, sexual arousal difficulties, loss of libido, and hyporgasmia. Other drugs frequently associated with sexual complaints include beta-blockers and some diuretics. Consequently, the effects of current medication used should be considered in the sexual health assessment.

In the last years, there is a more and more growing evidence suggesting that lifestyle factor (particularly physical activity, eating right, not smoking, getting enough sleep, and balanced diet) may offer some protection against sexual problems, frequently associated with health concerns. In this regard, Derby et al. reported that obesity status was associated with ED, with baseline obesity predicting a higher risk regardless of follow-up weight loss, whereas physical activity status was associated with ED, with the highest risk among men who remained sedentary and the lowest among those who remained active or initiated physical activity [9].

50.4 Assessment of Sexual Function in the Elderly

A diagnosis should be made when symptoms cause distress or interpersonal problems.

The assessment of SD in elderly should include a sexual history, a discussion of how sexuality has been experienced over time, laboratory testing, health conditions (presence of comorbidities), concurrent medications, and psychological and neurological evaluation [1]. Moreover, in males particular attention must be given to patients with cardiovascular disease, following the algorithm for determining the level of sexual activity according to cardiac risk in patients with ED [10]. Actually, older males who present with complaints of ED should be screened for cardiovascular disease because comorbidity often exists even though most men are asymptomatic prior to the onset of an acute cardiac event. The rate of ED in older adult men with coronary artery disease (CAD) is increased compared to those without CAD. ED typically presents about 3 years prior to onset of CAD symptoms, and older men with ED have a 75% increased risk of developing peripheral vascular disease.

In the medical evaluation of older female patients with sexual problems, it is important to inquire about early sexual experiences, including childhood sexual abuse, that impact greatly on their sexuality in later life. Other clinical factors that impact on older women's sexuality include breast surgery, urinary incontinence, and hysterectomy. With regard to this, it is necessary to assess pelvic floor dysfunction, particularly pelvic organ prolapse, chronic pelvic pain, and urinary incontinence: all these conditions significantly bother the sexuality. When SDs are related to the menopause, customized hormone replacement therapy is the treatment of choice.

50.5 Physical Activity as a Treatment Modality of Sexual Dysfunction in the Elderly

Sedentary lifestyle predisposes to metabolic syndrome (MetS), a clustering of metabolic disorders: visceral obesity, hypertension, dyslipidemia, and DM. MetS comprises a high risk for CVD events even in the absence of DM. Mechanisms that link MetS to increased CVD risk are, however, incompletely understood. Many of the physiological changes of aging as well as those secondary to physical inactivity are reversible or retarded by exercise. Bone density, muscle mass, aerobic conditioning, and flexibility can also be increased through an appropriate exercise program. Physical activity and strength/flexibility exercises can also reduce the fatigue and improve quality of sleep, stress, depression, weight control, gastrointestinal function, and sexuality.

Regarding this latter, many studies report a clinical evidence of benefits induced by physical activity on ED and, in general, on sexual responsiveness both in men and women. The literature shows that ED in middle-aged men is often an early event in endothelial damage and has been associated with cardiovascular diseases [11]. Physical activity (in association with Mediterranean diet) is able to improve both sexual responses and overall cardiovascular health in men and women [12].

There are conflicting data regarding the effects of exercise on androgen or estrogen status, but in clinical practice it would be recommended to add regular physical activity to balanced diet and drugs to achieve better therapeutic results. Regarding the ED in males, besides the well-known phosphodiesterase type 5 (PDE_5) inhibitors, it is recently reported that statins could be considered as adjuvant or alternative therapy, because of their protective effect on the dyslipidemia and reduction of endothelial damage [13].

In men and women with pelvic floor dysfunction (overactive bladder, urinary incontinence, pelvic organ prolapse, constipation and fecal incontinence, chronic pelvic pain), it is mandatory also to organize a correct pelvic floor muscle training, in association with other pelvic floor treatment modalities (as biofeedback, functional electrical stimulation, and behavioral modifications) and pharmacological therapy.

50.5.1 Physical Activity

Many authors stated that it is never too late to start an exercise program or a generic physical activity. To stay healthy or to improve health, older adults need to do two types of physical activity each week: aerobic and strength exercises.

Patients aged 65 or older, who are generally fit and have no health conditions that limit their mobility, should try to be active daily in accordance with the recommendations from the American College of Sports Medicine (ACSM) and the American Heart Association (AHA) [14].

The older people should do:

- At least 150 min of *moderate aerobic activity* such as cycling or walking every week
- *Strength exercises* on 2 or more days a week that work all the major muscles (legs, hips, back, abdomen, chest, shoulders, and arms)

Two alternatives are possible in the context of aerobic activity, in association with *strength exercises*:

- 75 min of *vigorous aerobic activity* such as running or a game of singles tennis every week
- A mix of *moderate and vigorous aerobic activity* every week (e.g., two 30-min runs, plus 30 min of fast walking, equates to 150 min of moderate aerobic activity)

A rule of thumb is that 1 min of vigorous activity provides the same health benefits as 2 min of moderate activity.

Examples of activities that require moderate effort for most people include walking, water aerobics, ballroom and line dancing, riding a bike on level ground or with few hills, playing doubles tennis, canoeing, and volleyball.

Instead, examples of activities that require vigorous effort are jogging or running, aerobics, swimming fast, riding a bike fast or on hills, singles tennis, energetic dancing, and martial art.

Moderate activity will raise the heart rate and make breathe faster and feel warmer; exercising at moderate level signifies that people can still talk, but cannot sing the words to a song. Daily chores such as shopping, cooking, or housework do not count toward the 150 min of moderate activity, because the effort is not enough to raise the heart rate, but they are important nonetheless, as they break up periods of sitting.

Older adults at risk of falls, such as people with weak legs, poor balance, and some medical conditions, should do exercises to improve balance and coordination on at least 2 days a week (yoga, tai chi, and dancing).

Vigorous activity makes the breath hard and fast. Working at this level, the people will not be able to say more than a few words without pausing for breath. In general, 75 min of vigorous activity can give similar health benefits to 150 min of moderate activity, and there is a good evidence that vigorous activity can bring health benefits over and above that of moderate activity.

Regarding activities that strengthen muscles, whose good function is necessary for all daily movement, maintaining strong bones, regulating blood sugar and blood pressure, and maintaining a healthy weight, they include carrying or moving heavy loads, dancing, heavy gardening, exercises that use body weight for resistance (such as push-ups or sit-ups), yoga, and lifting weights. There are many ways for strengthening muscles, whether at home or in the gym; in these programs also, flexibility exercises are recommended.

Muscle-strengthening exercises are not an aerobic activity; then they have to be done in addition to 75–150 min of aerobic activity. It is possible to do activities that strengthen muscles on the same day or on different days as aerobic activity.

Some vigorous activities count as both an aerobic activity and a muscle-strengthening activity and include circuit training, aerobics, and running.

Moreover, to maintain the flexibility necessary for regular physical activity, older adults should perform activities that maintain or increase flexibility on at least 2 days each week for at least 10' each day. Balance exercises are also indicated to reduce risks of injury from falls.

Obviously modifications of the exercise prescription are advisable in selected aging-related chronic conditions, as degenerative joint diseases, CHF, diabetes mellitus, low back pain, osteoporosis, chronic obstructive lung disease, hypertension, and orthostatic hypotension [15]. Many randomized controlled studies have shown that physical activity and exercise have a beneficial effect on physical performance, pain, and disability; there is also a strong evidence that resistance training is the most effective strategy to counter and prevent age-related muscle weakness.

50.5.2 Physical Activity and Sexual Function

Many studies demonstrated the presence in men of ED and METs. Physical activity is a strong and independent predictor of normal erectile function among all as well as among only MET subjects. Thus, especially MET patients presenting with ED should be considered at high risk for CVD. Consequently, physical activity is very important in the management of METs, ED, and concomitant diseases, leading the researchers to conclude that enhanced sexuality is directly correlated with the improvement in physical fitness [11].

Obviously, balanced diet, reducing stress, cessation of smoking, and getting enough sleep are all important for having a satisfying sex life, but physical activity determines the release of endorphins, opioids, and sex hormones, elevating the mood and lowering hearth rate and blood pressure. These positive effects of regular physical activity are seen on menopausal women through an increase of synaptic transmission of monoamines, which supposedly functions in the same manner as antidepressants [16]. Active elderly women obtained the highest total scores on all Female Sexual Function Index (FSFI) domains (desire, arousal, lubrication, orgasm, satisfaction, and pain), compared to moderately active and sedentary subjects.

Conclusions

Aging continues to rise in the USA and in all Western countries. Older people are at risk for several chronic conditions that interfere and, sometimes, exacerbate SD both in men and women.

Many studies demonstrated that adopting or increasing regular physical activity may be beneficial to sexuality of elderly people improving cardiovascular fitness, flexibility, mobility, mood, and self-image. Physical activity consists of moderate or vigorous aerobic and strength exercises (see guidelines suggested by American College of Sports Medicine), in association with pelvic floor rehabilitation, when necessary [14].

Most studies suggest also that physical activity and exercise training are associated with better QoL and health outcomes. Therefore, assessment and promotion of physical activity may be beneficial in achieving desired benefits across older people, including a satisfying sexuality.

Understanding the effects of physical activity on sexuality can potentially have a positive influence on the clinical practice of physicians. Physicians rarely recommend that their older patients exercise more, despite the documented advantages of systematic physical exercise. This could possibly promote a more satisfactory QoL and prevent SD.

Key Points

- Sexuality continues to be an important aspect of life for many adults throughout midlife and into old age. Unlike men, whose sexual performances generally decrease after early adulthood, women do not show such a consistent pattern over the life span.
- Physical activity (in association with Mediterranean diet) is able to improve both sexual responses and overall cardiovascular health in men and women.
- Physical fitness is very important in the management of patients with metabolic syndrome and erectile dysfunction and is related to enhanced sexuality.

References

1. Montorsi F, Basson R, Adaikan G et al (eds) (2010) Sexual medicine: sexual dysfunctions in men and women. In: Proceedings of the 3rd International Consultation on Sexual Medicine, Paris
2. Araujo AB, Mohr BA, McKinlay JB (2004) Changes in sexual function in middle-aged and older men: longitudinal data from the Massachusetts Male Aging Study. J Am Geriatr Soc 52(9):1502
3. Addis IB, Van Den Eeden SK, Wassel-Fyr CL, Vittinghoff E, Brow NJS, Thom DH (2006) Sexual activity and function in middle-aged and older women. Obstet Gynecol 107:755–764
4. Bretschnider JG, McCoy NL (1988) Sexual interest and behavior in healthy 80- to 102-years-olds. Arch Sex Behav 17:109–129
5. Taylor A, Gosney MA (2011) Sexuality in older age: essentials considerations for healthcare professionals. Age Ageing 40:538–543
6. Lindau ST, Schumm LP, Laumann EO, Wendy Levinson W, O'Muircheartaigh CA, Waite LJ (2007) A study of sexuality and health among older adults in the United States. N Engl J Med 357:762–774
7. Basaria S, Dobs AS (2004) Safety and adverse effects of androgens: how to counsel patients. Mayo Clin Proc 79:S25–S32
8. Hichey M, Davis SR, Sturdee DW (2005) Treatment of menopausal symptoms. What shall we do now? Lancet 366:409–421
9. Derby CA, Mohr BA, Goldstein I, Feldman HA, Johannes CB, McKinlay JB (2000) Modifiable risk factors and erectile dysfunction. Can lifestyle changes modify risk? Urology 56:302–306
10. Hatzichristou D, Rosen RC, Derogatis LR et al (2010) Recommendations for the clinical evaluation of men and women with sexual dysfunction. J Sex Med 7(1 pt 2):346
11. Pohjantähti-Maaroos H, Palomäki A, Hartikainen J (2011) Erectile dysfunction, physical activity and metabolic syndrome: differences in markers of atherosclerosis. BMC Cardiovasc Disord 11:36. doi:10.1186/1471-2261-11-36
12. Belardinelli R, Lacalaprice F, Faccenda E, Purcaro A, Perna G (2005) Effects of short-term moderate exercise training on sexual function in male patients with chronic stable heart failure. Int J Cardiol 101:83–90
13. La Vignera S, Condorelli R, Vicari E, D'Agata R, Calogero AE (2012) Physical activity and erectile dysfunction in middle-aged men. J Androl 33(2):154–161
14. Nelson ME, Rejeski WJ, Blair SN, Duncan PW, Jo J, King AC, Macera CA, Castaneda-Sceppa C (2007) Physical activity and public health in older adults: recommendation from the American College of Sports Medicine and the American Heart Association. Med Sci Sports Exerc 39:1435–1445
15. Capodaglio P, Narici MV, Rutherford OM, Sartorio A (2000) Physical exercise in the elderly: its effects on the motor and endocrine system. Eur Med Phys 36:205–219
16. Cabral PU, Canario AC, Spyrides MH, Uchôa SA, Eleuterio Juniorn J, Giraldo PC, Gonçalves AK (2014) Physical activity and sexual function in middle-aged women. Rev Assoc Med Bras 60:47–52

51 Rehabilitation Treatment in Older Cancer Patients

Antonella Brunello, Giuseppe Lombardi, and Vittorina Zagonel

Cancer is one of the most common and disabling health-care conditions affecting people. Progress in diagnosis, treatment, and supportive care in the last years has raised the 5-year relative survival rate for all cancers to about 67% [1].

Median age at cancer diagnosis, for all cancer types, is 67 years, and by the year 2020, about 60% of new patients diagnosed with cancer will be aged 65 years and older, with estimates for the *oldest old* (patients aged 85 years and older) rising from the actual 9% to 17% [2].

The general improvement in survival rates observed in the overall cancer patient population has also been seen for the older ones [3].

Older individuals may present different issues unrelated to cancer; therefore supportive care along with rehabilitation measures is an essential step in the management of elderly cancer patients.

One of the main issues for cancer patients is physical disability, and this probably may also be one of the leading causes of emotional distress in cancer survivors.

The goals of cancer treatment in older cancer patients therefore must include, along with prolongation of life expectancy, the prevention of functional dependence.

Indeed, disability in older patients, and consequent impairment in functional status is strongly associated with frailty, which in turn is associated with higher mortality [4].

For older patients, "standard" oncological outcomes which are normally pursued in the adult population such as increased overall survival or progression-free survival may indeed be not a major goal if they come at the price of losing independence [5].

A. Brunello • G. Lombardi • V. Zagonel (✉)
Department of Experimental and Clinical Oncology, Medical Oncology 1, Veneto Institute of Oncology - IRCCS, Padua, Italy
e-mail: antonella.brunello@iov.veneto.it; giuseppe.lombardi@iov.veneto.it; vittorina.zagonel@iov.veneto.it

© Springer International Publishing AG 2018

S. Masiero, U. Carraro (eds.), *Rehabilitation Medicine for Elderly Patients*, Practical Issues in Geriatrics, DOI 10.1007/978-3-319-57406-6_51

Rehabilitation for older cancer patients may be needed in two major settings, namely that of curable malignancies and a palliative setting in which incurable malignancies have an indolent clinical course.

For most localized tumors, in addition to surgery and/or radiation treatment, the optimal management often involves the use of adjuvant systemic therapy. This consists of endocrine therapy, cytotoxic therapy, or targeted therapy administered in order to reduce the risk of recurrence and death in patients at high risk of relapse after local treatment.

The rehabilitation of older cancer survivors is largely unknown, and several issues related both to the needs and interventions indeed deserve further studies.

As for rehabilitation needs for advanced tumors, we must acknowledge that some forms of advanced stage lymphoma, especially large cell lymphomas, are curable. Also, some incurable malignancies with an indolent clinical course may benefit from rehabilitation, and these are mainly low-grade lymphomas and breast or prostate cancer with bone metastases only.

Most older patients treated for cancer will likely experience some toxicity which may hamper their quality of life and, in some cases, mine their autonomy.

In this light, it has long been known that older patients with a cancer diagnosis are best managed by means of a Comprehensive Geriatric Assessment, with a thorough evaluation of several domains pertaining their functional status, cognitive status, mood, nutritional status, social and living conditions, and polipharmacology.

A progressive decline in one or more of these domains leads to reduced life expectancy and functional reserve [6, 7].

Cancer may increase the likelihood for older patients to need rehabilitation.

Cancer itself may worsen baseline conditions which are common in older subjects, such as malnutrition or sarcopenia. Also, cancer may cause and/or increase fatigue.

Moreover, both acute and chronic complications of cytotoxic chemotherapy increase with age [8].

Among the acute complications, myelotoxicity, mucositis, cardiotoxicity, and peripheral neurotoxicity are the most common.

Of the chronic complications, some conditions in particular may increase the need of rehabilitation for older cancer survivors, and these are fatigue, dementia, deconditioning, chronic cardiac dysfunction, and chronic polyneuropathy.

51.1 Fatigue

Fatigue is defined as a condition of exhaustion that does not improve with rest [9].

Fatigue is both an acute and a chronic complication of cytotoxic chemotherapy that is more common with increasing age [10] and may represent a major cause of functional dependence.

In older individuals, fatigue is a cause of deconditioning [11], functional dependence [12, 13], and increased mortality [14].

Any serious attempt to rehabilitate older cancer patients should include a plan to prevent and overcome fatigue.

The causes and the mechanisms of fatigue are largely unknown. It is clear that fatigue is associated with chronic inflammation and sarcopenia and may be improved with the correction of anemia in some patients [15].

Beside the cancer itself, which is one of the causes of fatigue in those patients with active disease, among other presumptive causes of fatigue, there are chemotherapy, as well as polipharmacy and sleep disorders [16].

The management of fatigue is paramount to the functional rehabilitation of older patients. This involves both prevention and timely treatment.

As some recent studies highlighted, fatigue is associated with functional dependence [12, 13] and death [14] in older individuals. Thus the management of fatigue is critical to rehabilitation.

51.2 Cognitive Decline

Another important concern in older patients undergoing chemotherapy is the possible role of chemotherapy as a cause of dementia. Though the evidence supporting this association is inconclusive [17, 18], it is well known that chemotherapy may lead to some form of cognitive decline and that older people are at particular risk for this complication [19, 20].

51.3 Deconditioning

Deconditioning is a common complication of prolonged hospitalization and prolonged inactivity in elderly individuals [11]. Older cancer patients are at particular risk of prolonged hospitalization from surgical and medical complications as well as of prolonged at home inactivity due to fatigue and malnutrition. Several controlled trials have assessed the prevention of deconditioning with exercise and home interventions, in particular the role of exercise and nutrition [21, 22].

51.4 Other Chronic Treatment-Associated Toxicities

Older individuals are at increased risk for long-term toxicity of chemotherapy. Among others, we acknowledge and include chronic cardiomyopathy from anthracyclines [23] and peripheral neuropathy [3].

Both sensory and motor neuropathies are a common complication of the treatment with platinum salts, vinca alkaloids, taxanes, and eribulin. Such complication is more frequent in older patients, and it may become chronic and irreversible.

At present an empiric approach to such problems includes careful cardiological baseline and follow-up evaluations, discontinuance of chemotherapy in the presence of early signs of toxicity, cardiological treatment for cardiomyopathy, and early rehabilitation of neurologic deficits.

51.5 Conclusions

It is of utmost importance to adopt all supportive measures in order to successfully treat vulnerable and unfit elderly patients with cancer and to reduce the risk of functional impairment.

In particular, it is important to rule out anemia and possible causes of anemia and correct them whenever possible in order to reduce anemia-associated fatigue and to choose cytotoxics according to expected acute and chronic adverse events [24].

Several important issues still need to be addressed in the field of rehabilitation of older cancer patients, in particular whether cancer and its treatment accelerate the physiologic aging of a person and whether nutritional interventions, exercise, and management of anemia have a role in preventing the long-term complications of cancer and its treatment and the long-term social implications of cancer and its treatment.

51.6 Rehabilitation Treatment in Neuro-oncology

Primary brain tumors account for 1% of all cancers in adults and affect 5–13 per 100,000 population worldwide annually. In the last years, the overall incidence of brain tumors has increased, especially in elderly patients in which the incidence has doubled; moreover, 20–40% of patients with cancer develops nervous system (NS) metastases [25].

A wide variety of impairments of nervous system function may result from cancer, either by direct effect at the primary or metastatic tumor site or as a treatment consequence, such as neurosurgery, chemotherapy, radiation therapy, and corticosteroids, alone or in combination. Some of the most adverse effects associated with these treatments include fatigue, myopathy, insomnia, and mood disturbance. Anticonvulsant medications may further accentuate fatigue and somnolence.

Among side effects of chemotherapy drugs, peripheral neuropathy is the most frequent (50–60% of patients treated with taxanes). Peripheral neuropathy may be characterized by losses in sensation and proprioception with postural instability. And so, interventions have to focus on patient education about foot care and balance training [26].

However, most patients with NS tumors have multiple impairments depending on tumor location and size and the volume of tissue excised. In an Australian study with brain tumor patients treated with integrated multidisciplinary rehabilitation, the most common neurologic deficits included ataxia/incoordination (62%), seizures (47%), paresis (47%), cognitive (45%) and visual impairment (47%), dysphasia (40%), dysarthria (29%), sensory-perceptual deficit (26%), and bowel/bladder dysfunction (21%) [27]. In another study, the most common neurologic deficits included pain (56%, which included a 42% incidence of headaches), ataxia (44%), seizures (43%), paresis (37%), cognitive dysfunction (36%), and visual impairment (35%) [28].

All of these neurological impairments may significantly impact the individual's physical, cognitive, and emotional capabilities, which significantly compromise the quality of life (QoL). Yet, brain tumors can be associated with significant costs and socioeconomic implications for health-care and social services. And so, NS tumor is a complex and challenging condition requiring integrated multidisciplinary care and services such as multidisciplinary rehabilitation.

Nevertheless, rehabilitation after brain tumor resection has been shown to result in better outcomes, including gains in functional status. In fact, Khan et al. [27], in a controlled clinical trial, analyzed the effectiveness of integrated multidisciplinary rehabilitation in primary brain cancer. The inclusion criteria for intensive multidisciplinary rehabilitation were stable medical course after surgery, radiotherapy, and chemotherapy; a total of 106 patients were recruited for the study, and all patients were allocated either to the treatment (53 patients) or control group (53 patients). The treatment group received comprehensive individualized multidisciplinary rehabilitation (for up to 6–8 weeks) incorporating a wide range of elements, such as education and health promotion for patients mildly affected to intensive mobilization program for the more severely affected patients. The primary outcome, Functional Independence Measure (FIM), measured "activity limitation" while secondary measures included depression, anxiety, and cancer rehabilitation evaluation system. Assessments were at baseline 3 and 6 months after program completion. In the intervention group, there were patients with low-grade glioma (46%) and high-grade glioma (54%). About 60% of patients performed radiation therapy and 45% chemotherapy. At 3 months posttreatment follow-up, there was a significant difference between treatment and control group patients in all FIM scale (sphincter, self-care, locomotion, mobility, communication) and FIM psychosocial subscale. At 6 months follow-up, there was a significant improvement in the treatment group for the FIM sphincter, communication, psychosocial, and cognition subscales.

In another study, Zucchella et al. [29] analyzed the effectiveness of cognitive rehabilitation for early post-surgery in patients affected by primary tumor in a randomized, controlled trial. They enrolled 53 patients with cognitive impairment after surgery for brain tumor. These patients were randomly assigned to the treatment group (25 patients) or to the control group (28 patients). The cognitive rehabilitation program was designed in accordance with the recommendations of Cicerone et al. [30] and was administered by two neuropsychologists. Analyzing the baseline and post-treatment outcome measures (within-group analysis), there was a statistically significant improvement in all the neuropsychological measures at the end of the treatment period in the study group; on the contrary, there was no improvement in the control group. Comparison of the outcome measures of the two groups showed a statistically significant difference only in the domains of visual attention and verbal memory in favor of the study group.

Among brain tumors, glioblastoma multiforme has the worst prognosis (12–15 months), and therefore there is a great need to improve the quality of life of both patients and caregivers, in particular, to the end of life period. The neuro-oncology group of Pace et al. [31] performed a prospective study to analyze the benefit of palliative care at home. This strategy is becoming important in oncology, both to improve the quality of care for cancer patients and to reduce costs for the health-care system. Home assistance included neurologist, nurses, psychologist, rehabilitation therapist, and a social worker. Clinical conditions were periodically evaluated by Barthel Index, Karnofsky Performance Scale, and Mini Mental State Examination. A positive impact for rehabilitation at home was recorded in 92% of cases, and 72% of patients had an improvement in their quality of life scores due to rehabilitation.

In addition to the brain, injuries to the spinal cord may be due to primitive and metastatic tumors or to medical complications. However, spinal cord metastasis occurs up to 5% of all patients with cancer [1]. Most frequent symptoms can be weakness (74–76%), autonomic dysfunction (52–57%), and sensory loss (51–53%). It is important to accurately assess the patient before starting the rehabilitation planning because it may result in pathologic fracture and cord compression. However, in a few studies, it showed interesting and positive results following rehabilitation in patients with disability from spinal cord tumors, in particular for patients with important neurological deficits [32].

Moreover, there are various studies establishing the efficacy of appropriate exercise in counteracting physical impairment such as fatigue and functional decline, cognitive impairment, depression, and anxiety in patients diagnosed with neurologic malignancies [33].

In conclusion, rehabilitation treatment has to be an important part of the multidisciplinary oncological therapy for patients with NS tumors; indeed, rehabilitation therapy showed to result in better outcomes and improvement in the quality of life. Noteworthy, rehabilitation measures need to be personalized for each specific patient depending on histological type of tumor, tumor location, type of surgery, and neurologic deficits to obtain the greatest benefit.

Key Points

- Rehabilitation treatment must be part of cancer treatment in older cancer patients
- In elderly cancer patients some conditions may increase the need of rehabilitation for older cancer survivors, such as fatigue and deconditioning
- Elderly patients with nervous system tumor can show neurological impairments impacting the individual's physical capability
- Nervous system tumor is a complex condition requiring integrated multidisciplinary care and services such as multidisciplinary rehabilitation

References

1. Silver JK, Baima J, Mayer RS (2013) Impairment-driven cancer rehabilitation: an essential component of quality care and survivorship. CA Cancer J Clin 63(5):295–317
2. Hayat MJ, Howlader N, Reichman ME, Edwards BK (2007) Cancer statistics, trends, and multiple primary cancer analyses from the Surveillance, Epidemiology, and End Results (SEER) Program. Oncologist 12(1):20–37

3. Hoffe S, Balducci L (2012) Cancer and age: general considerations. Clin Geriatr Med 28:1–18
4. Balducci L, Dolan D, Hoffe SA (2015) Palliative care in older patients with cancer. Cancer Control 22(4):480–488
5. Yang Y (2008) Long and happy living. Trends and patterns of happy life expectancy in the US, 1970–2000. Soc Sci Res 37:1235–1252
6. Mitnitski AB, Song X, Rockwood K (2004) The estimation of relative fitness and frailty in community dwelling older adults using self-report data. J Gerontol Med Sci 59:M627–M632
7. Yourman LC, Lee SJ, Schonberg MA, Widera EW, Smith AK (2012) Prognostic indices for older adults: a systematic review. JAMA 307:182–192
8. Balducci L, Extermann M (2000) Management of cancer in the older person: a practical approach. Oncologist 5(3):224–237
9. Heins MJ, Korevaar JC, Rijken PM, Schellevis FG (2013) For which health problems do cancer survivors visit their General Practitioner? Eur J Cancer 49(1):211–218
10. Alcock M, Chilvers CR (2012) Emergency surgery in the elderly: a retrospective observational study. Anaesth Intensive Care 40:90–94
11. Gillis A, Mac Donald B (2005) Deconditioning in hospitalized elderly patients. Can Nurse 101:16–20
12. Luciani A, Jacobsen PB, Extermann M, Foa P, Marussi D, Overcash JA (2008) Fatigue and functional dependence in older cancer patients. Am J Clin Oncol 31:424–430
13. Hardy SE, Studenski SA (2008a) Fatigue predicts mortality in older adults. J Am Geriatr Soc 56:1910–1914
14. Hardy SE, Studenski SA (2008b) Fatigue and function over three years among older adults. J Gerontol A Biol Sci Med Sci 63:1389–1392
15. Balducci L, Fossa SD (2013) Rehabilitation of older cancer patients. Acta Oncol 52(2):233–238
16. Hardy SE, Studenski SA (2010) Qualities of fatigue and associated chronic conditions among older adults. J Pain Symptom Manag 39:1033–1042
17. Baxter NN, Durham SB, Phillips KA, Habermann EB, Virnig BA (2009) Risk of dementia in older breast cancer survivors: a population based cohort study of the association with adjuvant chemotherapy. J Am Geriatr Soc 57:403–411
18. Heck JE, Albert SM, Franco R, Gorin SS (2008) Patterns of dementia diagnosis in the surveillance, epidemiology and end result breast cancer survivors who use chemotherapy. J Am Geriatr Soc 56:1687–1692
19. Ahles TA, Saykin AJ (2007) Candidate mechanisms for chemotherapy induced cognitive changes. Nat Rev Cancer 7:192–201
20. Argyriou AA, Assimakopoulos K, Iconomou G, Giannakopoulou F, Kalofonos HP (2011) Either called "chemobrain" or "chemofog" the long-term chemotherapy induced cognitive decline in cancer survivors is real. J Pain Symptom Manag 41:126–139
21. Courtney MD, Edwards HE, Chang AM, Parker AW, Finlayson K, Hamilton K (2011) A randomized controlled trial to prevent hospital readmission and loss of functional ability in high risk older adults. BMC Health Serv Res 11:22
22. Fairhall N, Aggar C, Kurrie S, Sherrington C, Lord S, Lockwood K (2008) Frailty Intervention Trial (FIT). BMC Geriatr 8:27
23. Pinder MC, Duan Z, Goodwin JS, Hortobagyi GN, Giordano SH (2007) Congestive heart failure in older women treated with adjuvant anthracycline chemotherapy for breast cancer. J Clin Oncol 25(25):3808–3815 and peripheral neuropathy
24. Brunello A, Loaldi E, Balducci L (2009) Dose adjustment and supportive care before and during treatment. Cancer Treat Rev 35(6):493–498
25. Dolecek TA, Propp JM, Stroup NE et al (2012) CBTRUS statistical report: primary brain and central nervous system tumors diagnosed in the united states in 2005–2009. Neuro-Oncology 14(Suppl 5):v1–49
26. Kannarkat G, Lasher EE, Schiff D (2007) Neurologic complications of chemotherapy agents. Curr Opin Neurol 20:719–725
27. Khan F, Amatya B, Drummond K et al (2014) Effectiveness of integrated multidisciplinary rehabilitation in primary brain cancer survivors in an australian community cohort: a controlled clinical trial. J Rehabil Med 46:754–760

28. Khan F, Amatya B (2013) Factors associated with long-term functional outcomes, psychological sequelae and quality of life in persons after primary brain tumour. J Neuro-Oncol 111:355–366
29. Zucchella C, Capone A, Codella V et al (2013) Cognitive rehabilitation for early post-surgery inpatients affected by primary brain tumor: a randomized, controlled trial. J Neuro-Oncol 114:93–100
30. Cicerone KD, Langenbahn DM, Braden C et al (2011) Evidence-based cognitive rehabilitation: updated review of the literature from 2003 through 2008. Arch Phys Med Rehabil 92:519–530
31. Pompili A, Telera S, Villani V et al (2014) Home palliative care and end of life issues in glioblastoma multiforme: results and comments from a homogeneous cohort of patients. Neurosurg Focus 37:E5
32. Eriks IE, Angenot EL, Lankhorst GJ (2004) Epidural metastatic spinal cord compression: functional outcome and survival after inpatient rehabilitation. Spinal Cord 42:235–239
33. Cormie P, Nowak AK, Chambers SK et al (2015) The potential role of exercise in neuro-oncology. Front Oncol 5:85

Cancer and Physical Activity

52

A. Musumeci and S. Masiero

52.1 Physical Activity and Cancer Prevention

The relationship between physical activity (PA) and tumor has been subject to many studies; one of the most studied malignancies is colon cancer.

PA may influence the development of colon cancer by acting on the energy balance, on hormone metabolism, and on insulin regulation, by reducing the exposure time to potential colon carcinogens, and by increasing the speed of intestinal peristalsis. PA can also modify a number of inflammatory and immune factors that are involved in the genesis of colon cancer [1].

More than 50 scientific papers have examined the association between colon cancer and PA, and many of these have found that adults who increase their PA, in intensity, duration, or frequency, can reduce the risk of 30–40% of colon cancer regardless of their body mass index. In addition, the greatest reduction in risk was in more active individuals [2].

The protective effect also appears to be higher in those who perform high-intensity activities, although the exact level of training has not been established. According to some authors, 30–60 min of moderate-intense daily PA has a protective effect against colon cancer [3, 4]. Whether PA has a protective effect on rectal cancer, adenomas, or recurrence of intestinal polyps, it is still a matter of debate (www.cdc.gov/nccdphp/dnpa/physical/pdf/PA_Fact_Sheet_Adults.pdf).

The scientific literature documented that both premenopausal and postmenopausal active women have a lower risk of developing breast cancer than sedentary ones. However, data on risk reduction percentages vary greatly among studies from 20 to 80% [2, 3, 5]. PA can prevent tumor development by lowering the levels of

A. Musumeci (✉) • S. Masiero
Rehabilitation Unit, Department of Neuroscience, University – General Hospital of Padua, Padua, Italy
e-mail: alfredomusumeci@yahoo.com; stef.masiero@unipd.it

© Springer International Publishing AG 2018

S. Masiero, U. Carraro (eds.), *Rehabilitation Medicine for Elderly Patients*, Practical Issues in Geriatrics, DOI 10.1007/978-3-319-57406-6_52

insulin and insulin-like growth factor 1 (IGF-1), improving the immune response, and contributing to the maintenance of an adequate body weight [4, 6, 7].

The risk of breast cancer would be inversely correlated with the increase in the frequency and duration of physical exercise, and despite the fact that women who increased PA after menopause may experience a reduction in risk, it is better to engage in physical training during the whole life. Thirty to sixty minutes a day of exercise at moderate to high intensity are sufficient to reduce the risk of breast cancer [3, 8].

Several studies have examined the relationship between endometrial cancer risk and PA and found that physically active women have a 20–40% reduced risk of endometrial cancer [3]; this risk does not seem to vary by age [8]. Change in the body mass index (BMI), level of sex hormones (e.g., estrogens), and metabolism appears to be the main biological mechanisms that connect PA and endometrial cancer.

An inverse association between PA and lung cancer risk has also been hypothesized: the most active individuals have a 20% reduction in risk [3, 8]. High levels of PA would have a protective effect against cancer, but exercise is not able to counteract the negative effects of smoking or respiratory diseases [3, 9]. The relationship between PA and risk of lung cancer is less noticeable on women than it is on men [10].

52.2 Cancer and Physical Activity

Two observational studies examined the relationship between levels of PA before and after the diagnosis of colon cancer, demonstrating how the pre-diagnosis levels of PA were not related to survival after diagnosis. However, participants with higher levels of PA after diagnosis of nonmetastatic colorectal cancer had lower mortality. The biological mechanism for this association is still unknown; it was hypothesized that PA may decrease the tissue insulin and insulin-like growth factor (IGF) levels and increase IGF binding proteins, thus influencing their action on micrometastases [11].

Regular (≥3 h a week) and intense sport activities, such as biking, tennis, jogging, or swimming, can slow prostate cancer progression [12, 13].

PA also improves quality of life and metabolism, reducing fatigue in patients with breast cancer [4, 14]. Currently, it is not possible to draw definitive conclusions about the relationship between PA and survival of breast cancer; some studies documented that the women who have engaged in moderate exercise after a diagnosis of breast cancer (3–5 h of walking, every week), particularly those who had tumors responsive to hormonal therapy, had better survival rates than those who were sedentary [15, 16]. However, a home exercise program has a beneficial effect not only on physical fitness but also on psychological well-being of previously sedentary women [17, 18].

In conclusion, further studies are needed in the future to understand the positive biological effects of physical activity on cancer, the type of tumors that mostly benefit from exercise, and the frequency and intensity of training that can improve quality of life and survival of oncologic patients.

Key Points

- Physical activity can prevent colon, breast, endometrial, and lung cancers.
- Physical activity can improve survival of nonmetastatic colon cancer patients and quality of life of women affected by breast cancer.

References

1. McTiernan A, Schwartz RS, Potter J, Bowen D (1999) Exercise clinical trials in cancer prevention research: a call to action. Cancer Epidemiol Biomark Prev 8(3):201–207
2. Lee IM (2003) Physical activity and cancer prevention—data from epidemiologic studies. Med Sci Sports Exerc 35(11):1823–1827
3. Lee I, Oguma Y (2006) Physical activity. In: Schottenfeld D, Fraumeni JF (eds) Cancer epidemiology and prevention, 3rd edn. Oxford University Press, New York
4. McTiernan A (2006) Cancer prevention and management through exercise and weight control. Taylor & Francis Group, LLC, Boca Raton
5. Monninkhof EM, Elias SG, Vlems FA et al (2007) Physical activity and breast cancer: a systematic review. Epidemiology 18(1):137–157
6. Friedenreich CM, Neilson HK, Lynch BM (2010) State of the epidemiological evidence on physical activity and cancer prevention. Eur J Cancer 46(14):2593–2604. doi:10.1016/j.ejca.2010.07.028
7. Friedenreich CM, Woolcott CG, McTiernan A, Ballard-Barbash R, Brant RF, Stanczyk FZ, Terry T, Boyd NF, Yaffe MJ, Irwin ML, Jones CA, Yasui Y, Campbell KL, ML MN, Karvinen KH, Wang Q, Courneya KS (2010) Alberta physical activity and breast cancer prevention trial: sex hormone changes in a year-long exercise intervention among postmenopausal women. J Clin Oncol 28(9):1458–1466. doi:10.1200/JCO.2009.24.9557
8. WHO (2002) Weight control and physical activity. In: IARC handbooks of cancer prevention, vol 6. IARC Publications, Lyon
9. Tardon A, Lee WJ, Delgado-Rodriguez M et al (2005) Leisure-time physical activity and lung cancer: a meta-analysis. Cancer Causes Control 16(4):389–397
10. McTiernan A (2003) Intervention studies in exercise and cancer prevention. Med Sci Sports Exerc 35(11):1841–1845
11. Meyerhardt JA, Giovannucci EL, Holmes MD et al (2006) Physical activity and survival after colorectal cancer diagnosis. J Clin Oncol 24(22):3527–3534
12. Giovannucci EL, Liu Y, Leitzmann MF et al (2005) A prospective study of physical activity and incident and fatal prostate cancer. Arch Intern Med 165(9):1005–1010
13. Kenfield SA, Stampfer MJ, Giovannucci E, Chan JM (2011) Physical activity and survival after prostate cancer diagnosis in the health professionals follow-up study. J Clin Oncol 29(6):726–732
14. Carter SJ, Hunter GR, McAuley E et al (2016) Lower rate-pressure product during submaximal walking: a link to fatigue improvement following a physical activity intervention among breast cancer survivors. J Cancer Surviv 10:927–934
15. Holmes MD, Chen WY, Feskanich D, Kroenke CH, Colditz GA (2005) Physical activity and survival after breast cancer diagnosis. J Am Med Assoc 293(20):2479–2486
16. Irwin ML, Smith AW, McTiernan A, Ballard-Barbash R et al (2008) Influence of pre- and post-diagnosis physical activity on mortality in breast cancer survivors: the health, eating, activity, and lifestyle study. J Clin Oncol 26(24):3958–3964
17. Wilson DJ (2017) Exercise for the patient after breast cancer surgery. Semin Oncol Nurs 33:98–105
18. Pinto BM, Frierson GM, Rabin C et al (2005) Home-based physical activity intervention for breast cancer patients. J Clin Oncol 23(15):3577–3587

53 Rehabilitation for Palliative Care and End-of-Life Management

Sophie Pautex

53.1 Introduction

Diseases with a long end-of-life trajectory such as cancer, cardiovascular disease, or neurodegenerative diseases such as dementia have largely replaced unexpected deaths [1]. Treating these patient's complex medical, social, psychological, and spiritual needs requires adequate structures and state-of-the-art geriatric palliative care [2]. Palliative care is an approach that improves the quality of life of patients and their families facing the problem associated with life-threatening illness, through the prevention and relief of suffering by means of early identification and impeccable assessment and treatment of pain and other problems, physical, psychosocial, and spiritual [3]. More importantly, palliative care should offer a support system to help patients live as actively as possible until death and enhance quality of life and may also positively influence the course of illness. Therefore, palliative care should be applicable early in the course of illness. Indeed several clinical studies have demonstrated that the introduction of early palliative care programs improve quality of life of patients, particularly with cancer [4].

Deteriorating physical function is a significant problem for people approaching the end of life. Patient's dependence in self-care increases during the last months or weeks of life, with leisure activities affected just as much as household or activities of daily living [5]. Some particularly older frail patients can have a low physical functioning during the years. The loss of ability to participate in desired daily activities is among the most distressing concerns for patients [6]. It leads to unwanted dependence on others and threatens dignity and autonomy [7]. It can have severe consequences on social interaction and can contribute to depression and anxiety and sometimes a wish to die. That is for even in the context of a life-limiting illness,

S. Pautex
Community and Geriatric and Palliative Care Unit, Primary Care Division,
University Hospital Geneva, Geneva, Switzerland
e-mail: Sophie.pautex@hcuge.ch

© Springer International Publishing AG 2018

S. Masiero, U. Carraro (eds.), *Rehabilitation Medicine for Elderly Patients*,
Practical Issues in Geriatrics, DOI 10.1007/978-3-319-57406-6_53

where deterioration is inevitable, rehabilitation offers a major route to improving patient's quality of life, no matter how long or how short the timescale. The definition of rehabilitation, "enables people affected by illness or disability to regain function, to live independently, and make decisions for themselves process that aims to maximize physical and emotional well being, enhance social participation, and minimize caregivers' distress," perfectly matches the needs of palliative care patients [8]. The interest for rehabilitation in cancer patients has increased in recent years. These principles must also be deployed in the domain of palliative care and end-of-life care, in particular for patients with non-oncological disease [7, 9].

Understanding end-of-life care from a holistic perspective should allow the interprofessional team, including the rehabilitation team, to intervene appropriately in order to improve quality of life in the final days, year, or months of a patient.

53.2 Palliative Care and Rehabilitation

Different studies relate some discrepancy between patient's existing needs, their adequate assessment, and support provided [10]. Indeed, often health professionals have tendency to assume what factors and issues affect patient's quality of life. This assumption is then translated in specific interventions based on the health-care professional assumption and not on the needs of the patients. Incongruities between patient's view and their ability to pursue their activities can result in frustration and sense of meaningless [11]. The role of health professionals working with palliative care or end-of life patients is to improve their quality of life through physical interventions in order to reduce gap between patient's expectations and hope and actual experiences. They should assist the patient to live as fully as possible within the limitation of the disease [12]. Indeed they should define reasonable goals to support the hopes of the patients as much as possible (e.g., "I would like to go back to my house in the mountain"). Maintaining patients at home as long as possible can also be in some situations a very important goal. Therefore, each health professional should assess the symptoms and the needs of patients, including physical functioning and activities of daily living to identify patient's functional difficulties in all different settings (hospital, nursing home, or home) and to implement the most adequate support. In addition of the limitation in the functionality, fatigue is a very prevalent symptom as the management is still suboptimal and that there is an urgent need for improvement [13] The benefits of exercise on fatigue in patients with cancer could maybe also be translated in palliative care and therefore integrated in the care planning of these patients [9, 14, 15].

Finally, anticipating for the needs and planning for future needs is paramount in the management of these patients.

The rehabilitation team is often trained to improve or restore function and to assist individuals to return to their prior level. However, objectives need to be modified by setting more modest goals whenever patient's health begins to deteriorate. Health professionals should reframe patient's condition in a positive perspective, in order to encourage the patient to use his residual energies and to avoid frustration of the team. Health professionals' beliefs, hopes, and positive attitudes that will be communicated can have some positive impact, and patients may feel encouraged. Patients need to know that it is always possible to do something.

Therefore, the role of the rehabilitation team in this particular context should be in all different settings:

- The symptom control: pain relief, improvement of fatigue, alleviation of respiratory symptoms, and edema control
- Providing material to minimize efforts and energy expenditures and to improve physical function
- Educating patient and relatives regarding safety issues, positioning, pressure relieve, and relaxation
- To promote staying at home, if desired by the patient and his relatives

Conclusion

Rehabilitation medicine and palliative care share many common goals. They strive to maximize physical function and emotional well-being to the highest extent possible given the nature of the underlying disease process. Working with patients at the end of their life is challenging but also rewarding. Understanding many issues that impact quality of life of the patient will enable health professionals to give some meaningful care to these patients, thereby enhancing their quality of life.

Key Points

- The primary goals of palliative care for patients in advanced stages of disease are to improve or maintain the patient's health-related quality of life and to allow patients to live as actively as possible and relieve symptoms.
- The rehabilitation team must be part of the palliative care team that take care of the patients in all different settings.
- The rehabilitation must be based on patient's specific goals.
- Health professionals should reframe patient's condition in a positive perspective, in order to emphasize remaining physical strengths of the patient, despite the deterioration.

References

1. van der Heide A, Deliens L, Faisst K et al (2003) End-of-life decision-making in six European countries: descriptive study. Lancet 362:345–350
2. The Lancet Oncology (2004) An ageing problem. Lancet Oncol 5:459
3. http://www.who.int/cancer/palliative/definition/en/. Accessed 12 July 2016
4. Kelley AS, Morrison RS (2015) Palliative care for the seriously ill. N Engl J Med 373:747–755
5. Fyllingen EH, Oldervoll LM, Loge JH et al (2009) Computer-based assessment of symptoms and mobility in palliative care: feasibility and challenges. J Pain Symptom Manag 38:827–836
6. Singer PA, Martin DK, Kelner M (1999) Quality end-of-life care: patients' perspectives. JAMA 281:163–168

7. Elmqvist MA, Jordhoy MS, Bjordal K, Kaasa S, Jannert M (2009) Health-related quality of life during the last three months of life in patients with advanced cancer. Support Care Cancer 17:191–198
8. Wade DT, de Jong BA (2000) Recent advances in rehabilitation. BMJ 320:1385–1388
9. Cramp F, Daniel J (2008) Exercise for the management of cancer-related fatigue in adults. Cochrane Database Syst Rev 2:CD006145
10. Harrison JD, Young JM, Price MA, Butow PN, Solomon MJ (2009) What are the unmet supportive care needs of people with cancer? A systematic review. Support Care Cancer 17:1117–1128
11. Helbostad JL, Holen JC, Jordhoy MS, Ringdal GI, Oldervoll L, Kaasa S (2009) A first step in the development of an international self-report instrument for physical functioning in palliative cancer care: a systematic literature review and an expert opinion evaluation study. J Pain Symptom Manag 37:196–205
12. Cheville AL, Beck LA, Petersen TL, Marks RS, Gamble GL (2009) The detection and treatment of cancer-related functional problems in an outpatient setting. Support Care Cancer 17:61–67
13. Oldervoll LM, Loge JH, Paltiel H et al (2006) The effect of a physical exercise program in palliative care: a phase II study. J Pain Symptom Manag 31:421–430
14. Stricker CT, Drake D, Hoyer KA, Mock V (2004) Evidence-based practice for fatigue management in adults with cancer: exercise as an intervention. Oncol Nurs Forum 31:963–976
15. Cheville AL (2009) Cancer-related fatigue. Phys Med Rehabil Clin N Am 20:405–416

Part III

Inpatient Rehabilitation Units: Age and Comorbidities Are Not Relevant if Admission Fits the Mission

54

Luigi Tesio

54.1 Aging, Disability, and Inpatient Rehabilitation

Inpatient rehabilitation is a growing need. In Italy (about 60 million inhabitants) in the first semester of 2015, there have been 3,178,661 hospital inpatient admissions for a total of 21,790,190 days. Inpatient rehabilitation accounted for 4.9% of the cases but for 19% of the days (http://www.salute.gov.it/portale/temi/p2_6.jsp?lingua=italiano&id=1237&area=ricoveriOspedalieri&menu=vuoto). The disability epidemics have at least three acknowledged causes: (a) the increasing capacity of intensive and acute care to provide survival, though with residual impairments; (b) the growing sensitivity of the general public toward disability, and (c), of course, the increasing population aging, involving high risks for the most various disabling conditions, most of them chronic.

The booming rehabilitation costs are forcing health-care politicians to invent optimal criteria for allocating resources, with special emphasis on expensive hospital-based rehabilitation programs. "Appropriateness" (admitting the right patient to the right facility, for the right cost) is the key criterion appealed to by most stakeholders.

L. Tesio, MD
Department of Biomedical Sciences for Health, Physical and Rehabilitation Medicine, Università degli Studi di Milano, Milano, Italy

Department of Neurorehabilitation Sciences, Istituto Auxologico Italiano, IRCCS, Milano, Italy
e-mail: luigi.tesio@unimi.it

© Springer International Publishing AG 2018

S. Masiero, U. Carraro (eds.), *Rehabilitation Medicine for Elderly Patients*, Practical Issues in Geriatrics, DOI 10.1007/978-3-319-57406-6_54

Table 54.1 Diagnostic vs. functional classification systems

Diagnosis (ICD terminology)	ICD 9 cm coding	DRG coding	Disability
Flaccid hemiplegia and hemiparesis caused by a lesion of the dominant hemisphere	342.01	12	?
Multiple sclerosis	340	13	?
Hip joint replacement	V43.64	256	?

Examples of the confluence of ICD (9-cm version) into DRG codes. Neither coding system takes into account the disability of the patient

Classifying individual cases is the premise to any selection policy. In all Western countries, except for the USA, cases are still coded according to the International Classification of Diseases (ICD) logic (https://www.cms.gov/medicare/coding/ICD9providerdiagnosticcodes/codes.html) and/or the aggregation of ICD codes known as Diagnosis-Related Groups (DRG) (http://www.rch.org.au/rchhis/coding_casemix/DRG_and_Casemix_funding/): i.e., coding and reimbursement are ultimately based on a "disease" diagnosis [1] (see Table 54.1).

By "disease," reference is made here to a biological alteration considered as lowering the person's health status. It is well known that this biological diagnosis tells little about the disability associated to (or following, in case of subacute conditions) the disease itself, due to the intricate pathway leading from biology (ultimately, an alteration of body parts) to disability (ultimately, a decreased capacity of interaction of the whole person with the outer world) [2, 3]. On the other hand, disability itself [4] is the very reason for admission to an inpatient rehabilitation unit.

Various models of prediction of resource consumption have been proposed. Indirect costs, uniform across patients, prevail in rehabilitation units. Therefore, quite pragmatically, most models target the summary indexes of costs, i.e., the length of stay (LOS). Models have been realized (Table 54.2) in order to estimate also the expected outcome of hospitalization, in terms of severity of residual disability and/or of discharge destination (mostly, home vs. long-term institutionalization). A predictive model implies the possibility to compare observed and model-expected costs and/or outcomes, thus providing a relevant cue to the definition of both an "appropriate" admission and an efficient care.

Not surprisingly, the most predictive models (not in force in the European Union but active in the USA) are those encasing not only a diagnostic coding but also the disability level at admission [5].

A harsh debate exists on the opportunity to include also age and comorbidity in the predictive models. The latter is a position strongly supported by gerontologists, whereas physiatrists, in general, do not agree (the reason will be given below).

Table 54.2 Functional grouping systems adopted in post-acute care, in the USA

Grouping system, acronym	Name	First author	Date of proposal (subsequent versions)	Dependent variable, variance explained	Main applications
FIM—FRG	Functional independence measure—function-related groups	Stineman MG	1994, 1997	Length of stay, days (log-transformed), 30%	Efficacy/efficiency study of rehab facilities. Research through National US and affiliated foreign databases
CMG	Cost measurement group	Carter J – RAND Corp. Study for the Health Care Financing Administration (now CMS), USA	2001	Total cost of inpatient stay, 30%	Prospective payment system, rehabilitation, MEDICARE program, USA
RUG	Resource utilization groups	Fries BE	1985, 1994	Nursing and therapy costs, 55%	Per-day payment, nursing homes, USA

A sketch of the main classification systems adopted in the USA for case-mix classification in the "post-acute" area. The CMG has been used since 2001 for prospective "per capita" payment (Medicare-covered admissions). The RUG system is used for per-day payment of nursing homes, only. The variance explanation summarizes the reliability of the predictions that can be made, based on the independent variables and specific algorithms, with respect to the dependent variable (e.g., days of hospital stay, cost of the whole stay, cost per day). Empirically, a 30% variance explanation is recognized as suitable to warrant an equitable reimbursement of a facility. In the EU (and, to the author's knowledge, in all other countries), inpatient rehabilitation is still paid on a per-day basis. The same holds true for nursing homes. Local governments adopt various adjustments (based on diagnosis, functional scales, time since disability onset, and the like) aimed at taking into account the severity (hence, the expected costs) of different cases. Unlike the classification models in the USA, these adjustments do not stem from large-scale epidemiologic studies, nor they are uniform even within single countries

54.2 Classification Systems in Rehabilitation

54.2.1 The FIM-FRG System

The widest and oldest application of a specific classification system to inpatient rehabilitation in the USA is the "CMG-cost measurement groups" system. With only minor adaptations, this is a variant to the original FIM-FRG system [6]. The FIM™ [7] (Functional Independence Measure) is the most popular (and validated) scale of independence in daily life (Fig. 54.1).

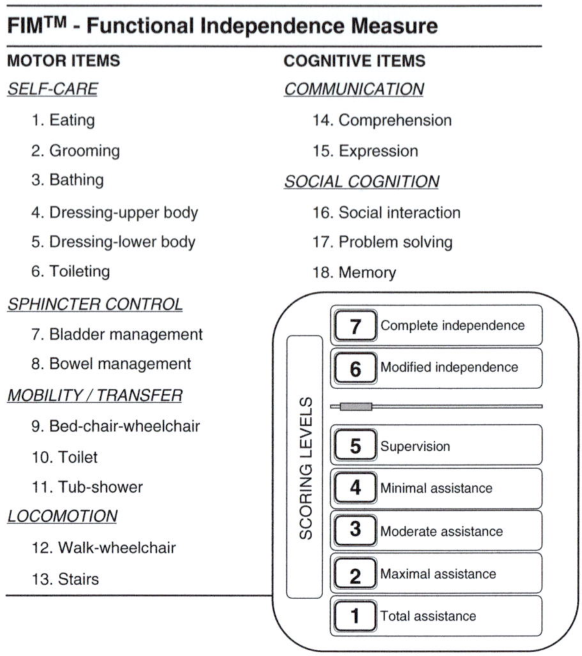

Fig. 54.1 The FIM™ scale. It rates independence in 18 activities of daily living (score 0–7, the higher the score, the better the condition). The 13 motor (total score 13–91) or the 5 cognitive (total score 5–35) items can be grouped into a "motor" and a "cognitive" subscale. Several national validated versions exist. Official teaching and credentialing procedures and authorized national data banks are foreseen, in order to preserve the national and international standardization of measures and to foster cross-cultural research

As shown in Fig. 54.1, the FIM rates 13 neuromotor (such as bladder management and locomotion) and 5 cognitive activities (such as communication and social interaction), scored 1–7, the higher the score, the greater the subject independence from aids (e.g., canes or orthotic appliances) and someone else's help. The FIM is a worldwide standard, including rigorous scoring procedures, validated translations in several languages, dedicated courses, and a centralized credentialing exam releasing a "competency certificate." The system also includes the diagnostic coding system RIC (Rehabilitation Impairment Codes), comprising approximately 70 macro-diagnostic categories which are function-oriented, like some codes for "stroke" or for "spinal cord lesion," with no reference to the specific underlying pathophysiology (to compare, there are approximately 600 DRGs and almost 12000 ICD codes).

How can "diagnostic" or "functional" classes generate outcome predictions and/or indexes of appropriate admission to a health-care unit? Technically, a "decision tree" must be built. The most famous clinical decision tree is perhaps the one giving rise ("triage") to the colored priority codes in the first aid departments. The idea is combining the patient's biomedical "class" with other relevant information available at admission: for instance, in the case of rehabilitation, this can be gender, age, time since onset of the present disability, etc. The suspect "independent variables" may or may not be relevant determinants of the dependent variable. If they are, homogeneous "groups" can be identified, sharing a given value of that variable and presenting different values from the other groups (e.g., length of stay can be similar in patients below a given age cutoff and very different from the length of stay

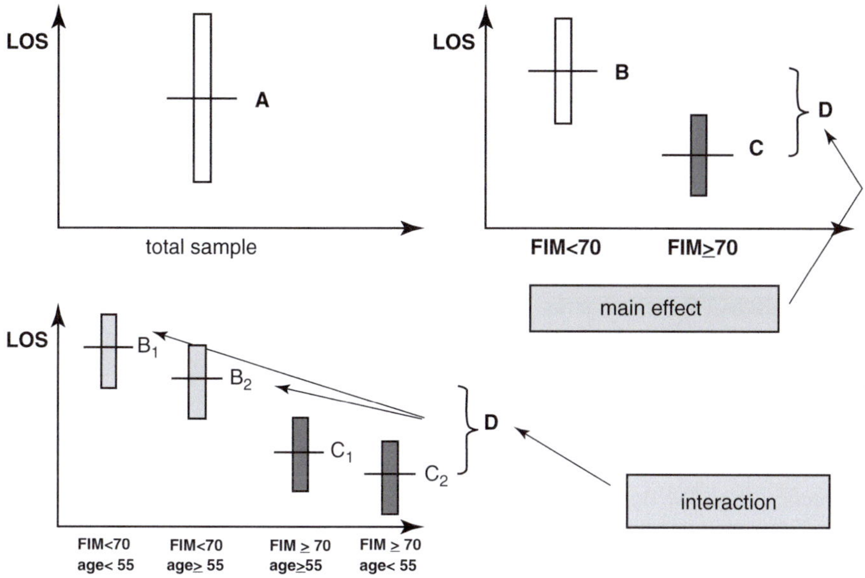

Fig. 54.2 A sketch of the "decision trees" leading to case-mix classification in inpatient rehabilitation units (after Tesio L [8]). Let us imagine that one aims at building a "classification system" predicting the length of stay (LOS, on the ordinate) based on patient's age and his/her FIM total score at admission. In the *upper left panel*, the vertical bar represents the distribution (or, if one so prefers, the variance) of the observed LOS in the total sample of patients (A), the horizontal bar giving the mean. There are no "explanations" for the variance referring to the mean, which must be accepted and ascribed to chance. In the *upper right panel*, the sample is split into two subsamples, B and C, on the basis of the patient's FIM score at admission (the ideal cutoff is 70 out of 126; see the abscissa). It can be seen that a large difference (D) exists between the two means, and, most importantly, that uncertainty around the mean (i.e., the variance) across each subgroup is decreased (or: some variance is now "explained"). The FIM score alone is a determinant of LOS (it represents a "main effect"). In any case, one can do better. The *bottom panel* shows a further splitting of the sample, based on the combination ("interaction") of the FIM cutoff (70 out of 126) and the age cutoff of 55 years. The variance around the mean across the four subgroups is furtherly decreased. Given the FIM and the age at admission, one can reliably predict the expected LOS of the patient. If the observed LOS does not match the expectation, a diagnostic procedure can be established. The cutoff values are taken from real epidemiologic studies. Their definition and the interaction rules require dedicated statistical modeling and software [1, 8]

recorded in patients at or above the same cutoff). As a rule, however, the variables interact with each other in complex, unpredictable ways, thus giving rise to unsuspected homogeneous subgroups of patients. Figure 54.2 exemplifies (in a very simplified model) the concept of "classification systems" based on the interaction between two independent variables.

Numerous and extensive studies both carried out in the USA [5] and Italy [9] used a particular decision tree algorithm (Classification and Regression Tree, CART). For an application to another field, see [10]. The FIM-FRG system includes only the RIC, the FIM score at admission, and age—the latter for a few groups only—and succeeded (in terms of variance explanation) in predicting the patient's LOS. More precisely, it could assign each case to one of few FRGs (function-related groups) sharing the same LOS within groups and showing a significantly different LOS between groups. Once "groups" have been defined, they can also be assigned to an expected "gain" of FIM scores between admission and discharge. The ratio of FIM "gain" to LOS is an index of "efficiency" of the inpatient stay. The efficiency of different facilities, or even of different units within the same facility or institution, can thus be compared with respect to any given FRG (so-called efficiency pattern analysis, EPA [11]). Periodic FIM-FRG reports, specific for major impairment categories, are issued in the USA, showing that the introduction of the FIM-based system led to a moderate, yet constant, decrease in LOS, whereas FIM levels at discharge and consistent relationships in LOS across the FRGs [12] were unaffected. Two points must be emphasized. First, in such "predictive" classification systems (both in the USA and Italy), the independent variables that are *not* included because not predictive are worth being considered not less than those that *were* included. Perhaps counterintuitively, age and comorbidities play only a minor role in these systems. Second, a FIM-FRG system can be effectively produced also for predicting the FIM outcome or the discharge destination, based on the admission parameters. Again, the RIC and the FIM are the strongest determinants of the expected outcome, with only a minor role (and often an unexpected one; see below) played by age. In the CMG system (the official US federal system, a close variant of the FIM-FRG system), a few comorbidities may enter the algorithm but only in extreme cases (e.g., bacterial meningitis and the like). Since 2001, the CMG grouping system, based on the FIM-FRG algorithm, is adopted as a prospective payment system in the USA (i.e., a *per capita*, not *per diem* payment), for all rehabilitation admissions covered by the Medicare program (i.e., over 65% of cases).

54.2.2 Rehabilitation Units and Nursing Homes: Which Is Which

Before adopting the FIM-based classification system, the US Federal Regulatory Agency (Health Care Financing Administration, HCFA, now Centers for Medicare and Medicaid Services, CMS) imposed the experimentation of a hybrid instrument to be shared by all "post-acute" facilities, including rehabilitation units and nursing homes. The experimentation failed, mostly due to the vigorous (and motivated) protests arising from the rehabilitation field. The FIM-based system was approved for inpatient rehabilitation, and dedicated systems, the most famous of which is the Resource Utilization Groups (RUG) [13], were adopted in nursing homes (see Table 54.1). Actually, nursing homes are just one of the many types of "long-term care facilities" available both in the USA and other countries; yet, this issue goes beyond the topic of this chapter.

54.2.3 The Diverging Perspectives on Classification: Disability Seen from Rehabilitation Units and from Nursing Homes

The conceptual points of the lively debate finally leading, in the USA, to distinct instruments for the diverse "post-acute care" inpatient settings can be summarized as follows.

First, in nursing homes the admission criteria do not include—like it happens in rehabilitation units—a prognosis of functional recovery nor the patient's capacity to sustain specific exercise procedures (in the order of 1–3 h/day). Second, the provision of rehabilitation interventions is the core mission of rehabilitation units, while it is an optional service in nursing homes. Unlike the FIM-FRG grouping, the algorithm of CMG includes the provision or rehabilitation services and of life-supporting procedures (e.g., tracheostomy, gastrostomy, etc.) as independent variables leading to a more rewarding reimbursement "group," clearly, a fee-for-service logic. This incentivizes a medically oriented attitude of nursing homes, but it does not incentivize specific efforts toward the reduction of the guest's disability. In short, although both types of facility intervene in the "post-acute" phase of a disabling illness, and provide various rehabilitation services, their mission is entirely different.

It is of interest that the aforementioned debate across stakeholders and HCFA—fully accessible through the web—included a deep reflection on the "specificity" of rehabilitation units. From the rehabilitation side, the successful claim for a specific classification system (fully endorsed by the author [8]) was atoned for by a robust "slimming" of the set of clinical conditions admissible in "true" rehabilitation units allowing a prospective *per case* payment through the CMG algorithm. At least 75% of the inpatient admissions, irrespective of patient's age, had to represent either severe neurologic conditions (stroke, brain injury, etc.), burns, or traumas, and a few others. The frequent cases of arthritic knee and hip joint replacement were not included in this "golden list." Most importantly, "cardiac," "pulmonary," "oncologic," and any non-neuromotor post-acute conditions were not considered as appropriate for "rehabilitation units," although they were judged as fully entitled to receive also rehabilitation interventions within their specific organ/disease-based units. The key argument was that both the main competences and resources dedicated to these patients, and the logic of admission and discharge, were disease- and organ-specific and not specific of the physical medicine and rehabilitation discipline.

The emphasis placed in the USA on the specificity of neuromotor inpatient rehabilitation with respect to chronic care and in general, elderly care, is a stimulating lesson for rehabilitation in Europe.

54.3 Outcome Studies in Inpatient Rehabilitation Units: The (Non)-Predictive Role of Aging and Comorbidity Indexes

Not surprisingly, age is not a relevant predictor of the functional status at discharge from rehabilitation units. This emerges from all the FIM-based classification studies conducted in the USA and, according to the author's experience, in Italy [12, 13, 14, 15]. The above considerations should clarify why this is the case.

Age and its related groups of comorbidities and risks for complications may surely limit the patient's potential recovery, whatever his/her main underlying neuromotor impairment is. However, rehabilitation units must select ("creaming" or "skimming") the admission cases according to two main criteria: (a) the prognosis of meaningful functional improvement (not necessarily a great one) and (b) the prediction of the capacity to tolerate exercise programs (not necessarily a motor one; for instance, the program can be focused on cognitive, swallowing, sphincter impairments). Admissions *must* be subjected to these selection criteria: hence it is clear that, downstream a correct admission, age and comorbidities play a little role in predicting the functional outcome of the inpatient stay. It *must* be this way, if the admission fits the unit's mission. Age in itself must not prevent admission to a rehabilitation unit. Let us rephrase the reasons: first, because after the specialist's functional screening, age is playing only a marginal role in determining the predicted outcome and, second, because age may even work in a counterintuitive way. An unexpected finding emerged from all classification studies in the USA and Italy. Elderly patients (mainly, above 70 years) with various impairments may paradoxically have a shorter stay, compared to their younger counterparts. The reasons are not yet fully elucidated. However, there may be at least four good reasons, not mutually exclusive: (a) elderly people may have a lower potential for recovery, encouraging their earlier discharge; (b) their recovery may show an earlier plateau; (c) in rehab units physicians tend to discharge elderly patients earlier in the attempt to minimize their risk for side effects of hospitalization (infections, disorientation, depression); and (d) at least in the cases of brain vascular accidents, elderly people may recover faster, thanks to a collateral circulation developed along the previous years in order to compensate for chronic hypoxia.

54.4 Concluding Remarks

It does not seem convenient to considering age, nor its related various comorbidity indexes, as criteria for admission to rehabilitation units. Such a criterion would encourage a discriminating adverse selection, and it could dilute the highly specific mission of rehabilitation into one of a more generic "elderly care."

The correct response to the challenge of the disabled elderly is rather the establishment of rehabilitation units tuned on high- or low-intensity rehabilitation, the latter to be reserved to those patients who cannot tolerate (perhaps temporarily) an intensive rehabilitation regimen [16]. Again: the setting selection should follow functional criteria, not privileging age and/or comorbidity. The mere fact that elderly may represent the majority of these "low-tolerance long stay" cases must not cast shadows over the specific mission of a true neuromotor rehabilitation unit.

Key Points

- The majority of patients suffering from disability of acute onset or acute worsening are elderly and affected by various comorbidities.
- Old age and comorbidities themselves must not prevent the patient's admission to an inpatient rehabilitation unit.
- In fact, a prognosis of functional recovery and of tolerance to exercise is the main criterion for appropriate admission, whatever the patient's age.
- Epidemiologic studies based on functional/diagnostic classification of patients demonstrate that age and comorbidities, downstream an appropriate admission to a rehabilitation unit, are not relevant determinants of the outcome.

References

1. Tesio L, Rota V (2005) Function-based case-mix in rehabilitation medicine: the Italian experience. In: CLADAG. Meeting of the Classification and data Analysis Group of the Italian Statistical Society, Università di Parma, June 6–8, 2005, free download at https://www.researchgate.net/profile/Luigi_Tesio/contributions
2. Gresham GE, Granger CV, Linn RT, Kulas MA (1999) Status of functional outcomes for stroke survivors. Phys Med Rehabil Clin N Am 10(4):957–966
3. Tesio L (2004) Bridging the gap between biology and clinical medicine. Some help from Rasch measurement theory. J Appl Meas 5(4):362–366
4. Tesio L, Franchignoni F (2007) Don't touch the physical in physical and rehabilitation medicine. J Rehabil Med 39:662–663
5. Stineman MG, Granger CV (1997) A modular case-mix classification system for medical rehabilitation illustrated. Health Care Financ Rev 19(1):87–103
6. Tesio L, Granger CV, Perucca L, Franchignoni FP, Battaglia MA, Russell C (2002) The FIM™ instrument in the United States and Italy: a comparative study. Am J Phys Med Rehabil 81:168–176
7. FIM is a trademark of the University of Buffalo Foundation, State University of New York at Buffalo-NY; http://www.udsmr.org
8. Tesio L (2003) Case-mix classification systems. The specific case for rehabilitation. Eura Medicophys 39:201–204
9. Tesio L, Francescutti C, Genetti B (2009) Misure di disabilità nel percorso riabilitativo dopo ictus cerebrale. Studio epidemiologico e gestionale della Regione Autonoma Friuli-Venezia Giulia. (Disability measures along the rehabilitation path after stroke. An epidemiologic and managed-care study with Regione Autonoma Friuli-Venzia Giulia-Italy). Aracne Editrice
10. D'Alisa S, Miscio G, Baudo S, Simone A, Tesio L, Mauro A (2006) Depression is the main determinant of quality of life in multiple sclerosis: a classification-regression (CART) study. Disabil Rehabil 28(5):307–314
11. Stineman MG, Goin JE, Hamilton BB, Granger CV (1995) Efficiency pattern analysis for medical rehabilitation. Am J Med Qual 10(4):190–198
12. Granger CV, Karmarkar AM, Graham JE, Deutsch A, Niewczyk P, Divita MA, Ottenbacher KJ (2012) The uniform data system for medical rehabilitation: report of patients with traumatic spinal cord injury discharged from rehabilitation programs in 2002–2010. Am J Phys Med Rehabil 91(4):289–299. doi:10.1097/PHM.0b013e31824ad2fd
13. Carpenter GI, Ikegami N, Ljunggren G, Carrillo E, Fries BE (1997) RUG-III and resource allocation: comparing the relationship of direct care time with patient characteristics in five countries. Age Ageing 26(Suppl 2):61–65
14. Franchignoni FP, Tesio L, Martino MT, Benevolo E, Castagna M (1998) Length of stay of stroke rehabilitation inpatients: prediction though the functional independence measure. Ann Ist Super Sanita 34(4):463–467
15. Tesio L, Franchignoni FP, Perucca L, Porta GL (1996) The influence of age on length of stay, functional independence and discharge destination of rehabilitation inpatients in Italy. Disabil Rehabil 18(10):502–508
16. Crimaldi S, Porta GL, Vaccari A, Springhetti I, Tesio L (1999) Comparison between low- and high-intensity inpatient rehabilitation. FIM measures as an index of appropriateness and effectiveness. Eura Medicophys 35:177–183

55 Healthcare and Rehabilitation for the Elderly in Italy

Paolo Boldrini

55.1 Demographics and Healthcare Organization in Italy

Italy is the sixth largest country in Europe and has the second highest average life expectancy: in 2011, it was 79.4 years for men and 84.5 for women (compared with 77.4 years for men and 83.1 years for women for the EU as a whole).

Italy has also one of the lowest fertility rate in the world: 1.4 births per woman in 2011. As a result, the population growth rate is very low (0.35), one of the lowest in Europe [1].

One of the major aspects of demography in Italy is therefore the growing number of elderly people: 6% of the country's total population are over the age of 80, and the estimate for 2016 is that people of 65 years and over will reach the 21.3% of population. By the year 2050, this figure is expected to rise to 34% [2].

There are marked regional differences for both men and woman in most health indicators, reflecting the social and economic differences between the North and South.

The Italian health system has been ranked the second best in the world by the World Health Organization, with only the French system ranked higher. The Ministry of Health is ultimately responsible for the administration of the health service, but much of the control has been passed to the regional and the local health authorities known as ASL (azienda sanitaria locale). The whole system includes 21 regional health authorities and about 200 local authorities.

The Italian national healthcare service (SSN) was created in 1978 to replace a previous system based on insurances. In 2001, a reform increased the role and responsibility of the regional authorities in ensuring the basic healthcare services (livelli essenziali di assistenza, LEA) which must be provided to all citizens.

P. Boldrini, MD
Department of Rehabilitation Medicine, ULSS9 Treviso – Ospedale Riabilitativo di Alta Specializzazione, Motta di Livenza, Italy
e-mail: pboldrini@ulss.tv.it

© Springer International Publishing AG 2018

S. Masiero, U. Carraro (eds.), *Rehabilitation Medicine for Elderly Patients*, Practical Issues in Geriatrics, DOI 10.1007/978-3-319-57406-6_55

Therefore, the SSN covers all necessary treatments, providing universal coverage and free healthcare at the point of delivery. It should be noted, however, that there are variations in the quality of services between the regions; in general, with better coverage and quality in the North with respect to the South and Islands.

Local health units (ASL) are responsible for the management of all health services in their area, and private providers can also operate within the SSN.

The SSN is mainly funded through national taxes, with a relatively small co-payment for pharmaceuticals and outpatient care. In 2012, the health expenditure accounted for 9.2% of GDP. Public sources account for the majority of healthcare spending: private spending being about 18%, mainly in the form of out-of-pocket payments. Private insurance covers only about 1% of total expenditure [3].

Hospitals are reimbursed by the SSN according to a national diagnosis-related group (DRG)-like system. National-level tariffs cover the cost of public hospital admissions throughout the country. Private hospitals are reimbursed to the same DRG-specified level and additional costs borne by patients—through private insurance schemes.

55.2 Rehabilitation Services for the Elderly in Italy

The prevalence of chronic conditions, most of which determine disability, increases with age, reaching 75.6% in people between 65 and 74 years [4].

The 1998 Guidelines for Rehabilitation Care issued by the Ministry of Health [5] established general rules for the organization and delivery of services, concerning inpatient, outpatient, and home- and community-based rehabilitation. Rehabilitation medicine specialists, together with other healthcare professionals, would provide services to people affected by various disabling conditions through the definition and implementation of an individual rehabilitation program, based on a comprehensive multidisciplinary assessment of each individual's health and social care profile in order to outline the required treatments and the most appropriate treatment setting(s) for an active recovery.

In 2011, the Ministry of Health issued a strategic plan for rehabilitation (piano di indirizzo per la riabilitazione) [6], in which rehabilitation is seen as an integrative component of prevention and therapy within an effective integrated patient pathway. The plan proposed the establishment of rehabilitation departments within ASLs to uniformly coordinate the provision of care and guarantee better integration with providers. To date, implementation still differs from region to region and from ASL to ASL.

As for the specific rules and laws addressing the needs of the elderly persons, in 1992 a national plan for senior citizens was issued with the name "Objective: Ageing Persons" aimed at better coordination of medical and social services, which can be integrated within a person's home care service system.

Most of the users of inpatient and outpatient rehabilitation services are elderly. Services provided in the post-acute care are usually delivered in hospitals (in rehabilitation wards of general hospitals as well as in public or private rehabilitation hospitals).

Inpatient rehabilitation is classified as "intensive" or "extensive" according to the number of services and hours of specific therapy.

In 2014, the "intensive inpatient rehabilitation" accounted for about 300,000 hospital admissions (12% of the total number of hospital admissions), while the "extensive inpatient" accounted for about a third of these figures [7].

Most of the conditions requiring inpatient rehabilitation typically affect the elderly persons: stroke, hip fractures, neurological degenerative diseases, and complex multimorbidities.

Rehabilitation admissions are classified into "Major Diagnostic Categories"; the majority of them fall into the "neurologic" and "orthopedic" categories.

Rehabilitation care for the elderly is also provided in long-term hospitals, outpatient ambulatory settings, nursing homes, and residential and semi-residential homes. These settings deliver services for frail or chronically ill people not requiring an acute hospital setting. These types of care involve a range of services designed to link primary care, acute care, and social care in an integrated patient pathway. ASLs are responsible for coordinating and delivering such services and coordinating a set of multidisciplinary activities aimed at switching the care setting from hospital to home care, reducing the length of hospital stay, as well as preventing hospitalizations and inappropriate readmissions. When the local units are not able to directly deliver the set of services required, they can make agreements with public or private hospitals to provide them. In practice, services have been developed differently by the regions, with marked variations in how such services are organized.

Rehabilitation is also delivered in the long-term care settings. This area is still characterized by multiple providers and delivery methods. Historically, local municipalities have been in charge of providing social care services, and ASLs have been considered responsible both for healthcare services and some social care. Thus, in the provision of long-term care, many different models are implemented in the different regions; in general GPs play a pivotal role in selecting the different options and in referring the persons to the different settings.

The residential settings for the elderly are usually classified as residential or semi-residential facilities (residenze sanitarie assistenziali—RSA) or community nursing homes. RSAs generally care for patients who require healthcare resources in terms of nursing and medical consultations, whereas more "stable" patients are directed toward community nursing homes.

As for the home-based rehabilitation, service delivery is usually based upon the home care model (assistenza domiciliare integrata—ADI), which is part of the LEAs.

The ADI care model is based on the formulation of a Personal Care Plan (Piano Assistenziale Individualizzato—PAI), which may include rehabilitation interventions (in such case a Personal Rehabilitation Plan is also defined) according to an individual's care needs. A multidisciplinary unit (unità di valutazione multidimensionale—UVM) of different healthcare professionals (GPs, medical, nursing, and rehabilitative staff) is activated to assess the patient's needs. Nationally, 597,151 people received home care services in 2010; 990 cases per 100,000 were patients receiving services under ADI, representing an increase of 11.7% compared to 2009. Some regions or municipalities established financial supports and vouchers for both home care and residential facilities (including disability support and in some cases rehabilitation services).

It must be said that in Italy, there is still a lot of emphasis on family support. Looking after the older members of the family is regarded as a responsibility or a "social duty," especially by the women, and this also includes taking care of extended family. A large part of the population, mainly family members, provide informal healthcare without receiving any kind of subsidy from the government and professional support. Many patients' organizations try to cope with this deficiency by collecting funding and delivering services to patients and informal caregivers.

A relatively new phenomenon is the care for the elderly or the disabled provided by immigrants or women on very low incomes. Some cash benefits for disabled people, including the elderly, to support care at home, are delivered by the social care authorities or by local municipalities. In recent years, a strong emphasis has been put by some regional and local health authorities in programs aimed at promoting healthy lifestyles among disabled and elderly people, usually through a referral made by the rehabilitation professionals or GPs after the phase of formal medical rehabilitation. Such programs are defined under the umbrella term of adapted physical activity (attività fisica adattata—AFA).

Key Points

- Italy has the second highest average life expectancy.
- Regional and the local health authorities known as ASL (azienda sanitaria locale) administer the health service in Italy.
- The Italian national healthcare service (SSN) provides universal coverage and free health service for all citizens. Private providers can also operate within the SSN.
- There is a better coverage and quality of services in the North Italy with respect to the South and Islands.
- In the provision of long-term care, many different models are implemented in the different regions.
- In Italy family is very important in providing healthcare without receiving any kind of subsidy.

References

1. Eurostat (2014) Statistics database. European Commission. http://epp.eurostat.ec.europa.eu/portal/page/portal/eurostat/home/
2. Central Intelligence Agency: The World Factbook. https://www.cia.gov/library/publications/the-world-factbook/geos/it.html
3. Ferré F, de Belvis AG, Valerio L, Longhi S, Lazzari A, Fattore G, Ricciardi W, Maresso A (2014) Italy: health system review. Health Syst Transit 16(4):1–168
4. National Institute for Statistics (ISTAT). http://www3.istat.it/dati/catalogo/20100513_00/arg_09_37_la_disabilita_in_Italia.pdf
5. Conferenza permanente per i rapporti tra lo Stato le Regioni e le Province Autonome di Trento e Bolzano – 7 maggio 1998 – Linee-guida del Ministro della Sanità per le attività di riabilitazione – GU 30 maggio 1998, n. 124
6. Ministero della Salute. Piano di Indirizzo per la Riabilitazione. 23 maggio 2011
7. Ministero della Salute Rapporto annuale sull'attività di ricovero ospedaliero (Dati SDO 2014). http://www.salute.gov.it/portale/documentazione/p6_2_2_1.jsp?lingua=italiano&id=2396

Healthcare Rehabilitation Organization for the Elderly in Greece

56

Xanthi Michail

List of Acronyms

EKA	National Center of Rehabilitation
EOPYY	National Organization for Healthcare Services Provision
ESY	National Health System
IKA	Social Insurance Institution
KAAKYAMEA	Center of Recovery, Rehabilitation and Social Support for People with Disabilities
KAAMEA	Center of Rehabilitation of People with Disabilities
KAFKA	Center for Recovery, and Physical and Social Rehabilitation
KAPI	Open Care Center for the Elderly
KEKYKAMEA	Centers for Social Support and Training for People with Disabilities
KEN	Closed consolidated medical expenses based on diagnosis-related group (DRG)
LTC	Long-term care
MoH	Ministry of Health
OAEE	Agency Insurance Self-Employed
OECD	Organization for Economic Co-operation and Development
OGA	Agricultural Insurance Organization
OPAD	Agency Insurance Public Servants
PHC	Primary healthcare
SEYYP	Inspection, Ministry of Health and Social Community

X. Michail, MD, PhD
Emeritus Prof. of Rehabilitation Medicine, Faculty of Health & Caring Professions, Technological Educational Institute of Athens (TEI-A), Athens, Greece
e-mail: xanthimichail@gmail.com

© Springer International Publishing AG 2018

S. Masiero, U. Carraro (eds.), *Rehabilitation Medicine for Elderly Patients*, Practical Issues in Geriatrics, DOI 10.1007/978-3-319-57406-6_56

56.1 Introduction

56.1.1 Greek Population's Health Status

Greece, till the beginning of the twenty-first century, is facing a considerable aging of its population. According to the 2011 Population Census, the resident population of Greece is 10,816,286, of which 5,303,223 are male (49.0%) and 5,513,063 are female (51.0%) [1]. According to the data of the National Statistical Service of Greece, in 1991 the percentage of the population over 65 years old was near to 14%, while in 2001 this percentage rose to 17% and is expected to reach 24% by 2030. Approximately 18.7% of the Greek population is aged over 65 (OECD average 15%) with 4.3% of the population over 80 (OECD average 4%) [2].

The majority of patients consist of elderly people (over the age of 65). One out of two persons (49.7%) aged 15 years and over reports suffering from a chronic illness or health problem. In comparison to the other age groups, the elderly account for 60% of ambulance calls, 80% of homecare users, and 49% of inpatient care, and 85% of the patients are suffering from chronic diseases [3].

Self-perceived chronic morbidity and limitation in activities of the population on account of health problems are two basic health indicators. In Greece, chronic illness or a health problem is reported by five out of ten women (54.1%) and by four out of ten men (44.8%). According to the data recorded, one out of two persons aged 65–74 years and almost eight out of ten persons aged 75 years and over are limited in their activities due to health problems [4].

56.2 Healthcare Organization in Greece

In 1983, Greece established a national health system (ESY) in which the Government must, under the Constitution, "guarantee that all citizens enjoy the benefits of a complete range of services of high quality, free at the point of service" (The Greek Constitution, 1975). The Greek health system is characterized as a dual system. The supply side is organized largely along Beveridge lines, with state-provided hospital care and a network of rural health centers covering almost one-third of the population. On the demand side, the system functions mainly along Bismarck lines, with health insurance provided traditionally by 39 health funds, up until 2012 when the various funds merged into one fund, called EOPYY (National Organization for Healthcare Services Provision), covering the entire population [5].

Health services for inpatients are systematically provided by hospitals that are placed all over the country—there are over 130 secondary and tertiary hospitals—which are state run (there are seven public university medical schools). Primary healthcare (PHC) is provided by health centers run by the National Health System (ESY) and social insurance funds. In these centers, physicians often have a very small role, limited to prescribing and referring. In addition to the ESY, there are also healthcare services provided by the private sector, both at PHC level and hospitals.

In 2010 the first step was taken toward the unification of the social health insurance funds, and a year later, Law 3918/2011 introduced a major restructuring of the health system. More specifically, the health sectors of all major social insurance funds (IKA, covering employees and workers in the private sector; OGA, farmers; OAEE, self-employed professionals; and OPAD, public sector employees) formed a single healthcare insurance organization (the National Organization for Healthcare Services Provision (EOPYY) which henceforth acted as a unique buyer of medicines and healthcare services for all those insured. EOPYY also became the country's main new body tasked with managing and providing primary healthcare (PHC), which also undertakes the operational coordination and the cooperation between (public and private) healthcare units and health professionals constituting the PHC network [6].

In terms of rationalizing the hospital payment system, the former reimbursement method based on a fixed per diem charge was abandoned in 2012, and a new payment system (called KEN-DRGs), based on the German version of diagnosis-related-groups (DRGs), was developed [7].

The fragmentation and non-unification of the primary healthcare sector means that data on the use of primary healthcare services are very limited, though some indications exist that the major PHC centers are heavily used by older people. The lack of general practitioners has implications in the continuity of care, particularly important for older people with functional limitations, since there are no permanent medical records kept in the public primary healthcare sector. There are no specialist geriatric services, as this is not a recognized specialty in Greece, and there is only limited geriatric and gerontological training for health and social care personnel. Current doctor-nurse imbalances imply that the division of tasks in delivering health services is not optimal with twice as many doctors as nurses [8].

56.3 Rehabilitation Care Organization in Greece

In Greece, rehabilitation services are provided within the healthcare sector and the social sector, by both public and private institutions.

Rehabilitation is partly provided by public hospitals' departments of physical medicine and rehabilitation and the National Center of Rehabilitation (EKA) with inpatient and outpatient treatment facilities. There are four public hospitals with such departments and two departments of PRM in the EKA (which is the most complete rehabilitation center in Greece), all of which are located in the wider area of Athens. The capacity of all these departments does not exceed 200 beds.

In addition, there is a university clinic with 40 beds that has been partly operating since 2006 in the Medical School of the University of Ioannina and a second one with 22 beds that has been suboptimal operating since 2013 in the Medical School of the University of Patras. A children's rehabilitation outpatient department has also recently been established in relation to the Children's Hospital in Athens offering evaluation and rehabilitation treatment services to outpatient disabled children. Moreover, there are private physiotherapy clinics, throughout Greece, which cover fully or partly the needs in physiotherapy of outpatients, adults, or children, financially covered by contracts with state funds.

Greece has a long way to go toward adequate rehabilitation services, since a total of 200 public rehabilitation beds is insufficient to cover the spectrum of rehabilitation needs from people with injuries to people with strokes or other problems within LTC (long-term care). Although not all of the cases need inpatient rehabilitation, the need is still not covered by the existing structures, and out-of-the pocket payment is necessary as social security covers only part of the expenses. Finally, it is worth mentioning that during the last 15 years, private sector profit-making activities in the provision of physical rehabilitation have increased due to the gaps in ESY services and the inefficient operation of public facilities owing to staff and equipment shortages. These profit-making centers enter into contracts with insurance funds to provide services. In rural areas, about 20 private rehabilitation centers, with in total around 1800 beds, cover the needs of the population, and the social security fully or partly covers the cost. There is no age or disease discrimination and older people with strokes constitute a big proportion of the patients. Both public and private rehabilitation services are functioning with limited quality control from the Ministry of Health (MoH), and the number of PRM doctors responsible for the scientific supervision of rehabilitation offered in the private structures is extremely limited.

There are about 240 specialists practicing physical and rehabilitation medicine (PRM) and 33 trainees.

Within the social sector, rehabilitation is offered by two structures. The first structure comprises a network of 24 Centers for Social Support and Training for People with Disabilities (KEKYKAMEAs), established according to the provisions of Law 2646/1998 for the development of the national system of social care, and of 17 Centers for Recovery, and Physical and Social Rehabilitation (KAFKAs). These are independent public entities supervised by the Ministry of Health and Social Solidarity. The aim of these centers is to offer early diagnostic services, psychosocial support, education, and training to provide disabled people with the tools they need to attain independence and self-determination. The intention of creating KEKYKAMEA and KAFKA was to deinstitutionalize and regionalize the provision of care and to supply open services allocated across the whole country. However, their operation has fallen short of expectations, mainly due to inadequate staffing (scientific, administrative, and auxiliary personnel) and equipment (reports of SEYYP 2005–2015) [9].

The second social sector structure providing rehabilitation to adult disabled persons includes a variety of different forms of the so-called "rehabilitation centers" for LTC (long-term care), with a more residential-oriented character. These are:

(a) Centers of Recovery, Rehabilitation and Social Support for People with Disabilities (KAAKYAMEAs)
(b) Centers of Rehabilitation of People with Disabilities (KAAMEAs)

All of these centers cater for people with disabilities and, more specifically, support people with congenital disorders, or temporary or permanent muscle, respiratory, circulatory, and nervous system problems, as well as those with mental disability. They offer services mainly to resident-disabled patients.

56.4 Community-Based Care

The aging of the population and the increase of the incidence of chronic diseases and disabilities, combined with the limited financial health resources, forced the reorganization of the National Health System toward the development of primary healthcare system. As a result of this development and considering that 80% of the users are elderly people, priority has been given to the establishment of community-based care.

In Greece, the most important care network for older people is the Open Care Centers for the Elderly (KAPI). KAPIs are multidisciplinary centers (>1000 throughout Greece) which, from their outset in the early 1980s, offered locally provided combined social and health programs, with the aim of supporting older people to remain independent in community-based settings and avoiding the need for more intensive long-term care (LTC), including family provided care and admission to institutional forms of care. They typically consist of a social worker (who is the team leader and coordinator), a nurse or health visitor, a physiotherapist, an occupational therapist, and a family assistant. The service aims to detect any unmet medical, social, or mental health needs and to promote independence. The Open Protection Centers of the Elderly (KAPI) are open programs involving the elderly over 60 years without socioeconomic criteria, in order to integrate and socialize all members of the community. They provide all forms of organized recreation, medical care, physiotherapy treatment, occupational therapy, social work, provision of hospital care, and all kinds of material and moral services to the elderly. These Elderly Care Units supply the elderly with their services continuously, as long as they live there. The day care centers of the elderly provide their services several hours a day, so as to help the family to care for the elderly. Most health promotion programs are applied in KAPIs.

In 1996, the Ministry of Health, in cooperation with the Ministry of the Interior Affairs, in order to cover the need for health services, developed the so-called "Help at Home," healthcare programs which provide health and social care services at home. The program "Help at Home" is part of the primary social care services, providing nursing care, social care services, and domestic assistance to older people who live alone continuously or at certain times of the day and cannot sufficiently take care of themselves and also to disabled people who face situations of isolation, exclusion, or family crisis. Its aim is to support and care for the elderly in their home, to enhance the quality of their life, to inform the society, and to attract volunteers [10].

The Help at Home services (implemented under the responsibility of the local authorities in municipalities throughout the country and usually associated closely with the local KAPIs,) provide a range of essential services to support dependent older people at home, focusing on those with limited financial means and no family help. However, recent studies have shown that their insecure funding has seriously undermined their capacity to function effectively. Nevertheless, with a planned policy for operation and adequate funding, the combined KAPI and Help at Home network could provide a model for the integrated provision of long-term care.

Key Points
- The lack of a well-distributed primary healthcare
- The unbalanced distribution of medical staffs in the different regions of the country
- The limited number of rehab beds and specialists in the public hospitals
- The incomplete and disorganized long-term care and community-based care for the elderly

References

1. Organisation for Economic Co-operation and Development (OECD) health data [Internet]. Greece. https://data.oecd.org/greece.htm#profile-health
2. Colombo F et al (2011) Help wanted? Providing and paying for long-term care. OECD Publishing, Paris. https://www.oecd.org/els/health-systems/47836116.pdf
3. Kalokerinou A, Adamakidou T, Damianidi M et al Overview on health promotion for older people in Greece. HealthPROelderly, National report—Greece. http://www.healthproelderly.com/pdf/National_report1_Greece.pdf
4. Hellenic statistical authority [Internet]. http://www.statistics.gr/en/home/
5. Siskou O, Kaitelidou D, Papakonstantinou V, Liaropoulos L (2008) Private health expenditure in the Greek health care system: where truth ends and the myth begins. Health Policy 88(2–3):282–293. https://www.clinicalkey.com/#!/content/journal/1-s2.0-S0168851008000900
6. Karakolias S, Polyzos N (2014) The newly established Unified healthcare fund (EOPYY): current situation and proposed structural changes, towards an upgraded model of primary health care in Greece. Health 6(9):809–821. http://file.scirp.org/pdf/Health_2014032813434550.pdf
7. Polyzos N, Karanikas H, Thireos E, Kastanioti C, Kontodimopoulos N (2013) Reforming reimbursement of public hospitals in Greece during the economic crisis: implementation of a DRG system. Health Policy 109(1):14–22
8. Altanis P, Economou C, Geitona M et al (2008) Quality in and equality of access to healthcare services-country report for Greece. http://ec.europa.eu/social/BlobServlet?docId=5086&langId=en
9. Economou C (2010) Greece—health system review. Health Syst Transit 12(7):1–180. http://www.euro.who.int/__data/assets/pdf_file/0004/130729/e94660.pdf?ua=1
10. Sissouras A, Ketsetzopoulou M, Bouzas N et al (2002) Providing integrated health and social care for older persons in Greece—National Centre for Social Research (EKKE). http://www.euro.centre.org/procare/body_reports_natreps/procare_Greece_NR.pdf

Long-Term Care for Older People in England

57

Raphael Wittenberg

57.1 Introduction

Long-term care is crucial for the well-being of the rising numbers of older people with personal care needs and younger people with disabilities. Despite its importance, there is no single internationally agreed definition of long-term care. In the UK, the term long-term care, or care and support, tends to be used to refer collectively to a range of health, social care, supported housing, disability benefit and other services which help disabled younger and older people live an independent life. The emphasis is generally on help with personal care tasks such as dressing, bathing, feeding and toileting but extends to help with domestic tasks and to some forms of professional support.

57.2 Structure

Health, social care, and housing (but not social security) are all devolved functions within the UK. This means that the administrations in Scotland, Wales and Northern Ireland are responsible for these services within their countries. Since there are some differences in policies and practices between countries within the UK, this chapter concentrates on England, which contains over 80% of the population of the UK.

Local authorities are responsible for assessing needs for social care and arranging care for those with eligible needs in their areas. They set eligibility criteria for publicly funded care for their areas within national guidance. They are also responsible for public health, education, and housing. Their services are funded through a combination of revenues from local taxation, grants from central government, and income from user charges for services.

R. Wittenberg
Personal Social Services Research Unit,
London School of Economics and Political Science, London, UK
e-mail: R.Wittenberg@lse.ac.uk

© Springer International Publishing AG 2018

S. Masiero, U. Carraro (eds.), *Rehabilitation Medicine for Elderly Patients*,
Practical Issues in Geriatrics, DOI 10.1007/978-3-319-57406-6_57

Clinical commissioning groups are responsible in England for assessing needs, setting priorities, and commissioning most healthcare services for their local populations. NHS England however is responsible for commissioning primary care services and some specialist services. It sets the overall priorities for the National Health Service (NHS) in accordance with a mandate from the Government. The NHS is funded from general taxation and is mostly free at point of use.

The Department for Work and Pensions (DWP) is responsible throughout Britain for cash disability and carer's benefits. The main cash benefit for older people with disabilities is Attendance Allowance which is a non-means-tested cash payment which recipients can use as they wish. The main cash payment for unpaid carers is Carer's Allowance which has a number of eligibility criteria including a provision that the carer provides at least 35 hours of care per week. Social security benefits are funded through general taxation.

57.3 Unpaid Care and Formal Services

Unpaid care is crucial to the care and support of older people: the majority of community-based care is unpaid care by family and friends. This means that the future sustainability of adult social care will depend heavily on the future supply of unpaid care over the coming decades. This may in turn be affected by a range of economic and social trends as well as by social security and other policies on support for carers and on employment laws and practices relating to carers.

Around 2.1 million older people in England receive unpaid care from relatives and friends, mainly from spouses, daughters and sons, and some 5.2 million people provide unpaid care to an older relative or friend, according to estimates based on recent Health Survey for England findings. The difference between these figures is likely due mainly to differences in perceptions between caregivers and care recipients about whether the help and support provided be regarded as unpaid care. Around 875,000 of the carers provide unpaid care for 20 or more hours per week, comprising 325,000 spouse carers, 200,000 other coresident carers, and 350,000 providers of care to an older person in a different household.

Most formal social care is provided by the independent sector, both for-profit and not-for-profit providers. Local authorities' direct provision of services is fairly limited in most areas: they now provide less than 10% of care home places for older people and less than 10% of home care hours. Local authorities commission services from a diverse but mostly competitive market of mainly relatively small providers. This does not mean however that the care market meets all the characteristics of a classic competitive market. Local authorities mostly have considerable monopsony power as the dominant purchaser.

Around 325,000 older people live in care homes, slightly over 3% of the older population. This is down from around 5% in the early 1990s. Around half of these care home residents are funded by local authorities, under 10% are fully funded by the NHS, and over 40% fund their own care privately. The majority are female and aged 85 and over, lived alone before they entered residential care, are cognitively impaired, and have a high level of functional disability.

Over 400,000 older people receive long-term support funded by their local authority [1]. As at 31 March 2015, 157,000 received support in a care home and comprised around a half of all older care home residents. The remaining 254,000 received support in the community. This includes recipients of home-based and recipients of cash payments in lieu of services. An estimated further 100,000 older people purchased home care privately.

Local authorities' gross current expenditure on adult social care in 2014/15 was £17.0 billion, and their net current expenditure on adult social care (net of income from user charges) was £14.4 billion [2]. Around half of the gross expenditure figure relates to care of older people. Adult social care accounts for some 15% of the local authorities' overall net current expenditure.

The rising numbers of older people and rising real costs of care mean that public expenditure on care and support for older people will need to rise in real terms to keep pace with the expected demand pressures. Public expenditure on social services for older people, net of user charges, is projected to rise by 155% from around £6.9 billion (0.43% of GDP) in 2015 to £17.5 billion (0.69% of GDP) in 2035 at constant 2015 prices [3]. This is on the basis of constant disability rates (by age) and unchanged patterns of care and an unchanged funding system.

There is a mixed economy of finance of adult social care. The majority of the costs are in effect borne by unpaid carers in terms of the opportunity cost of their time, and a minority of the costs are borne by the funders of formal services. The services are funded by a combination of central taxation, local taxation, user charges for publicly subsidized care, and out-of-pocket payments by service users and their families. Insurance for long-term care needs is not available commercially in England other than immediate needs annuities.

Social care in England, unlike healthcare, is not free of charge to those needing support. People with savings above a specified capital limit (currently £23,250) are generally ineligible for publicly funded social care, and those with savings below this threshold may still have to pay part, or all, of their care costs, depending on their wealth and income. A person's home is counted as part of their savings if they enter residential care (with some exceptions) but is not counted if they receive home-based care. This means that it is not unusual for care home residents to need to sell their former home to fund their care and not uncommon for those with long stays to exhaust their savings down to the level of the capital limit for public support.

57.4 Reforms

The Coalition Government set up shortly after its election in spring 2010 a *Commission on the Funding of Care and Support* to produce new recommendations on the vexed issue of reforming the funding system. Its main recommendation was that there should be a lifetime cap of between £25,000 and £50,000 on the liability of service users to meet the costs of their care [4]. This would in effect be a form of social insurance subject to a large excess. The Government decided to implement a lifetime cap in April 2016 but at a higher level of £72,000. It subsequently decided, however, that because of the costs, implementation would be postponed to 2020.

The Coalition Government published in November 2010 a *Vision for Adult Social Care* [5]. The vision was based on seven principles: prevention, personalization, partnership, plurality, protection, productivity, and people. The vision for prevention focuses on empowered people and strong communities working together to maintain independence and the state, where needed, supporting communities and helping people to retain and regain independence.

In July 2012, following a public engagement, the Government published a white paper *Caring for Our Future* with substantial proposals for reforming the system of care and support in England [6]. Among its priorities, it advocated "re-ablement services and crisis response to help people regain their independence at home after a crisis." This white paper was followed by the publication of legislation which was enacted in the Care Act 2014. The Act gives local authority responsibility to promote well-being when carrying out any of their care and support functions. The Act covers a wide range of reforms including assessment and care planning, national minimum eligibility criteria, support for unpaid carers, funding reforms, market shaping, and information and advice. Most of the provisions of the Act came into force in April 2015, but implementation of the funding reforms has been postponed to 2020.

Local authorities have increasingly established re-ablement services, sometimes jointly with the NHS. These are short-term services, for a typical duration of 6 weeks, and are generally not subject to user charges. The aim of these services, which may be provided on discharge from hospital, is to help the service user to regain confidence and skills to perform personal and domestic care tasks and to regain or retain their independence. Research suggests that re-ablement services can reduce need for longer-term support [7].

During the period October to December 2014, 44,000 older people in England were discharged from hospital to rehabilitation where the intention was for them to go back home. Eighty-two percent of these 44,000 older people were still living at home 91 days after hospital discharge [1, page 24].

Conclusion

The majority of long-term care for older people in England is provided by unpaid carers and only a minority by formal services. Adult social services are the responsibility of local authorities, and health services are the responsibility of clinical commissioning groups with the NHS. While healthcare is funded from general taxation and provided almost entirely free at point of use, adult social care is subject to a means test of savings and incomes and is funded from a combination of central and local taxation and out-of-pocket payments by service users and their families. While health services are provided mainly by public sector providers, social services are provided mainly by independent sector providers. Considerable reforms to the system of care and support were implemented in April 2015 but reform to the funding system has been postponed to 2020.

Key Points

- The majority of long-term care for older people in England is provided by unpaid carers and only a minority by formal services.
- While healthcare is funded from general taxation and is almost entirely free at point of use, social care is subject to a means test of savings and incomes and is funded from a combination of sources.
- While health services are provided mainly by public sector providers, social services are provided mainly by independent sector providers.
- Considerable reforms to the system of care and support were implemented in April 2015, but reform to the funding system has been postponed to 2020.

References

1. Health and Social Care Information Centre (HSCIC) (2015) Community Care Statistics: Social Services Activity, England 2014–15, final release, November 2015
2. Health and Social Care Information Centre (HSCIC) (2015) Personal Social Services: Expenditure and Unit Costs England 2014–15, final release, November 2015
3. Wittenberg R, Hu B (2015) Projections of demand for and costs of social care for older people and younger adults in England, 2015 to 2035, PSSRU discussion paper DP2900
4. Commission on Funding of Care and Support (2011) Fairer care funding: the report of the Commission on Funding of Care and Support
5. Department of Health (2010) A vision for adult social care: capable communities and active citizens. 16 November 2010
6. HM Government (2012) Caring for our future: reforming care and support. Cmnd 8378, July 2012
7. Glendinning C, Newbronner E (2008) The effectiveness of home care reablement – developing the evidence base. J Integr Care 16(4):32–39

MIX
Papier aus verantwortungsvollen Quellen
Paper from responsible sources
FSC® C105338

If you have any concerns about our products,
you can contact us on
ProductSafety@springernature.com

In case Publisher is established outside the EU,
the EU authorized representative is:
Springer Nature Customer Service Center GmbH
Europaplatz 3, 69115 Heidelberg, Germany

Printed by Libri Plureos GmbH
in Hamburg, Germany